HOT YOGA
MasterClass

Discover A Beautiful Hot Yoga Practice

Precision Techniques For Beginners To Advanced

Gabrielle Raiz

Hot Yoga MasterClass: Discover a Beautiful Hot Yoga Practice – Precision Techniques for Beginners to Advanced
Raiz, Gabrielle
ISBN 978-0-9805319-5-4
Third edition: Full color
Published by Colete Pty Ltd.

Design and layout by Jana Rade of Impact Studios, jrade@impactstudiosonline.com

Photography: All indoor and most outdoor images (725 in total) taken by Greg Gardner www.greggardner.com.au except for those taken by Debra Livingston (on pages, 15, 22, 41, 46, 49, 69, 93, 103, 123, 133, 149, 173, 181, 191, 227, 243, 293).

Clothing supplied by Lorna Jane

Models: Amber Werchon, Carlos Azcarraga, Gabrielle Raiz, Jess Fleming, Lauren Power, Racheal Gaunt, Scott Woodward and Sumi Dorairaj.
Makeup by Marina Passalaris

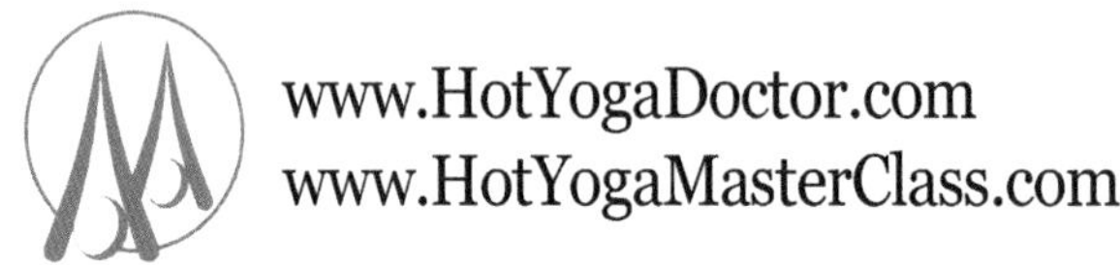

For Robert
My adored and cherished husband

For Isabelle
You are my “favourite girl in the world”

Acknowledgements

Thanks go to many people when writing a book of these immense proportions. Thank you to my students and friends for posing for the photographs. While the indoor studio shots were taken fairly quickly, a long spate of poor weather spanning over 6 months, meant even more longstanding commitment from my models. Thank you Amber, Carlos, Lauren, Jess, Scott, Sumi, and Racheal for injecting your enthusiasm and your beauty whenever you willingly turned up to be one of my stars. Thank you for always saying ‘yes’ when it would have been so easy to say ‘no’. Thank you Greg Gardner for your commitment to taking great photographs – indoors and out. Thanks Marina Passalaris for allowing us all to put our best faces forward. I would like to acknowledge Debra Livingston for taking some of the beautiful ‘arty’ shots on her own time and for nothing but for the joy of taking wonderful photographs.

Extra special thanks to Jana Rade of Impact Studios for creating the beauty in print of this enormous tome. Thank you for making my project ‘our baby’. Your dedication to excellence in design is evident in your personal pride and willingness to do whatever it takes ‘til it works. Our friendship means a lot to me.

Part of the beauty of this book is due to the generosity of Lorna Jane. There is no other yoga or sports gear that I would rather wear. Nothing beats it for comfort, style and practicality. I hope you enjoy looking at the wonderful clothing as much as we love wearing it.

This book would not be possible without my passion for this yoga fuelled by the enthusiasm of millions of hot yogis the world over who inspired me to write this book. Thanks to my mother, Raymonde Raiz for continual support, encouragement and love. My greatest inspiration is my own cherished family. Our beautiful, wise, loving and intelligent daughter Isabelle is not only the light in her parents’ eyes but a constant source of my joy, inspiration and learning. My family constantly reminds me of the joys of life, that to ‘be’ in this moment, every moment is my most worthwhile pursuit. Thank you both for always being there with me and for me. Robert is my other bright and shining star. Thank you for encouraging greatness without compromise, living a fun and baggage-free existence, your inspiring intellect, playful banter, smiling eyes, passionate spirit and unconditional love. Thank you for being you.

Contents

Warming up

Standing balancing poses

Warrior poses

Transitioning to the floor

Belly-down poses

Spine strengthening poses

Completing and integrating your class

★★★★★

Lorna B - Australia

I recently purchased the Hot Yoga Master Class complete set and I love it. I have practiced Bikram Yoga 4+ days a week for almost a year and a half and have had limited luck clearing up confusion or misconceptions about certain postures with many of the teachers. The photos and descriptions clearly let me see what I was missing and how to fix it. I am finally making progress in the postures I thought I would never get and my body is really opening up. This set is definitely worth the money, I'd recommend it to anyone practicing Bikram or other Hot Yoga.

★★★★★

Amany I - Saudi Arabia

My Dear Gabrielle, I am writing you from Jeddah Saudi Arabia. I found you through the net and I joined your group and have been enjoying your emails. And now I have your wonderful manual. I can't believe the tiny things you mention that we should notice and when I teach it to my yoga members WOW, I can't believe the big difference these teachings do to the poses. You manual is a must have book regardless if you do hot yoga or any type of yoga in general. Thank you sooooo much for all your teaching, you truly made a difference in my practice and in my classes.

★★★★★

Tom R - USA

I've been practicing Bikram for eight years and have constantly searched within my own abilities to move my practice to a "higher level". I felt the difference from the very first class after I got the book, dvd, cd and poster; now I feel that I've started over with a fresh outlook with these materials as my road-map. Great stuff and I recommend it to my closest friends!

★★★★★

Steve C - USA

As beginners in yoga my wife and I were looking for a definitive guide to yoga starting from the ground up, the way we would build our knowledge and understanding of the yoga poses. The Hot Yoga Master Class is exactly what we were looking for. It dispels the rumours and myths and has enabled us to really enjoy and get the most out of our yoga practice. My wife has already thought about further studies in yoga and even perhaps teach it further down the line. The Hot Yoga MasterClass is fantastic and I would recommend it to anyone who is starting their yoga practice or a more experienced person looking for something that will help them get even more out of their practice.

★★★★★

Neil E - Philippines

A great benefit! I am new to yoga, in my sixties, and have now done about twelve classes. This Hot Yoga MasterClass does three things really well: it shows me how to do things and, more importantly, how NOT to do them; it helps me focus on the form of the poses and not just the end position; and finally its beautiful format and illustrations provide the inspiration for me to keep practising. I love the email reminders too. I couldn't recommend it more highly.

★★★★★

Rosie M - USA

I am fairly new to hot yoga and have been practicing for about 3 months. The biggest challenge for me was getting the most out of the poses which I could not perform correctly nor completely being a newbie. The Hot Yoga package is of tremendous help in breaking down the poses and modifying them for practitioners of all levels. I am already starting to see improvement in my ability to complete certain poses. This is exactly the kind of instruction I needed and was not getting in my classes. Many thanks. Namaste

★★★★★

Cathy E - Canada

The ability to communicate information is a very power tool. Bikram yoga needs to be practised correctly in order to achieve the benefits and success in the poses. I found this out the hard way. My lower back was in so much pain after my first 2 classes that I had to make a weekly visits to an Osteotherapist. Rather than give up yoga ('cause isn't it supposed to be good for yourback?) I googled and came up with your website, ordered the book and videos and 'voila'- pain has disappeared. The book now sits proudly on my coffee table and is frequently read by family and friends. Very informative. Congratulations and thank you!

★★★★★

Mary D - USA

The Master Class is just what I was looking for. It is perfect, just like being in class! Definitely worth the investment. The book is so beautiful and so helpful in helping me perfect and understand each pose. Thanks so much, Gabrielle. Namaste.

★★★★★

Mikaela M - United Kingdom

No stone is left unturned - so much information and really clear photos. Since I have been practising along with Gabrielle's instruction, I fall out of poses far less (and no more bad language!), I feel calmer during the class and I even smile sometimes! Be warned though this Hot Yoga thing is addictive! So only buy this course if you want to change your life, feel happier and be in the best shape you can possibly be!

★★★★★

Kate M. -USA

I have your wonderful, beautiful, Hot Yoga Master book and love it. I own a hot yoga studio in the US. Your book has become my bible for my own personal practice and in teaching hot Yoga. Thank you so much for writing it. It's by far is the best I have ever seen! I think you are right on in your philosophy and teaching approach in the hot yoga world! Keep Writing!!!!!!! See you on the mat someday..... Sincerely Katie - Intentional Yoga

★★★★★

Denise H - Canada

After taking a different Teacher Training course, I purchased the Hot Yoga MasterClass products. I wish I had them before and during training. It has given me the information I wish I'd received during my intensive course. Beautifully photographed, perfectly illustrated, clear and concise, this is a MUST HAVE for anyone who is interested in the Classic 26 Hatha postures in a traditional Hot Yoga class. Quite simply, it is the best book/manual I've ever seen, and I was a complete skeptic before I purchased it. Thank you, Gabrielle. It is truly invaluable.

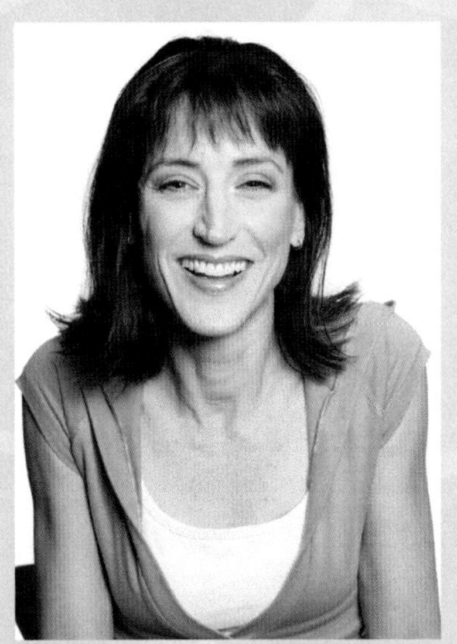

Gabrielle Raiz BDS

Foreword

Chances are you have heard many amazing claims about the power of hot yoga. It has a remarkable reputation for healing, reducing symptoms of chronic illness, regulating all the body's systems to function more effectively, and for generally enhancing wellbeing. Many of these seem far too good to be true.

I am happy to report there is no need to doubt! Since I began teaching,
I have witnessed and helped facilitate some incredible miracles.

They range from the seemingly trivial to the downright unbelievable.

Students under my watch have dodged neck, back and knee surgery, have stopped taking medication, have cheated injury, chronic illness and healed at incredible rates.

Some of my favorite stories are of people on chronic pain medication for 20 years or so.

They come to only two or three classes and incredibly, they get up for their morning walk and can't believe that they have literally 'forgotten' to take their pain tablets. One lady told me she 'forgot' her cane!

All true stories.

Frequently arthritic conditions all but disappear. Diabetics reduce or eliminate medication, as do those with hypo or hyperthyroidism. Several students' longstanding backaches have disappeared after only one, two or three classes.

More than a handful of women that I know have had miraculous conceptions.

Yet for me, the most heartening stories are those where people tell me that they feel happy for no reason whatsoever. They tell me that they walk around with a smile on their face, that they walk upright with shoulders back, that there is a general feeling of satisfaction with themselves, and everything that they do.

Wow.

Can you ask more than that?

Warm wishes

Gabrielle

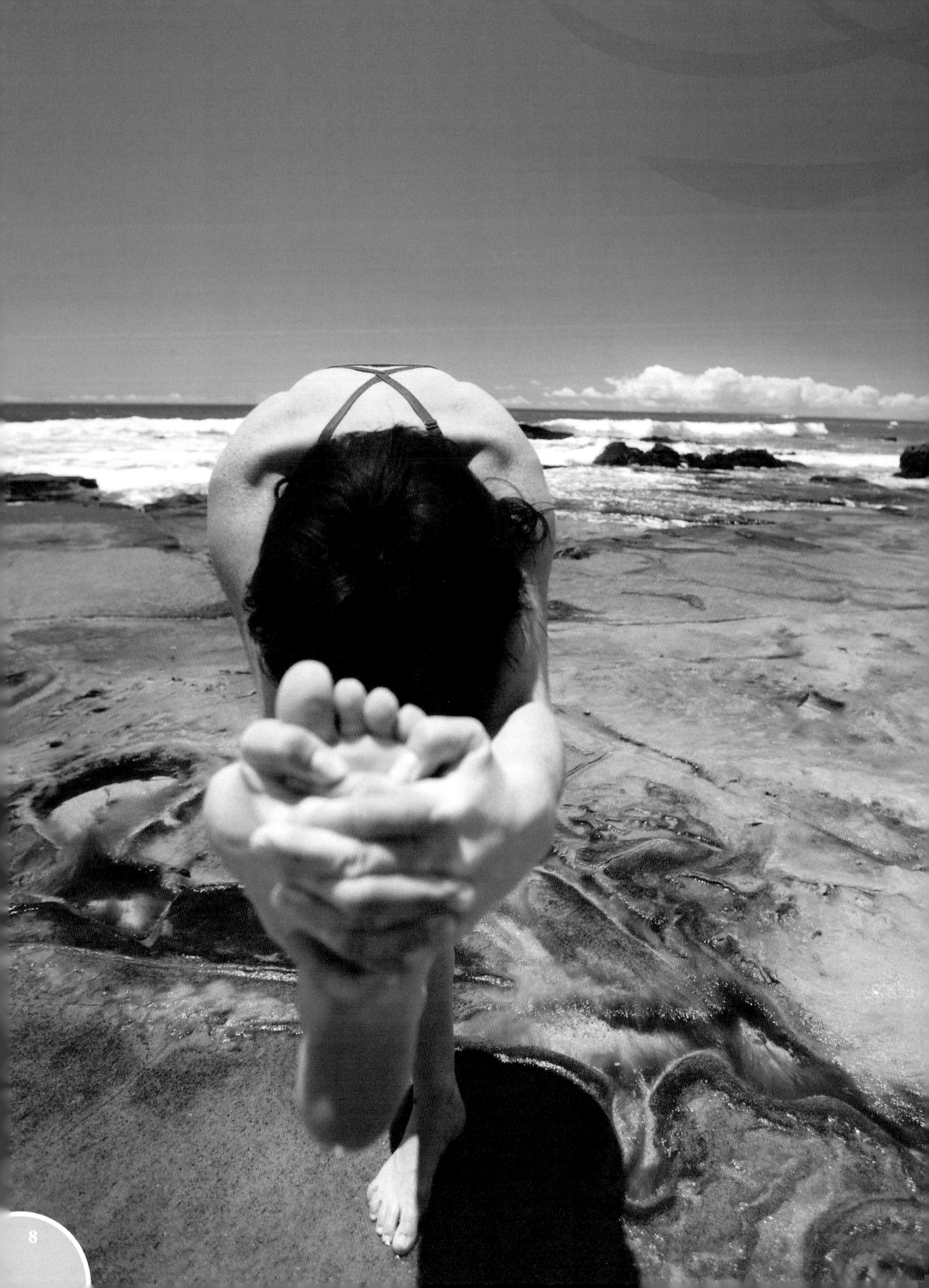

Introduction

Welcome to the Hot Yoga MasterClass

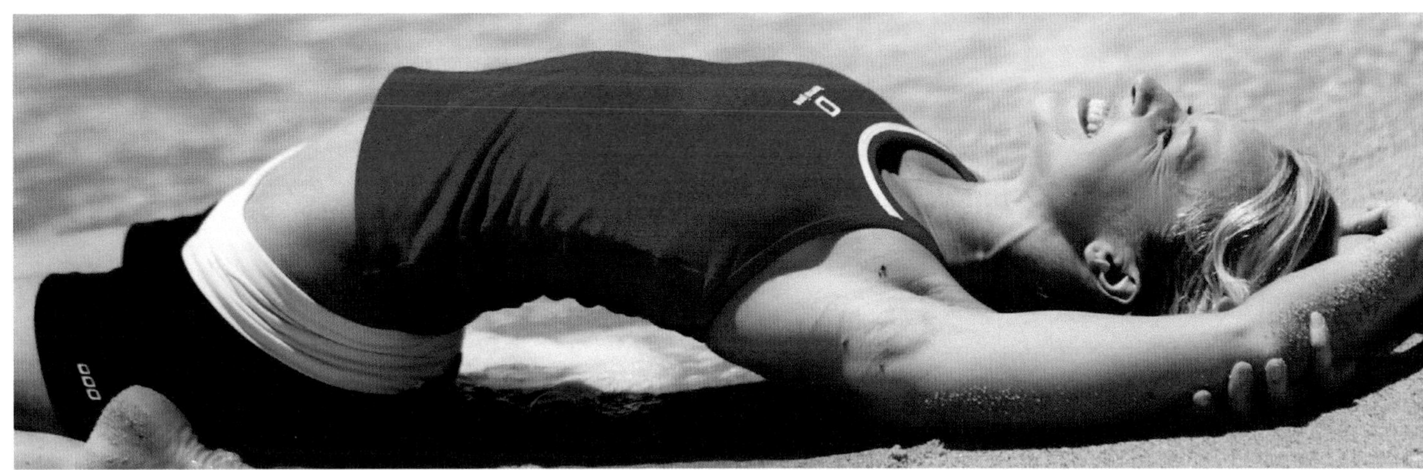

It must have been only a week or two after beginning my own hot yoga practice before the teachers at my studio were trying to persuade me to go LA to attend teacher training – but in the beginning all I wanted to do was practice yoga!

Like many thousands of hot yoga students I was astounded by the countless benefits I experienced in a very short time. I was having such astonishing and obvious physical and mental benefits from even the first week, that my husband suggested I take a few months 'time-out' to continue to explore this as I was at the end of a work-contract. It was an opportunity too good to pass up, so I made the most of it.

I practiced at least six times per week and often went eight times. Within two weeks I had lost two dress sizes and 10 pounds (5 kilos).

I felt vital and energetic. My food choices unconsciously became health-driven rather than cravings-driven. I became strong and happy.

And how about this for the icing on the cake – my back stopped aching. This was just the beginning, for within 5 months my moderately severe scoliosis almost disappeared.

Right from the very beginning I loved discovering new and interesting distinctions about each pose. I could see that becoming a hot yoga instructor would be truly rewarding for me as a vocation – but more importantly, to share these amazing benefits with anyone who would listen!

Since then I have taught thousands of students. I also started what became, within weeks, and remains the world's most popular and highly respected hot yoga forum. My way of teaching hot yoga challenges those who sanctify a solely script-based class: Its strengths lie in the solid logic of working with the body, its physiology, its natural and automatic reflexes.

I believe that yoga should never cause struggle but should definitely challenge you to grow, open, breathe, and live fully. If you ever feel struggle then your body is signaling you that something must change. My techniques give you practice in mindfulness which awakens sensitivity, trust and intuition making your practice safer and more effective. My students report breakthroughs they have been searching for, for years.

I have incorporated my study of human anatomy and medical training as a dentist to provide very accurate instructions. I have now personally interned and coached many certified teachers, sharing with them my knowledge. In turn they help their own students gain even more from their hot yoga practice.

Hot yoga has become very popular all around the globe for people from all walks of life. They love the heat, the poses, the glow and the way they feel. Some who say they hate it during class, can't keep away. Something happens to you, your body craves the attention, the cleansing and the healing. No one can deny the incredible satisfaction that they feel after class. There is simply nothing else like it – guaranteed.

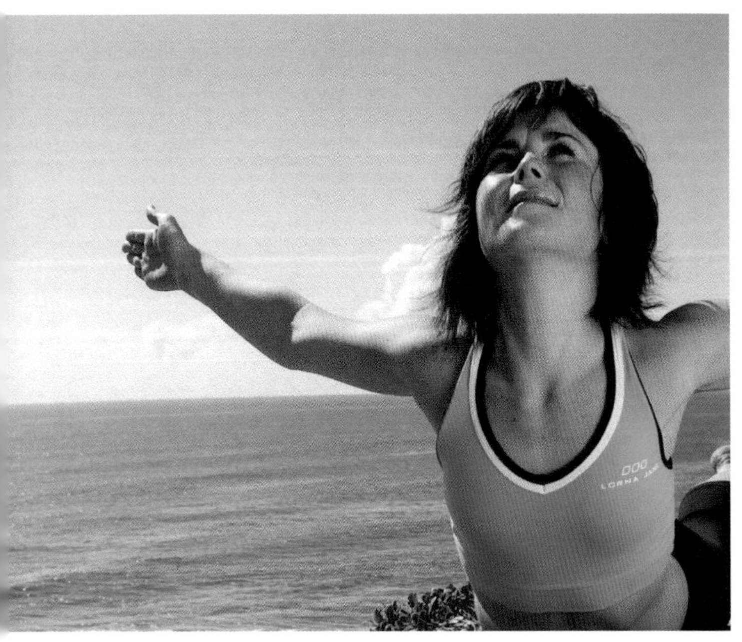

You will discover how to find the sweet spot in each pose, how to set up the right alignment, the twists, the organ compressions, the way to lengthen and strengthen, how to find power and precise subtle movements of muscles or limb movements.

A detailed, practical, guide to hot yoga

There are already a few books available on hot yoga, so why on earth write another? In my opinion there was nothing that a student could take off the shelf and use it exclusively, without having professional instruction. I changed that.

Hot Yoga MasterClass is a comprehensive off-the-shelf reference guide that breaks down each and every step of the hot yoga poses. I systematically take each pose and dissect its main aims, its challenges, every single detail from beginning to end.

You'll also discover a huge range of small adjustments and modifications for every mistake and condition you can bring to the table.

It is likely that you are familiar with different series of hot yoga poses but want to know much more about each aspect of practice. It is possible that you have never had a satisfactory standard of teaching. You may not even have questioned whether you were getting the best quality because there is something you love about the postures and the way you feel.

Whatever your motivation, the Hot Yoga MasterClass will help you deconstruct each and every pose to reveal so much more. It may challenge your understanding and provide you with finer distinctions, so you can take yourself to a higher level. I discuss the different - and sometimes controversial - approaches to poses and provide recommendations. I hope you find it both provocative and motivating.

My approach to this practice has always been pragmatic and sensible. I want you to get the best outcome in terms of personal benefits, all the while satisfying the foundational principles of yoga - physical, mental, emotional and spiritual.

I want the directions to be so crystal clear that a blind student in my class can manage as easily as a sighted person.

In fact, one of my very first students was blind. The printed script from my original training would never be enough for Cheryl to understand everything. With a class full of students it was difficult to be with her all the time and guide her body into the right forms.

Thanks must go to Cheryl for opening my eyes many years ago to the difference between quality professional instruction and just reciting a script.

I want the directions to be so crystal clear that a blind student in my class can manage as easily as a sighted person.

The way I teach reflects the accuracy required for anyone to learn. I teach a technically precise class, accessible by all, but detailed enough for the most hard-core yogi.

Everyone has a different body. You may be flexible. Or maybe you suffer from sciatica. This guide will help you find the right approach, respecting a multitude of circumstances. For most students the principles will remain the same. You will discover how each pose should look and feel. Ideally we should all look fundamentally very similar in these postures, but your flexibility or strength may determine your personal depth and what specifically you will be working on.

My training and previous career as a dentist and my strong body intuition have helped me understand, nurture and grow an intimate knowledge of hot yoga. My passion was sparked years ago and has grown from the very first lesson. Join me so I can guide you through your whole practice and I will personally walk you through each and every step of every pose.

Is Yoga physical or spiritual?

The western mindset usually makes the first visits to a yoga studio based purely on the desire for physical benefits; weight loss, a toned, slim body with healthy looking skin and getting exercise.

On the surface hot yoga fits this mold, appealing to those with a competitive spirit, a need to strive for success and to fit their frantic lives into neat boxes with almost zero free time. We turn up to pack a solid physical workout into 90 minutes. But if that were all it did then it wouldn't be the great success story that it is. I tell my students that coming to hot yoga is like exploring your spirituality through the back door.

The wonderful thing about these rigorous poses is that spirituality and all the corresponding non-physical benefits are there for all to benefit from. They do not need to be pushed down anyone's throat.

With deep breath work and the stillness and calm of your practice, you will find peace. Along with this will come your own realizations, your own spirituality and your own truth. Talk of Chakras, reincarnation and god or gods is not necessary (and certainly outside the scope of this book).

Sometimes students who come to hot yoga start as yoga skeptics – or perhaps they are even skeptical of anything 'new-age'. They shy away from new-age or spiritual philosophies. Yoga has been around for thousands of years and could hardly be called 'new-age', though its popularity has grown dramatically in the western world over the last few decades.

To respect this desire for 'yoga without the chanting', I've learned over the years to ensure my instruction style is technique-driven. I use metaphors, life-stories and meditation concepts to invite each student on their own path of self-discovery. This allows students to discover for themselves the less obvious, but equally beneficial 'non-physical' benefits of yoga. I have been delighted to witness the emotional and spiritual benefits present themselves to the student when they are ready to receive them.

My hope is that you too discover the many 'non-physical benefits' through your personal dedication to your practice.

Why hot yoga is also a deep and powerful meditation

In most hot yoga classes the teacher talks and the student responds. It is one of the only yoga styles where the instructor 'works the room' but does not generally demonstrate the poses.

The constant stream of instruction from the teacher has the effect of fully occupying your conscious mind. Many students don't recognize the great importance of this mechanism, and how it also allows your mind some rest and helps restore mental balance.

The effects can be immediate. Random thoughts quickly minimize. The 'monkey mind' (or mind chatter) starts to slow down, and when your mind slows down, you are freer to encounter the 'here and now'. Burdens of the past or imaginings of the future are lessened. You get to be 'one' with your body.

In practical terms, over time you will recognize the effects that flow over from your class to your 'real' life. You'll find that events that used to trigger poor reactions won't provoke bad behavior anymore, if at all. You notice that you are becoming calmer, more balanced, more good humored.

Hot yoga (and indeed yoga asana in general) is a tool to create varying states of enlightenment, inner truth, peace and calm which deepen with continued and regular practice. There is a synergy of physical asana and meditation.

In class, whether teaching or practicing I want inspiration, I want discovery, I want to explore the body, mind and soul's limitless possibilities ... and I want that for you too.

Your own practice can become an extremely restful experience despite being physically rigorous – and perhaps because it is. This is why stress reduction is one of the most qualitative benefits of the hot yoga class. Over-active minds simply don't have the time in class to get into 'out-of-control' stress patterns. The more frequent your regular practice becomes, the more you can create the stillness.

Your body is a storehouse for emotions and past events.

Your body has memory, which can be triggered by movement. The asanas move your body into all sorts of positions, and your circulation breathes life into stagnant areas. Just as impurities move, so do crystallized emotions dislodge. Your body and mind are cleansed holistically and your reactivity to stressful situations lessens.

We already know that simple meditation based on breath and/or visualization is effective. The physical asanas used in hot yoga are also very effective. Combine the two and you'll access some of the deepest, most calming meditation possible.

How to use this guide

Perhaps you are reading this because of one or more of the following:

- You want an effective series of beginner poses to practice at home;
- You are a new student of hot yoga;
- You are too far away from a studio to attend regular classes;
- You have been attending classes for some time but there are some poses that, despite instruction, you still don't 'get';
- You love your practice but are unsure why you still experience struggle, pain or difficulty;
- You are a regular yogi and want to deepen your practice with real practical tools and information to gain finer distinctions of the poses;
- You are thinking of attending some yoga training and want more pose information and refinements.

Whatever your stage of practice, your ability, your flexibility, your level of health, my goal is for you to be pleasantly surprised by the level of detail that you will find as you work through this manual.

My aim for you is that you use this reference guide as your own hot yoga Bible. It is designed to be referred to for general learning as well as for specific needs. Perhaps you will take a pose and digest it fully and take your new awareness to each class as you inspire yourself with new distinctions.

All poses with a couple of exceptions are practiced twice. In broad terms, the first set is a 'warm-up' and the second set, which is usually identical in approach, allows you to explore more depth. Each chapter on each pose generally has a similar layout:

1. **The Essentials** is a broad brush stroke introduction to the elements of each pose.
2. **What Makes This Pose So Difficult To Get Right?** discusses difficulties either experienced from understanding the instructions from the teacher, or idiosyncrasies of your own approach. These issues range from teaching, mechanics or body geometry. This section may even highlight the areas of a pose that are commonly incorrectly taught.
3. **The Technique** breaks down the entire pose step-by-step, from the entry till the last moments before releasing. This section does not deal with errors at all. All the information is geared toward positive action, the 'what to do', 'when' and 'how'. All the steps are positive commands and are numbered. You will also find some advanced distinctions and tips within these points. After you have digested the technique section you will be able to access the information at a glance because of the bolded subheading on each point.
4. **Common Mistakes And How To Fix Them** covers all the 'what ifs' and the 'what not to do'. These are subtitled in a bold text and not numbered, so that you can skim the text for a mistake you may want to research that may be specific to your practice.
5. **Second Set And Release.** Any important extra information about each pose will be placed next and prior to any special differences of the 'Second set' and 'Release' sections.

Please commence your journey by reading this entire introductory section. Some aspects of your practice are relevant to many or all poses. Rather than discussing repetitive elements in detail every time the issue arises, I explore them in detail in this introductory section and cross-reference them in pose chapters.

I believe some elements of hot yoga have been completely misunderstood, wrongly interpreted and incorrectly trained for years. Sometimes this is because the passage of time has diluted the technique. To support my methods I have provided as many evidence-based procedures and experiments as possible. They represent strong anatomical accuracy and scientific reasoning. Once you have a broad understanding of these principles you are ready to embark on your own journey of discovery.

If you have some kind of condition, illness, tightness or injury you will probably find the way to overcome your difficulties in the pose. At the very least you'll be confident to approach it with integrity and in a manner that contributes to healing, opening and cleansing rather than exacerbating your condition.

In class, whether teaching or practicing I want inspiration, I want discovery, I want to explore the body, mind and soul's limitless possibilities ... and I want that for you too.

What this guide is not about

This is the commonsense guide to hot yoga. It is designed to be accessible to everyone. Using my medical training, I have translated the jargon often used in anatomical references and provided anatomically precise, but easy to understand steps and movements for you to follow.

Most people, after all, don't need to know specifically about supraspinatus. However they may want precise methods to resolve all muscle tension in the head, neck and shoulders, or to know in which specific way to rotate the arms or shoulders.

This book is based on my years of experience of refining that which is required to get into, stay in, get out of the poses safely and with accuracy.

I operate on the principle of measuring twice and cutting once. In other words, set yourself up properly, maintain the conditions throughout the pose and benefit from the get-go till you let go. This book is also not about Chakras, reincarnation or kundalini energy. I will not discuss the 8 limbs of yoga – you can find masses of free information on the internet and there are hundreds of books. See the resources section at www.HotYogaDoctor.com. It is not about the benefits of each and every pose. Even though I will occasionally discuss benefits, I have deliberately not taken up valuable space in the book on information already in the public domain.

What you will find are down-to-earth principles of yoga practice and how to approach your hot yoga with safety and precision. You will discover how to find the sweet spot in each pose, how to set up the right alignment, the twists, the organ compressions, the way to lengthen and strengthen, how to find power and precise subtle movements of muscles or limb movements. You will learn the skill of relaxation and meditation by paying attention to the right things.

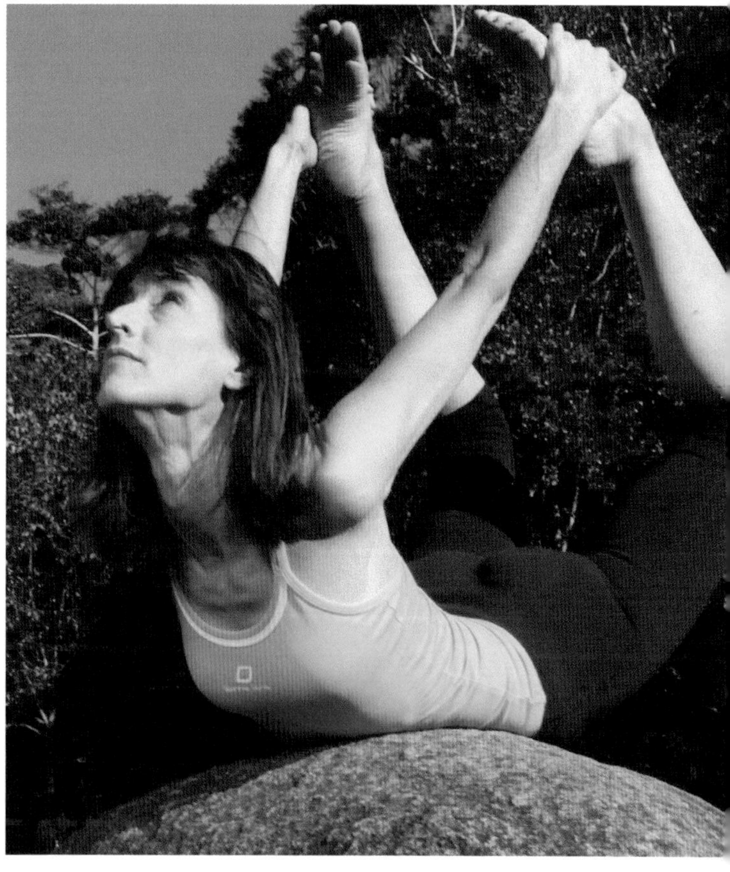

You'll find that events that used to trigger poor reactions won't provoke bad behavior anymore, if at all. You notice that you are becoming calmer, more balanced, more good humored.

Learning About Learning

How Hot Yoga Can Transform Your Life

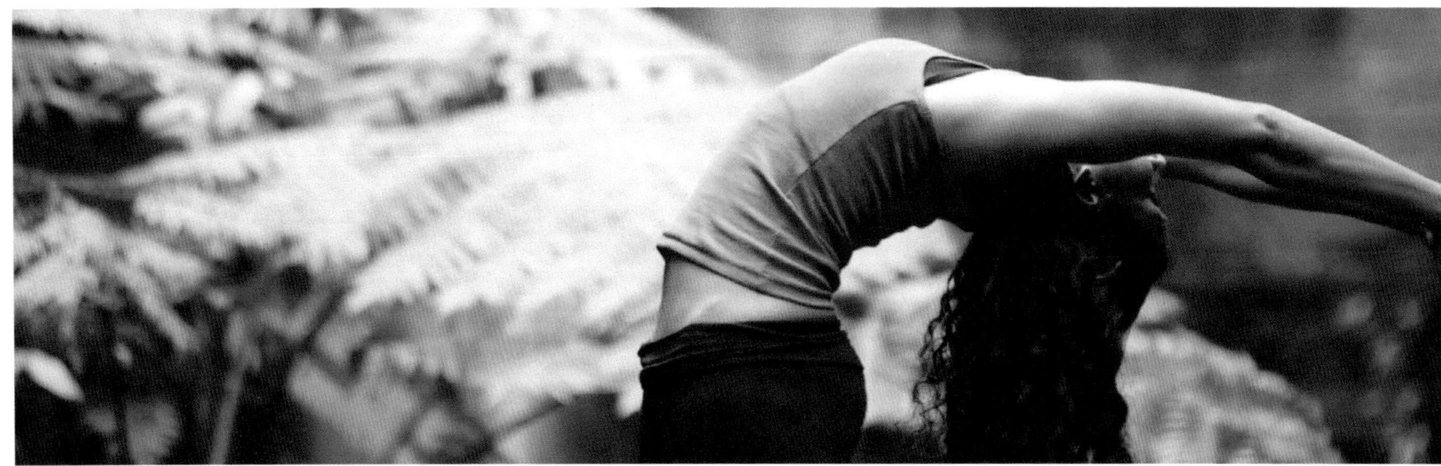

Hot yoga is a moving meditation combining asana, breath work and heat.
All are needed to get the best results.

Repetition is the parent of wisdom

The fact that we repeat the same class each time creates perfect conditions for deep learning.

Unlike other yogas where it could take years to learn 100s of poses, an effective hot yoga practice may only take a number of classes to gain sufficient familiarity.

This offers you a great opportunity to stand back from the process and be the observer. A beautiful side-effect of this is a corresponding deepening of the meditative qualities of your practice.

Use this repetitive element wisely to learn and grow, not to judge progress.

By simply being the observer, you don't need to attach any meaning to success or failure, losing energy, falling out of poses, or losing balance. What you did last class – or plan to do next class – has nothing to do with yoga and can prevent you observing and learning.

Equally, when things go badly the tendency is to try to work out why. However, if you try to attach meaning to an action or reaction you will rob yourself of objective learning.

Repetition can also create your worst enemy in hot yoga: Habits.

The ability to be unattached to your sensations means you can deepen the meditative effects of your yoga practice.

I recommend you avoid practicing poses on 'auto pilot', because by doing this you are simply exercising your body and nothing more.

For example, if you know that your next action will be to lift your leg off the floor to enter Eagle Pose, then have the humility to wait for your instructor's command. If you proceed earlier it could mean so many things:

- That you are anticipating difficulty in balance or leg wrap;
- That you are not listening and are allowing your thoughts to take control;
- That you might be overly attached to your ability to get into the pose.

Treat every second of your practice as Yoga, not just the poses themselves. If you find your mind is wandering, then observe your breath and bring yourself back to the present moment.

Hot yoga is a moving meditation combining asana, breath work and heat. All are needed to get the best results.

A useful thing to remember, is to breathe with mindfulness and approach each class, each teacher, each pose and each moment as if it were your first.

Be aware of your learning process

There are thousands of details involved in learning new skills. Coming to your first hot yoga class can be a great challenge. Your ability to manage will be dependent on your conscious attention. What you are able to pay attention to is determined by your state of mind, your emotions, your memory, your level of tiredness and health. Your ability to learn can be variable.

I like to offer an analogy to all my new students – you might find it useful too. Let's imagine that you only have a certain amount of headspace available for conscious attention. Research shows that the number of items you can typically pay attention to at any given moment is between 5 and 9. For the purposes of example we will imagine that you can pay attention to 10 things and I will give you 10 conscious-awareness-dollars. In the following scenario we'll pretend that you can only spend this allowance in whole dollar multiples.

Imagine now that you are learning to drive a car for the first time. You slide into the seat, your instructor beside you. After a little orientation she says to pull away from the curb, drive up to the intersection, stop and when the road is clear, turn right. That sounds easy. Well, maybe because right now you most likely know how to drive.

But as a total beginner this is completely overwhelming. You have to pay attention to (and not necessarily in the following order):

1. Putting your key in the ignition
2. Putting your belt on
3. Checking your rear vision mirror
4. Adjusting your mirror
5. Locating and adjusting your side mirrors
6. Working out how to decipher what you see in reverse in terms of distance and location
7. Starting the car
8. Finding and operating the turn signals
9. Looking over your shoulder
10. Finding the gear shift
11. Locating the brake pedal
12. Locating the accelerator pedal
13. Being able to hear your instructor.

We have not even moved the car yet. We have already busted your $10 limit. This is when you can feel lost, overwhelmed, often unable to act – or act with any degree of skill.

At times like this, you might be very aware of your driving incompetence. As you progress along the path of your learning process, certain elements start to become engrained and automatic (conditioned responses). Gradually you don't have to spend your precious conscious-awareness-dollars on the basics and you are left with plenty of headspace for that which requires your attention.

Using this driving example might mean that you now drive home from work and you can happily think about shopping lists or what's for dinner, all the while automatically observing stop signals, other vehicles on the road and so-on.

Translate this to your yoga practice and as you progress through your first few classes, you'll be able to pay more attention to the basics. Then, with the basics handled, you can start to embrace new and more advanced distinctions.

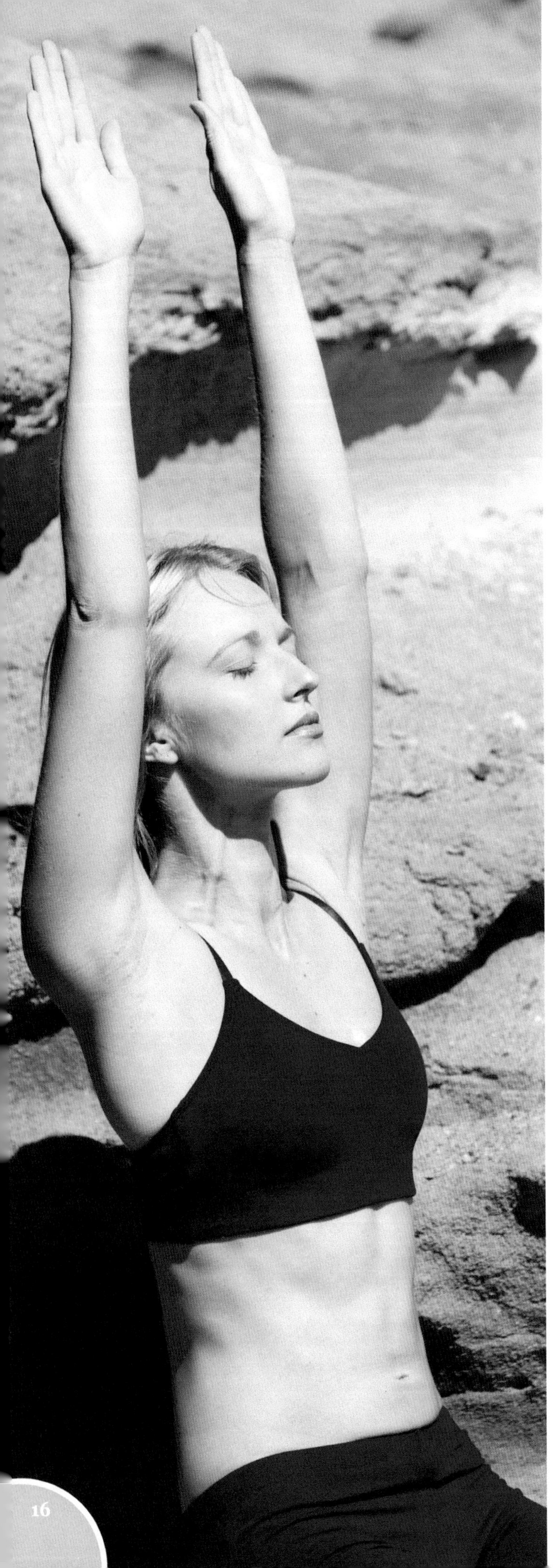

There are 4 stages of learning:

1. Unconscious incompetence (you don't even know what you don't know).
2. Conscious incompetence (when you arrive at your first yoga class, you know you are going to learn yoga but don't know the poses or the order of practice).
3. Conscious competence (when you are starting to embrace the techniques and have space to take on new information, but still need to think about most aspects of your practice).
4. Unconscious competence (gaining a flow state where thinking about your skill or craft is unnecessary).

Once you are familiar with your practice you will cycle between stages 3 and 4 as you start to hear, learn, understand and embrace new distinctions. Bringing understanding to your learning process means you can disregard the things that may have previously drawn your attention. Being disappointed because you fall over when trying to balance, or being elated because you are successfully balancing, can now become fascinating observations that you can let go of and be totally unemotional about. The ability to be unattached to your sensations means you can deepen the meditative effects of your yoga practice.

Understanding your own learning process and response to taking on new information and skills will be a journey in itself. It requires you to remove judgment and avoid defending your own behaviors. Allow yourself to invite new ways of looking at what may even appear to be simple.

There is more to skill acquisition than meets the eye. Often we are protective of what we have learnt as the correct way.

It will take some humility to take what is an unconscious behavior and make that skill conscious again for the purposes of gaining deeper understanding. This is cycling between stages 3 and 4 of learning. Don't assume you know it all. If you do, you rob yourself of learning.

When you read the Hot Yoga MasterClass, there may be times when the information is quite detailed and takes time to understand and absorb. I recommend occasionally adding a physically active component to your reading. Get up and try something out. Doing just one thing is often enough to get momentum and understanding.

Act out the pose and demonstrate to yourself the difference between the best-practice techniques and those of the mistakes. Get conscious about your behaviors and discover better, more effective techniques.

...stay inside the depths of your body without paying attention to anything that occurs outside of yourself. This is 100% meditation.

I hope you will surprise yourself with new realizations and wonder why you haven't done it this way before. You are after all, aiming to get the most out of your practice and your life. With these techniques your physical asanas will be better and your meditation will be more effective. You will be delighted to discover that the positive effects from your yoga practice are manifesting throughout all areas of your life.

Feel the feeling ... and let it go

Unless you are doing a silent class (for example at home without CD or DVD instruction) then part of your yoga experience will be to stay-in-the-moment. Specifically, this means listening to everything your teacher says.

You're probably familiar with the cliché, 'take each moment as it comes'. This means that you neither expect, anticipate, or even dread your next move. This attitude is extremely useful for improving the quality of your yoga.

Your best meditative results will issue from your ability to do as is instructed - without embellishment and without omission, with humility, and avoiding ego.

In this way you can see each moment as unique: To truly observe the breath, the feelings, the emotions – all your sensations, your ease, your challenge, your yoga.

Some of these sensations may be of frustration and impatience, yet it's your job to notice these feelings, and then let them go. Other times you will experience ease and calm. Once again, observe, but do not attribute any reason for these differences.

Some students have a love-hate relationship with hot yoga. They can't stand it in the studio, but they can't bear to miss the tremendous elation they feel after finishing every class. The sublime sense of satisfaction that comes from doing a hot yoga class is what brings students back, again and again and again.

On your journey you will discover something amazing: The power of 'sameness'. In each class you will most likely complete the same postures, you have the same body, you work in the same temperature. The only thing that truly changes from day-to-day is YOU, and your ability to do/cope/practice.

When you fall, you learn

Naturally, there will be times when you have more 'going on' in your life than usual. This may be reflected in a class where you can't as easily switch off your thoughts. This may manifest in your poses and you may find balancing difficult, or you are irritable or easily annoyed. These are the times when you can demonstrate the effectiveness of your yoga practice. Let go of your thoughts. Abandon ego and focus your attention on your breathing. Be happy if you fall. After all, falling, is learning how not to fall.

The phrase 'falling is learning' encapsulates a spirit of non-attachment to both your success and your fear of failure. Having either a 'success or failure' mindset can hinder your own progress, but achieving non-attachment can produce undreamed of results.

For example, if you like the way you look or feel in a pose, you may be reluctant to try something new. Perhaps you fear you'll lose concentration and have to go back in and try again. Perhaps your unwillingness to go beyond your 'comfort zone' (for example, kicking harder in Standing Bow and thereby risking discomfort or overbalancing) is a metaphor for the way you run your life.

Think about it. If you don't fall sometimes, you might not really be pushing your edge. Perhaps the 'edge' you are pushing may not even be a physical one.

It all boils down to not caring one way or the other about results.

Do the yoga. Use the physical principles of the asana, breathe through whatever intensity occurs (whether physical, mental or emotional), observe the responses of your body and mind, and the magic will follow.

Reacting to what happens will only take you out of your body and into your mind, into the area of judgment and fault-finding. Lots of students openly criticize themselves, sometimes even curse. It is a sign of being ruled by the mind and its collaborator, the ego. What you must always do in yoga is stay inside the depths of your body without paying attention to anything that occurs outside of yourself. This is 100% meditation.

Breaking out from habitual anticipation can liberate you from paralyzing life patterns. Facing your fears works better in the long run.

Do it, already! A look at procrastination and anticipation

Going into a pose too slowly is a sneaky distraction technique, called procrastination. Progressing too leisurely through the stages of a pose is another form of procrastination. Often, students prolong the entry time and minimize finished pose time – for example I see this typically in Balancing Stick and Toe Stand. Or they won't explore their limit in the pose until the last couple of seconds (in poses such as Eagle and especially Standing Bow or Standing Head to Knee).

My question to those students would be, what breakthroughs are you missing out on by just hanging out right until moments before release?

Follow this 75% rule ...

I have a clear guideline for this which I call my 75% Rule:

Spend 75% of the time in the final part of the pose.

Yes, spend 75% of the time in the pose – and no more than 25% of your time 'getting into it'.

Don't submit to mediocrity. As soon as you are able to access the pose, then do so – don't procrastinate! Don't waste precious time. Get there and grow.

Even if you can only get to the first stage of any pose – spend 75% of your time in this stage. You will find details of the application of this rule on page 115.

Beware of habitually approaching your poses in stages

You may be approaching the physical technique perfectly. However, taking too much time to get to your regular depth, makes your yoga too easy. In fact, it is a 'cop-out'. If you don't push your edge, you are just coasting.

So if you are in the habit of breaking your pose entries down into deliberate stages to make it 'easier', this might be robbing you of significant benefits. Once you know how to enter a pose ... then do so efficiently without pausing to regroup.

Remember: Get there, STAY there at least 75% of the time, and work there.

A note of caution regarding speed of entry: Some poses incorporating long and deep stretches require a smooth and sustained approach – so be mindful that while you want to move quickly and deliberately into a pose, it is not a race to see who gets into it first.

Your body has a natural intelligence to allow movement into long duration stretches with safety. Your muscles become more compliant in a stretch when you give them time. This is why you can feel your body opening in great stretches such as Head To Knee Pose (floor) and Intense Stretching Pose.

Anticipation is the 'cousin' to procrastination

Just as you can delay getting into a pose, you can anticipate its end by releasing early. Anticipation is damaging to your yoga practice. It clearly takes you away from the 'now'. It has you either going in early (through impatience) or coming out early.

Procrastination and Anticipation usually result from 'fear'.

You may fear, for example, experiencing the perceived difficulties of the long protracted hold of Half Moon, Triangle, or Floor Bow. So you engage your mind, think too much and either consciously or unconsciously neglect to observe the teacher's timings. Maybe you release half way, and contrive some reason for the early exit, e.g. bend over and rub a thigh, adjust your shorts or pick up a water bottle – all obviously urgent activities! Sound familiar?

Breaking out from habitual anticipation can liberate you from paralyzing life patterns. Facing your fears works better in the long run.

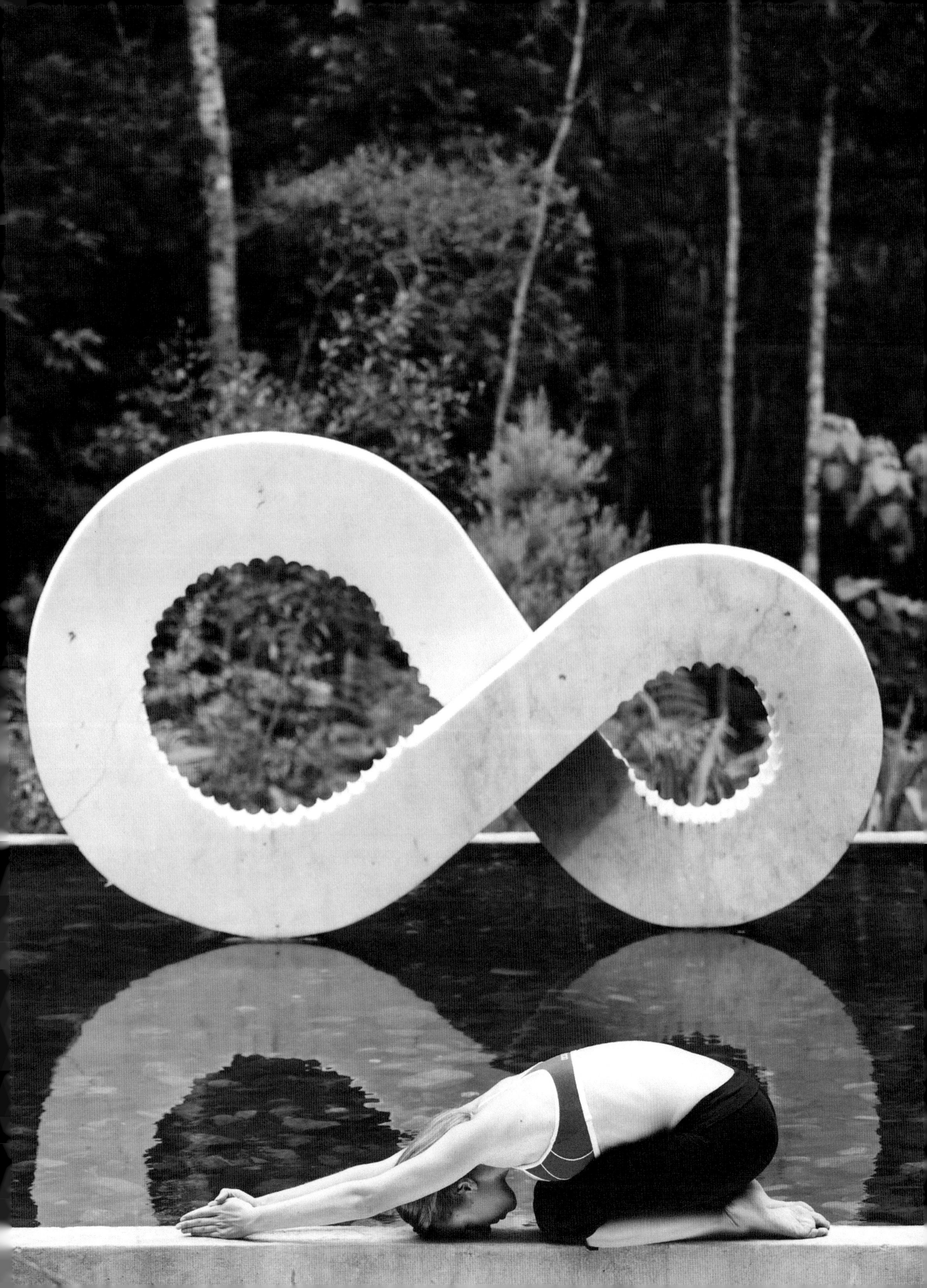

Uniquely Hot Yoga

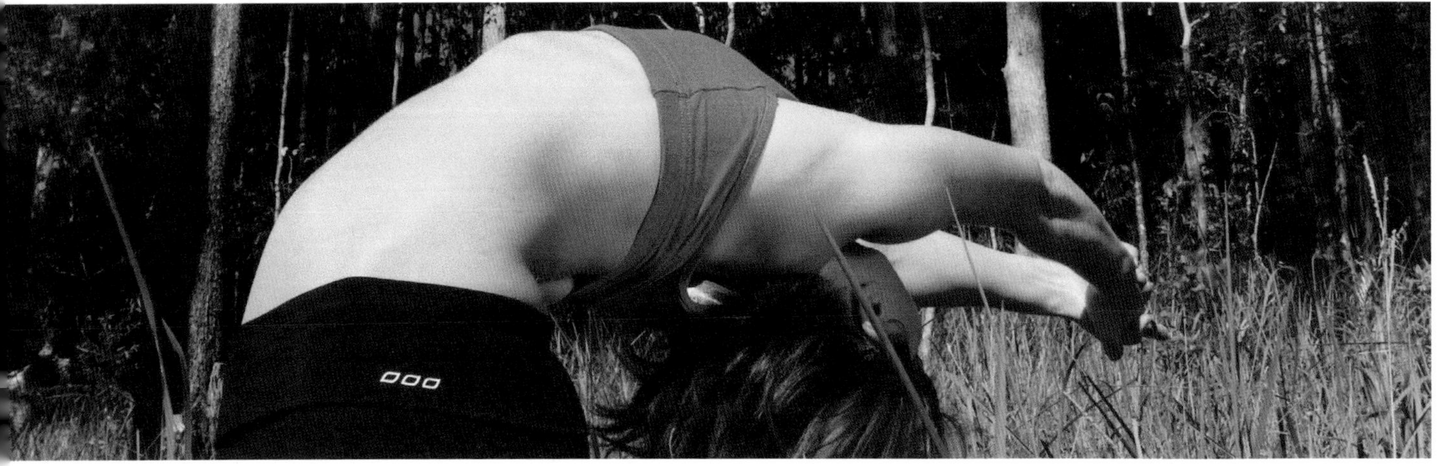

The heat seems to accelerate the benefits beyond logic or expectation making it more holistically satisfying than any other type of yoga.

Creating balance in your life

Life is full of forward bends. We do practically nothing else. We are getting into and out of beds and cars, getting up and down from tables and chairs, bending over, lifting up, reaching for things. The spine however, is designed to bend in all directions! It takes conscious awareness to open the body up in ways that everyday life doesn't cater for.

Balance is very important to a deeply satisfying life. We often relate balance to our lifestyle, eating habits, work schedule and activities. Curiously, finding balance in your life reflects in your yoga practice.

In your life, challenges may present themselves as difficulty in standing on one leg or constantly falling out of poses (even those on two solid legs!). The more you practice yoga the more you will find balance and equanimity in your mind. Then if you do encounter hard times you are less easily distracted or thrown off center.

Your hot yoga practice is a great balance of forward bends, backward bends and twisted spine movements. However they are not in equal doses. Everyday life has us rarely performing backbends. It is no surprise that there are few forward bends and most poses encompass the other movements. This focus on backbends, stretches and twists creates the balance that will result in restoring your natural range of motion.

You don't have to be flexible to do yoga. In fact conversely – it helps to be stiff to practice yoga. You learn to work, and balance your strength and flexibility.

Which is better? Flexibility or strength?

Part of the magic of hot yoga is that the more you know, the deeper and harder you can work. The more distinctions you discover, the more you can work your edge and achieve our outcomes. It is a great balancing act, literally.

If you are strong (typically men, or athletes of either sex) then chances are that you need to work on your flexibility.

If you are flexible (typically dancers and gymnasts, non-athletic students who haven't tightened their bodies up with exercise over the years) then no doubt you will need to work on your strength.

Who has it harder, the strong or the flexible?

Typically, students with great strength appear to be having a harder time balancing themselves out. They have to lengthen and become more supple and soft in their muscles. They have to surrender more, give up the fight and relax into themselves. They often have more obvious difficulty getting into the poses with any depth. However, these people usually have more immediate and measurable success in balancing themselves because they are used to physically demanding work.

The flexible noodles actually have a harder time finding their flexibility/strength balance. Why? Because they find it easy to get into most postures. What's more, they find that they look good in the postures (and they do). Why else do they call them poses? Just kidding!

Let's explore how every student can work to their own edge ...

How do you find your edge?

Initially every student has to learn their practice. You can definitely benefit from the very first class and you will certainly grow to love coming to class, feeding your soul and banishing stress. But you must balance your need for accomplishment, and humility, with your requirement for being in the moment. That being said, it takes knowing the poses sufficiently well to know HOW to work them hard. The most experienced yogi in the room could be working harder than anyone despite the appearance of effortlessness to an outsider.

Anyone however, can 'hang out' in a pose and just go through the motions. Here is how to avoid that happening to you ...

I'm using Standing Bow (Dandayamana Dhanurasana) as an example pose for the following two scenarios:

The strong man in Standing Bow

Let's imagine these students have attended sufficient classes to know what is required of them. They have balance and can lock out their legs and they know how to kick into this pose. The strong man may have difficulty in holding his foot. His shoulders and latissimus dorsi are so tight that it is hard to hold his hand above his head, with an activated arm at the same time as keeping his chest open and chin up.

Still, with very few classes his flexibility starts to return. His steady persistence and strength allows him to open his body. The kick backward and up may be difficult but it is strong and serves to actively stretch his body.

The ballerina in Standing Bow

The ballerina easily launches herself into Standing Bow and almost effortlessly approaches the standing splits. But her arm may not even be engaged and often her standing leg will not be locked out the whole time. She has her leg up over her head but she needed almost no kicking power to get it there.

Typically you will hear your teachers saying that everybody gets the benefits. True to an extent. But in this example, unless our ballerina brings energy to her arm in trying to extend it, activate it and lift it up high, and unless she tries hard to press her leg strongly back and up towards the ceiling, then it is the 'strong man' who is getting more out of this pose.

You don't have to be flexible to do yoga. In fact conversely – it helps to be stiff to practice yoga. You learn to work, and balance your strength and flexibility.

Stiffer bodies enjoy so many benefits from the traction and active stretching that it is almost an advantage to be tight!

I hope this enthuses you to find your edge and work it no matter what your 'body type'. Give yourself the time to learn what you need to do to make this the most satisfying workout of your body and mind.

Why developing core strength is essential

Anyone can have weakness in their core, which is the stabilizing network of muscles in the lower torso and pelvic region. This network provides strength, stability and balance to your whole body for everyday functioning. Your core strength is sometimes referred to as your center of power. The stronger your core, the easier your everyday activities will be. You will also be less likely to have back pain, urinary incontinence and general back weakness. Strengthening your core is part of any sensible exercise routine. Oh – and a better sex life.

Some have a love-hate relationship with hot yoga. They can't stand it in the studio, but can't bear to miss the tremendous elation they feel after every class. The sublime sense of satisfaction that comes from doing a hot yoga class is what brings students back again and again.

Practicing hot yoga will improve your core strength - though importantly and critically, only by observing precise technique. Gains in core strength will make the mundane aspects of life easier; bending over, picking things up, getting into and out of bed or a car, picking up a toddler or a box!

There is no particular group of people who have weak cores. Abdominal strength is NOT equal to core strength. You may be aware that women are often reminded to exercise their perineal muscles. These muscles may suffer stretching and weakness as a result of giving birth. It is common for women to need to give conscious attention to restoring perineal health.

Men too can benefit. It may surprise you to learn that men who can retract their perineum are less likely to have prostate problems and urinary issues.

Throughout your hot yoga practice it is important to engage your core muscles. This does not mean simply sucking in your stomach. Correctly drawing in your abdomen helps core strength and provides a trigger for contracting or sucking 'upward' the muscles deep within your pelvis, between your genitals and anus. In yogic terms this is called your mula bandha (or root lock). Read the following example.

The 40-something year old man with weak core muscles who can't do a forward bend

I have taught literally hundreds of men who have difficulty with their core strength. These are men who are apparently strong – perhaps in their 40s or 50s – for whom brute strength in their upper body can no longer compensate for their lack of core strength.

These men can appear to have abs of steel, lovely defined shoulders and pecs but have weak core muscles. They complain of their inability to bend forward without pain in their lower spine. They often cannot do a sit-up. Their strength is often only surface deep, or confined to their shoulders and legs.

These men have survived with their upper body strength compensating for an underlying weakness. And then all of a sudden one day they bend over forward to pick something up, or get into or out of the car and they collapse with painful spasms. If this sounds like you (whether male or female) then try hot yoga with conscious intent to improve your core strength.

There are specific poses that will, when approached correctly without short cuts, develop your core. Most importantly, an integrated hot yoga practice works well for holistic health and strength.

Why is the heat beneficial?

Somewhere along the way (whether it is the first, 10th or 50th class) hot yoga students consciously notice that they are calmer, more stress- or pain-free, more self-actualized, healthier and happier. If they don't notice it consciously, often someone close to them will point it out!

What does this have to do with the heat?

The heat seems to accelerate the benefits beyond logic or expectation making it more holistically satisfying than any other type of yoga.

The changes can be very quick and sometimes instant. Unconsciously you may find yourself making better life choices; such as eating healthily, or quitting smoking.

Maybe you will just FEEL better for no apparent reason or you will feel impervious to stress. With a quietening of your extraneous thoughts you get increasing control over your own mind. You find a depth of calm and stillness within. You discover your limitless energy and potential.

The alchemy created by the hot yoga sequence, the mirrors and the heat, starts a deep operation in your mind and soul, quickly reversing years of physical and mental baggage and peeling back layers to reveal a truer, more compassionate, loving self. The mirrors bring you face to face with your own reality. You can face it or even walk away.

When you persist you will find yourself working towards true self-acceptance and love.

Important facts about sweating

Sweat is an integral part of your hot yoga experience. It is important to understand it doesn't just happen because the temperature is high. For optimum conditions you need a balance between heat and humidity. The most satisfying conditions are when you feel warm, have a good sweat and your movements feel deep and safe, facilitated by the heat.

Quite a number of students may feel stressed out by the heat, and sometimes they even struggle. They often blame the heat

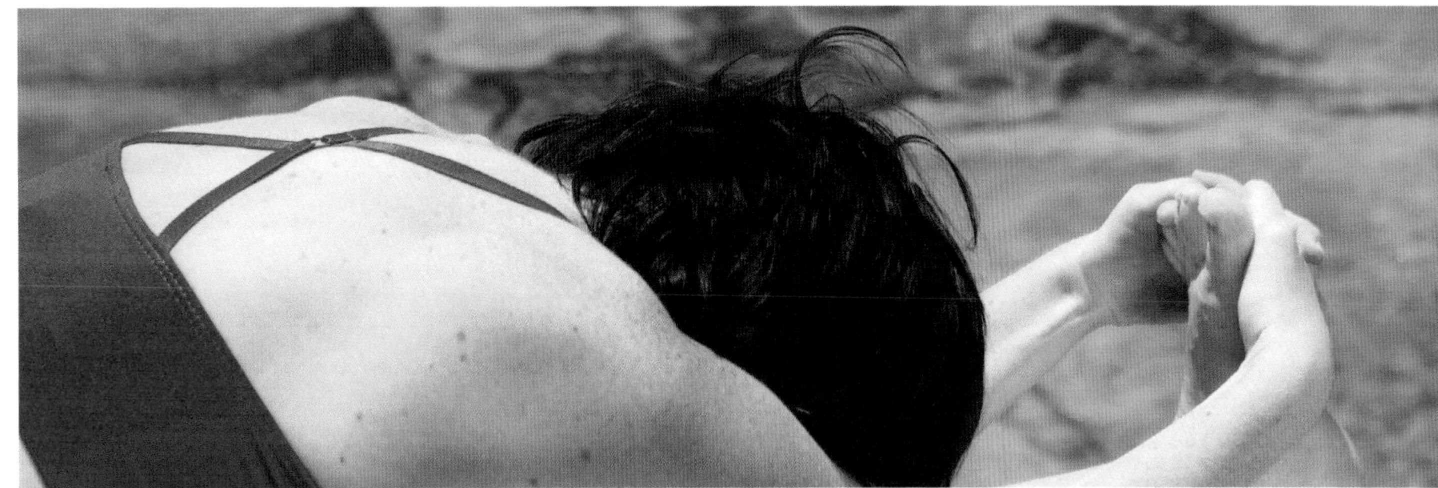

for their difficulties. Yet struggle in yoga is usually more about your mind rather than your body's reaction to physical effort and environment.

The body can take up to two weeks to physiologically acclimatize to the heat which strengthens the body's cardiovascular system amongst other positive benefits. The heat is not generally to blame when it comes to initial difficulties. Remember your mind does play huge tricks on you. It will come up with excuses to haul you away from your challenges if you are not careful.

Let's remove the mind's games from the equation and simply look at humidity and heat as physical conditions. Your perception of heat is going to be affected by the humidity in the room.

The lower the humidity the lower your perception of the heat. In fact in dry weather you may feel the room is 'cooler' because you are not sweating to your satisfaction. If the humidity is about 20%, the temperature can reach 105°F (41°C) and hardly cause a sweat. Students commonly ask to the have the heat turned up! This is why an accurate thermometer needs to be in the studio.

The converse is true, if the humidity is very high (at around 70% or higher) then the temperature need only be about 95°F (35°C) for a good sweat. Humidity levels will also depend on the number of students and how well the room is ventilated. The more students, the more humid breath, the more sweat and moisture in the atmosphere. The less well ventilated the higher the humidity.

Sweating alone does not cool the body. Evaporation of sweat is only one mechanism that lowers body temperature. Movement of passing air across your body also acts as a cooling mechanism as does your body heating the air around it which will then rise, carrying the heat away.

Humidity however, also increases sweat and fluid loss. I have to remind students (especially new ones) you cannot cool the body by wiping sweat. Wiping it off actually removes the body's vital 'evaporative cooling' mechanism. Body temperature rises and more and more sweat is produced. Repeatedly wiping sweat may lead to massive fluid and electrolyte loss where basic body functions are detrimentally affected (making this a life-threatening problem).

This is why you must be very well hydrated before class. Your normal daily intake of over 2 liters of water must increase when you go to hot yoga. But water is not enough. Electrolytes must be replaced.

I recommend generously using sea salt (never table salt) in your diet. Try a pinch in your water with a few drops of lemon juice. You don't need to buy expensive branded electrolytes. Pure sea salt is the way to go. Simplistically, your body is a big battery and needs electrolytes to keep charged.

Drink if and when you need to during class. Avoid inappropriate times such as mid-pose, or habitually at the same time(s) every class. If you are truly thirsty then you have not been hydrating enough prior.

Many reach for the bottle because of 'sudden thirst'. This impulse to drink can be an unconscious avoidance tactic, so be mindful. Often the standing poses can be very confronting. Enduring your own reflection and accepting what you see can be hard. Time, experience and honesty will help you determine your real hydration needs.

Approached with care and understanding you should never experience any of the problems associated with heat, fluid or electrolyte loss. You too will appreciate the heat as both the magic and necessary ingredient for your yoga experience.

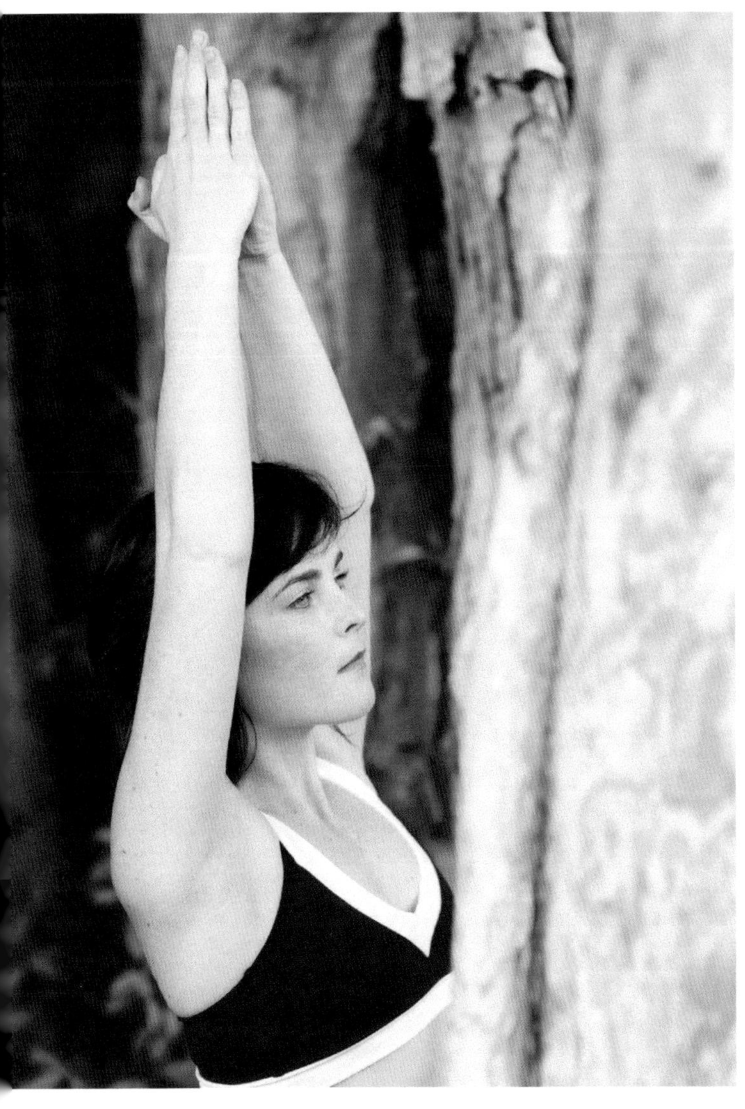

Whenever a student returns after a practice interruption we hear the same song again and again: "I feel so great. Why was I so scared of returning? I will never do that again. I wish I had never stopped coming."

Why not air-conditioned comfort?

You can go to other less structured hatha yoga classes in unheated or un-mirrored rooms and know that you're doing something great for yourself. You may discover like many others that the hot yoga experience feels more powerful and refreshing and perhaps more satisfying than other styles.

I have attended structured Iyengar and Ashtanga classes as well as ad hoc yoga classes where the pose selection changes at the whim of the teacher. Although I really enjoy Ashtanga yoga and I have gained some (mild) enjoyment or benefits from other styles, nothing beats hot yoga, period.

You wouldn't go running a marathon without a thorough warm-up. You wouldn't dream of performing stretches in a walk-in fridge. Logically we know we have to warm up for our workout. Still many find the idea of the warm room foreign.

How on earth could exercising in an air-conditioned gym be better for you? Your body will end up in a tug-of-war between getting warm enough for exercise and cooling down too much because of the pumped cold air risking undue damage.

In hot yoga, the body starts and stays warm. The stretches are deeper and safer. Your body's systems work more efficiently when warm. The fact is, your body loves the heat. It's only your mind that may behave differently.

There are many thousands of great hot yoga stories yet very few that are more than anecdotal. However, these are just too numerous to ignore. There does not seem to be much if any solid scientific evidence that hot yoga does what it claims. Yet the huge wave of enthusiasm for these contentious series is overwhelming.

You simply cannot deny that it creates magic in the lives of many. My own life changed for the better the day I walked in to the heat. It is my personal hope that it does the same for you.

How often should you practice?

You either love hot yoga or you hate it – maybe during class anyhow! But how many times per week should you go? This is a question asked by just about every new student.

Do the yoga more intensively if you are searching for clarity; if you are working on a problem; if you need space in your head, if you have aches and pains. It is the closest thing to a panacea.

That is a difficult question to answer. You may need to balance your practice with a hectic lifestyle or a full active timetable. I have many students for which hot yoga is their only form of exercise. They now use it as their body workout and base their other activities around it to the virtual exclusion of other formal exercise. Partly because it is so incredibly satisfying and partly because you feel its comprehensive nature – a whole body and mind workout.

Other students supplement their training or dance schedule with it to get the stretch that they don't get elsewhere. High level athletes – triathletes, Olympic athletes, professional footballers, basketballers, swimmers and surfers – all use hot yoga to give them a physical and psychological edge.

Consider your goals. By when would you like to achieve them? Do you want gradual or quick change? This style of yoga can bring you an incredible and remarkably fast makeover.

My husband uses an analogy. Like butter in the fridge, the more often you take it out, the easier it is to spread; the less time it has to set back solid. The more classes per week the more effective, profound and long lasting the change will be. So, here are some suggested guidelines to approaching your practice:

The first two months:

Take your pain early. Well that's just an expression. I suggest you initially commit for a finite time. A couple of months is ideal. Make sacrifices. Cut out other commitments, even your other exercise until you pass this initial phase. If you do this, you will only have to do it this one time. Just like the butter in the fridge analogy, you want to make changes to your physical being, and your mental and emotional state. Frequency creates sustainable changes. Get some traction and benefit from your hard work so that you stay motivated.

Four times per week is where the magic starts to happen ...

A hot yoga practice brings amazing benefits. The effects of exercising with added heat seems to accelerate the changes you can make in your life and physical body, mentally, emotionally and spiritually. Practicing with best technique and with the right frequency can make this a most life changing and satisfying yoga workout. Many people feel they have a healthy addiction!

Coming once a week is fine if supplementing your main exercise regime, but on slim pickings like this it feels like you are starting again every week. You get a good stretch, provide good cross-training and help counter tight muscles from running and cycling. Three times a week, if you can, is a fantastic maintenance regime. The majority of students practice three times.

But ... if you want to change any part of your life, commit to two months at least 4 times per week (more if you can, 5 or 6). Let the other things slide. Miss that television program (record it), give up some or all other sporting pursuits to get to these classes. After two months if you can't see and feel changes then I would be extremely surprised. With your commitment and your intention you will feel and look and act differently.

With your solid introduction and with some tangible results it's time to settle into your own maintenance program. When I started I was practicing 6-8 times per week. After five months, I settled in to a 4-5 times a week practice. Now that I have a family and business if I cannot manage to practice four times, I have lots of cumulative benefits that tide me over. It is important to take a day off each week for rest and recovery.

Do the yoga more intensively if you are searching for clarity; if you are working on a problem; if you need space in your head, if you have aches and pains. It is the closest thing to a panacea.

When you can't drag yourself to class

Often the reasons that keep us away from the warm room are THE exact same reasons we should be getting there. A stressful lifestyle, difficulties with coping with a job or the kids can make it hard to get to yoga. But paradoxically, given the two hours or so that it takes out of your day, our students find that they have more to give to their family, friends, workmates and their jobs and lives. Your practice becomes more of an investment in yourself than just another time-draining activity.

One of my regular students is a building contractor and a specialist in laying of concrete slabs. Decades of playing football has tightened his body into a coil of muscles. Stuart finds physical difficulty with much of the class just hauling his muscular body into position. A regular practice has a great payoff. What he does love is the focus he develops. Previously stressful situations are a breeze. Over the years he has continued to practice regularly, with a few breaks here and there. Sometimes he is overseas on building jobs. Sometimes the breaks from yoga extend further. You may be familiar with what happens: You get into a routine and somehow after a break it is harder to get yourself back into the swing of things.

What brings Stuart back? Well, his employees have told him point blank, several times that he is a far better boss, more balanced, calm and fair when he does his yoga.

No matter what the excuse is, one thing is for sure, whenever a student returns after a practice interruption we hear the same song again and again: "I feel so great. Why was I so scared of returning? I will never do that again. I wish I had never stopped coming."

Practicing hot yoga at home

Some think practicing in a purpose-built studio is the ideal option, others prefer to do their own thing. There are several reasons why studio practice may be impractical:

- You live or work too far away from a studio to get there as regularly as you would like.
- There is no studio within a reasonable distance.
- You need to be at home for logistical reasons to run your home or business.
- You are away on business, or on holidays where there is no studio or you have limited time to get to a studio.
- You don't have a full 90 minutes and need to practice for a shorter time.
- You don't have 90 mins practice time available and the additional travel time to and from the studio.
- You prefer practicing on your own terms, due to temperament, illness, injury or simply because you prefer practicing solo.

Hot yoga is typified by the presence of mirrors and heat. You can simply set up a mat and start doing your asana. I did exactly that when I first started. I set myself up near a sun drenched window in the lounge room. I didn't have a mirror but I worked up a great sweat and I was doing yoga.

If you can't practice in the heat then better to do some yoga than none at all. There is also no rule that 90 minutes is the only way. There are plenty of options to practice shorter classes if you are time-poor.

Here, are some guidelines to create a dedicated hot yoga space and to get the most out of your home-practice.

Where to practice

Energetically, it is better to have a space that is dedicated to your practice, even if it serves other purposes at other times. You may still need to do a little furniture moving. The size of the room will determine the number and position of mirrors and the strength of the heaters. The floor covering will also be important.

The classic minimum requirement is a mirror on one wall. Aim to heat the room to body temperature. It is best to be able to close off the space to confine the heat.

Setting up your space:

- Insulation is probably the most important consideration and if done well your heating costs will be vastly reduced. Insulate the ceiling particularly well. We always over-insulate our studios (aim for a high R-value). All walls are heavily insulated. We place insulation film on the windows or use special insulating glass or thicker panes.
- Use the right heater for the job.
- Install good mirrors, lined for safety.
- Use a temperature/humidity monitor.

Mirrors

You must at least be able to see yourself in the mirror. Your poses will be better, more easily corrected and your meditation and self-connection will deepen. Think about having mirrors along a wide expanse or if space is limited either one mirror on one wall or on two separate walls in case you have to do your warrior poses stepping out along the length of your mat.

Heaters

Not all heaters are created equal! Most domestic heaters have a thermostat that cuts off the power long before your room is heated to body temperature. You may find it difficult to heat your room past 90°F (30-32°C). This means that it doesn't matter how many heaters you have on in the room you will be hard pressed to get the room super-heated. You will have to research the best heater for your space.

Remember that insulation is a prime consideration. Take into account what surfaces are present. We converted a garage once, the hard cold floor prevented the temperature rising sufficiently and necessitated full carpet coverage, which yielded immediate results.

Never overheat a room. Many studio owners use this next trick, but it is dangerous and is not recommended. They place the thermostat outside of the room to 'trick' the system into super-heating the room. The heater never cuts out because the trigger temperature is never reached. The problem is that you have no control. The temperature could rise above safe levels and you may not know it. Moisture levels can alter your perception of how hot a room really is.

If the temperature rises above 104°F or 40°C, then this could be dangerous because the body may not be able to cool its core temperature sufficiently, especially if the humidity is high or ventilation is very poor. No matter which heating system you choose, ensure that your yoga space is removed from drafts,

I practiced at least 6 times per week and often went 8 times. Within two weeks I had lost 2 dress sizes and 10 pounds (5 kilos).

though it must never be airtight. Radiant (infrared) heaters can remove the need for completely closing off the space.

If there is no carpet:

- The room could take longer to heat due to lessened insulation.
- The floor will be more slippery if your sweat lands on the floor.
- It is easier to keep clean and smelling fresh.
- You will probably have to face one of the side walls and step out from the narrow end of your mat for your warrior poses. This is an important non-slip safety consideration.
- You may choose to have two mats placed at 90° in a 't' configuration so you can continually face the mirrored wall.

For rooms with carpet:

- Thick carpet or carpet with underlay may challenge your balance.
- Ensure the room can be aired to get rid of the smell of sweat and to dry any moisture.
- Make sure you sweat on your towel and not on the carpet. The smell can be very persistent and necessitates professional carpet cleaning. We learned this the hard way. Our house stank after only two classes. Try our trick of placing your towel at 90° across your mat in a 't' configuration to start your class. Realign your towel lengthwise just before you get to the floor for the first time for "Corpse Pose" (Savasana).
- Consider indoor/outdoor carpet because it is washable and much more hygienic.
- Domestically laid carpet usually has underlay. The extra layers and the difficulty in drying it out fully, makes it a health hazard. Another good case for using a 't' configuration with a towel or extra mat.
- In our first home studio we used an edged piece of regular carpet that could be lifted and aired.

Understand the conditions

Have moisture and temperature gauges visible at all times. You can buy these on one neat little unit that also show the time. Position it for an average reading, about half way up in the room; not on the floor, because hot air rises.

Use electric rather than gas because of ventilation problems with gas in a small enclosed space. Also recommended are circulating oil and infrared heaters. Fan and infrared heaters are responsive so you can alter conditions quickly.

Ideally you want a reliable, controllable heat. You don't want to be sidetracked by frequently monitoring the temperature. You want yoga with minimal distraction.

An appropriate heater should only take 30-40 minutes to get up to temperature. If it takes over an hour and is still struggling to get to temperature then use a more powerful heater and consider better insulation to stop losses.

You may need to introduce a vaporizer to control the moisture in the room. You are aiming for between 45 and 80% humidity (optimal humidity is 60-70%). Less than 30% and you will never feel that the temperature is high enough, even when it gets to over 105F (41C). Conversely if the humidity is 75% and higher you may find that heating to between 90-95°F (33-35°C) is enough to warm your body up and sweat.

Your mirror doesn't need to be very wide because there are only very few poses that have a wide stance. Make do with whatever mirror you can and maximize your view. If it is not wide enough to see yourself in triangle pose then don't fret, you can change your position from class to class, step out from the narrow end of your mat and use your developing inner eye, or proprioception.

Generally you will want a good quality sticky mat of around 1/8" or 3-4mm thick. I'm personally quite happy with them even thinner than this – it all depends on your floor surface. If you have carpet then you can have a very thin mat, if you have a hard floor then you will probably want more padding in your mat. I don't recommend anything thicker than 1/4" (6mm) as this can affect your balancing poses.

Clothing: Don't wear loose, comfortable clothing as many studios recommend. When you sweat, you'll find that loose gear will stick to your body and make some poses more difficult. This is unpleasant. Anything other than gym gear such as sports bras, singlets, bike shorts or capris tend to ride up during many poses. Too much time and attention is paid to what I call 'modesty checks'. Remember you will have a better chance of activating your leg muscles if you can actually see your knees' reflection.

Before You Begin

Hot Yoga Essentials

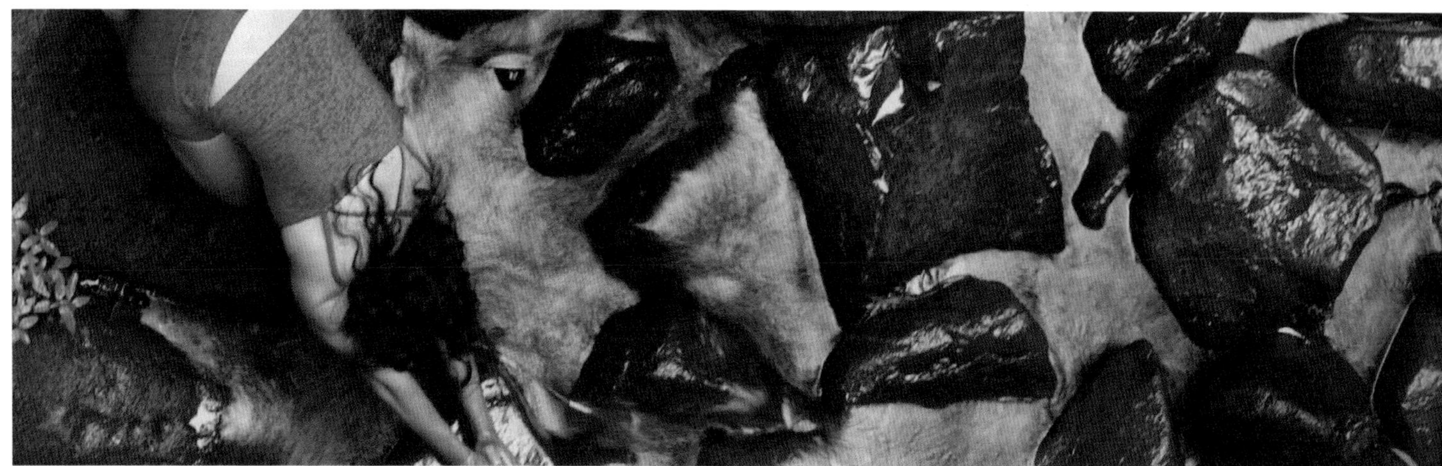

Whenever you are not doing an asana you are in Savasana.

There are aspects of your hot yoga practice that influence every moment of your class. The way you breathe; your habitual focus; the way you hold your body to name a few.

There are things you must do and things you must not do. I've outlined the key principles and 'hot yoga essentials' that, once you follow them, you will wonder why you didn't do them before.

Savasana: The key to unlocking all the benefits

Savasana means Corpse Pose. A pose literally all about doing nothing at all. Nothing, that is, except breathing. While Savasana seems like the easiest pose in the whole yoga world, it could in fact be the hardest.

Here's a key point to remember: Whenever you are not doing an asana you are in Savasana.

There are standing and lying Corpse Poses in a hot yoga practice. On the floor you will take Savasana on your back or on your stomach. Interestingly, some of the key principles of Savasana will make a difference regardless of the position you find yourself in.

...creating calm and relaxation and stillness in the body and mind is a skill that can be practiced. After each pose you stand or lie in a certain way to trigger your Savasana state of relaxation and calm full body breaths.

The longest Corpse Pose during class takes place between the standing and the floor poses, and is the first thing you do when you finally get to the floor. It is worth underlining the importance of Savasana. Anyone can stand still, or at least relatively so. Savasana encompasses a far broader definition of stillness that transcends physical inactivity. One of the great benefits of hot yoga is its power as a moving meditation. Your body moves, but the mind's conscious attention is taken up by an almost continuous stream of instructions. There are so many things to do that for the most part you simply do not have enough time to think.

It is little wonder that with this rigorous and demanding style of instruction that students are seldom bored. They find themselves in a zone of calm. Even students new to hot yoga discover this very early on. Some students report better sleep, better skill accomplishment and better concentration in their 'normal life' after as little as one single class.

By using these carefully constructed poses in the prescribed way, the mind has little else to do than to succumb to a certain quietness, and the mind chatter fades. Not all yogas are created equal. And by this I mean styles of yoga asana (or physical pose yoga). I find no greater satisfaction than with hot yoga. Personally I find the less physical and slower styles of yoga fail to distract the conscious mind sufficiently to allow slowing of the mind to create a growing calmness.

I find this particularly in yoga styles where the class flow is constantly interrupted by calls to grab this strap or that block or go and get a chair, a blanket, or stand next to the wall. Each and every command that takes you out of your zone dilutes the positive effects of an otherwise flowing practice. But during hot yoga asana your body's movements and the stream of instructions serve to distract your conscious mind and lull it into calm. You find a retreat, a sanctuary.

Each and every class, you continue to train your conscious mind to accept this calm zone and begin a deep operation to remove distracting, disturbing or damaging thoughts and deep seated emotions.

It is suggested that the body's emotions could be stored in a 'crystalline' form manifested in the body. The yoga reaches the deep recesses of the body in a cleansing way, sweeping out emotional cobwebs as well as physical impurities.

You can learn to still your mind while you move the body. You can learn to still your mind while you stay completely motionless. When you can accomplish deeper and deeper stillness of mind and body you are more in tune with yourself and your interaction with your environment. You are on your path to enlightenment.

When you are in Savasana it is time for total body stillness. You no longer have the body's movements to occupy your thought processes and still your mind. Now you are on your own – no distractions and no reprieve. You have to have discipline to stay physically still. And learn the discipline to avoid engaging your mind. Perhaps at first you will find it difficult to stay still.

Students suddenly find themselves adjusting their clothing, their hair, finding a nail to groom, removing a nagging thread on a hem, wiping away a dissolved bit of eyeliner, adjusting a little bit of podge hanging over their shorts, taking a drink, looking around or at the floor or the ceiling or anywhere else they shouldn't. Anything at all outside of breathing and keeping still can be a distraction. Preventing yourself from dwelling on a passing thought is the hardest thing to do when physically still. I offer my students an extremely useful visualization: If you are on a train of thought, get off the train and let it continue on without you.

This acknowledges that you are aware of your thoughts, even your sensations but you don't identify with them. You simply observe them, but you remain attentive to your breath. You don't get attached to them, nor do you fear them. You let them run their course like background music all the while focusing, concentrating your mind on the fine distinctions of your breath.

This will help you create the ideal circumstances for meditation and reap the benefits through diligent observation and awareness. Recognize that creating calm and relaxation and stillness in the body and mind is a skill that can be practiced. After each pose you stand or lie in a certain way in order to trigger your Savasana state of relaxation and calm full body breaths. Continually revisiting the same physical circumstances of your Savasana each and every time you enter it is key to recreating and deepening your experience.

The tourniquet effect

We have all heard of a tourniquet. It works to isolate fluids to one part of the body. Typically we hear about their use in spider or snake bite victims. In this case we are attempting to isolate the venom to the site of injury. A tourniquet occurs when pressure is applied in a circumferential band on the skin to a part of the body. It serves to limit venous or arterial circulation to that part for a period of time. Tourniquets have different applications. Used in surgery they allow operations to be performed in a bloodless area. In emergency situations it can prevent blood loss from limb trauma or venom spread in insect or reptile bites. Similarly a tourniquet-like effect occurs when you hang a heavy bag from your arm or wear clothing that is too tight. So how is this relevant to yoga?

Each and every class, you continue to train your conscious mind to accept this calm zone and begin a deep operation to remove distracting, disturbing or damaging thoughts and deep seated emotions.

Research into the term 'tourniquet effect' will yield many references to describe the benefits of hot yoga. However you can see by the tourniquet definition that every style of yoga can potentially have this same effect. It is not unique to hot yoga. In yoga asana or physical yoga we enter poses or body positions which create specific pressures in varying locations, or mini tourniquets. While the tourniquet is applied during the pose, it is the 'tourniquet effect' which happens when the pose is released and you immediately and swiftly attain Savasana. The success of the effect will be determined by two factors:

1. How diligently the tourniquet is applied.
2. How quickly and economically you can access stillness in your Savasana.

The effect involves pressure and release. The greater the pressure then the greater the force of the release. It is as if water is building up behind a dam. The barrier is released and the water floods through the opening, flushing away anything in the way. If we choose to let the water build up behind but let a little out at a time, when the barrier is opened it cannot be as explosive or have the same flushing effect. In hot yoga we can maximize this important effect using two key principles:

1. **Hold The Pose With No Interim Release Of Grip Or Position**: When you enter into a pose, keep the effort continuous without gaps. Don't apply pressure and then let it go by adjusting and readjusting your grip. If you don't hold your effort, or you inconsistently vary the forces (in pulling, pushing, kicking or twisting) you will only create a partial tourniquet. Consequently the build up behind the 'blockage' or flow limitation will be variable. The release of the pose then brings a less forceful flush. So maintain constant effort – or better yet, steadily increase it right up to the end of the pose and maximize the flushing, cleansing and healing effects.

2. **Release Straight Into Savasana With No Interim Poses Or Actions**: When you release make sure you mindfully let go and enter Savasana without reversing the effects of your pose. Here are some practical examples:

- From a backbend, release and neutralize your spine, don't fall into a forward bend.
- From a forward bend, don't release past neutral to relieve your lower back with a little backbend.
- When releasing legs from Wind Removing Pose simply let the bent leg pivot from the hip and fall to the ground with no effort. Lifting the leg up to the sky and bringing it down with control, although providing some exercise to your abdominal and spinal muscles completely negates the compressive effects on your abdominal area by stemming the free flow of blood. It uses different muscles to that which you used during the pose and you markedly dilute your 'tourniquet effect'.

There are certainly conditions for which tourniquets are not recommended. One of these is in patients who have varying stages of lymphedema. This is a condition that commonly occurs in post-operative cancer patients where lymph nodes have been removed. Protein rich lymph which is unable to be removed from the body gets stuck between the layers of connective tissue.

It has not been clinically studied whether all patients with this problem can benefit from yoga poses that create a further flow limitation. You may want to try hot yoga and see if it is beneficial. I have taught a number of students suffering from this who found this style beneficial. After practice they have gone home and elevated the limb in question to further drain any potential build-up. If you have lymphedema you need to get as much information as you can.

Where do I look? Or, how to distract yourself from what is really going on...

You've heard it said: "Where the eyes go, the body follows". If you want to change lanes when driving, if you look over your shoulder to the lane into which you want to cross, you will most likely already be moving towards it. When you are riding a bike it definitely helps you to look where you are going, particularly when cornering for example.

When you are practicing yoga asana you are often told to look where you are going. If you are in a backbend, then looking back will deepen your pose. If you are in a rounded forward-bend it may help to look to your chest or at your abdomen, or 'into your heart'. Little wonder that standing and balancing on one leg will be unsuccessful, if you are focusing on the floor in front of your toes.

If you want to balance then looking forward-and-out is the key.

Where you look can also be a challenge to your physical posture. As I have already illustrated, it can affect your balance and the execution of your pose – but I believe there is more to the movement than just achieving the pose. There is a deeper connection with your own soul possible – but how? Perhaps one of the most confronting elements of a hot yoga practice can be looking at yourself in the mirror. The mirror is not simply about checking or refining your poses. You have an inbuilt mechanism called 'proprioception' that does that for you.

Proprioception helps you identify where your body is in space without actually having to look. Although, a mirror is rarely used in yoga, it is frequently used in hot yoga. It is one of the key aspects to helping you create personal change.

When you are standing in Savasana look forward and try to meet your eyes in the mirror. If that is difficult, then your third eye (between the eyebrows) or at the base of the throat are very good alternatives.

You can look out at your left eye in the mirror, then your right eye, and back again. You may at times have to break through some personal barriers in order to do it, but with practice you will leave that weakness behind and expose yourself to more of the real 'you'. Observe whatever surfaces for you and let it 'float away' to leave you feeling lighter, with a heightened sense of self-acceptance.

In backbends and forward-bends the rule is to 'look where you are going'. Up and back, or down and in. For twists, your eyes lead the charge. For one-legged balance poses, keep your chin up and look forward.

If you cannot bear to look into your own eyes, then ensure that your chin is up and that you look no lower than the knee of your standing locked-out leg. It is then your mission to, over time, climb your eyes back up your body. Eventually, you will settle on a level of comfort for looking into your own eyes.

While practicing the floor poses, without the added distraction or difficulty of looking directly into their own eyes, students are less likely to fall out of poses. Balancing is less of a problem. There are far fewer visual distractions.

On the floor, lying on your back in Savasana, naturally you won't be looking into your own eyes in the mirror. Instead you will find it best to look at one point on the ceiling forward of your toes. Without burning a hole in the ceiling, soften your gaze and focus on your breath.

On your stomach, you turn your head and look just to the edge of your towel, and no further.

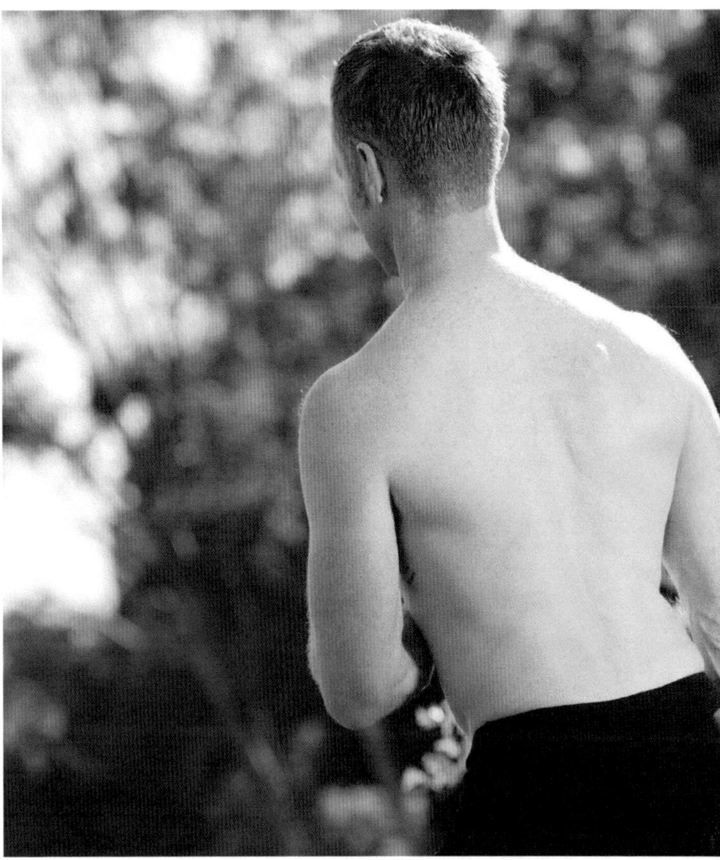

If you want to balance then looking forward-and-out is the key.

Don't react to your surroundings

One of the classic 8 'limbs' (or philosophies) of yoga is Pratyahara - learning to control and withdraw the senses. This is non-reactiveness to your surroundings.

The less reactive you are, the more you can focus on your breath and keep your gaze steady. A steady gaze does not mean totally immovable eyes. That would be unnatural. Eyes by their nature don't stay perfectly still. A steady gaze involves the exclusion of visual distractions so you can focus on your yoga.

It can be especially confronting to look into your own eyes in the mirror. However this is a major aim of your meditation. It can be intense to experience the feelings that arise, either derived from your body's physical movements, or your mental or emotional state. All wonderful breakthroughs that become possible when you work with a mirror.

Whatever your intense feelings, you will move through them more easily by simply breathing deeply. Typically though, many students will avert their eyes, or distract themselves by doing one of the following typical behaviors:

1. Looking at the floor;
2. Looking at another part of their own body;
3. Looking at other people;
4. Talking or sub-vocalizing (talking out loud to themselves);
5. Moving their body around; shaking out their shoulders, legs or arms, doing little backbends. (Let's not get coy here, they will say they have to iron out some pain or tightness. Really it is because if they stay still, they'll have to face their truth.);
6. Checking the position of their feet, hands or body before or during a pose;
7. Adjusting their clothing, their hair, their nails;
8. Taking a drink, or drinking at the wrong times;
9. Bending over, the legs taking the weight of the body through their hands (while looking down);
10. Shallow breathing (to avoid the intensity of deep breath);
11. Wiping sweat.

And so the list goes on.

If you are a regular at hot yoga, keep 'position checks' to a minimum. Too much constant checking and you'll begin to second guess yourself, losing the ability to confidently monitor the way your body feels in the correct position. 'Checking' distracts your practice and your meditation, so learn to minimize it.

- Remember that wiping sweat can be dangerous.
- Do not allow yourself to be distracted.
- Let the sweat drip. It is cooling your body's core temperature.

You will get used to the sweat and wetness. Your strength will improve and make it unnecessary ever to wipe sweat. The only time you need to wipe is when sweat is stinging your eyes. Otherwise work through it, be calm, and breathe.

You are attempting at all times to limit your bubble of existence, to allow you to maintain inward attention. Block out that which occurs outside of your own space. Bringing other people into your focus or view, (students or the teacher) will distract you and enlarge your sphere of attention. This makes it hard to focus on just your inner being. So, always keep your eyes to yourself, literally.

To blink or not to blink?

Blinking happens automatically and consciously trying to control it will not deepen your yoga practice. So take your attention off the way you blink your eyes. Just stop your eyes from wandering around the room. Keep your gaze to yourself and work on bringing your gaze to rest softly, easily and acceptingly on your own eyes. Breathe through the experience and 'be'.

Over time you will feel comfortable in your own presence and be accepting of yourself. You will take on feedback that comes from within and from your teacher and from the progressively more refined knowledge you have of your own body.

Drinking as a distraction

Recognize that you are avoiding confronting your issues if you consistently distract yourself. Drinking water at the wrong times is one of the most common distractions. Avoid ritualizing the times that you drink, simply make it a question of physical necessity. If you have to stop a pose to take a drink then this is a dead giveaway that you are avoiding confronting yourself.

For many new students falling out of a pose has them suddenly reaching for their bottle. Why? Did they all of a sudden get thirsty? Hardly.

... you are aware of your thoughts, even your sensations but you don't identify with them. You simply observe them, but you remain attentive to your breath.

It could be the inability to accept their failure to get through a single pose without stopping. If it is not a question of ego, then perhaps it is stamina, or simply not able to stand still and 'be'. If you are not doing a standing pose, then you should be standing in Savasana, doing absolutely nothing.

Perhaps you ritualize your water drinking in another less harmful way. Every time you finish Eagle or Toe Stand you reach and drink. If that describes your habits then observe your capacity to stand still and make eye contact. You will soon work out if you really need a drink or if you can cope with a little quiet time, discomfort or intense sensations. Try taking a drink later on at another less utilized time! Maybe you will find you can get through the whole class not needing water at all.

Conversely, I don't recommend being a martyr. If you need to drink, you drink.

A few words of safety. Make sure you are hydrated before class and you continue drinking afterward. Take electrolyte supplements with a regular practice. Your best, most inexpensive choice is pure sea salt. Be as mindful of your drinking as you are of other important yoga principles. Try not to drink at precisely the same time every class. Take every opportunity to stand without distraction observing yourself, accepting yourself, doing nothing but breathing.

Mat placement recommendations

Fussing around with anything that does not add to the deepening of your yoga experience, is effectively a distraction. Whether a mental distraction (thoughts) or physical (moving around unnecessarily), it is still a distraction from your meditation. Unfortunately for some, their mat becomes their distraction.

There are many students who fuss with their yoga mat, continually fixing the ripples, flicked corners, squaring off slight misalignments and even changing the direction that it faces.

Mat placement varies depending on your venue. If you are practicing in a professional yoga space with instruction, chances are it will be set up with a whole wall of mirrors and appropriate floor covering. In this case you will set up your mat perpendicularly to the mirror and then leave it there for the entire class.

If you are practicing at home you may have limited space and only a small mirror span. You may also have domestic carpet that is slippery or want to avoid any chance of dripping sweat on it.

Some hot yoga studios have timber floors. Although more hygienic because they are easily cleaned, wooden floors are slippery when wet, which poses significant physical danger.

Here are some recommendations for maximizing safety and hygiene.

It is not easy to keep high levels of hygiene in a studio where there are lots of students sweating. If the sweat remains in the carpet then smells can linger and micro-organisms can breed.

I used to have a personal studio at home and invited up to a dozen people to practice with me and my husband. It was great fun to have a fully equipped studio but so many sweating bodies on a carpet in a confined space was not pleasant.

We came up with a solution for home practice. Mats are placed at 90 degrees to the mirror (as is usually the case at hot yoga studios). Then towels are positioned at 90 degrees to the mat in a 'T' or 't' formation. This means that the student stands in the middle of the 'T' and simply steps to the left of the towel for all the warrior poses. The sweat drips onto the towel. At the end of the standing poses the towel is realigned lengthways on the mat ready for the floor poses. This completely solved the hygiene problem and virtually eliminated lingering odors in our home carpet.

At my public studio we installed an excellent carpet that was impervious to sweat, could be washed easily, and was always well sanitized. This is a wet and dry carpet, or an indoor/ outdoor carpet. The two biggest factors in keeping a fresh studio have been ventilation after each and every class, and placing the towel at 90 degrees to the mat.

Be your own best teacher

Whether you practice hot yoga at home or in a studio, or to a CD, or even a silent class, you ultimately have to rely on yourself. For those of you attending class for the first time, you will generally follow teachers' directions and use visual observation to learn from others. In this way, you will learn to pay attention to yourself.

The tools you will use are:

- The mirrors
- The external feedback from the teacher
- Visual cues from fellow students
- Internal feedback from your own body intuition
- Your accumulated knowledge of the poses
- Your proprioception.

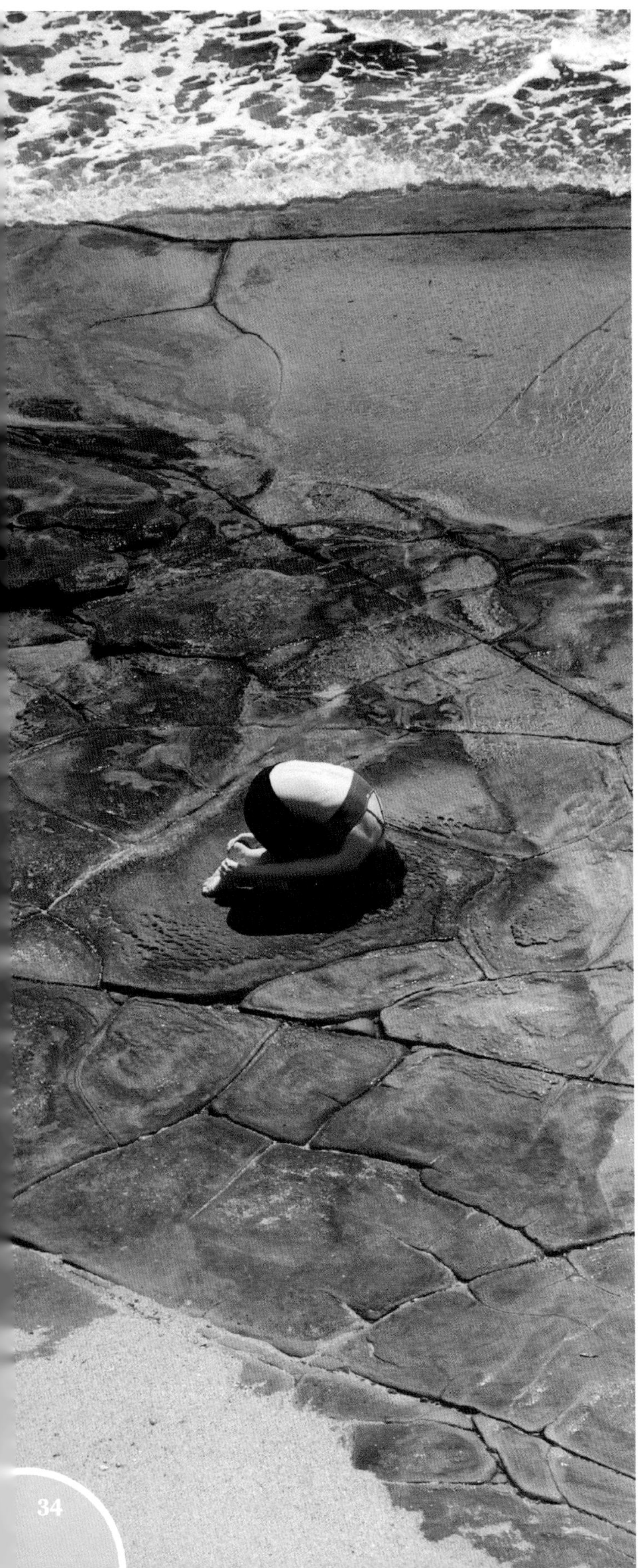

When you attend any kind of class regardless of location, developing self-reliance is the key to being your own best teacher.

1. Use your non-judgmental observation skills and unbiased assessment of each and every aspect of your class.
2. Remove your ego and attachment to a particular result, feeling, or look.
3. Become more sensitive to your responses and remain attentive not reactive.
4. Delve deeper into your own experience in a balanced, impartial and objective way.
5. Learn to create a profound moving meditation.

Personal responsibility

While being your own best teacher is definitely about taking responsibility, there is even more that you can do for yourself.

You will learn best by practicing humility. With that you must let go of your ego, and be 'teachable'. Be prepared to learn something from every teacher you meet, regardless of their level of knowledge or physical ability. Listen to your teacher and follow directions with personal safety as a prime concern.

In hot yoga, you strive for a balance between humility, intuition, skill and the directions of your teacher. This balance will be different for everyone.

What if you disagree with a teacher's method?

Sometimes a teacher's skill doesn't coincide with your own understanding of yoga philosophy, and you think you could teach them a thing or two. If that is the case and you feel that they teach a potentially damaging move or position, or neglect to include a vital safety precaution, then I do not recommend blindly following them.

Whether this error is through omission or ignorance doesn't matter. Don't go against your intuition by doing something risky or you know to be wrong just because a teacher tells you.

Part of your responsibility is to select a teacher who shows respect for the souls in their class, and is trying to keep everyone safe. Only when you feel safe and respected, can you nurture your skills.

You must always listen to your body. You must also use your growing knowledge to perform the poses in the safest way possible. And you must do this while showing the utmost respect for your teacher. This is where humility comes in.

You could find yourself awash with emotion, extra oxygen, and new found possibilities.

Take responsibility for your reactions or prejudices. Make these reactions a personal lesson in emotional management.

Breathwork

Breathing is important to life! Conscious breathing is paramount to the practice of yoga. Your greatest gift to yourself is your ability to consciously breathe deeply and fully. It seems funny to some that you can actually learn to breathe. But getting past your physical and emotional limitations can depend on this skill.

While holding a posture, we have heard it a thousand times - focus on the breath. It may be the biggest and most important key to your progress in your yoga.

In my personal practice, I had to learn how to breathe from scratch. My lungs had a tiny capacity and I had limited emotional health. I felt very stressed particularly in my chest, solar plexus and diaphragm. For five whole months when I started yoga and was practicing 6-8 times per week, I neither had the capacity to breathe deeply enough, nor to hold my breath at any significant volume for the beginning Pranayama exercise. I had to sneak in extra breaths in a few of the cycles.

As you practice more and more, you will find that the poses that constrict your airways - necessitating shorter shallower breathing - will transform with your growth in breath capacity.

Typically your ability to breathe will be constricted or limited in any pose where you are in a big forward or backbend. You may often hear your teacher say "take short shallow breaths". But as your practice develops you will find that you can dare to breathe far more deeply.

Remember to let 'struggle' be your guide. This means that you never let struggle into your practice. If you are struggling then this is your body's sign to do something differently. Find the challenge but lose the struggle.

Push your edge to continually grow your breath. Most obvious in the physically demanding poses, anxiety manifests in short shallow breathing, and tension will shortly follow. If you notice your breath is short and sharp, calm it, slow it down and deepen it. It may take courage to do so.

For example, whenever I suggest students to slow the breath in Floor Bow, the results are astounding to them. The whole class is quiet and determined. The breath is deep and the bows are incredible. And the 20 seconds seem to fly by without notice. Amazing. No struggle, just yoga.

Deep breathing in a warm and humid room

Doing this yoga in the heat can be a revolutionary experience. The breath work and especially Pranayama have students breathing deeper than they may have ever done. The physical expansion of the lungs during class, allows oxygen to reach right down into the depths of the two and three lobes of the lungs. For many people this brings up feelings of distress. They put it down to NOT having enough air in the room.

In fact, if they are breathing through their noses, then the opposite is surely happening. They are deepening their breath, they are accessing a better gaseous exchange and they are unlocking incredible potential.

The availability of previously untapped lung volume, is like breaking new ground or exploring uncharted territories of your limitless nature. You could find yourself awash with emotion, extra oxygen, and new found possibilities. It is as if your body is trying to get used to the new space, the new expansion. It can be scary and exciting. Allow these emotions to come to the surface. Stick with it and within a short amount of time this new volume of lung expansion will become the 'norm'.

Equally your breath may tighten when you look in your eyes. But don't let your breathing become a distraction from your practice. Panting or a shallow breath is an anxious panic breath. It lessens oxygen supply and robs you of energy. Slow and calm your breath enough to stop the panting, and to break through the intensity.

An emotional 'bubble' burst in class is one that leaves you and (with continued work) doesn't come back. How your bubble emerges makes no difference. Your body's physical manifestations of stress are the same whatever the trigger - emotional, physical or mental. Your trigger might simply be your breath, the heat, looking into your own eyes, reacting to an emotional event, or perhaps a hip opening pose. Whatever manifests, if you manage to breathe through it and observe it, positive changes occur through your calm response to stressful stimuli.

How far do you go in each pose?

There may be a point in a pose beyond which everything you are trying to achieve just unravels or falls apart. It is at that point that you fall out, or your body no longer holds its proper position. Benefits are lost when you are not correctly aligned, so let's look at a hierarchy of priorities on which to focus during your class. They can be summed up as 'breath, alignment and then depth'.

Breath, alignment and then depth

Breath is the most important component of your practice. It must precede all other activities. In the hot yoga room we are only practicing yoga asana or physical yoga. It is but one step on your own journey towards some kind of enlightenment.

The physical yoga combined with good breath work, and your own attitude of calm, produces an incredible moving meditation that goes way beyond physical exercise. Neglect one of these elements and you lessen the power of your yoga. Here are my guidelines ...

1. Firstly pay attention to your breath.
2. Then you allow yourself to enter into the pose with correct alignment.
3. Then, and only then, do you allow yourself to explore the depths of the pose.

You may always be caught up trying to get the right alignment. Remember, depth is relative. In fact, every time you find new depth in a pose you will likely find that your alignment needs renewed attention, which brings us to ...

'Measure twice, cut once'

I recommend placing sufficient attention on your alignment from the beginning of a practice session to the end. Think how ridiculous the reverse would be - i.e. measure once and cut twice.

Remember yoga means unity of mind and body. Going in and out of focus on your attention to the breath, body and pose means you fragment your practice and dilute the benefits.

'Measure twice, cut once' also takes on an added dimension for me. It means having an attitude for which ego has no bearing. What does ego have to do with it? Students may not be conscious of this but I see it happening all the time.

Usually, it happens because a student forms an attachment to getting the pose 'right'. And 'right' for a new yogi usually means that they go as deep as the people around them. Who could blame them? They have examples all around them paving the way, showing how the pose should look - and they try to emulate that. Reflected in the mirror they see how the body should look.

But, the poses are new to them, and they are overwhelmed by the number of things that demand their attention. They get lost with too many instructions, and their bodies collapse into all sorts of deformed shapes that hold poor physiological alignment. Fortunately it doesn't take long for these students to improve, given consistent precise instruction.

'Measure twice, cut once' can help drive your commitment to participate fully in the class regardless of your ability or flexibility.

Start with great alignment and you have a real body-understanding of the pose. Start with slapdash alignment, then when you move into the pose you will spend precious time correcting it. Poor alignment is much harder to correct in the midst of a pose. Typically, the body is already in various degrees of collapse. Usually, the student needs to back out completely, and restart. However, if you take a second or two of extra time to set up the pose correctly (more for some poses), then your conscious and unconscious mind will pay attention to the things that matter.

There will always be improvements to make, but they will be smaller, and the pose will start earlier for you. You will have better focus and be able to work harder, and deeper on refinements and better distinctions.You'll also enjoy more benefits from having a longer and more precise pose.

Using 'struggle' as your guide

Struggle is your body's way of telling you that you have gone too far. In terms of our principle of 'breath, alignment and depth', struggle relates to depth. It may also result from depth in an incorrectly aligned pose; for example, if something is excruciatingly painful, or if you can't breathe or your breathing is shallow and fast. Or, if you have stopped breathing completely. Then, not only are you no longer doing yoga, you have probably gone beyond your design capabilities!

You will need to back off and get yourself to where you can work into the pose correctly. Sometimes you will have to surrender, or just let go of something that's hindering you. And sometimes you will just have to regulate your breath again.

...take a second or two of extra time to set up the pose correctly. You will have better focus, work harder and deeper on refinements and enjoy more benefits from having a longer and more precise pose.

Backing off is not just about coming out of the pose. Let's look at some examples.

Surrender: Often men can get caught up in the whole macho thing. They are used to running their lives by muscle. They come to hot yoga and have to 'let go'. They have to strive for balancing their strength with improving their flexibility. And this means to surrender-to-the-pose. In other words, you don't need to be tense to have strength. Poses are not muscled into, they are entered with care and awareness. Typical examples are Half Moon, Standing Separate Leg Stretching Pose.

Breathe: Often, we get caught up in the activity and either forget to breathe, or we pant with a shallow stress-ridden breath. Typically affected poses are any kind of backbend, Half Moon, or Eagle.

You will have to start breathing again (and stay in the pose). Or you will have to come out and re-enter with precision. Pay attention to breath, then alignment, and then depth.

Reassess: In the example of Camel Pose, it may be that you start to feel 'struggle' because you get caught up in your own emotional reaction to this very deep back bend. You won't necessarily need to come out, but you will need to address your breathing and where you are looking, to calm the effect.

Never go past a point of pain, into struggle and excruciating pain. Yes, you may have some pain in your poses, but it should be more of a discomfort. Classically, students will talk of 'comfortable discomfort'. If you are wincing (not just for show but out of real pain) then you have gone too far. Your facial expressions should also reflect your accepting attitude; not caring, not minding, just observing.

When backbends throw you off balance

You may be thrown off balance particularly when you are practicing backbends. Why does this occur? Why don't students exit early or 'fall out' out of forward bends? Surely they are just as challenging!

Typically if someone is scared (or feeling vulnerable) they curl up, or bring their arms in across the chest or abdomen, hugging themselves to feel safe. Little wonder that you find relatively more comfort in 'curling up' poses (forward bends), despite the hard work and your intense effort.

It is when the arms open and the head drops back that you can really feel at risk and open to the elements. Your soft underbelly is exposed, as is your heart center and all your major organs. Until you can work through it, logic will not override the intensity. You may at first resist surrendering to your backbend and have to come out early.

Essentially you are being distracted by your thoughts and emotions. While you are in the throes of backward bending, you are supposed to look up and behind you; looking where you are going, leading with your eyes.

On a neurological level when you look up, you are aware of your sensations and your breath as an observer.

However, when your eyes look down you connect more directly and associate with your sensations. This accounts for why students exit backbends early if they are looking down their noses, because they are no longer being objective about the experience. Instead, they are directly stepping into their feelings.

You may ask why this doesn't happen on a forward bend. It is very seldom that students come out of Rabbit Pose or Head To Knee Pose early, or even Hands To Feet Pose.

Why does looking down in the forward bends not engender the same intense emotions, sensations or thoughts? The reason is that, although you are still aware of the apparent or imagined dangers when curling up in a ball or bending forward, you are, for the most part, feeling physically protected.

Generally, if you exit early from Eagle Pose or Standing Head To Knee Pose, it is due to loss of balance and not vulnerability.

In contrast, the most commonly early exited poses are Half Moon Backbend, Standing Bow, Floor Bow and of course Camel. You could say that exiting Standing Bow could be about balance, and you would be half right. The reluctance to go back into it would suggest that there is more going on, and that the challenge is not simply physical.

How do you resolve neck and shoulder tension in each and every pose?

How to override the counter-productive self-protection mechanism during backbends

A dog or cat who encounters a stranger is less likely to bare their tummy to them for a tickle. It certainly won't do it if it senses danger. But in the sanctuary of your yoga studio, you can allow yourself to be physically vulnerable because logically you know you are safe. In a group class situation, even though you try to practice alone, you know that there are people there to support you.

Here are the keys to help you work through this:

- When doing backbends, keep your eyes looking back.
- Allow your eyes to settle on the ceiling, or better, the wall behind you.
- Always look further, for the next place. If you can see the wall, try to see the floor. If you can see the floor, try to see your mat. Your mat. Your heels.
- Continually look back, re-correcting any upward eye movements.
- As you come across an interesting sensation make sure you keep breathing.
- Breathe as deeply as your position will allow.
- Deepen the breath sufficiently to deliver plenty of oxygen to your body.
- Avoid shallow short sharp breaths.

Apply these principles to all your backbends.

As you stumble upon intense sensations you have choices. A new yogi's first impulse is to try to dampen or stop this sensation. This is usually because they are still identifying with feelings and still learning to be the observer. When they do, they stop looking back, look up to the ceiling or worse, down the nose. Neurologically, they step more fully into their emotions and associated responses, and inevitably exit the pose.

There are real physical dangers to looking down the nose. The chin drops toward the chest and the neck is no longer soft. The head is prevented from simply resting back in a safe position. The muscles around the neck, head and shoulders (and down the front of the body) tense and engage, and may cause strain, pain and damage. This is less dangerous in Floor Bow, but you will definitely find more lift and strength when you look up and not forward.When you make the choice to stay in your backbend, you breathe through the intensity. You will delight in discovering what it means to be the observer of your practice. Your sensations run their course in the background, and you learn how not to be reactive to troubling feelings. You are not denying your feelings, you are working through them to a positive end. This ability paves the way to a deeper meditation through calm and acceptance.

How to use your arms to best advantage in hot yoga: WARNING – Controversial!

Throughout our lives our experiences manifest themselves in our bodies. These have the potential to produce illness, stress and tensions which occur in many key areas of the body according to their cause. Yoga and other bodywork can help flush out, remove, cleanse, heal – or at the very least reduce their effects.

One important key area is the head, neck and shoulders. Most humans hold a significant amount of stress in this very complex network of joints, nerves, blood vessels, muscles, tendons and ligaments.

Some people have incredible tightness in the shoulders. This problem has a multitude of causes including tight neck muscles, injured rotator cuff muscles, shoulder joint issues and tight torso muscles (including and not limited to the back's largest and most powerful; latissimus dorsi). People carry stress here and it is a habit that needs breaking.

All of which raises some interesting – and controversial – questions for your yoga practice.

- How do you hold your arms to facilitate relaxation through your head, neck and shoulders?
- How do you lift your arms up without hunching your shoulders?
- How do you get maximum length and stretch from the shoulders through to your fingertips in your yoga?
- How do you resolve neck and shoulder tension in each and every pose?

Good questions! In order to answer them we really need a little anatomy lesson, a simplified one where the focus is practical application and not on terminology and fine detail.

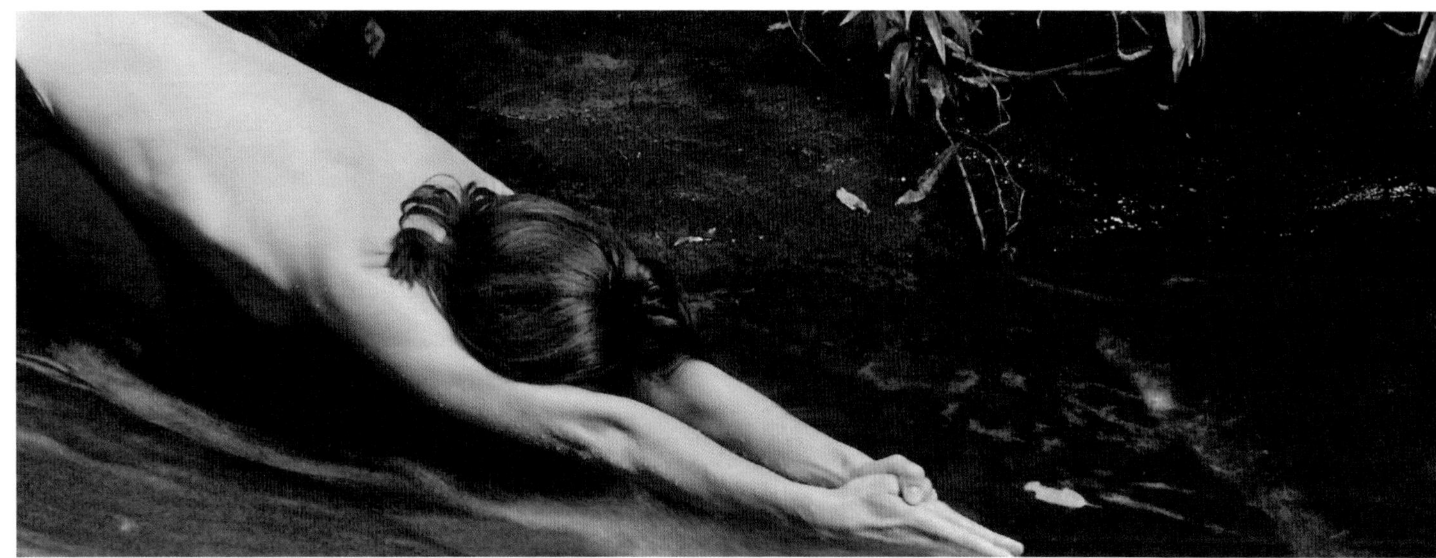

Many of the mistakes made practicing hot yoga revolve around the shoulders. The problem is so significant that a separate discussion here is warranted.

Every pose requires some attention being paid to your shoulders and neck; whether you are in a forward bend or backbend, setting up and twisting your arms in Eagle pose or moving your body into Half Spine Twist.

It is valuable to learn how to hold your head, neck and shoulders in space, to create ecologically sound movements which help resolve tension and not contribute to pain or dysfunction. Please note, you will find specific techniques in the chapters on each individual pose. Here I will discuss generalized ways to ensure your overall safety and progress.

If you are already a yoga student then you have probably seen others standing in Savasana holding their bodies in a variety of ways. In the beginning of my hot yoga journey I noticed people standing with arms just hanging down from their sides while others had palms facing forward. I did not know what was the best thing to do. It definitely plagued my mind for a time. And it certainly is a point of contention amongst yogis that I have met.

After several classes my mind came up with the answer. If you lie down on the ground in Savasana with your palms up to facilitate an open chest, wouldn't it be a good idea to do this when you are standing upright?

So what is the best thing to do? Well, after reading this chapter it will be up to you to decide. I will give my recommendations based on my knowledge, my intuition and years of experience. I am also going to reference other yogis' work.

The way you hold your arms is seen by some as a contentious issue. I remember a student at the LA teacher training I attended telling everyone he could that it was a waste of energy to stand in Savasana with one's palms facing forward. He wasted more energy getting into people's faces than we did standing like that. And then another student noticed my mildly slumping shoulders. Because I had been a dentist leaning over patients all day, this had become an engrained habit.

This same problem affects a massive amount of people, especially those who spend their time in an office environment or at some kind of terminal or bench. Some muscles strengthen while others weaken causing an imbalance that is potentially damaging. Before you know it your shoulders are in a permanent slump, your cervical spine is no longer upright, your weighty head is forward and your chest is no longer open.

The list goes on. Even the act of concentrating can introduce head, neck and shoulder tension which can carry over into your yoga practice.

My friend at that teacher training took me aside one day and gave me a bad-posture-antidote. He said that I should imagine that my 'elbows were in my back pockets'. I immediately latched onto this excellent tip and it changed my life. At training you attend almost 100 classes in 60 days. Bodies go through incredible change and the possibility for emotional release is huge. Every time I transformed my stance I felt years of emotional memory through my heart and solar plexus below the surface aching to be freed. Once I realized the potential for self-cleansing I encouraged it, I dared it to happen and it felt great. I felt physically lighter.

I immediately latched onto this excellent tip and it changed my life.

I took these physiological principles and applied them to every pose. I made distinctions for myself about how to release tension and relax through the whole upper spine and through the shoulders.

Not everyone will have the opportunity to create change on such a short schedule and there is a great deal more to this than simply 'putting your elbows in your back pockets'. It is a complete and transformational approach to the physical aspects of hot yoga that employs a far more correct and anatomically accurate approach than is generally found.

I've been teaching these and many other transformational refinements with great results. I am going to outline some very detailed and practical techniques within the pages of this manual so you can modify your approach (with both subtle and gross adjustments), deepen your practice and share in the benefits.

When I was writing my manual, I came across a couple of articles by Roger Cole, Ph.D. Roger is an Iyengar-certified yoga teacher, and Stanford-trained scientist. He specializes in human anatomy and in the physiology of relaxation, sleep, and biological rhythms. His writing encapsulated what I had already worked out. Roger has kindly given me permission to use his work which I will touch on in this chapter.

My desire is to present ways to get the best and most ecological movements out of your shoulders. It will benefit you in your yoga poses and your life in general. Here and throughout the manual I will give you distinctions in arm movements: How to stand in Savasana; how to manipulate your shoulders in class; how to initiate movement without holding or introducing stresses in your neck and shoulders.

Both in and out of class, 'elbows in the back pocket' triggers great habits. It helps you shorten the gap between your 'practice' and 'outside life'. You will quickly learn to counter the physical and emotional stresses which manifest in your body – many of which center around the head, neck and shoulders, caused by habitual slumping and just general stress.

The antidote to neck-ache and shoulder stress

Standing with palms facing forward for me and thousands of my students has been an amazing gift – a great posture touchstone in class. Out of the studio I recall my friend's words to get my 'elbows in my back pockets' and my posture opens up and I stand tall. It feels good.

This became even more obvious to me when I became a parent. Naturally I was continually picking up and holding my daughter, breastfeeding etc. A simple external rotation of the upper arms to move the shoulders down and away from the ears became one of the greatest little actions I did on a daily basis to relieve the muscular tension that had built up in my neck and shoulders.

When you try this for yourself it may initially feel forced because you have to train your tired, disused, or weakened muscles to do some work.

Inside the studio you externally rotate your upper arms. This is exactly what you need to do to 'pocket your elbows'! It is up to you whether you also externally rotate your lower arms. It is possible to rotate the upper arms independently of the lower arms. I leave it to you to decide whether you want to carry it through right down to your fingertips. When you extend the effect to your fingers your palms will be facing directly forward manifesting in your physiology a spirit of openness and receiving.

Note that in the 'real world' you won't be walking around with your palms in some crazy front-facing position but you will rather be paying attention to rotation of your upper arms as you lift your breastbone. By the way, try getting your elbows in your pockets from a slumped shoulder position. It is impossible. You have to lift up through your torso and chest to rotate your upper arms.

At first as you incorporate this into your life, you will have to think about it, but when it becomes automatic your posture will be transformed. You will stand tall and have less stress. You will physically have a greater capacity to breathe more deeply and draw in more prana, more life force, more oxygen.

Shoulder anatomy

There are many poses where the arms are brought from their position in Savasana to over the head. They either stay there for the duration of the pose, or it is an interim position (for example to get to the warrior poses). A greater understanding of how the shoulders behave as the arms travel upward, and how they should behave once the arms are there, will help you enormously.

Each shoulder is comprised of a shoulder blade (or scapula) plus a ball and socket (the gleno-humeral) joint formed by the head of the humerus (your upper-arm bone) articulating with the glenoid fossa (the shallow socket that is part of the scapula).

In the simplest of terms your shoulder blades are shaped as right angle triangles. The right angle corner is at the top and close to the spine (the midline). The longest side runs from the bottom extent of the bone near the spine to the outside shoulder. At the top outer corner is the acromion. It is a bony projection that forms a kind of protective cover over the top of the joint.

Together the blade and joint can perform a great many varied movements. Stabilization of this important joint is created by muscles, ligaments and tendons, but is primarily muscular. Perhaps you would already have heard the term 'rotator cuff'. This refers to a set of 4 muscles and you may have heard of them separately. You can remember them by the mnemonic SITS; supraspinatus, infraspinatus, teres minor and subscapularis.

This chapter covers enough information to give you tools for you to make practical changes to your posture and your poses. I leave it to you to decide if you want to research more anatomical details.

Probably the most important item to take note of is that the supraspinatus tendon goes from the superior aspect of the scapula under the acromion and down over the head of the humerus between these two bones. Without understanding or actioning proper arm and shoulder movement your supraspinatus tendon could be getting stuck between your acromion and humerus.

The most common rotator cuff injury comes from lifting the arm without firstly rotating the arm externally. The supraspinatus tendon gets jammed in the space between the arm (the head of the humerus) and the scapula (the acromion).

The way to avoid the damage is to use other rotator cuff muscles to draw the ball of the joint down away from the acromion process and then rotating the arm externally. Moving the head of the humerus down and out of the way has to happen to initiate full unhindered movement of the arm up over the head.

In order, this is what you need to do:

1. Rotate upper arms outward
2. Pull upper arms downward
3. Pull arms inward toward body during the outward rotation (this is akin to moving your elbows to your back pockets!).

For ecologically sound arm movement the above arm actions (which Roger calls 'cinching' down and rotation) should occur BEFORE the arm begins to lift. These principles apply both during and after the lift.

Lengthen the neck

Another published yogini and physical therapist, Julie Gudmestad says that learning to decompress your neck before you enter a pose is essential. These are the same muscles you will use to keep your shoulders down and maintain neck relaxation in your poses. Julie suggests learning which muscles pull your scapulae down with a simple exercise. Hold a 1-2 pound (1kg) object in each hand. Allow your arms to surrender to the weight, your shoulder blades to drop. Avoid collapsing forward by lifting your breastbone up. See if you can reproduce this without weighting the hands. This is your lower trapezius in action.

I have taught another exercise in class for years. Stand with your arms out to the side, completely horizontal. See in the mirror that there is a straight line from fingertip to fingertip through your shoulders. Another way to activate your lower trapezius is to rotate your arms so that your palms are facing the ceiling while maintaining a completely horizontal line.

Create the length in the neck and draw your shoulders down away from your ears. Maintain that activation and now return your palms to face down again by rotating your arms to starting position. You are ready for your pose and your muscles are working in beautiful balance.

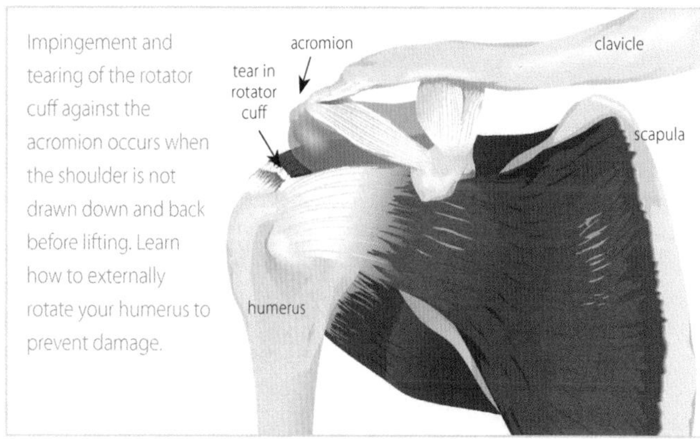

Impingement and tearing of the rotator cuff against the acromion occurs when the shoulder is not drawn down and back before lifting. Learn how to externally rotate your humerus to prevent damage.

These exercises along with placing your 'elbows in your back pockets' help you learn how to resolve stress. You externally rotate your arms, your palms now face the mirrors to some extent (the extent is determined by the degree to which you externally rotate the forearms). Your shoulders are back and down away from the ears. Although you hold your shoulders, your arms float down without any activation and could gently sway they are so relaxed. There is a slight bend in your elbows and a curl in your fingertips.

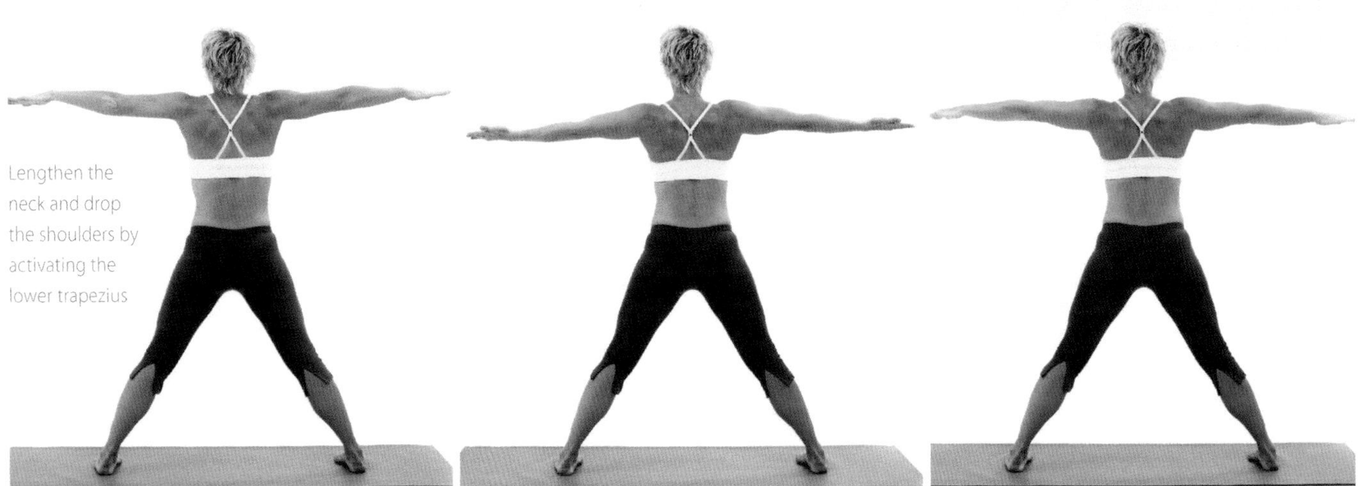

Lengthen the neck and drop the shoulders by activating the lower trapezius

Lifting the arms

Elevation of the arms is far more complex than you might think. This would be a short chapter if moving arms up involved the ball and socket joint alone. As touched on before you need to initially decompress your neck and rotate your arms externally before even starting your lift. For unhindered elevation the scapulae have to upwardly rotate. Let's break it down further.

Imagine you are standing in Savasana: Palms facing forward due to external rotation of the arms and shoulders drawn down and back. To lift your arms over the head takes them through a 180° arc. If you ignore the above principles and leave your arms simply hanging by your side, without any external arm rotation, when you lift your arms your acromion will already be hindering your movement at about the 20-30° mark.

But external rotation of the arms is only part of the story. Unless your scapula undergoes a rotation you won't be able to lift past the 2/3 point (120°). The supraspinatus tendon jams. Successfully reaching upwards and vertically means that the acromion process tips up out of the way of the head of the humerus. On the left side your scapula will rotate in a clockwise direction. Your right scapula will rotate in an anticlockwise direction.

So here are the two key elements to pay attention to when lifting the arms ...

1. pull the arms down and rotate then,
2. as you lift allow the outer side of your shoulder blade to draw up.

Don't use your neck or shrug your shoulders

You must always take steps to avoid shrugging or hunching. This mistake is mentioned in just about every individual pose chapter, so it definitely justifies an explanation and a solution. The shrugging movement is the upwards wholesale travel of the whole shoulder blade without any rotation. When lifting the arms, muscular tension is far better resolved with correct scapular rotation where the inner edge is tipped down away from the ears. This seems counterintuitive to students who mistakenly shrug the shoulders up in an attempt to lengthen the body or to get their arms up over the head more effectively. The benefits of the rotation are immediately sensed. You can feel the muscles in the neck and shoulders loosen and lengthen. Being a practicing professional dentist has certainly deepened my understanding of the importance of resolving stress in this area.

It is important not to use the neck muscles to lift the arms up over the head. The levator scapulae lifts the inner angle of the shoulder blade (and rotates the scapula in the opposite direction to that required for arm elevation). If levator scapulae is activated during arm lifts then it has the effect of hunching the shoulders. The neck gets stressed as muscles bunch up causing discomfort or pain.

The upper fibers of trapezius attach to the clavicle which attaches to the acromion process. When it contracts it has the effect of lifting the outer shoulder blade and causes rotation (and one that is useful for arm elevation). There are three parts of the trapezius. What all three parts do together is harmoniously rotate the scapulae. The shoulders neither hunch (wholesale elevation without rotation) or wholly move down.

Here's what to do in practical terms

The palms-forward position in class may be contentious but ultimately it is supremely useful in more than a physical way. You hold a mindful, more open stance and a spirit of willingness to receive from the bounty of the universe. This effect is deepened when you make eye contact with yourself in the mirror.

...learning to decompress your neck before you enter a pose is essential. These are the same muscles you will use to keep your shoulders down and maintain neck relaxation in your poses.

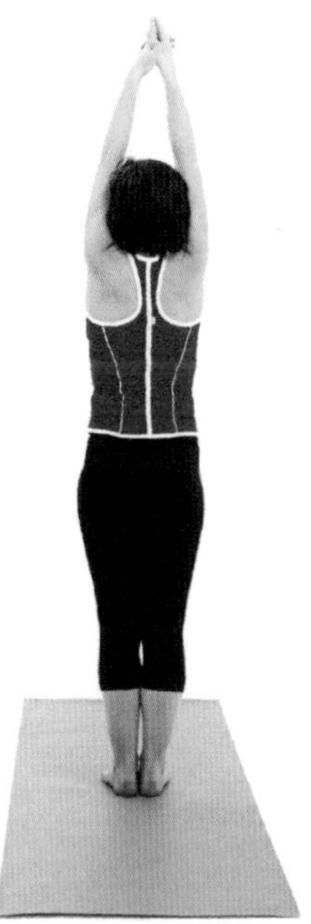

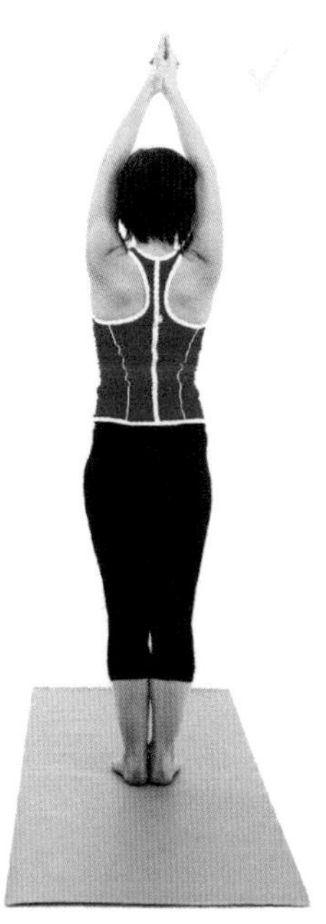

It serves no purpose however if the upper arms are not firstly rotated. What that trainee teacher said to me years ago never resonated with me. What he considered a waste turns out to be a great energy saver and encourages a beautiful posture and practice. One that adds value in and out of the studio. It removes the distraction of extraneous movement and reduces ritualization of your routine. No fuss.

Remember you can choose the extent to which you rotate your lower arms but your upper arms must be rotated externally to begin with. Without it you have to repeatedly lift yourself out of your disempowered partially collapsed chest position and manipulate your arms externally every time you are commanded into each pose. Each time you have to lift your breastbone as you decompress your neck and rotate your arms.

Clearly, you stand to benefit greatly by standing correctly to begin with. Those who don't, will simply have a harder time maintaining good alignment. Their shoulders more easily roll forward, their palms face in towards their bodies (or even face backward to a slight degree). Their shoulder blades will slide overly outward and forward towards the front side of the body. In this position it is hard to feel vital and is hardly a recipe for spinal and shoulder health.

Here is another very good reason to correct a slump

Neuro-physiologically speaking your moods are linked to your physiology. It is hard to be happy with shoulders slumped, head down and looking at the floor. Conversely it is hard to be depressed when you are standing tall and strong with head up, shoulders back, chest and body open with a deep invigorating life-giving breath. Practice good posture and experience how it transforms you at the deepest levels. The payoff is immediate.

When your arms are approaching each other overhead then you will broaden your shoulder blades. This further helps resolve tension in this complex area. The 'trick' is on full elevation relax the downward pull on your scapulae a bit, in effect surrendering to the stretch. You preserve the scapular rotation. In this way you are more likely to avoid over-engaging the hunching muscles (including levator scapulae). You get more height and you get more posterior freedom of movement.

I recommend that you take these principles and apply them to your whole practice. If your aim is to enter poses with mindfulness, remove chance of damage and not use any extraneous or abrupt movements, then surely having your body in open and ready position to begin your arm elevations is a wise thing. Introduce humeral external rotation before the lift (in your habitual stance) for safety and ease of movement, where the acromion and humerus are never in a position to collide and cause damage.

In this way your arms are in perfect position to execute any lift without further preparation. Don't waste precious time and energy and risk damage to your rotator cuff muscles by ignoring the principles of proper shoulder movement. To fully benefit from an unguarded and receptive yoga practice externally rotate your forearms too.

There are a number of people in the hot yoga world who believe that facing palms forward is wrong. Approach your practice and all your habitual movement from a practical and anatomical standpoint where your body is physiology safe and open, and you just might find yourself agreeing with me!

How to elevate arms, in a nutshell

Before you lift:

1. Cinch down and externally rotate your arms
2. Decompress your neck by dropping your shoulders down and back
3. Lift your chest and keep your body open.

As you lift:

1. Rotate your shoulder blades
2. Release levator scapulae.

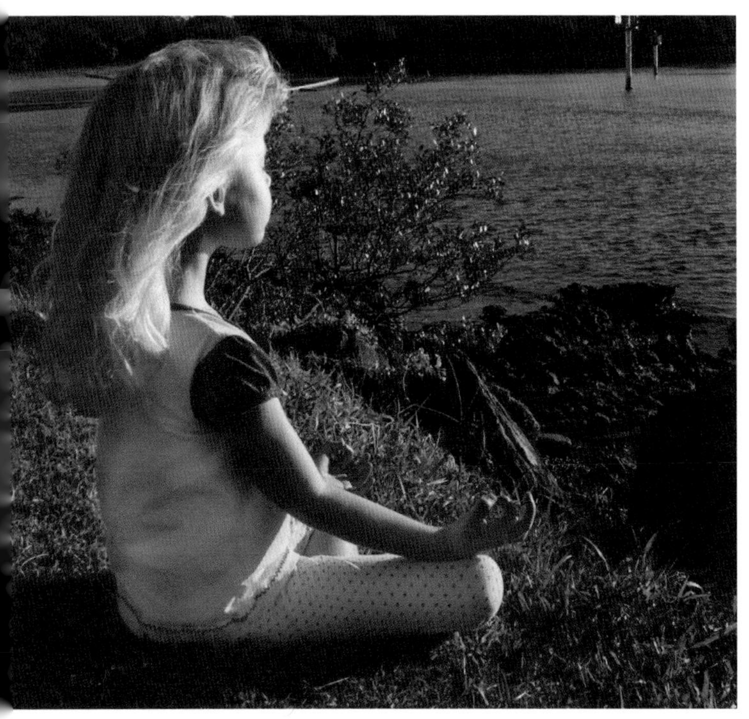

... your moods are linked to your physiology. It is hard to be depressed standing tall and strong with head up, shoulders back, chest and body open with a deep invigorating life-giving breath.

Should the teeth touch?

This is a simple question with a rather complicated answer. Having graduated in 1986 as a dentist and practiced for many years I feel I am qualified to give you a relevant opinion. I feel I need to explain why it even makes it into these chapters.

Many people experience headaches, backaches, neck aches and jaw pain. If you have regular aches then you are likely to go to your medical doctor. What many people don't realize is that it is a dentist who can help you resolve this pain. And not just the pain that occurs in the jaws. Grinding teeth is a sign of stress.

Teeth should only make contact when you eat and that is it. If you are aware of times when you are grinding more, or habitually finding your teeth together in normal circumstances, then you would be well advised to seek a dental opinion.

On a number of occasions when practicing hot yoga I have been instructed to bring my teeth together. The mistaken belief is that with the head back that biting the teeth together will enhance the stretch through the neck. Sure, you will feel the resistance. Your neck is stretched, and then when you occlude your teeth you actually engage muscles in your neck, this will contract them against the stretch. That in itself is counterproductive to create an effective elongating stretch. Even worse it can cause micro-muscle tearing.

Still, it is far more complex than that. The head and neck are an extremely intricate and complex network of muscles and nerves. The jaws do not approach each other with flat contacts like a closing book, because the teeth are present. To complicate matters further the TMJ (temporomandibular joint) is the most complex joint movement in the entire body. It is neither a hinge joint, nor a ball and socket joint. It is a combination of the two types creating movement of the lower jaw in all directions.

Because the teeth are irregular in shape and in collective form, the manner in which the jaws come together is determined differently in every single mouth. The teeth have cusps ('hills') or guiding planes against which the jaws slide to come into position. Even people with lovely looking teeth can have malocclusion, temporomandibular joint dysfunction or a number of other conditions which manifest pain in the head and neck, or simply cause asymmetric expression of the associated muscles.

When you bring your teeth together it recruits muscles in the face, the head and the neck, shoulders and upper back. Your neuromuscular conditioning occurs through repeated

Teeth should only make contact when you eat and that is it.

patterning determined by the way your teeth bite together. The moment that your teeth touch these habitual patterns take over and recreate with certainty the same conditions again and again. Most of us have some dysfunction whether conscious of it or not. Bringing your teeth together whether during practice or not, will only magnify the problems.

Biting together may be a much performed action but it is by no means a balanced one. It does not create stress-free conditions in the head and neck. Far from it. If you do find yourself clenching your teeth together routinely you may take a moment to work out what kind of stresses are present. Perhaps you have a headache, a backache, or some emotional stress, or illness. Remember nobody's occlusion is perfect.

I strongly recommend you remove this huge variable from your practice. Finally, let's look at what elite sportspeople do as a further example. Have you ever noticed that some sportspeople wear what appears to be a mouthguard? Chances are that if it is not a gladiatorial or contact sport (football, rugby) then it is not a mouthguard but an occlusal splint. It is typically worn on one arch, is often clear acrylic and clicks into place. It is fitted and adjusted by a dentist.

It removes all the harmful guiding influences of the teeth so that they come together in a ecological and harm-free fashion. The forces are then even on both sides of the arch when the jaws occlude. The muscles are lengthened in the head and neck and thus relaxation is enhanced.

This sets the scene for better performance, focus and concentration. These are not soft appliances that cushion blows to the face. These are precise instruments that must be professionally fitted. If you clench or grind or have tons of stress in your life which may or may not manifest as head and neck pain, then go get some professional advice.

Here's the solution: During class you might try the following approach to enhance your stretch when asked to bring your teeth together. Go into your back bend, relax your head back on a soft neck, open your mouth wide and then bring your lips together. At all costs avoid tooth contact.

Foot position

Ever wondered what you should do with your feet in any pose?

Perhaps you have bunions? Maybe years of wearing the wrong shoes have crowded your toes into each other? Maybe your toes lie passively at the end of your feet and don't really contact the floor (to ground you) in any meaningful fashion.

Small changes in foot position will affect ankle support. These changes will in turn affect knee relationship and hip position and therefore affect your spine and your posture.

The feet are your connection to the earth for most of your life and for a significant proportion of your hot yoga class. It needs to be strong and mindful. When standing you are usually asked to have your toes and heels come together. This is a generalized description that can be broken down further. Ultimately you want a foot position that will enhance symmetry and balance but also make you work for it! You want your knees and hips to face square on to the mirror if at all possible.

Look down at your feet when they are together and observe your geometry. If you have bunions or very triangular forms then if your heels touch, your toes will seem to fan out toward the corners of the room. This causes your knees and hips to turn out. To get the most out of your standing poses you should bring your heels out just sufficiently to have your feet, knees and hips facing the front in a neutral position. This can be a tiny space or could be as much as an inch or more.

This small change will translate to bigger effects through the body. It is very important to take this element into all your poses. When you lift one leg off the floor you are obviously left standing on one foot to balance. If that foot is not directly onto the mirror it will be to some degree positioned at an angle. Though this may help your stability, it removes from your practice the positive challenge of learning balance and improving ankle strength.

In more detail, if your foot is lined up correctly then when you stand on one foot you are creating the challenge to which your core muscles will rise. Your ankle muscles have to constantly correct and recorrect, seen and felt as a little wobble, as you learn finer and finer control and balance. You have to learn balance in multi-directions; back to front and side to side.

The moment you splay your toes out to the side you remove the side to side challenge, only preserving back to front oscillations. If you need to test this then stand on one leg with your foot square and then try again with your foot at a 45 degree angle.

Next time you are lifting one leg off the ground make a mental note to check how much automatic foot repositioning you are doing in an unconscious attempt to improve your balance. Your foot has to stay square to the room even if you find your foot shape necessitates a small gap between your heels.

Why don't you shift the weight to one leg before you lift the other up?

Many times you will hear a teacher say "shift your weight". Why shouldn't you do that? A very good question. What tends to happen is a weighting of the standing leg and a slumping of the other hip. The student is left standing lopsided. Hips that are uneven will certainly have an effect on your spine which should stay neutral in pose set-up.

Shifting the weight to your 'standing leg' is just not necessary. Your body is supported by many systems that work in synergy with your skeletal structure. You have muscles and connective tissues to hold your body in space. When you walk, your body makes the adjustments required to stop you falling over. Unless you are recovering from an injury you will probably never have to consciously take your awareness to shifting your weight to stop you falling when you lift one leg up.

In yoga asana we always have the intention of setting up correctly. We aim for excellence in alignment before depth to avoid wasting time, energy and attention recorrecting later - and worse still, diluting the great benefits of the pose.

My approach throughout this reference guide is to apply the principle of 'measure twice, cut once' so that your set-up is strong and pure. Carry an accurate set-up into your pose and you not only start your pose earlier on, your benefits start earlier and you have less work to correct mid-pose. You have more time available to continually recreate your set-up and find finer and finer distinctions in the position - you can work harder and smarter.

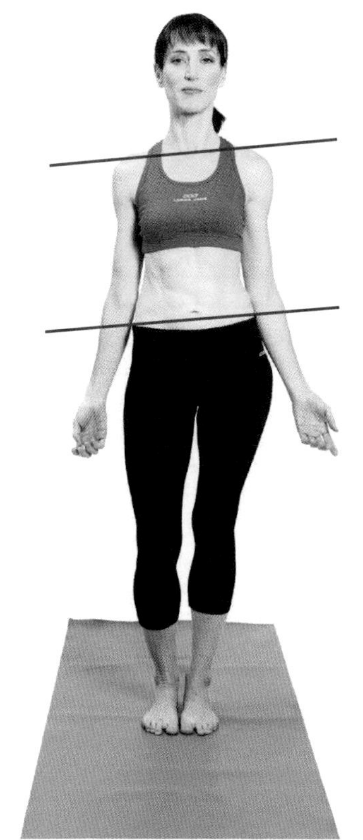

Shifting the weight affects whole body alignment

Modifications

Different Bodies – What To Do If You Can't Do A Pose, Have An Injury Or Are Restricted In Some Way

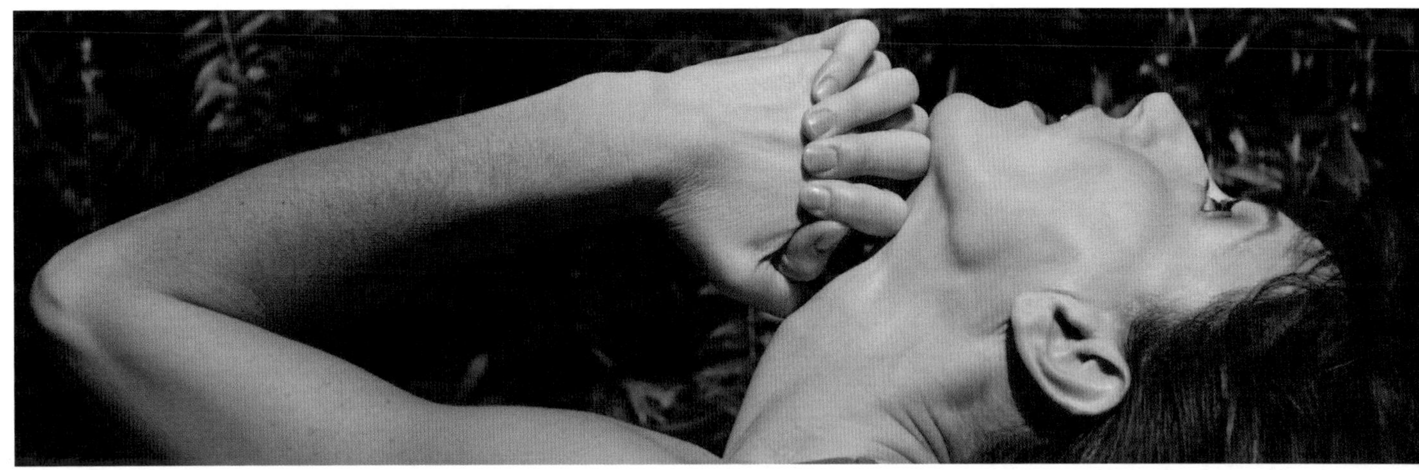

What do you do if you are not flexible or your body is less than perfect?

...it would be ridiculous to assume that a person with fused vertebrae will be able to approach their physical practice in the identical way to someone with normal and separate functional vertebrae.

Maybe you have been ill or injured? Your teacher should be able to help you find the right way to guide you in. Generally, for most students the practice principles will remain the same. Your flexibility or strength may determine your depth into a specific pose and what you work on but the principles will guide you to express your greatest depth in the pose.

Let's take a look at exceptions to general practice principles that become necessary due to specific conditions in the body.

For example it would be ridiculous to assume that a person with fused vertebrae will be able to approach their physical practice in the identical way to someone with normal and separate functional vertebrae.

The fulcrum points on a fused spine are going to change some of the foundational principles of a few of the postures involving forward and or backward bends.

Use the guidelines suggested here only after consulting your physician, surgeon, therapist and/or yoga teacher.

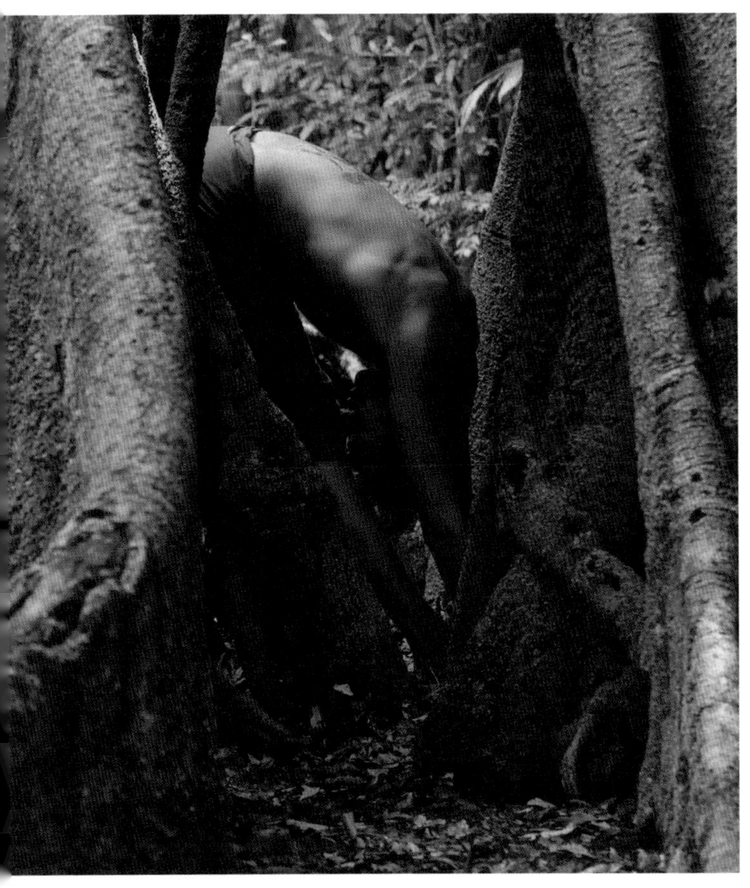

Your practice is useful for recreating juicy joints, giving back health to your shock absorbing systems and increasing circulation and movement.

You are unique and so is your body

When you attend your first class you will invariably have to fill out some kind of medical history form. As a teacher I am looking for unusual presentations such as fused vertebrae, neck, knee or back injuries that we have to monitor. However if it is a sore lower back, or sciatica, or sore knees or shoulders then usually all you have to do is follow directions by listening carefully for any adjustments or considerations for your condition.

For example in Standing Separate Leg Intense Stretching (Dandayamana Bibhaktapada Paschimottanasana), those with sciatica or acute lower back pain will keep their feet parallel and everyone else pigeon-toes their feet. This should be normal instruction for a hot yoga class.

Remember, a 'problem' pose is not just fixed by progress in THAT pose. Hot yoga works holistically to bring the entire body and mind into balance. It is like a reset button for the body and mind's better functioning. So if you find it hard to hold your foot in standing head to knee, working on that alone will not do it. The poses are of a complementary nature. Work on your practice. Maybe your head to knee poses will hold some of the answers, or maybe less obviously, the way you have to sit down in Awkward Pose (Utkatasana) will open your hips and ankles.

The information in this reference guide and associated resources is not intended to replace advice from your medical practitioner or natural therapies practitioner. Take responsibility, get the right advice for you, in tandem with using your own commonsense and body wisdom.

Let's take a look at some common problems and see how they need to be addressed for your practice. Use this list and short explanations and cross reference it with specific pose chapters relevant to your experience where appropriate.

Arthritis

There are many different types of arthritis. Huge numbers of arthritis sufferers have made incredible progress with a regular hot yoga practice. Many have reduced or completely eliminated medication. Your practice, and not just isolated poses, is useful for recreating juicy joints, giving back health to your suspension or shock absorbing systems and increasing circulation and movement.

Begin with gentle backbends and avoid the full pose. These are incredible heart opening poses – literally. They facilitate a growing of the chest and a stretch of your most important muscle.

Asthma

Asthma attacks can arise from panic and fear (as well as physical stimuli of course). Asthmatics are trying to reduce the reliance on open-mouth breathing and the effects of dry air. The humid room removes much of the danger. I have never had anyone have a problem with asthma attacks in the room, plus I am told that the problem is reduced outside too.

Back problems

Back problems present themselves in a multitude of ways. Naturally there is no one-size-fits-all solution in the yoga studio. If you happen to have general back discomfort (NOT caused by injury but possibly due to work, misuse, or lack of movement in all directions) then welcome to your body. You don't have to live with background pain. You may simply have to approach your practice with attention to the basics of breath and alignment. Perhaps things will appear to get worse some of the time as you begin to restore movement to your stiffened vertebral column.

Your condition may have been manifesting itself over the past number of years. So expecting it to magically disappear within a class or two may be unrealistic although it is entirely possible. It may take weeks or months to improve depending on how you presented to your first classes. I have several notable (and verifiable) cases of students whose longstanding backaches (of up to 20 years) have disappeared by the end of the first class. One woman in particular only participated in about one third of the class and yet she emerged elated and pain free. The pain did not return.

If you are experiencing spasms in your back then don't be a martyr. Exercise caution. Recognize that there are a number of poses where you bring your upright body to the floor from standing with a straight back. This may not only be painful for you, it could exacerbate or worsen your spasms. Muscles in the mid-back work hard to bring your straight back to the floor.

My recommendation is to come to the floor without engaging these muscles. Round your spine down from neck through your shoulders then through to your lower back.

- Drop your head and try walking your hands down your legs when you descend.
- Walk them back up the legs when you come up again.
- Let your chin come up last.

A similar modification occurs for hernia sufferers to modulate intraabdominal pressure, see next page.

Cardiovascular problems and poor peripheral circulation

Doing the yoga in the heated room increases your cardiac output and stroke volume. This means that the efficiency of your heart and the amount it pumps increases. The effects start to kick in from the first class. Luckily it is not all hard work for the entire 90 minutes (although it can feel that way).

The pose sequence is broken up by the Savasana Pose which not only provides rest and restoration of energy but flushes and cleanses the circulation allowing it to reach stagnant areas.

If you have labile (changeable) hypertension or cardiovascular conditions that are not controlled by diet, lifestyle or medication then it is advisable to enter backbends with caution.

Begin with gentle backbends and avoid the full pose as you allow yourself a process of discovery and gradual opening. These are incredible heart opening poses – literally. They facilitate a growing of the chest and a stretch of your most important muscle. Take it easy. Breathe.

In all backbends there is the potential to feel rather vulnerable because you are not acting in a way that protects your chest and organs. It is an innate reaction to act to protect it. If you are not feeling safe then you may feel like exiting the pose early. You will learn over time to breathe through the intensity of each pose at the same time as preserving all the basic alignment principles.

The poses to be careful of are Half Moon Backbend (Ardha Chandrasana), Floor Bow (Dhanurasana) and particularly Camel (Ustrasana). Allow your head to drop back on your soft neck. Make sure you look back and not up; certainly don't look down your nose when things get tough. Just don't go as far with your actual bend.

In Backbend stage your progress. Leave your arms above your head, drop your head back, look back. That's it. Next you can lock your legs and push your hips forward a bit. Then you can start to bring your arms back. Do this over a number of classes. In the meantime, keep checking your BP readings because if you are going regularly chances are your blood pressure will normalize and you may actually be taking too much medication!

In Floor Bow, depending on your flexibility, you can start by holding your feet and looking up to the ceiling. Soon you will be starting your kick.

You will learn over time to breathe through the intensity of each pose at the same time as preserving all the basic alignment principles.

You can stage Camel pose too. Start with hands on hips, just relax your head back, keep the eyes open and look back. Next steps will be to squeeze the bottom and push the hips forward while starting to go back.

Cramps

Cramps often occur during the first few days of an activity you're not used to. They may be a result of overexertion or dehydration. Usually only beginning students cramp during class. Sweating is part of your hot yoga experience. It leads to loss of electrolytes; magnesium, potassium, sodium or calcium which are vital to proper cell function. Sometimes drinking large amounts of water or fluids that lack salt can upset electrolyte levels. When cramping, you need to deal with your immediate discomfort and the underlying cause. You must rehydrate and restore electrolyte balance.

Imbalances can be fixed with diet or supplementation. The best electrolyte supplementation is hands down, pure sea salt; on your food or in your water. Sport drink quality varies tremendously. Many are just colored sweet drink with added table salt. Practicing in the heat does help resolve cramps, as does gentle massage. If cramps persist you need to investigate hydration, electrolyte balance and any underlying illness or condition.

Diabetes, thyroid and other endocrine problems

Coming to yoga regularly is like pressing a reset button on your hormonal systems. Let go, relax into the postures. Trust. Believe.

There are many stories of signs of diabetes both diminishing and reversing. Hypo- and hyperthyroidism healing. I have friends unable to conceive, 2 of those on IVF programs and one with an endocrine disorder told she would never have children. These women became pregnant after establishing a regular yoga practice in the hot room. No promises - but there is a better chance of natural conception.

Grip difficulties

Injury and inflexibility usually call for grip modifications. Poses most often requiring variation are Hands to Feet and the Intense Stretch poses as well as the Head to Knee postures. All grip problems are pose-specific and dealt with in the pose chapters. Sometimes sweat can make grip difficult but this is generally confined to those with a new hot yoga practice.

Hernia

There are many kinds of hernias. The types that affect your practice are usually the abdominal or the intervertebral ones. Inguinal and femoral hernias comprise 75% of all abdominal hernias. Incisional hernias are the result of incomplete abdominal post-operative healing. Umbilical hernias in adults usually affect pregnant or obese women. While inguinal and femoral present similarly around the groin, inguinal hernias affect men and femoral affect women.

Hernias range from painless to extremely painful. A hernia is the bulge that results from tissue that pushes itself through windows of weakness in the abdominal wall. The 'corset effect' of the muscles holding in the contents of the abdomen is lost. The gap itself is not the problem, it is the resultant movement of intestines or other organs through the space as a result of unrestrained pressure.

Hernias cannot heal themselves and are neither cured by yoga nor medicine. They need medical attention. If you have a hernia that worsens with increased abdominal pressure due to certain yoga moves then there are two things that need to happen.

1. You need to perform movements that remove the risk of worsening your condition.
2. You need medical intervention.

If you have a hernia that is yet to be resolved then pay attention to your body. If most of your practice is affected then you must consider breaking from yoga and other strenuous activity until you have received attention. I have had several students who had particular difficulty with deep forward bends that take them from standing down to the floor. To reduce intra-abdominal pressure tuck your chin and walk your hands down on your legs, rounding your body down to the floor. Reverse this to release. See previous instruction in 'Back problems'. Also see photos bottom right page 145.

Intervertebral disc hernias can cause back pain and sciatica. See below. Always consider your options carefully before contemplating medical intervention. Hot yoga is a very viable treatment alternative.

Herniated discs

Herniated discs are quite common and are a result of general wear and tear, constant sitting or (incorrect) lifting. The condition is not generally diagnosed unless it becomes painful. And then it ranges from uncomfortable to unbearable. The other labels used include ruptured, bulging or prolapsed disc, disc protrusion or degeneration, or sciatica. 'Slipped disc' is often incorrectly used and is neither possible nor descriptive of the problem.

A herniated disc is the bulging of the soft inner part of the body of the vertebra (nucleus pulposis) squeezing out through a hole in the outer part (the annulus fibrosis). Not always painful, you are aware of a herniation when the extrusion puts pressure on a spinal nerve. Because the vertebral bodies are on the stomach (ventral) side of the spine and a forward bend squeezes the front space closed while opening the back part wider, the extrusion pushes out backward, placing pressure on the nerve situated directly behind.

This is why forward bends cause the pain. And conversely why backbends are so very therapeutic. Mind you there is increasing evidence that shows that physical compression of the bulge against the nerve is not the cause of the pain. It seems to be the release of chemicals into the area as a result of inflammation. This is why anti-inflammatories can be helpful in treating the pain.

The position of the most common disc herniation is in the lumbar area at L4-5 or L5-S1. This is many times more common than a cervical or neck herniation at C6-7, which causes pain in the head, neck, shoulders, arm and hand. The lower spine herniation causes local pain and leg pain (often referred to as sciatica) and can radiate through the buttocks, thigh, foot and toe. The sensations can be pain, tingling or burning, muscular weakness and numbness. Pain is usually continuous and the problem is typically unilateral.

The risk reduces around the age of 50-60 years where the disc dries out, only to be replaced by osteoarthritic conditions and other causes of lower back pain.

In the non-yoga world there are only really three options for herniation; live with the pain; surgery; or permanent cortisone shots. But with care and patience hot yoga may be your answer providing a possibility for rehabilitation. Hot yoga restores mobility, flexibility, flushes damaging chemicals and impurities and brings nutrition to the area. Your discs become more nourished and less dry due to renewed circulation.

Once you make the decision to take your healing into your own hands then it is likely to be physically and mentally very challenging and may even be painful. The good news is that with continued practice you will feel relief. With enough frequency you can be pain-free.

Progress may be slow and require great persistence and patience over your healing journey. This may take weeks or months. I had a student who was coming for seven weeks with great progress in diminishing the pain. He actually achieved a pain-free status when he started coming twice a day for a two weeks, with a day off per week of course.

In the beginning you may not be able to participate in the whole class but over time you will do more and more. Your ticket to good back health is to increase your frequency of practice. The more classes you take the faster you can expect your recovery to be. Your range of motion will return and you will sleep better. The sacrifices are worth it if it gives you back your life.

How to deal with your condition in the studio:

Easy does it:

When forward bending make sure you take an 'easy does it' approach. You could try bending your legs to get to the floor. The forward bends of Hands to Feet, the Standing Separate Leg poses and even when coming forward in Rabbit and Tortoise may require you to 'walk' your hands down your thighs to add extra support and suspension. See page 145.

In Standing Head to Knee you may have to start with your thigh higher than parallel to the floor. Or, try to stand straight, bend up the leg without rounding down at all. It will be a great challenge to your stamina and strength.

Core strength:

Focus on creating support for your lower spine muscles. Work on your core strength to bolster your spine (maybe even seek extra professional help). The hydraulic pressure in your organs as you 'suck in your stomach' and activate your core muscles is always advised with any forward bending. See the free core strengthening video at www.HotYogaDoctor.com.

Increase mobility:

Focus on backbends and twists to create mobility in all directions. The increased movement will bring improved nutrition to the area through awakened circulation and make the joints 'juicier'.

Coming to yoga regularly is like pressing a reset button on your hormonal systems.

Know your limits:

You may not be able to go right into a pose to your 'ego's' satisfaction. Just stop before you get to excruciating pain. Work on alignment rather than depth and listen to your body, intelligently. For example you may have to lean on your thighs or knees with straight arms and body bent over at the waist if you really cannot get to the floor. If your pain is acute then you may have to temporarily suspend some of your forward bends. On some occasions you may have to avoid yoga altogether. Bed rest is a very temporary solution and never the answer to long term rehabilitation. Yoga will improve your posture, your flexibility and alleviate pain.

Infirm

Patience is required to gain progress. Your body will begin to open up. Sometimes the symptoms of your illness seem to increase as impurities could get flushed through. You may need to stand near a wall to help you with balance. I sometimes provide a tall stool for students so they can lean on, use for support or for getting to the floor or climbing back up. Take a look at the section on Injury below for further guidance.

Inflexible

Be careful to remove your ego from the equation. It simply doesn't matter how far you go in the pose. Proceed with care and precision before depth. Take a look at Triangle in particular for special alterations to standard practice. The heat is the best friend to inflexibility.

Many seemingly flexible students were very inflexible when they started – perhaps hot yoga could be your perfect exercise companion!

Injury

Make sure you record all problems and concerns on your medical history form. But take it further. If you are never approached by your teacher for clarification then you must go and talk with your teacher and each new one you encounter. It pays to remind teachers you may have only told once or twice. Remember, stay aware of your teacher's ability to give or remind you of appropriate modifications. Let your intuition also guide you to keep you safe.

Perhaps you have a new trainee teacher or someone who is not able to give advice in respect to your injury. Research the pose in question in this manual and take some responsibility for the way you do your yoga. Get advice where needed from health care professionals, knowledgeable yogis or yoga teachers who give really precise instruction and fixes. You may find some teachers will simply claim that the poses will fix everything without modification. This is simply not true for many of the poses. Sometimes it is a question of entering less deeply than someone without the injury. Other times – and especially with injury – you will have to consider other parallel techniques.

Knee problems and 'locking the knee'

The knee is a simple hinge, but that is where the simplicity ends. It is a complex system of ligaments and tendons, bone and cartilage with which millions have trouble. Always use caution with knee problems. They can take a long time to repair.

Thankfully there is every opportunity to strengthen the knee and supporting musculature by 'locking the knee' in many poses in both the standing and floor poses. The yoga technique of pulling the kneecap up with the help of the quadriceps is also recommended by physiotherapists to protect and heal the knees. This is why there is a strong focus on 'locking the knee'.

Building strength and stability and space in the knee will reduce many symptoms and help restore health. Many students have avoided knee surgery with hot yoga or it has given them better movement or helped in post-operative recovery. Be patient and push your envelope of comfort appropriately.

If you have knee problems then you will find a number of floor poses difficult. Fixed Firm Pose (Chapter 21) may be downright impossible, so kneel until you have no painful damaging twisting sensation in your knees. Keep knees, feet and heels together, hips over the heels. You may need padding. Use gravity, sit up very straight and focus on restorative healing. Allow the ligaments to stretch slowly. Over time gradually move your knees and heels apart.

Be careful of advice from 'armchair' experts to indiscriminately avoid locking the knee. You may hear people tell you to 'micro-bend' the knee instead of locking. The aim of modern treatment is to rehabilitate the muscles that support the knee. These include the calf, hamstring and quadriceps muscles in a range of movements.

Large bodies

There are some simple adjustments when your body just gets in the way. Some students will have to wait for the loss of shape from their girth or legs to manage the same grips or entries as their fellow students. Examples of affected poses are Hands To Feet, Standing Separate Leg Intense Stretching, or Standing Head to Knee. See specific pose chapters. There will be some poses where entry is more of a challenge and typically these are forward bending poses or those where you start seated on your heels – see Eagle (Garudasana), Rabbit (Sasangasana) or Head To Knee. Those with large abdomens or breasts may find the belly down poses a challenge.

Having a larger shape has little effect on your practice, you will still benefit greatly. Losing shape is usually fast and effective. Students find that doing this yoga starts to instill unconscious improvement in eating habits. Hormonal systems are reset and the body functions more effectively.

Neck problems

Fear is a major issue with those who have neck problems. To try to avoid pain, students in backbends drop the chin to the chest. This engages muscles in the head, neck and shoulders which in turn causes strain, damage and makes the neck problem even worse. A soft neck is arguably the safest place for your head in backbends but is clearly close to impossible without the right pose modifications or techniques.

Fear-affected poses are all backbends, including those performed belly-down and Pranayama breathing. As a first step try solely dropping the head back without any further action. You can go deeper into the pose another class. Perhaps ask a teacher to assist you. I place my stiffened hand along my forefinger with palm face down at the base of the neck to support the head. It allows the yogi to drop the weight and still feel supported. I keep it there till they release. Similarly I may support this same student in Camel.

Pay attention to your teeth and jaw in backbends, see page 44. It's OK for your lips to come apart – but you still must breathe through your nose.

There is a way to help students in initial Pranayama. They can interlock their fingers behind their neck. It makes the exercise a little more clunky and less straightforward but it does work. The inhales and exhales occur in the same way and the backward head movement is less far. Along with other backbends and the opening of the body the student learns to trust themselves and they can usually abandon the awkward neck hold after 2-3 classes.

Pregnant bodies

Whether or not you decide to do yoga, let the belly hang out about half way through pregnancy. Practice your perineal exercises. When I was pregnant with my daughter I was teaching hot yoga. I also loved being in the hot room for the 90 minute class.

You will need modifications to several poses. Sometimes it will be putting your feet and or knees further apart to avoid colliding with your belly (Awkward Pose and Half Tortoise). You should avoiding going too deep in Eagle. After about four months you will cease doing big forward curls like Standing Head to Knee or Rabbit. At that time too, you won't be lying down on your stomach.

For hot yoga pregnancy help please go to the forum at www.HotYogaDoctor.com.

My pregnancy and childbirth were both positively effected by my hot yoga practice. As the baby grows in the womb it pushes your digestive organs and diaphragm further up and back in the abdominal cavity. Eating has to occur in smaller amounts more often. Breathing can be very difficult. Lungs and diaphragm are cramped. Often just the act of walking or talking can have you breathless. However this was never a problem with my continued practice of Pranayama.

My energy and stamina were incredible. And I never had a backache the entire pregnancy. These are compelling reasons to do hot yoga when you are pregnant. The general rule of thumb when considering whether to do hot yoga is: 'Stick with what you know'. If you have never done hot yoga before and want to, then you have to follow your physician's advice and or your own intuition. You may feel more comfortable to wait until after the birth. There are plenty of alternative pregnancy yoga styles available.

Scars

The extent of healing will depend on your practice frequency and whether the scar occurred naturally or via surgery. Surgical scars generally take longer because of the way the scalpel cleaves through layers of connective tissue. They are not as 'reversible' as natural tear wounds.

The good news is that with continued practice you will feel relief. With enough frequency you can be pain-free. Your ticket to good back health is to increase your frequency of practice. The more classes you take the faster you can expect your recovery to be.

Internal and external scars equally benefit from your practice. Scar tissue can break down and impurities can be flushed away. Improved peripheral circulation visibly improves scar tissue. In hot yoga you are frequently bringing new nourishment to these discolored scars. They begin to soften in texture and color often changing from purple to soft pink.

Sciatica

Sciatica can be a very painful condition. It can be caused by problems with the site where the nerve emerges from the spinal column. It occurs somewhere along the distribution of the sciatic nerve due to pressure and inflammation and can occur in one or both legs. Depending on severity, it may occur from the lower back, through the buttock, over the thigh and may even extend to behind the knee, over the calf and to the foot. Many a student with sciatica has found incredible relief with hot yoga.

The ability to soften and work deeply into the affected areas makes hot yoga a better form of therapy than most other styles of yoga. I have known numerous students to find relief to longstanding conditions in only one to three classes.

All poses can be approached as prescribed in this manual. Particular poses that need technique review to avoid and heal sciatic injury include: Hands to Feet, Sit-Up, Head to Knee (floor), Intense Stretching (floor) and Standing Separate Leg Intense Stretching pose (where for example you step out then stay with feet parallel, pull with bent arms, straight back, not rounded). See the specific pose chapters for full instructions.

Using a strap, towel or mat

Although I am not a believer in using props for hot yoga there are a few exceptions. You may need to use a strap or small towel if you can't bend up your leg enough to hold the foot in Standing Bow (Dandayamana Dhanurasana), or if you can't bend up both legs for Floor Bow.

You won't need a strap for Head to Knee poses at all. Remember to take as much slack out of the strap or towel as you possibly can. Some people need a towel in Eagle Pose to simply have connection between the hands. Please see Floor Bow and Eagle for instructions.

You don't use a strap or towel for grips that you are trying to enhance. If you think you need a towel because your hand/s are slipping then using a towel doesn't help you build strength. Almost everyone has problems with sweat and slippage in the beginning. It is merely a problem with hand or finger strength. This builds over time so just be patient. (Note: There is one exception to this – Rabbit pose. See specific pose chapter for instructions.)

Yoga studios are generally carpeted with no underlay so there is little to no padding. For the most part you will only ever need your mat and no prop is necessary at all. However, you may have occasion to use your mat to provide extra cushioning for your body. See the list below for exceptions:

1. Providing padding for heels spurs. Place two mats in a 'T' if you have a severe case.
2. Roll or fold a towel or mat under knees provides cushioning for knee problems like injury, post-operative healing, missing patellas (kneecaps).
3. Roll or fold a mat or towel for seriously inflexible ankles. Allow protection or opening of your joints against the hard floor in a gentle way.
4. Cushioning for the neck when lying on your back.
5. You could even place your prop between hips and heels when sitting.

Vertebral fusions

Get advice, both professional and casual. It will help you to find another hot yoga enthusiast who also has a similar problem and find out their hints and tips. Be aware that fusions will affect your poses in different ways. The most dangerous fusions are of the cervical spine (neck). You won't be able to go into poses to the extent of an able-spined person. Rabbit Pose will need to be markedly different. Forehead to knee poses may have to be modified to be nose or lips or chin, to knee. Every body will be different and you need consultation with your teacher and your doctor. Let intuition be your guide when it comes to advice of your teacher – if what they are saying just doesn't seem right – seek further advice before proceeding.

Don't play around with your spine if it has a cervical fusion. Fusions lower down the spine have less effect on your safety but I always take each injury like this on a case by case basis.

If you have questions then take a look at the forum at www.HotYogaDoctor.com, the world's most popular and highly regarded forum for all things hot yoga.

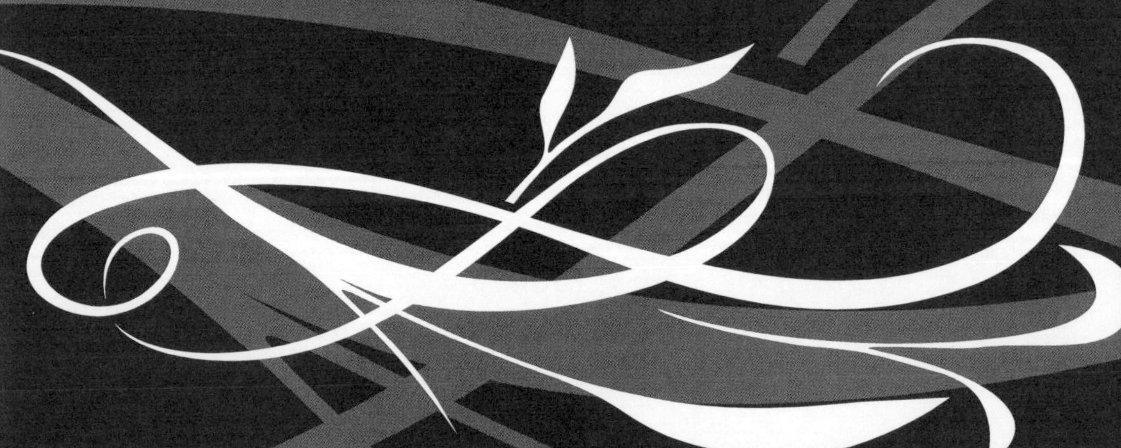

Pranayama Breathing

Every artist was first an amateur.
—Ralph Waldo Emerson

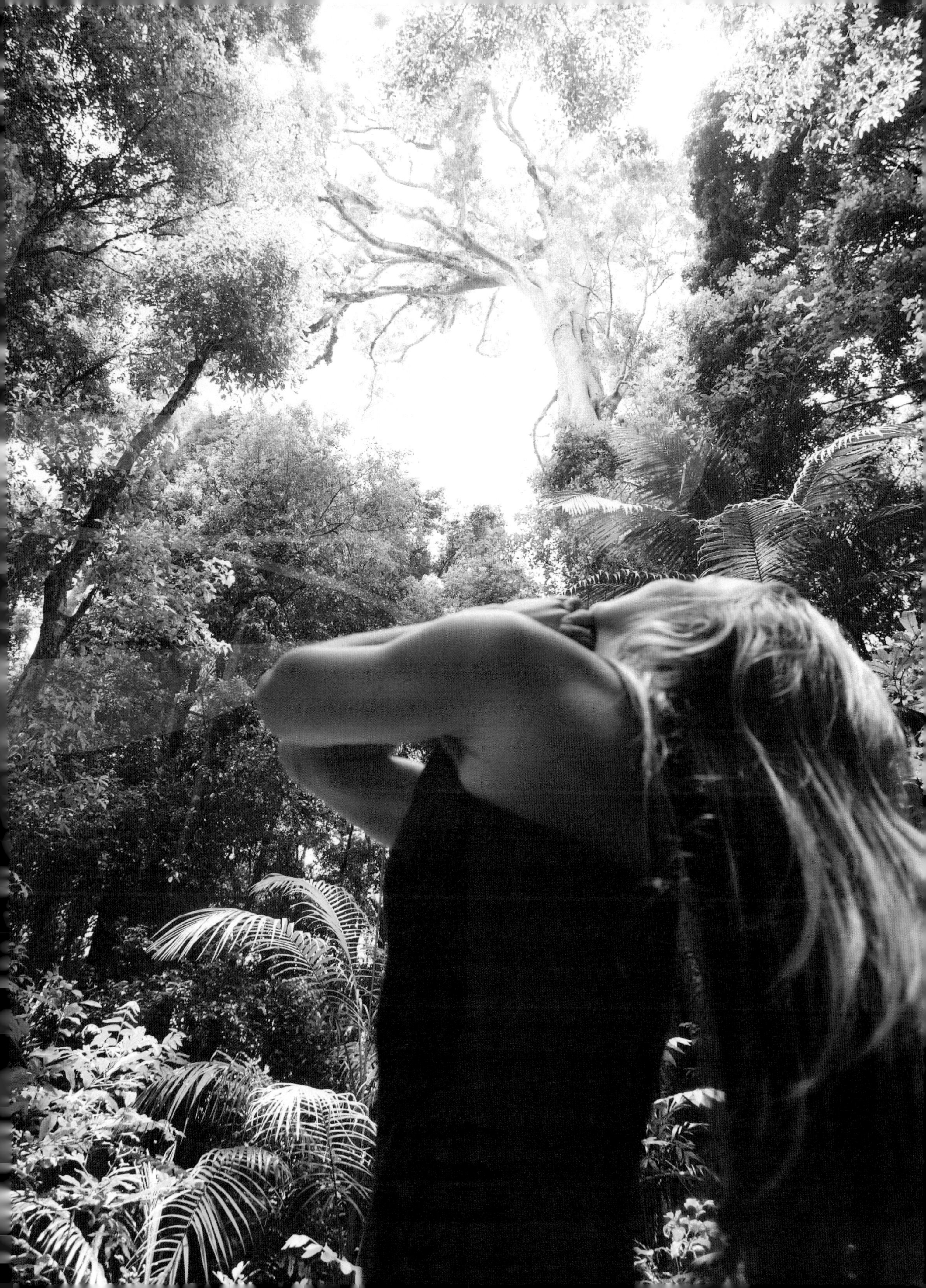

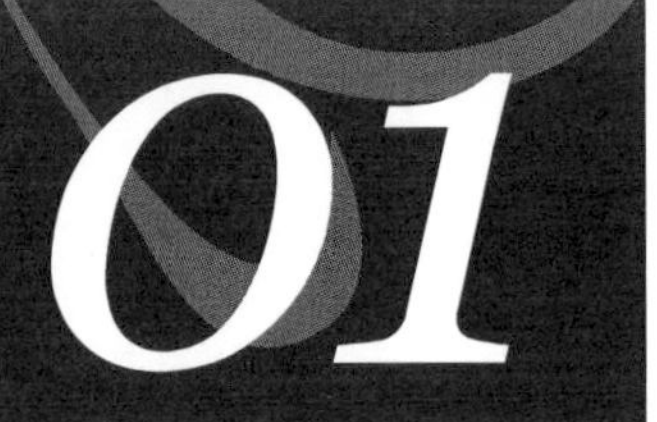

Pranayama Breathing

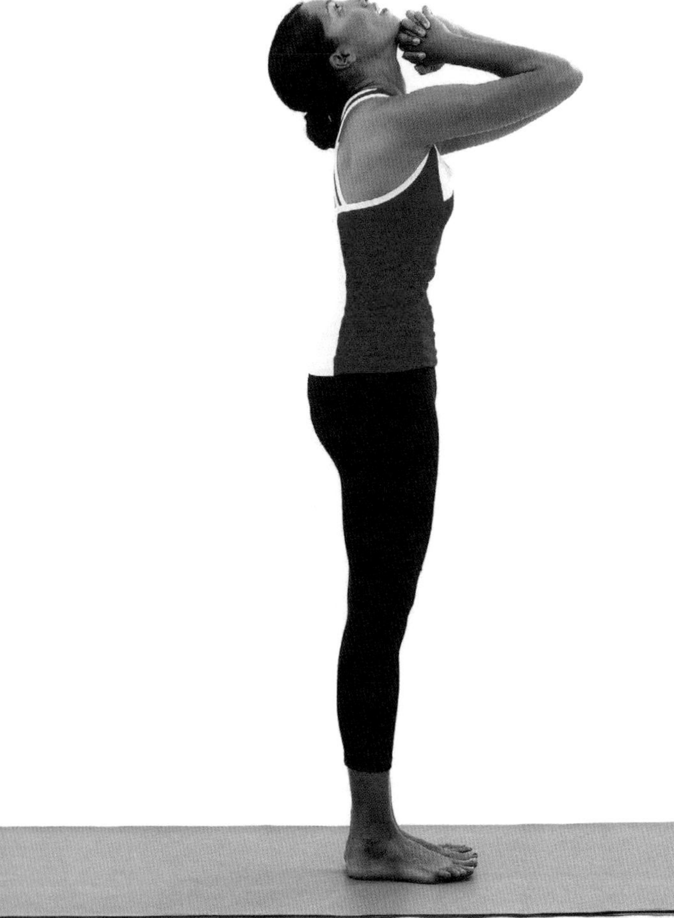

The essentials

Your class begins with this strong breathing exercise characterized by a deep conscious inhale and exhale. As the room is heated to body temperature (or more in many studios) the body is warm from the outside in, right from the start.

In essence Pranayama begins your process of meditation. It brings stillness to the mind by gaining a greater inner awareness through this complex movement. Ayama of Prana is literally the regulation of prana and is practiced by paying attention to the cycle of prolonged inhalation, retention and exhalation of the breath. Prana is present in all things and is universal life force, vital energy, power, oxygen, air or breath.

Where you may have just entered the room and may even have quite scattered thoughts about your day, or even the class to come, this exercise will definitely help empty your thoughts to some degree, calming you down and bringing you ever-presently into the room. Two sets of approximately 10 breath cycles occur to warm the body and focus the mind on the task at hand and therefore by the end you are ready to proceed.

What makes this pose so difficult to get right?

Forever improvable, Pranayama is indeed a work in progress. For the beginner this exercise is rarely fully grasped in one class. The student needs excellent listening and often excellent observation skills. If your teacher offers a physical demonstration prior to the class then this affords you a better launch on the path. You would be the exception if you have a) the coordination, b) the lung capacity and c) the shoulder, neck and wrist flexibility to get to the end without some difficulty. Make no mistake this is a very challenging physical undertaking. You will discover any barriers to deep breathing right here.

The good news is that you will begin to foster an enormous increase in your potential to simply breathe – and perhaps more deeply than you ever have before. Your diaphragm will strengthen enormously, helping you create a better life for yourself.

Your life is dependent on your breath more than anything else that you 'have'. Draw it in deeply here and create life and energy, finding within yourself almost boundless reserves. This amazing exercise can transform your life and take you from the oft-too-high-in-the-chest breath down to an invigorating and stress-relieving abdomino-diaphragmatic one.

The technique

There are two sets of approximately ten breaths each. This complex movement takes up so much of your conscious mind that it is easy to find yourself 'in the moment'. This makes it quite difficult to count an exact number of cycles, both for teacher and student. Surrender to the command of the teacher or, if practicing at home, work with your intuition and stop at around 10.

As there is a tremendous amount of coordination required, below, you will find a section on set-up and two other separate sets of instructions for the upper and lower body movements. Breaking it down like this will make it easier for you to comprehend.

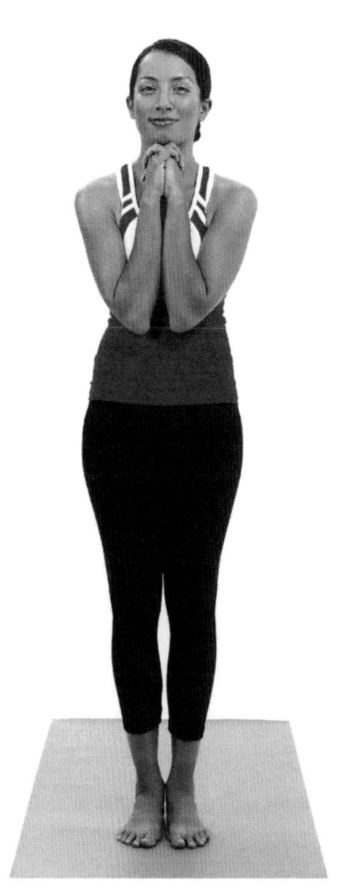

The set-up

Every standing pose starts with the same preparatory position – a type of upright Savasana or 'Corpse' pose where you center and ground yourself, calm your breath, and do nothing but breathe. Focus on yourself in the mirror. One of your greatest challenges, regardless of your yoga experience will be to stand still and look yourself in the eye. Your comfort will change as you encounter the peaks and troughs of life, especially at times of intense emotions or sensations.

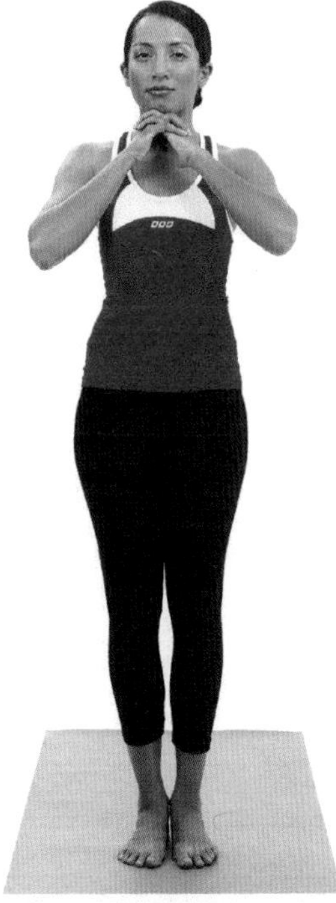

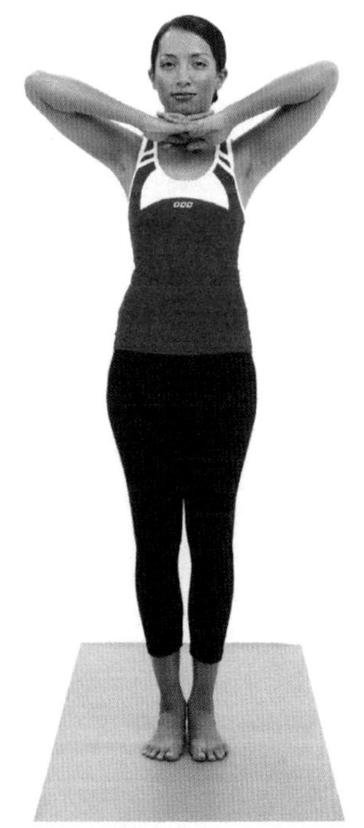

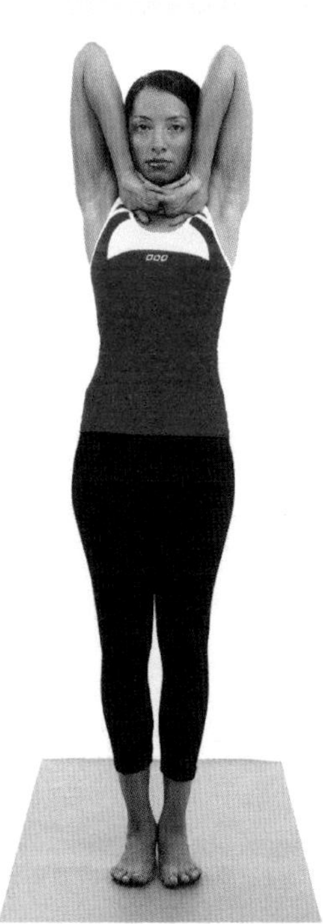

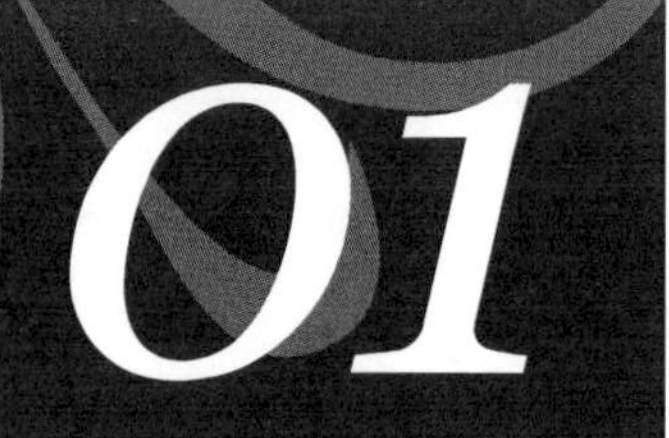

01 Pranayama Breathing

Stand with your feet together in the center of your mat. Please take a look at the chapter on feet position if you have bunions or other foot conditions like clawed toes or pronation. Square your knees and hips to the mirror. Ground yourself. Create more awareness of your earth connection by rolling the weight around your feet from side to side and back to front, lifting up and replacing your well-spaced toes. Now relax them, no gripping the floor.

Bring the energy up through your feet to your firm engaged legs. Now slightly tuck the tailbone under to lengthen and find space in the lower spine. Draw the energy up through your torso. As you find traction in your spine your chest will lift and open as your upper arms externally rotate. This corresponds to a simultaneous drop of the shoulders down and back away from the ears. Your neck extends further elongating your body and your chin is parallel to the floor. Your arms fall to your sides with your palms facing the mirror to some degree and you will find yourself physically able to breathe more deeply.

Practice this stance outside of your yoga class to improve your posture and enhance your wellbeing. This is particularly useful for those who do lots of lifting, especially Moms whose postures round terribly due to breastfeeding and child carrying. Now that you are physically and mentally in the room you are ready to set up for Pranayama breathing.

1.1 **Interlock Fingers**: Interlace your fingers together and cross your thumbs.

1.2 **Bend Your Arms**: Bring your hands to touch under your chin, thumbs in contact with your throat to start. Your elbows come together close to your abdomen.

1.3 **Your Chin**: Ensure your chin is parallel to the ground to start.

1.4 **Your Shoulders**: Hold your shoulders back and spine upright. Don't round the spine to bring your elbows together. Rather leave some space between them if you have tight or injured shoulders.

1.5 **Your Legs**: Legs do not lock out for the set-up. They are engaged and firm.

1.6 **Your Eyes**: Maintain focus for the moment in the mirror and gaze softly into your own eyes.

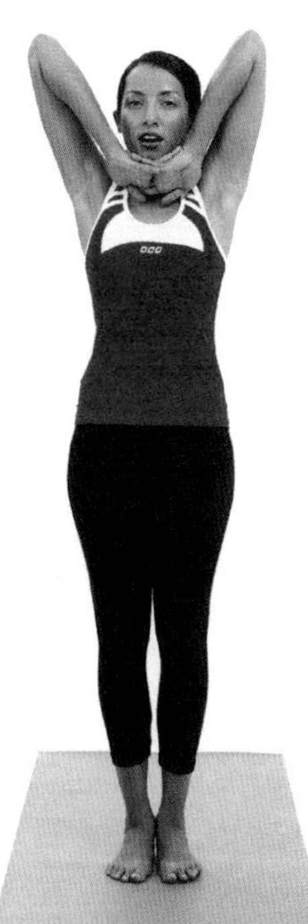

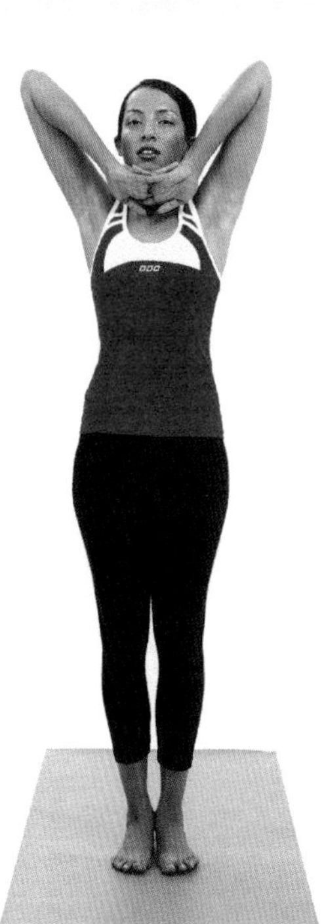

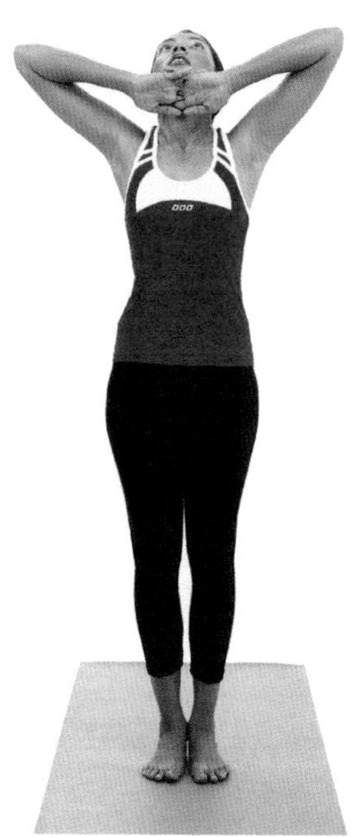

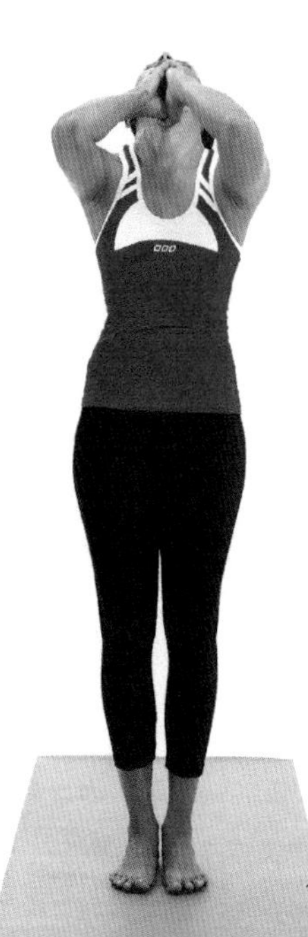

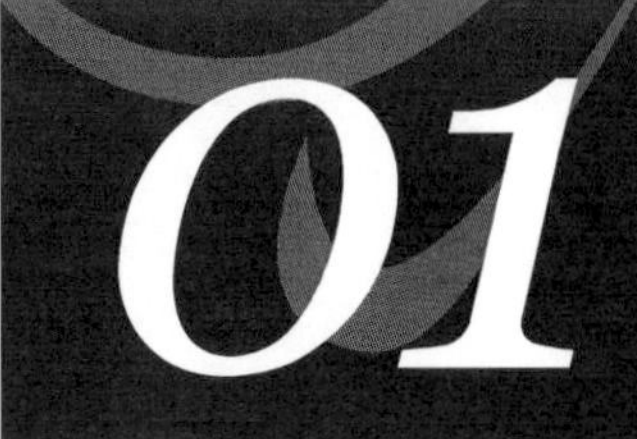

I always instruct students to start with an empty set of lungs. This definite start means energetically everyone begins at the same time in the same way, without getting left behind. In this vein I teach Pranayama as follows:

Your head, neck and arms:

2.1 **Empty Your Lungs**: Prepare for your first inhale by fully exhaling to empty your lungs. You are now not just mentally but physically ready to begin. The class starts with beautiful strong synergy.

2.2 **Your First Inhale, Elbows Up**: Keep your head still and inhale through your nose for around 6 seconds. For the duration continually draw your elbows apart, out and up in an arc toward the ceiling. If you cannot sustain such a long breath (which will undoubtedly grow over time) then you will hold it for the remaining time. Notice the stretch in your torso and under your arms, right down to your evenly grounded feet.

2.3 **Your Shoulders Down**: Even though your arms are moving up, keep your shoulders down away from the ears to avoid shrugging and muscular strain. As your elbows rise your shoulders stay 'behind' you even if this compromises the eventual reach of your elbows.

2.4 **Be Fit To Burst**: At the end of 6 seconds you are at the zenith of your inhale. Your lungs are full. Try taking another sip of air to help grow your lungs.

2.5 **Open Your Mouth, Force The Exhale**: Your relaxed mouth needs to open just enough to allow the passage of air. Draw in your abdomen and exhale fully over the 6 seconds. The best description I can offer is to sound like a hairdryer. You'll have to make a small constriction at the base of the throat which increases the flow in a similar way to a siphon. Your exhale is audible, forceful and way, way more complete. Increase the power of your 'hairdryer' and the benefits are greater and the exhalation more full.

2.6 **Arms Move Forward**: The length of your exhale fully accompanies a forward movement of the arms. Your first inhale brings your elbows up high. Maintain maximum elbow height from now on as you slowly move the elbows forward and together to meet high above the chest with forearms parallel to the ceiling.

2.7 **Your Head And Neck Move Back**: As you exhale and move your arms forward, your head will move backward to your neck's fullest backward flexion. Two factors will help you control this slow and deliberate cervical spine backbend. i) Move

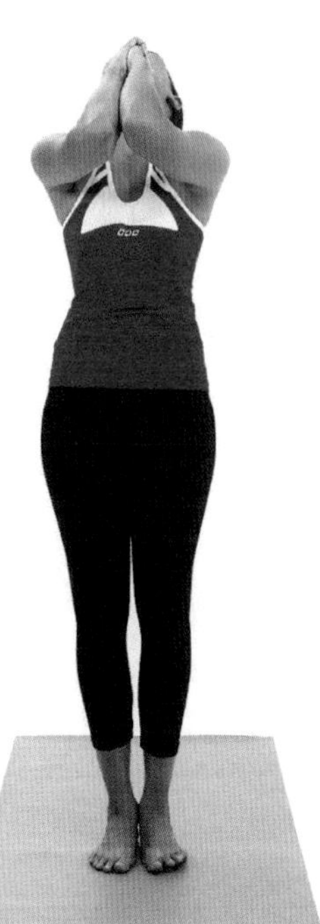

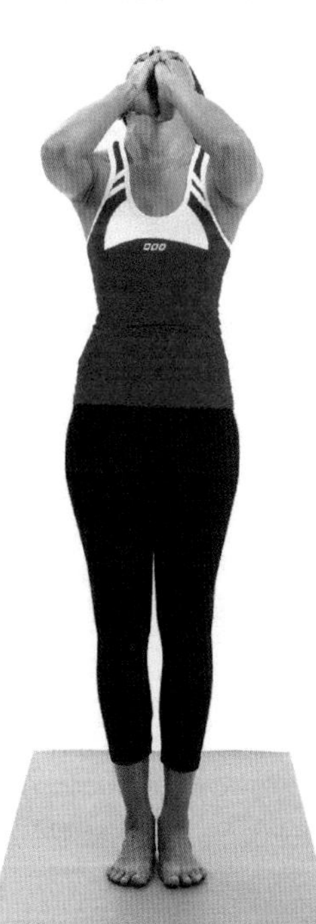

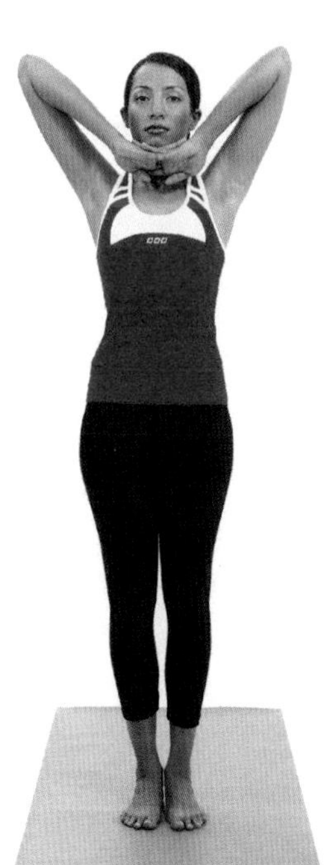

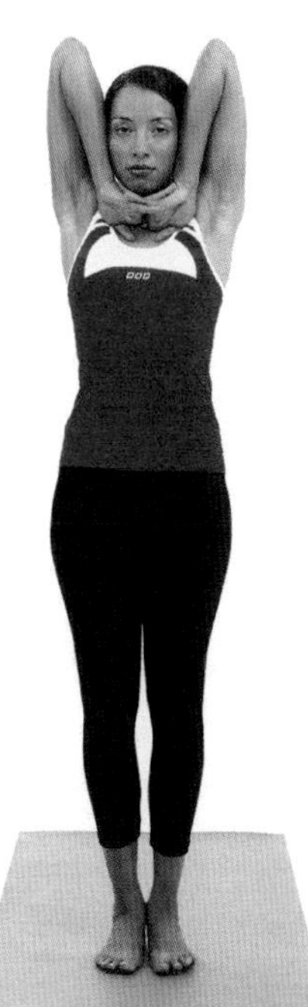

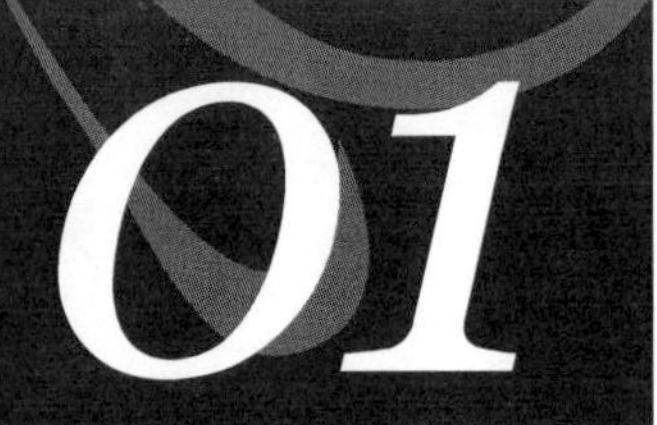

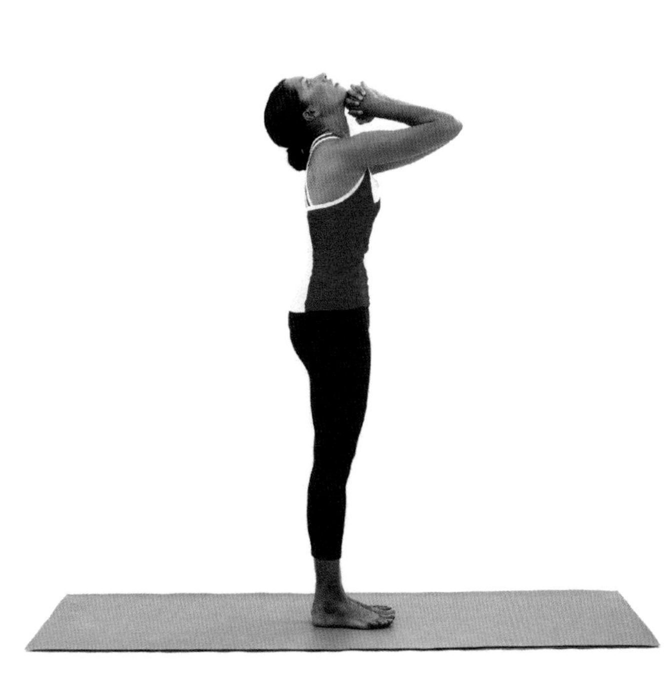

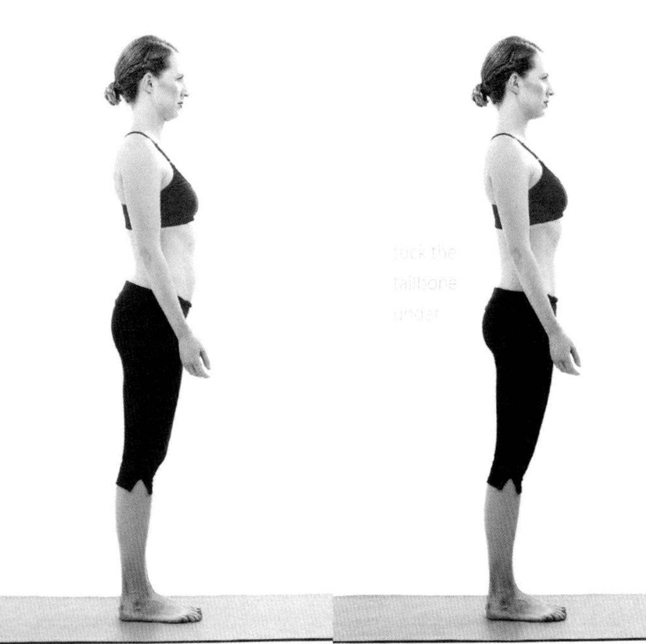

your head by 'walking' your eyes back across the ceiling as far as they will go. ii) Press your head back with the help of your fingers and resist this movement (in a sort of active stretch) by pushing back against your hands. The result is a smooth slow passage which safely opens the neck.

2.8 **Be Thirsty For Your Next Breath:** This is not regular breathing. Pranayama is forced and deliberate, growing your breath capacity, your chest cavity space, your lungs and strengthening your diaphragm. It helps to imagine your arms are bellows pumping air in and out. Squeeze your elbows firmly together to strengthen your shoulders and help you squeeze the last drops of air out of your lungs. So much that you literally cannot wait for your next inhale.

2.9 **The Rest Of Your Inhales:** From the second inhale your breath cycles start with your elbows squeezed together high above your chest and your head resting back on your shoulders, eyes to the back wall. As you inhale: i) Keep your elbows high as they move apart. ii) 'Walk' your eyes forward across the ceiling for the 6 seconds meeting your own eyes in the mirror iii) Push your head into your fingers as you lever your elbows out and up so that your chin finishes parallel to the floor. Every inhale finishes exactly the same way.

2.10 **The Last Couple Of Breaths:** Usually the teacher announces that 2 or 3 cycles remain. Bring as much focus to the maximum filling and emptying of your lungs as possible. When your elbows reach the top take extra sips of air so that you could not possible get any more air in. Similarly on the last exhales squeeze your whole body tightly to help the lungs empty right from the bottom. Be thirsty for your next inhale.

2.11 **Release And Savasana:** Take a small Savasana after each set. The shoulders and neck have had quite some workout. Don't jiggle or move them about to 'loosen' them. Release your arms by your sides, roll your shoulders down and back in a gentle opening movement which relaxes your neck, your palms facing forward. The magic of your Savasana and the sudden cleansing rush of blood through your joints will only happen when you stand absolutely still.

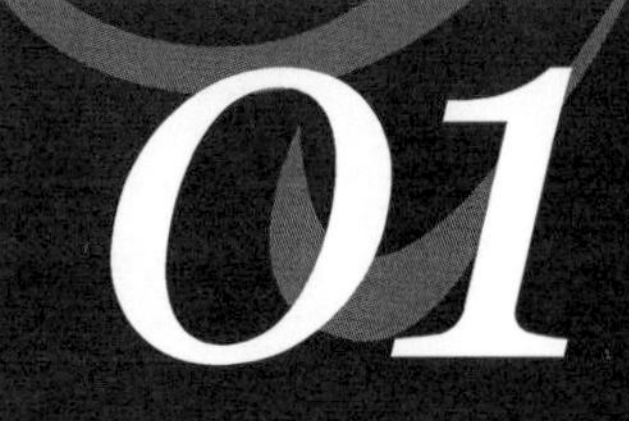

Your legs and spine during Pranayama breathing:

3.1 **Your Spine Straight**: Right from the get-go your spine has to be straight. This is easiest on the inhale. Your body loosens as you feel the traction of your spine extend and stretch between the floor and ceiling.

3.2 **Your Spine On The Exhale**: Your back remains straight on the exhale too. Lengthen the lower spine just as you begin your exhale, by tucking the tailbone under. Your bottom, hips and legs squeeze (see left) and your back and legs collectively form a straight 'plank' of firm strength. This will help you avoid 2 of the most common mistakes i) an upper torso backbend and ii) pushing hips forward towards the mirror. Any movement now is left entirely to your arms, head and neck and absolutely nothing else.

3.3 **Your Legs**: Your legs are always firmly engaged. For many people, especially when first practising, it is neither possible nor energetically realistic to lock the legs 100% of the time. On the inhale keep your legs engaged and focus on loosening and lengthening the body. This may mean the legs are not locked as solidly as they can be. Then, tuck the tailbone under, squeeze the hips and lock the legs fully on the exhale. Full exhalation is facilitated when everything you can squeeze, including the elbows, gets tightened on the exhale.

3.4 **Your Feet**: Your foot weighting changes on the inhale and exhale. On the inhale loosen everything upward against a firm even footprint to grow a physical space in your lungs. On the exhale when you tighten your plank of a body, lean the weight back into the heels (even allow your toes up off the ground with balls of the feet in contact with the earth). In an effort to stop your body falling over backward, the muscles in the front of your body will work hard, strengthen and tone.

A count of six

You are always asked to coordinate your movements and breath to a count of 6. This commonly equates to around 6 seconds. I believe the longer the breath, the stronger your diaphragm has to work, the greater the capacity to grow your lungs, the better the results. You are not exploring your breath's full potential if you are rushed through this exercise. I have on occasion attended others' classes where the teacher counts so fast I can barely keep up the fast arm movement.

Don't be concerned (in fact be thankful) if your teacher tends towards long breath cycles! Taking an extra breath now and then because you cannot manage any further is surely better than a Pranayama of quick shallow breaths. I have to admit some angst created by my physical reactions to the timings of my first teacher many years ago. The cycles would often be close to 10 seconds in and 10 seconds out. I thought this was normal and had no judgment. The growth of my breath and accompanying effects was absolutely the most life-changing skill I encountered in the early days. I attended 150 classes in as many days (some days off, but others with 2 classes per day) before I could stop sneaking an extra breath in the middle of the exercise. This would not have happened with a quick and easy Pranayama. Go deep, slow and long.

A note regarding pregnancy

This exercise could make an enormous difference for you. During pregnancy the fetus fills the space below the ribcage. In order to create this much needed space, the organs shift back and up and the diaphragm is squashed further superiorly. No wonder expectant mothers often pant, losing their breath performing even the most mundane of tasks (like talking!) and can only eat small amounts.

The stronger your Pranayama becomes the more vital and less tired you will feel during even the last weeks of gestation. More importantly your delivery should be far easier to cope with because of your increased capacity to breathe deeply along with the greater awareness of your body that yoga brings.

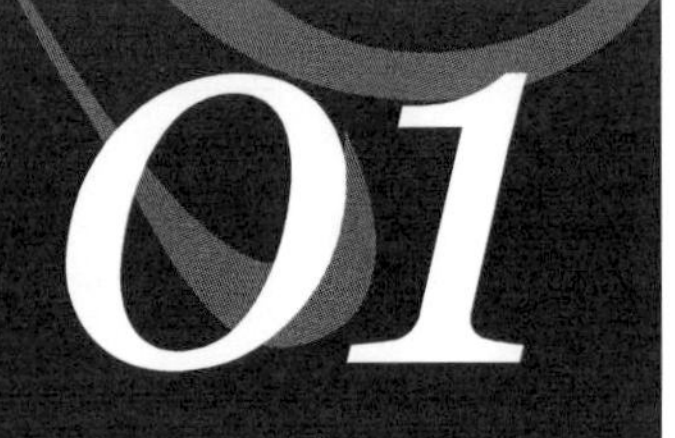

Pranayama Breathing

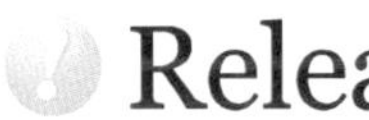

Release

You are standing with a beautifully straight strong body. Your muscles in your abdomen, arms and legs are strongly activated. The air has literally been squeezed out of your lungs. Your elbows are together, up high. Your head is back and your eyes are looking back. Keep the exhale force going until you literally cannot empty another drop of air. You are a completely empty cup and you are so thirsty for your next breath you can barely wait another moment. It is then that you remove the pressure from your chin, release your hands, start to bring your chin back down to parallel. Externally rotate your upper arms, rolling your shoulders back and down in one efficient movement. Meet yourself in the mirror in Savasana in total stillness, breathing.

Common mistakes and how to fix them

Dropping the chin: The chin may drop when you raise the arms. This happens often with students with tight shoulders or torso muscles. The chin stays at least as high as parallel to the ground and only moves higher through the cycle.

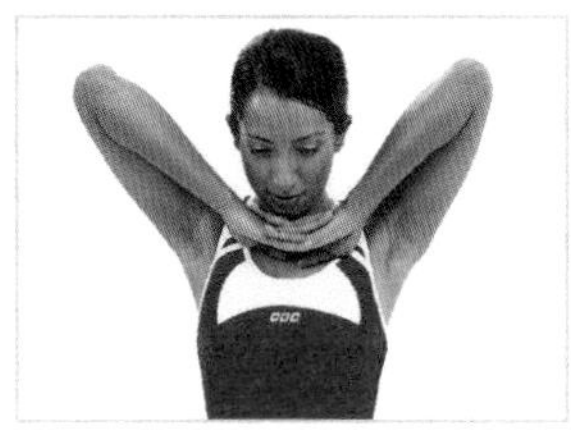

Jerky head movements: One of the most common errors is to move the head too fast in either or both directions. Most often students drop their heads back quickly on the exhale taking one second, and then leave their head stationary for the remaining count of five.

Coordinating movement of the arms and head is crucial. If at any time the hands lose contact with the head, no traction is created, the exercise is ineffective and you risk injury. Slow the movements to fill the 6 seconds by 'walking' the eyes across the ceiling. You should never be looking at the wall or into your own eyes for more than a second or two. Use constant contact of interlaced fingers under the chin to control the movements and open the neck safely.

Shoulders hunch up: Never squeeze the forearms to the side of the head (as instructed by most teachers). This movement raises the shoulders and introduces unsettling (and painful) tensions in the head and neck muscles (and you may notice your chin pulling down). Correct shoulder position will not create these tensions. Care must be taken to avoid hunching up the shoulders on the exhale too. Focus on the broadening stretch between the scapulae. Luckily you can correct this problem mid-pose by drawing your shoulder blades back down again and decompressing your neck. Your elbows may drop a little but the damaging forces will slacken.

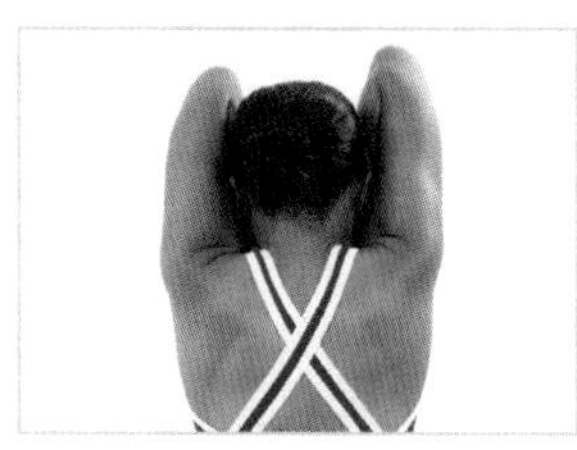

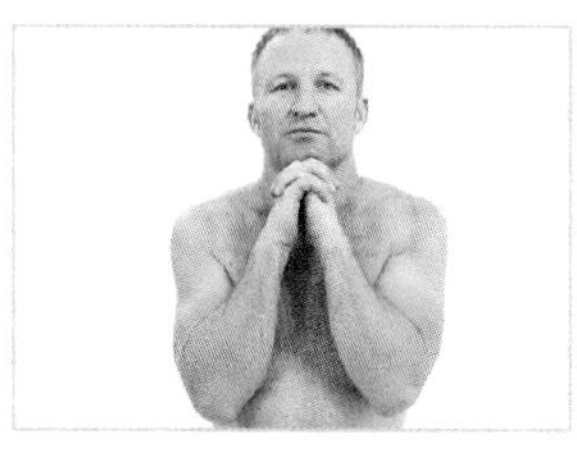

Eyes just look up: Often the travel of the head is limited by the focus of the eyes. Move your eyes slowly backward rather than tilting the head back and looking up to the ceiling. 'Walking' the eyes back slows the movement down for better coordination and with the eyes resting further back not only do your intra-ocular muscles work-out but your neck opens more with less resistance.

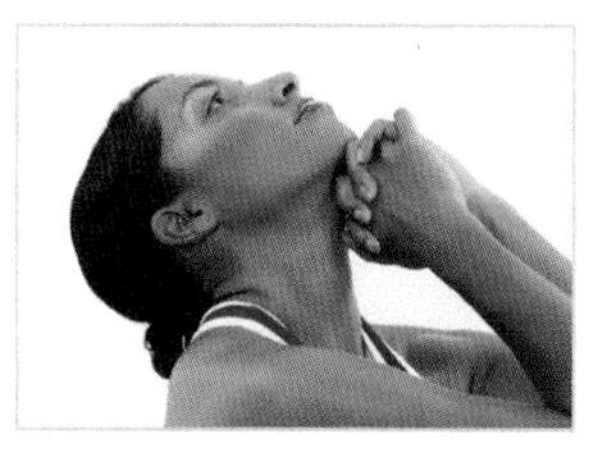

Weight falls into the toes: Sometimes students push the weight forward with a forward movement of the hips and even allow some (or all) of the weight to come off the heels. Tuck the tailbone under on exhale and lift the toes off the floor to fix this common mistake.

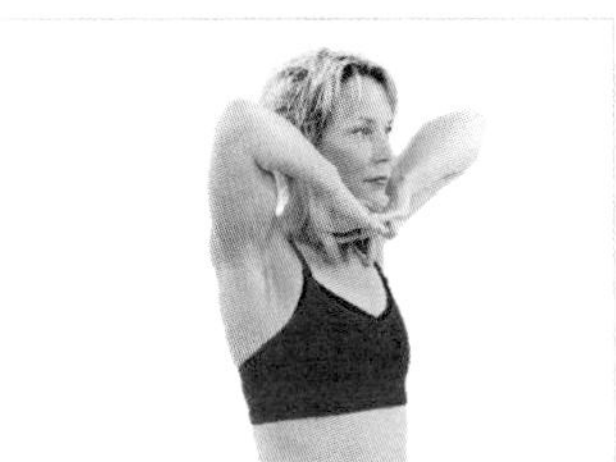

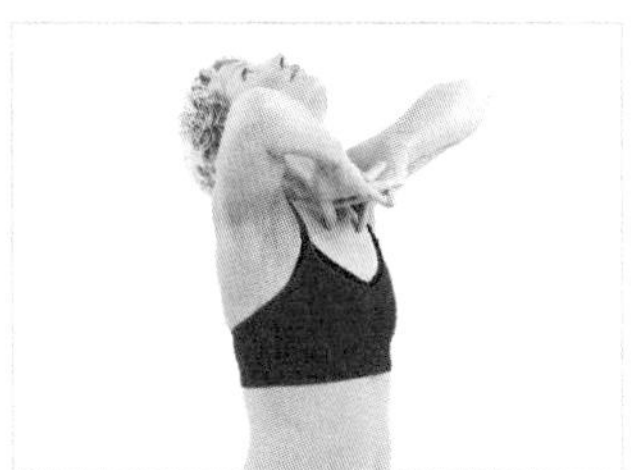

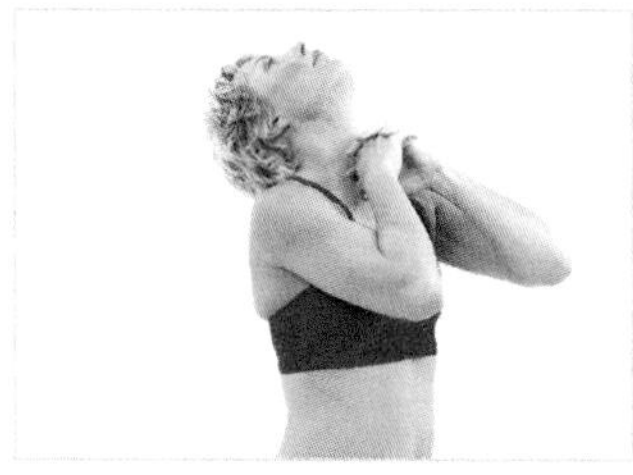

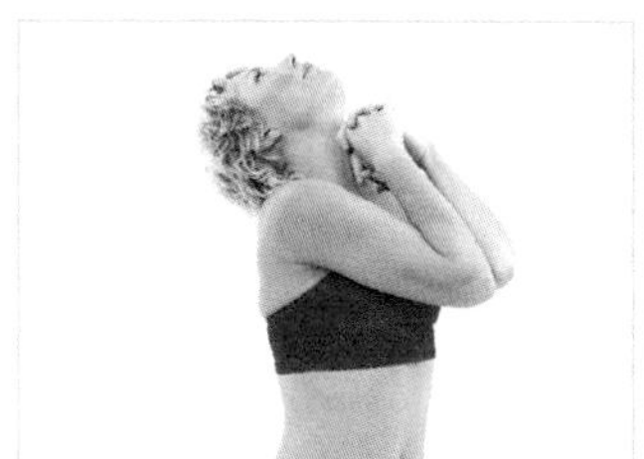

Pranayama Breathing

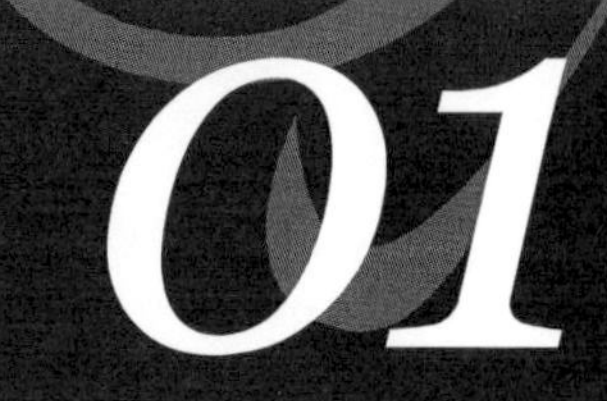

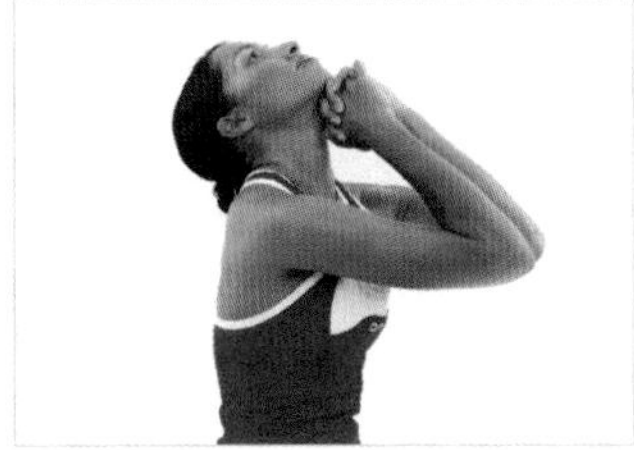

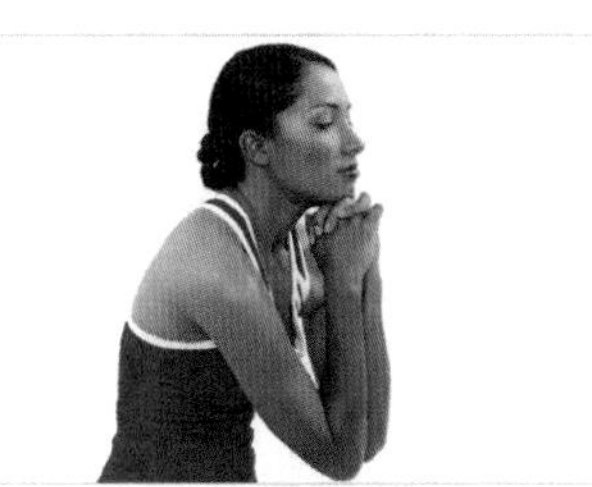

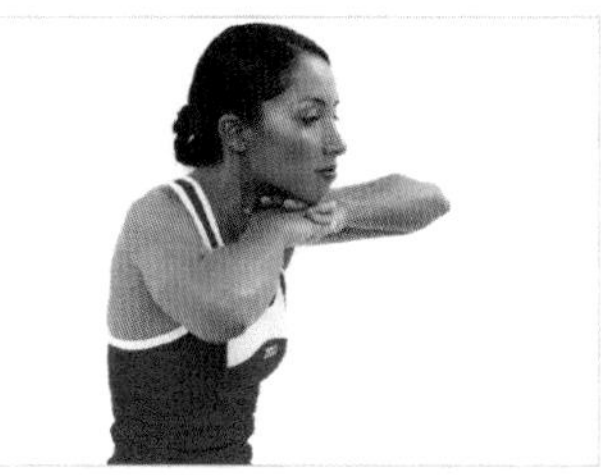

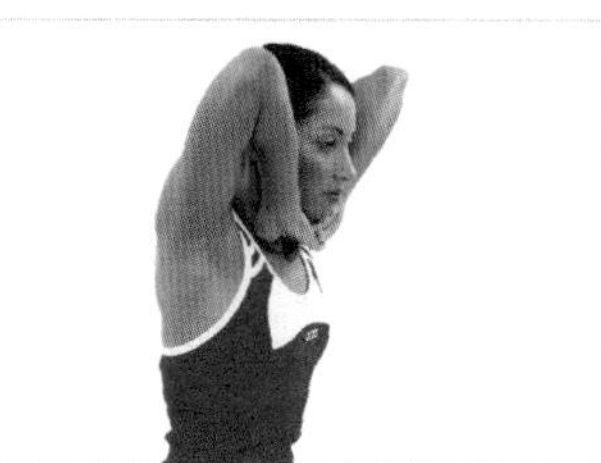

Elbows move down toward the sternum (or every inhale the arms start like the first breath): Most commonly this mistake occurs during the first second of the inhale. The student brings their chin and arms down with their elbows together and starts their inhale cycle as if they were taking their very first breath of the set. Often their hands and chin separate as a result, the chin drops lower than parallel to floor, the neck is moving very fast and the shoulders also tend to collapse. If this is happening to you, think of keeping the elbows high and pushing the jaw into the fingers to lever the elbows up. The arms move so that the elbows are at every moment and without exception trying to be as high as possible. Any time that they drop is an error.

Equally, on the exhale, students often skim the chest with their upper arms when bringing the elbows together. The head drops back in the first second, without control. The student either keeps the elbows down on the chest (and bends the wrists) or self-corrects them to shoulder height. The fix is similar: Focus on keeping finger/jaw contact, slow head movement and keep elbows high as they slowly come forward.

Hips forward: Often the hips are pushed forward during the exhale. The student leans into their lower back and does a back bend, deforming the straight line from heels to the bottom of the neck. Just before the exhale you need to tuck the tailbone under and squeeze the whole lower body solidly from the hips down.

Bent legs: The legs do not ever bend during this exercise. Mostly students allow their legs to bend on the exhale (while doing a backbend). The fix is easy: Lock the legs strongly on the exhale. Allow them to lengthen (and in effect rest) on the inhale. It is very difficult to lock them for the entire set of Pranayama. And locking them fully on the inhale works against the whole body stretch.

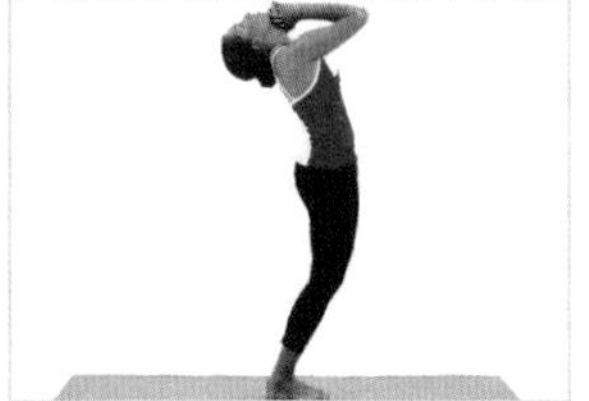

Closing eyes: You may get dizzy, disoriented and lose your balance with closed eyes. Commonly new students close their eyes on the exhale. Your eyes are a great tool to assist the controlled movement of your neck and determine the extent of flexion (where your eyes go, you go). Work on 'walking' your eyes back and forward rather than looking directly at your destination. Slow down the head movements and keep safe!

Fingers come away from the throat and chin: Often the hands and jaw separate. The movement of the neck becomes risky when the contact is removed. Use the leverage forces of the active stretch to slowly and mindfully open up the neck by using the pushing force of the chin against the fingers and fingers against the chin.

Wrists apart instead of straight: At the end of the exhale the elbows come together. New students often keep their wrists apart forming a diamond shape between the forearms and hands. Eliminate the space to squeeze along the whole length. Thankfully this mistake usually only happens the first class.

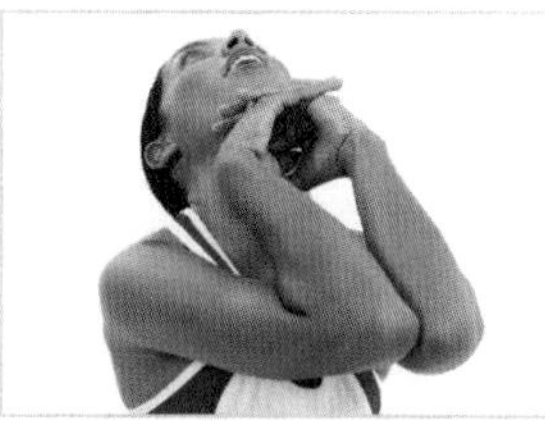

Not opening the mouth on the exhale: The force of exhale and degree of lung emptying (and therefore your maximum lung capacity) is greatly reduced if you exhale through your nose. You cannot create an adequate siphon effect and your next inhale won't be into empty lungs.

Mouth blowing on exhale: Some students blow air out on the exhale as if they were cooling food. The air may come out with loads of force but it emanates from the mouth only. Open your mouth without pursing the lips (relax them), slightly constrict your throat and create the force in your abdomen.

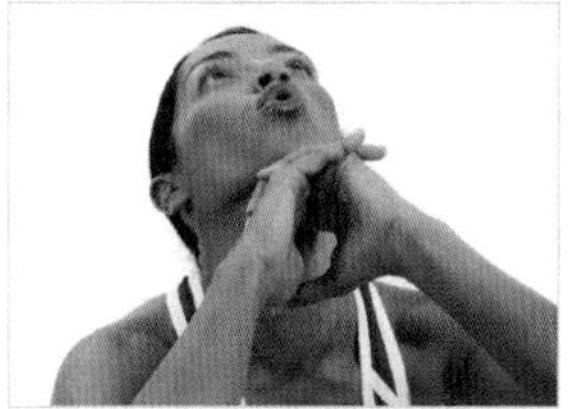

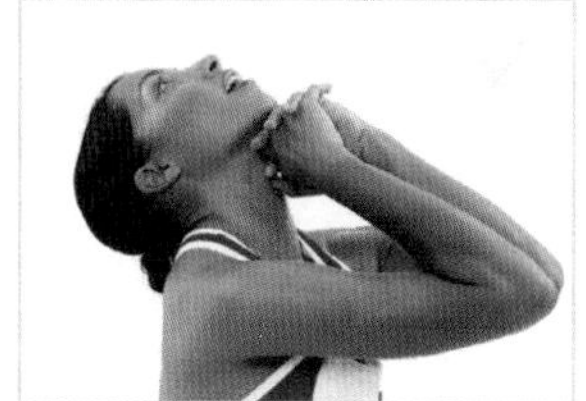

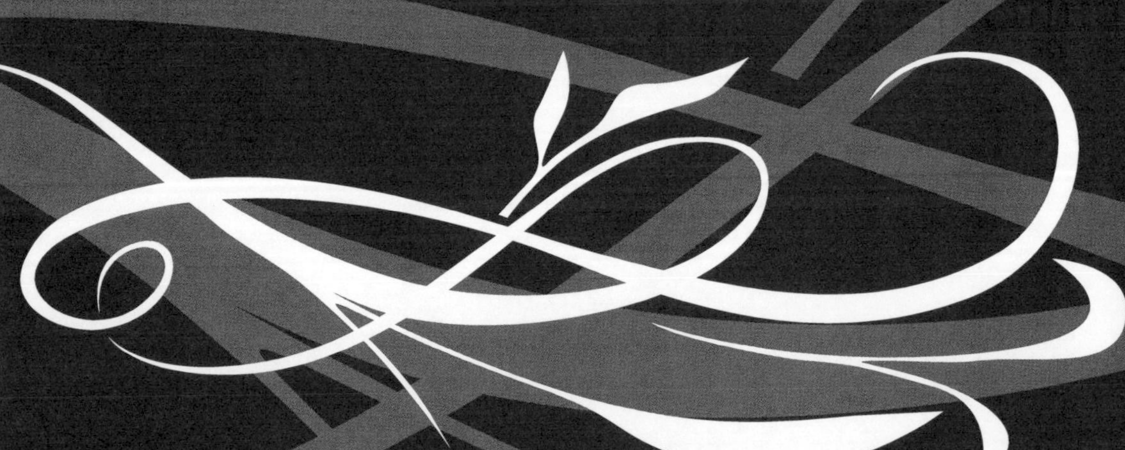

Ardha Chandrasana

I am always doing things I can't do;
that's how I get to do them.
—Pablo Picasso

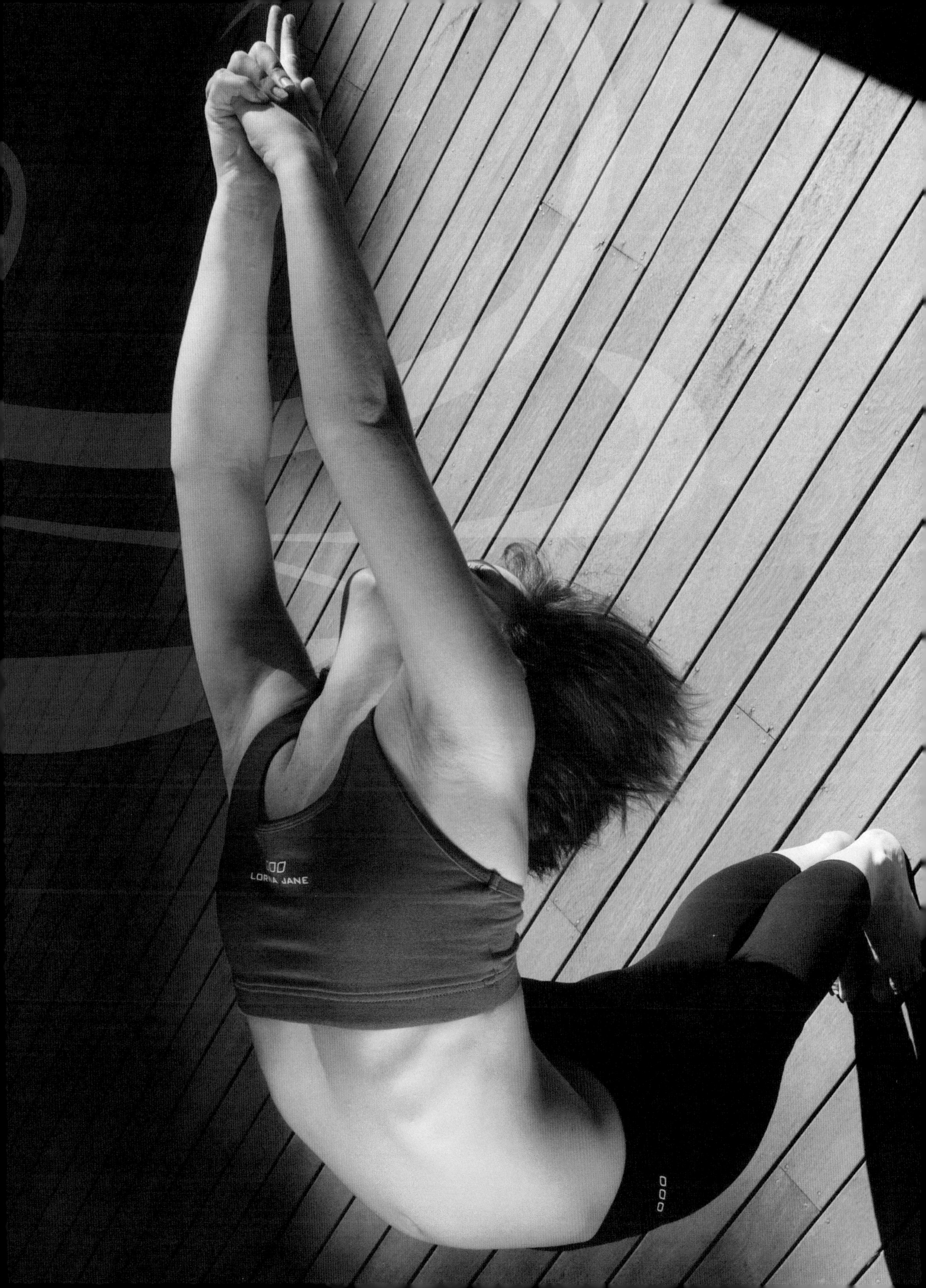
LORNA JANE

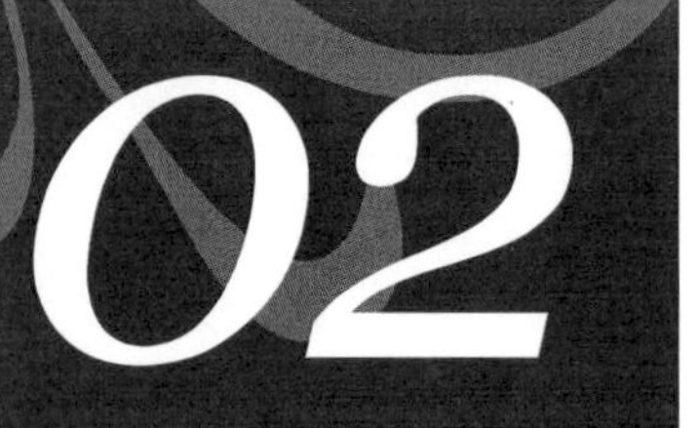

Ardha Chandrasana

HALF MOON POSE

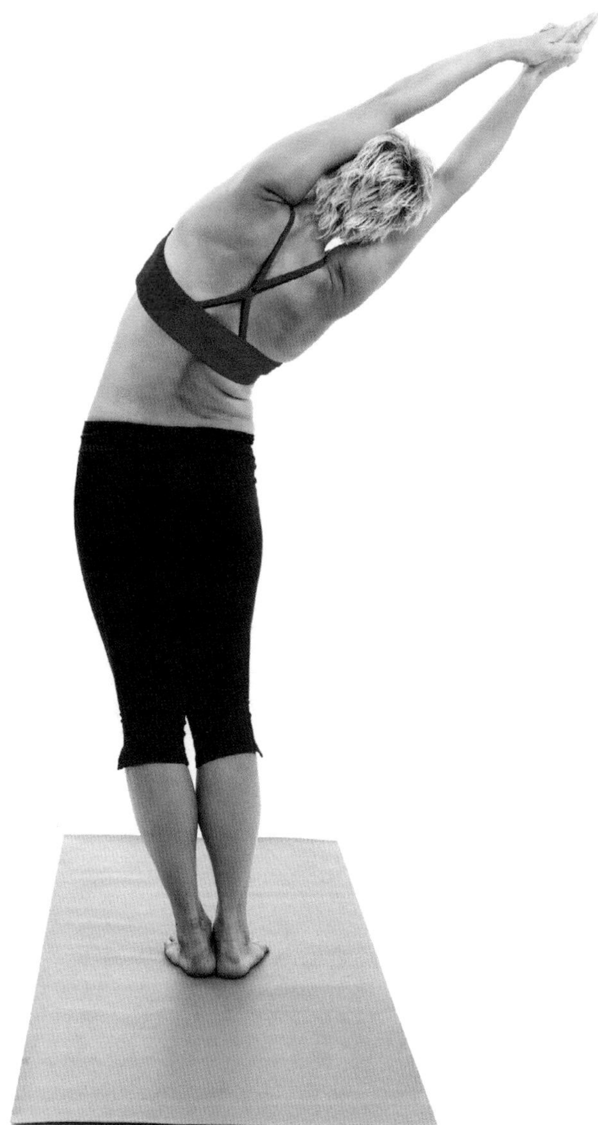

The essentials

This is our first 'real' down-to-business pose in the class. Where Pranayama breathing sets your focus and really brings you into the room, Ardha Chandrasana launches you headlong into some heavy duty yoga asana. Holding each part for a long time, you come face to face with your own perceived limitations. The intense focus really brings you into yourself. You will have to constantly self-correct to maintain the precision.

Half Moon is closely followed by, and made complete by its buddy, Hands to Feet pose. Together all four parts deliver deep stretches as you open your spine right to left, then backwards and forwards. Coming up out of your first Pada Hastasana you feel tremendously liberated; and not just physically. Your spine feels longer, stronger and more flexible. You feel relieved, refreshed and surprisingly ready to move on.

What makes this pose so difficult to get right?

The biggest challenge is keeping the shoulders and hips parallel to the mirror at all times in the two side bends. In the backbend, fear usually stops students from trusting that proper technique will keep them from falling over!

When the set-up and warm-up are sloppy, the pose is sloppy. Setting up mindfully, and then holding those same conditions in warm-up and throughout the pose is the key. This is referred to throughout this book as "Measure Twice, Cut Once". You will not only reap the benefits from the get-go, but you will have a lot less adjustments to make once you are in the pose.

Ardha Chandrasana

Half Moon Pose

The technique

The set-up

Start with your feet together, hips and knees face forwards (this basically means no turning out of the hips. You can refer to the chapter on feet).

1.1 **Your Stance:** Stand with firm contact with the ground, spread your toes, feel the balls of your feet and your heels take some weight. You can get some sense of your grounding with the earth and draw on those energy reserves during your pose. Stand tall with your shoulders relaxed, your tailbone tucked under to lengthen your lower spine and your palms face forward to the mirror. This action in itself facilitates the correct position of your shoulders and allows full unhindered movement in the arm-lift action that follows. This point in itself causes some contention. Please take a look at the section on healthy risk-free arm movement on pages 38-43.

1.2 **Your Gaze:** Your eyes are looking forward. It can be very confronting at times to meet your own eyes in the mirror. This is normal and does change even from class to class depending on your current levels of emotional wellbeing or feelings of self-acceptance.

1.3 **Straight Arms Next To Your Head:** As you inhale bring your arms up over your head and hands together. Establish a steeple grip with fingers interlocked, thumbs crossed and index fingers pointing upwards: One straight line from shoulders to fingertips.

Your ability to glue the hands from fingers to wrists and maintain strong, straight, energized arms will depend on many factors. These include (but are not limited to) the health and flexibility of your shoulder, elbow and wrist joints and muscles, (including latissimus dorsi and serratus anterior) your stamina, and your strength.

1.4 **Your Chin:** Lift your chin so that it stays parallel to the ground and so you can see your throat in your reflection.

1.5 **Your Lower Body Locked:** Lock your legs, squeeze your bottom tight and push your hips forward to the mirror (the most commonly neglected action).

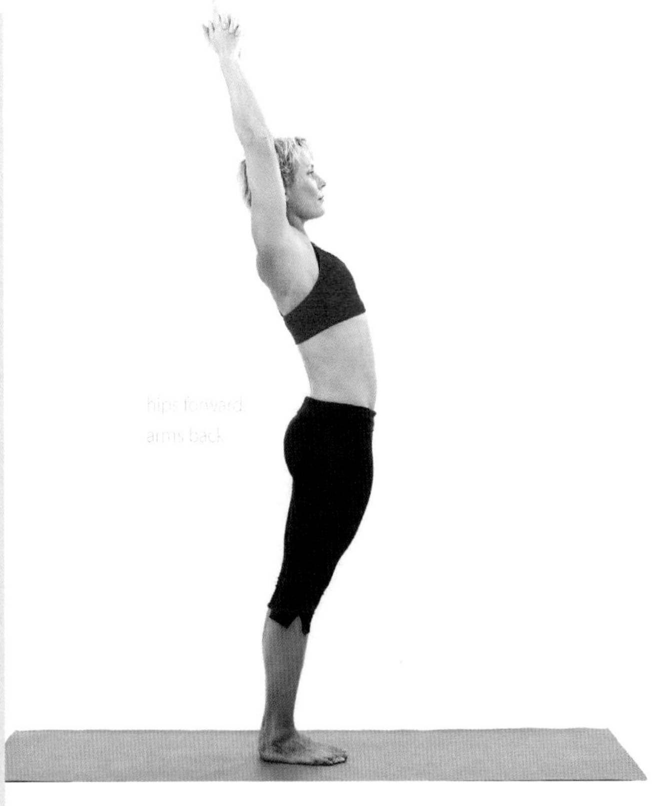

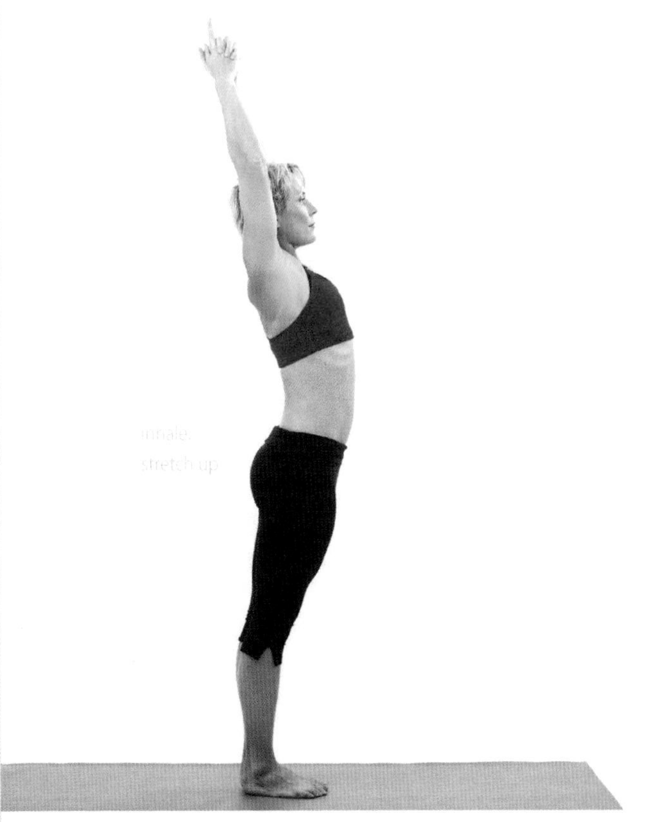

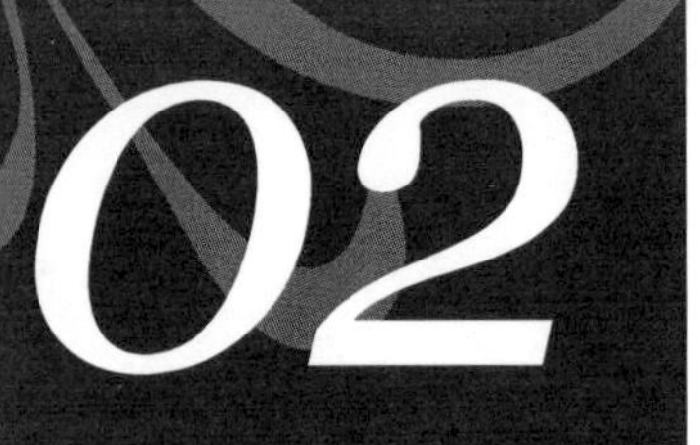

Ardha Chandrasana

Half Moon Pose

1.6 **Upper Body Position**: Recommit your strong straight arms. A tight neck, shoulders and upper body will cause your chin to drop and will work against you in the pose. Be careful to maintain your chin position parallel with the ground. As you move your arms back you will feel the weight transfer out of your toes toward your heels. Feel your torso lift up and lengthen delivering maximal opening in the chest and shoulders.

1.7 **Standing In A Slight Backbend**: It may feel strange, but when your arms are overhead, you need to stand in a little bit of a backbend. Your hips and shoulders will remain open when you continually and strongly push the hips forward and lift up through the breastbone.

Bring the weight back into the heels while grounding the balls of the feet. Maintain an arch from feet to fingertips through the body. All these actions require constant attention otherwise the forces quickly conspire to collapse the body. This position tones, firms and tightens all the muscles on the front side of the body which have to work very hard to stop you falling over backwards.

The warm-up

You have only just set up. Take your warm-up seriously. If you can keep the above conditions constant for the rest of your warm-up and also for the remainder of your Half Moon pose then you reap many benefits right from the get-go til you let go.

Your yoga class – your body-mind connection – begins when you enter the studio, not after you have entered your pose. When you pay attention to all these elements your mindfulness pays off in the deepening of your meditation. The Half Moon warm-up looks like you are swaying your body in an arc from right to left and left to right several times.

2.1 **Let Your Breath Guide Your Movement**: Inhale some length into your body, arms back, chin up, and as you exhale bring your body to the right staying long.

2.2 **Continue To The Left And Right**: Inhale again and move up through to the center again reaching up for the ceiling. As you exhale again bring your body to the left. Continue this movement for a few cycles – reaching the top of your inhale as you reach to the ceiling and exhaling (leaving some buoyancy in your chest) as you move to each side.

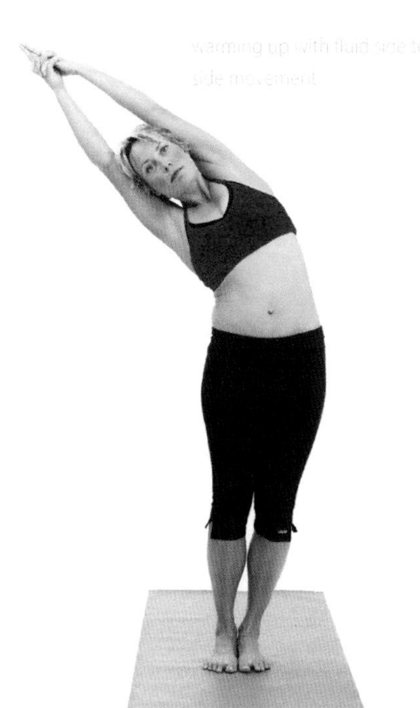

warming up with fluid side to side movement

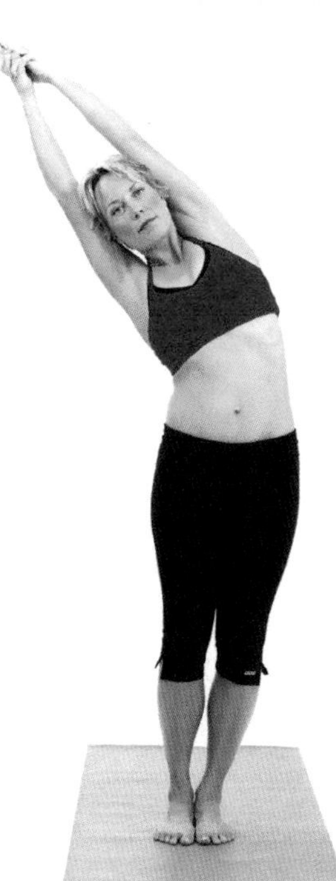

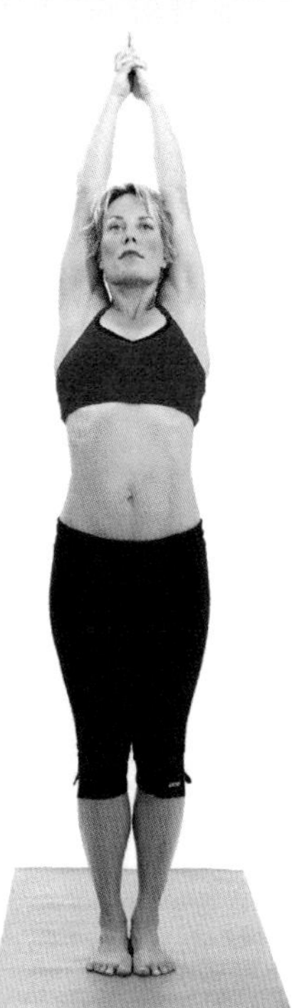

Ardha Chandrasana

Half Moon Pose

2.3 **Hips Move In The Opposite Direction**: As you move over to one side your hips move in the opposite direction.

2.4 **Lift And Lengthen**: Rather than swinging your body, lift and lengthen your body to create flexibility and space in your vertebrae. This is a stretch for the body and not just a bend – so aim to create space. This is not a flippant side to side action. The more attention you pay to the warm-up the more effective your pose. Don't be deceived by what appears to be a simple body sway.

2.5 **Observing Your Responses**: This movement is a great barometer for how you are feeling. Without judgment you are seeing how flexible you are, how strong or fragile you may be feeling emotionally, physically and mentally. You observe and don't judge. And at the same time you are creating space in your spine and warmth in your muscles before you get down to your real work.

2.6 **Constant Attention To Alignment**: Your spine is not able to move in one plane from side to side. The curves in your spine allow and create movement in a multitude of directions. The challenge is to move with the constant correction and re-correction that creates the impression of a simple side to side movement.

Your warm-up check list

Ensure that:

- your weight stays back in your heels
- your chin stays up
- your breastbone lifted
- your arms keep strong and straight if you can keep your shoulders down (otherwise a micro-bend can resolve any tension)
- your legs are strong, locked out and straight, hips forward
- your hips and your shoulders remain square to
- the mirror at all times.

Continually go through your warm-up checklist and apply it constantly. When you finish, come back to the center and stay in your set-up.

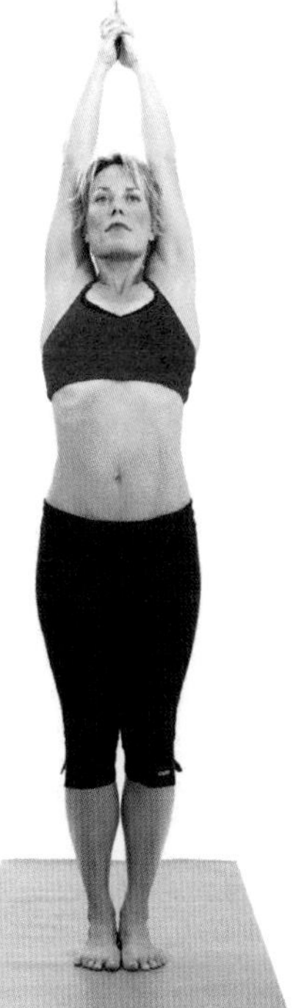

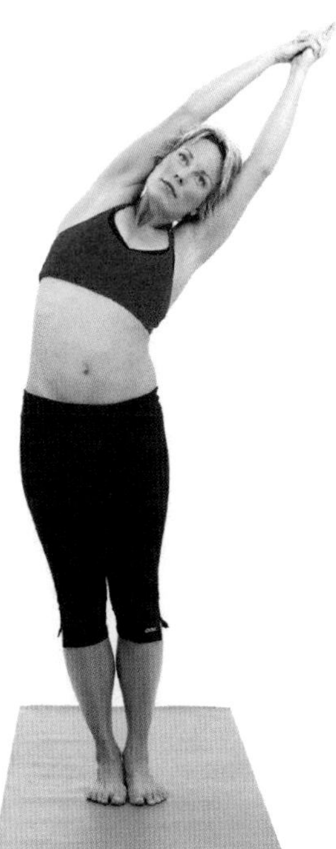

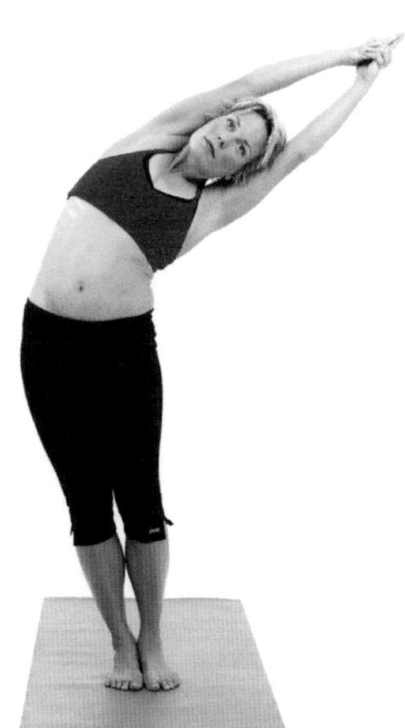

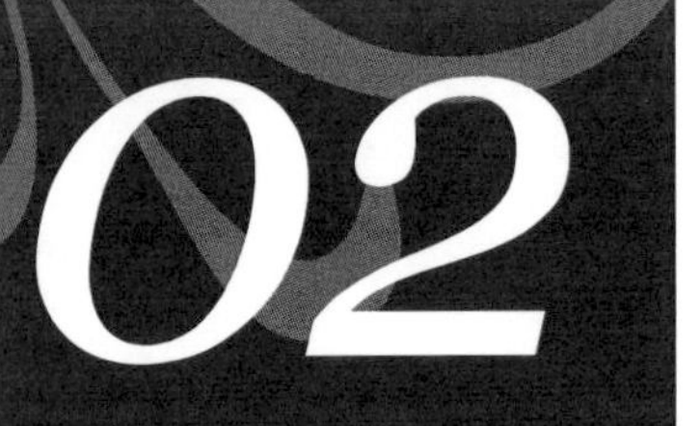

Ardha Chandrasana

HALF MOON POSE

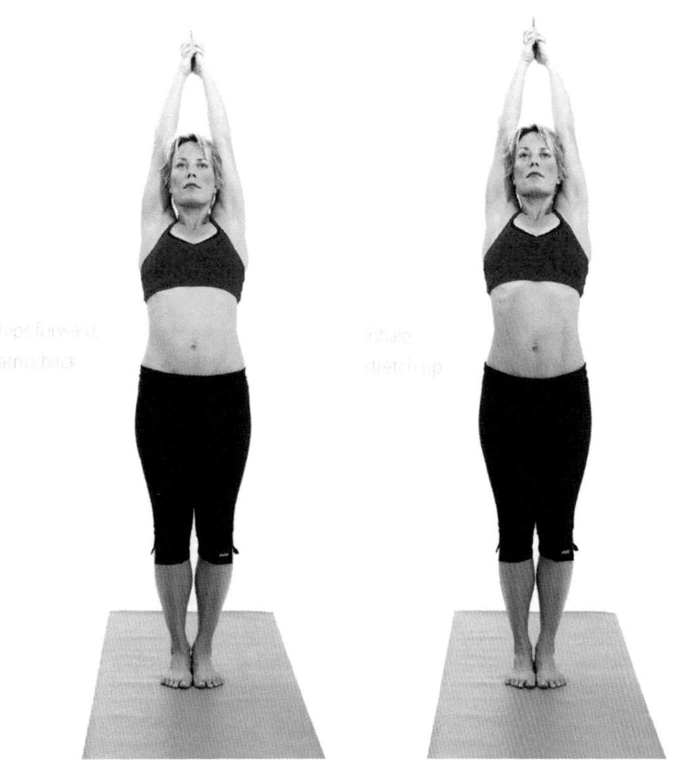

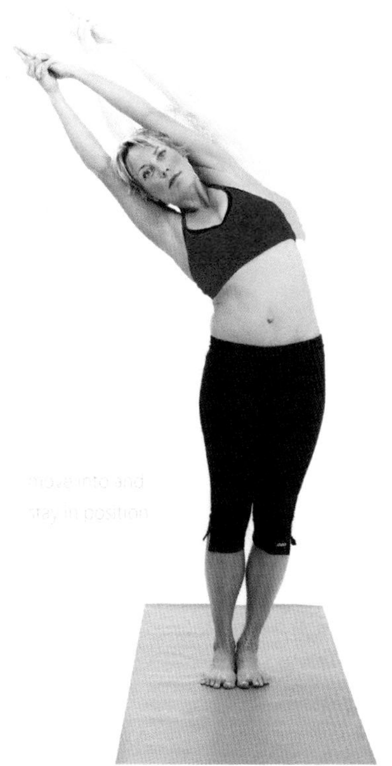

The pose

a) Inhale arms up.
b) Steeple grip. Arms straight (remember; relax those shoulders)
c) Lock legs, squeeze bottom and push hips strongly toward the mirror.
d) Arms back, chin up and then weight back so you are standing in a bit of a backbend. This stops you slumping forward in your pose.
e) Inhale length in your body as you stretch upwards and then AS you exhale slowly bring your body over to the right hand side.
f) Keep your arms, back and chin up and weight back.
g) At the same time move your hips over to the left hand side.
h) Keep hips and shoulders square to the mirror.

Holy moly! You are just getting me to do what you asked me to do before. Yes! That is correct. Do you see why I say "Measure Twice and Cut Once"? Here you are not correcting anything, you are going in with mindful alignment. This leaves you free for the entire time to work the depth, the finesse of the pose, the strength and form. The above points in set-up, warm-up and execution form the basis of this pose. Loss of alignment and therefore benefit, occurs when attention drifts away from any of the areas of focus.

Anchor with your feet, pull over with your arms: While you work this pose you are attempting to create increasing length on the inhale and more and more depth in the stretch on the exhale. Keep the breath moving for buoyancy. Avoid short shallow breaths. Recommit on all the above points.

Add an extra lengthening dimension by pulling yourself over to the side (and slightly backwards) with your arms. So on the first side pull your left arm over with the help of the right arm. Allowing the weight to fall forward also collapses the shoulders and chest. So, keep the arms and your weight moving back and your chin and breastbone up to help your alignment. Keep settling into this deepening stretch. Your last movement is on an exhale. Inhale as you exit with strength and alignment, keeping your body from twisting.

Checking your alignment

I like to start from the ground up. It provides a great way to cycle through your awareness of your proprioception: Constantly and mindfully bring yourself into alignment. This cycling trains your eye to scan the body in a logical fashion. In time this cycling happens automatically and then with an internal eye, sensing your body's position even without the mirror. When you cycle through, try starting with your footprint; your feet; your knees; your hips; your torso; your shoulders; your chin; your head; your arms and your fingers.

The second side

Each of the mirror-image side bends is held for of up to one minute. Usually one side is easier to hold in better alignment than the other. Skeletal and muscular problems and other conditions (like different leg lengths and natural asymmetries) may make it difficult to replicate the ease and depth on both sides. Simply take yourself to the point where all the foundations are addressed by paying careful attention to alignment.

Immediately following the side bends is the backbend. You simply exit your left side Half Moon to center.

Release

Finish this pose as deeply as you can. Take a full inhale as you use your hands to pull and stretch your upper arm up out of your torso. Deepen your pose as you exhale fully; literally pull yourself over while pushing hips in the opposite direction. Always exhale last, then inhale as you come back up to center. Reversing to center with strength and alignment takes great care and attention. Your eyes remain focused on yourself in the mirror.

Common mistakes and how to fix them:

Sloppy set-up: This results either from lack of attention or being misdirected into the pose. Teachers that don't provide precise set-up instructions spend most of the time making fundamental changes that would have been better handled just moments before. Each class they may rarely offer more than the basics. That is fundamentally not a bad thing, but approached systematically, the finer distinctions and the advanced stuff can be intelligently introduced to the whole class. This is particularly important to the more advanced students.

A few seconds setting up with your best possible alignment avoids sloppiness and guarantees a better pose and more benefits. Your reward will be less adjustments to do and more refinements to make regardless of your knowledge of the poses. Take full advantage of the mirrors to align yourself and to improve your proprioception.

Beginners in overwhelm, or maybe it's just ego: Everyone wants to do as well as they can. Beginners mostly take their cues from watching fellow students. They see the big side bend but may not see the whole body's square position relative to the mirror. They may easily get overwhelmed with all the unfamiliar instructions, and often go to a depth that is beyond the limits of their good alignment. As a result they unwittingly risk casting aside benefits in their eagerness to achieve.

So if this is you, then make sure you:

1) Keep breathing deeply yet calmly to maintain buoyancy in the chest and to stop you collapsing any further beyond help!
2) Retreat out of the pose somewhat and cycle your attention from the ground up through all the checkpoints listed above. Remember first comes breath, then alignment and then depth.

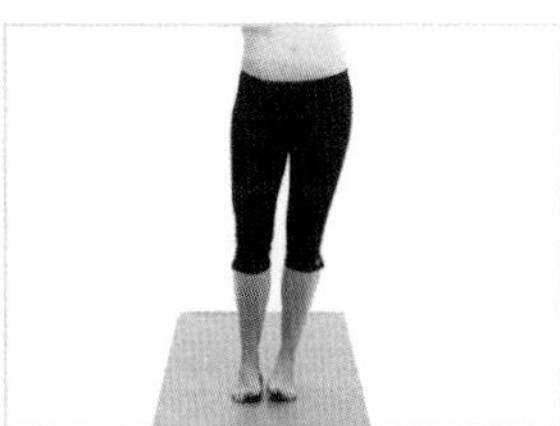

The inside or outside of the feet lift: One or both feet often become unevenly weighted with the heel or ball of the foot lifting. Plant the heels and bring the weight back (see 'toes take the weight'). In time your hip and ankle flexibility will improve to allow the side bends with both feet firmly planted on the ground.

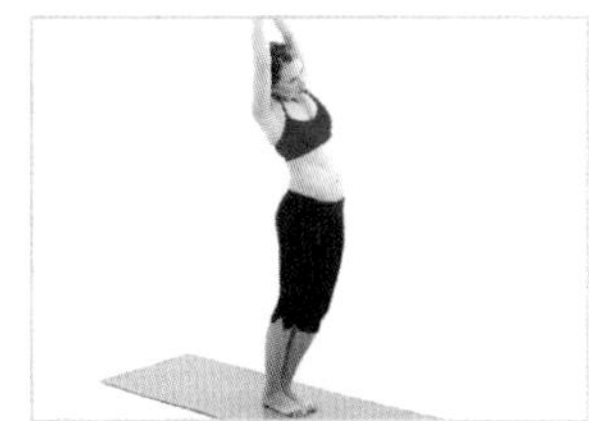

One or both knees bend: The inside knee usually bends more (the body twists). Plant your feet, straighten both legs and pull up your kneecaps with your quadriceps muscles.

Hips swivel: Generally one hip will have to come forward (as you lift your chest) to square both hips off.

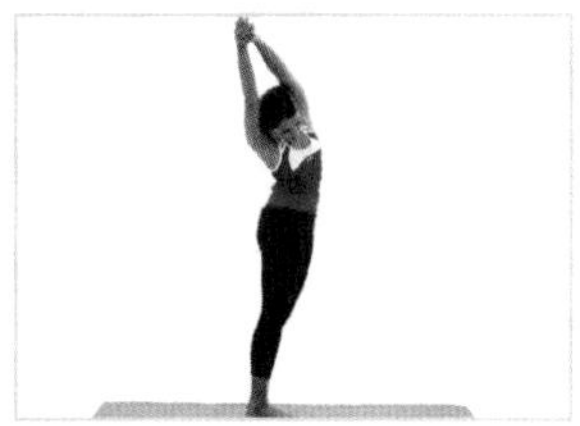

Shoulders swivel: Often it is the inside or lower shoulder that needs to come forward into correct position. If this misalignment is accompanied by a collapse in the torso what fixes this is bringing the upper shoulder back in a lifting movement to square both to the mirror. Bring the weight back, lift the chin and the breastbone.

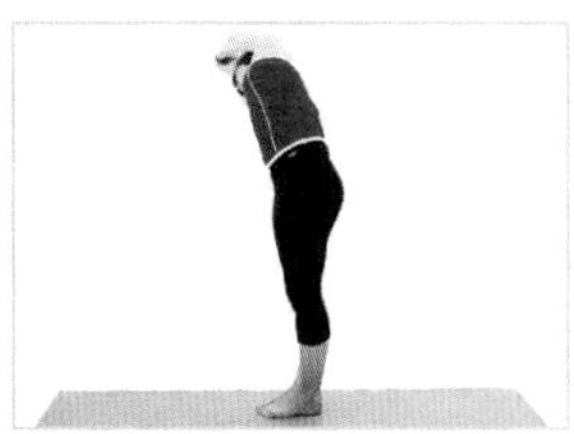

Torso swivels or sways forward: As the hips move to one side the body often adjusts by bending toward the mirror through the mid-torso. Lift up through the breastbone as you move the hips forward, chin up and arms back to create space in the chest. You will sense an opening at the bottom of the ribcage and your weight will drop back toward the heels.

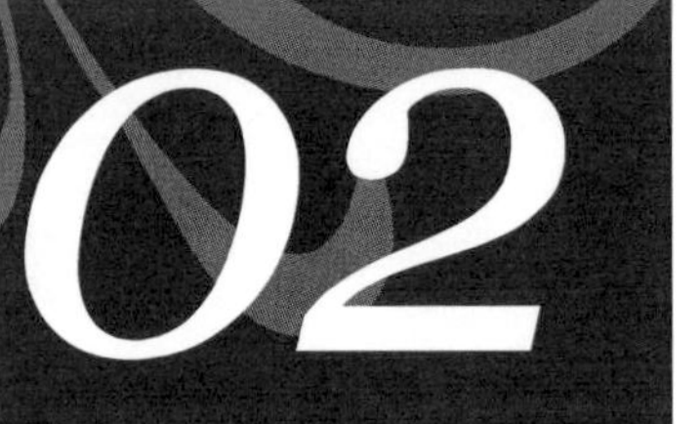

Ardha Chandrasana

Half Moon Pose

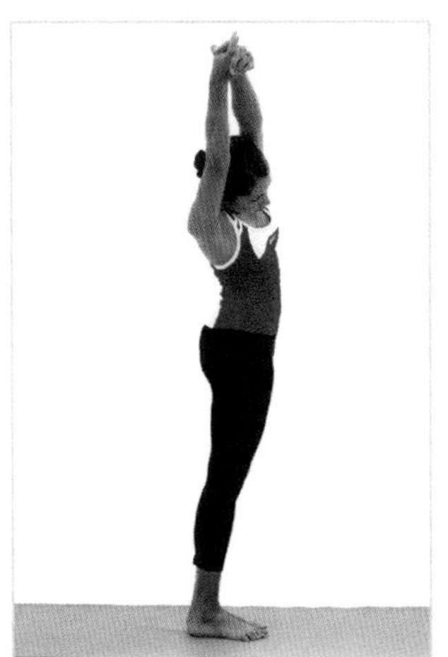

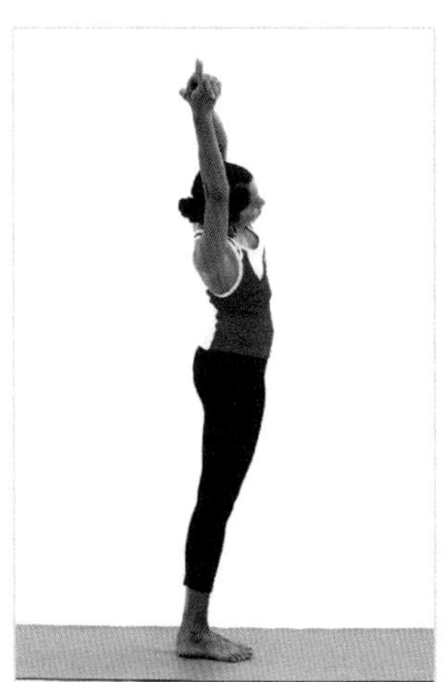

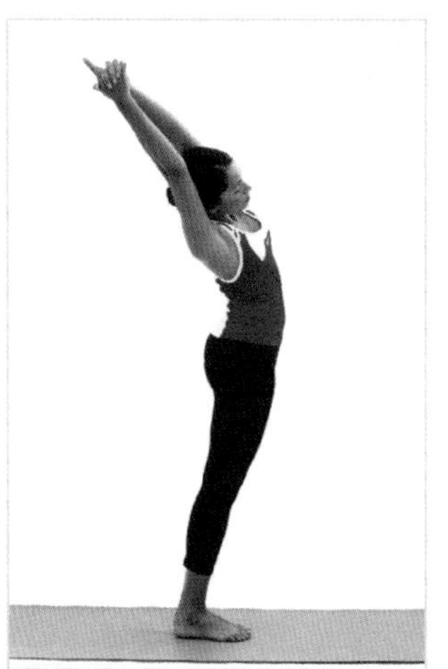

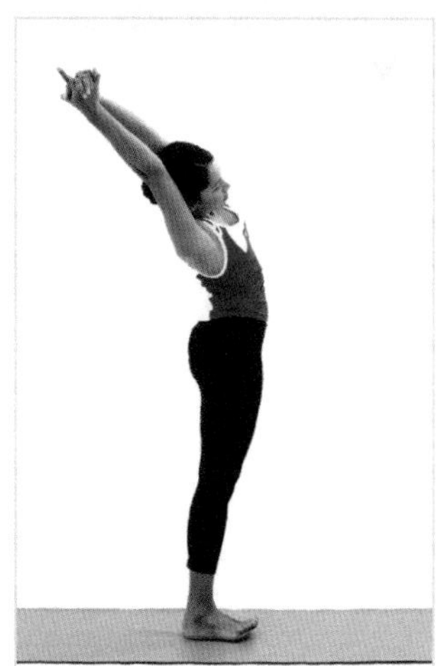

Your weight stays even in the feet: All standing poses start with strong active footprints. With arms up and back and hips forward, your weight shifts to your heels to produce a slight backbend. This allows your toes to lift off the floor, leaving the balls of your feet grounding down. You are right on track if this is happening (although with the weight back it is not necessary to lift your toes).

Toes take the weight: When you lack energy or awareness the body may slightly slump mid-torso and the weight moves to the toes. Two simultaneous actions bring you back on track; push the hips forward as you bring the arms back. The slight backward arching allows you to safely shift back the weight and keep the lengthening element in your sideways stretch. I find it helpful to imagine a gentle 'hook' under my sternum to lift the breastbone. The chest lifts and shoulders drop back at the same time.

Hips remaining in line with body and legs: A total vertical body-leg position will increase the propensity for the chin, upper body and arms to fall forward, and you will lose much of the toning and strengthening elements. Go back to basics; push the hips forward and lean back. Lift through the breastbone.

Collapsing into ribcage on concave side: Moving to the side you must avoid bringing the body down and forward out of alignment. Try extending your body up first finding length, taking it up, out and then over to the side as if over a giant ball. Don't just bend at the waist. Keeping hips forward and arms back will greatly help preserve the right position.

Let struggle be your guide: Struggle tells you that something is not right; it is all too hard, the breath is being held or it's shallow or ragged. Don't confuse struggle with the rewarding challenge of hard work. Struggle means you have sacrificed alignment for depth. Your job is to work on the basics. Your ability to breathe may change with your emotional tides or physical capabilities. Don't hold your breath, calm it, go with it, allowing it to flow rhythmically in and out as you make your adjustments.

Chin drops: Your chin tends to drop if you have tight shoulders or latissimus dorsi. Slacken off the arms to bring them back, decompress the neck and lift the chin. You will now be more able to bring the weight back. Take care to work on strong alignment before depth.

Shoulders hunch: Shrugging the shoulders to straighten and clamp the arms to your head is counterproductive and causes tension and alignment problems. Slacken off the arms to bring the shoulders down and back away from the ears and open the chest and shoulders. The tension is resolved when you introduce a small bend in the arms. Although not possible for everyone, ideally arms are straight and clamped in tight preferably behind the ears. The chapter on arm movement provides instructions for correct shoulder position.

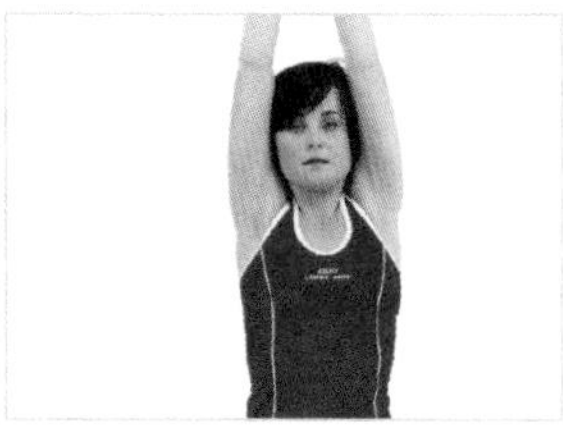

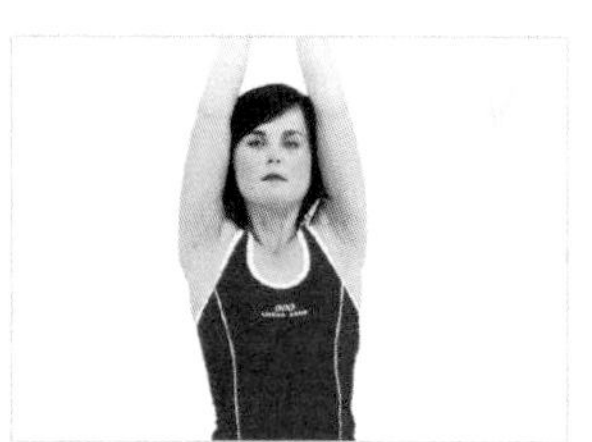

Wrists bend: Make sure your wrists are locked, not bent, and form a straight line from your shoulders through to your fingertips.

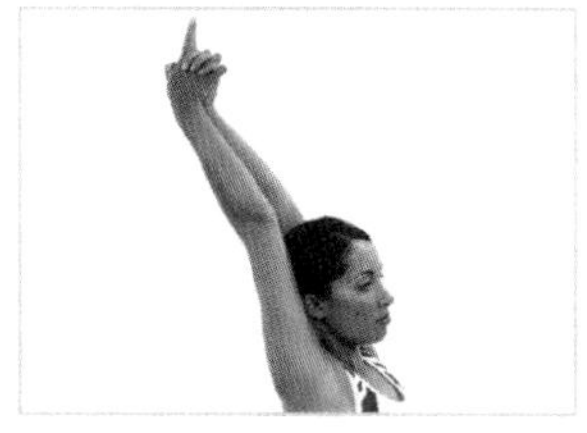

Getting tired: When getting tired your body may move toward the mirror setting off a cascade of events. The weight shifts into the toes; the body slumps; the chest closes and faces the floor to some degree; the chin drops and arms collapse forward. Keep attentive to any signs of your chin dropping toward your chest or eyes focusing on the floor. Lifting everything up and back is the answer.

Ardha Chandrasana

Half Moon Pose

02

The backbend technique

As with all backbends, this backward Half Moon is a compression of the back but a S T R E T C H for the front side of the body. Take this opportunity to open your chest, your heart and your lungs; literally and figuratively.

You will already be standing with your feet together. Your arms are already over your head with fingers interlocked, and you are looking forward in the mirror.

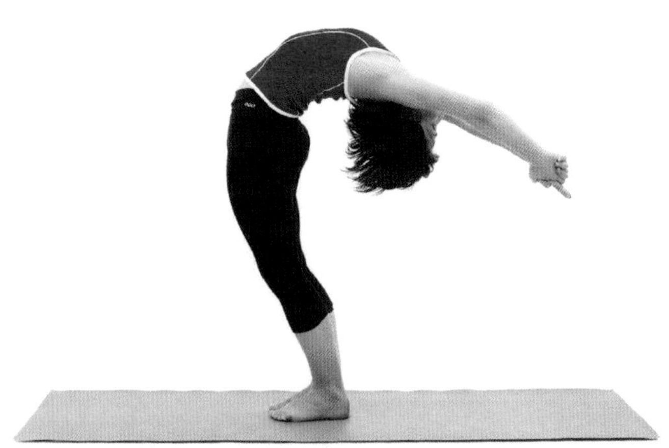

1. **Drop Your Head Back**: Take a big inhale and fill your lungs. Relax your shoulders; you may even put a slight bend in your elbows as they relax. As you exhale let your head move back on your soft neck. Take a couple of seconds to work these movements. It helps to look back to the wall behind you.

2. **Lower Body Set-Up**: Lock your legs fully, squeeze your bottom and strongly push your hips toward the mirror.

3. **Upper Body Set-Up**: Inhale again as you stretch your locked out arms up to the ceiling. Lift up out of the waist to lengthen your lower spine.

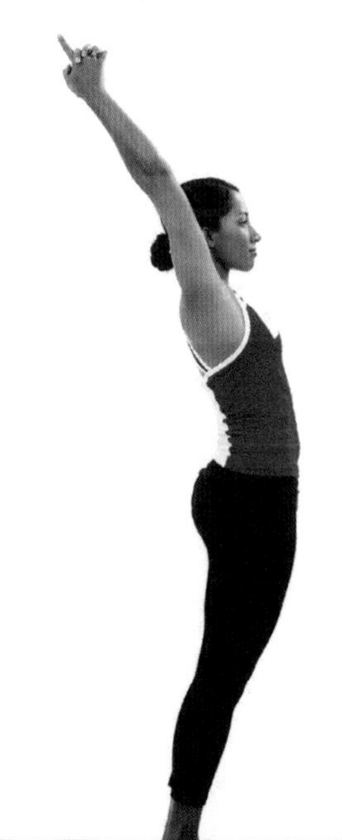

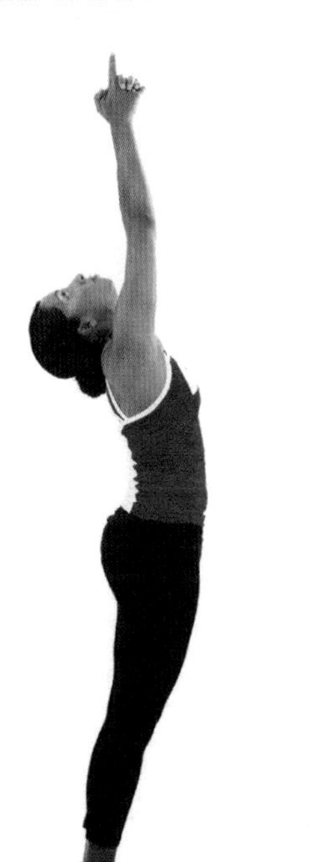

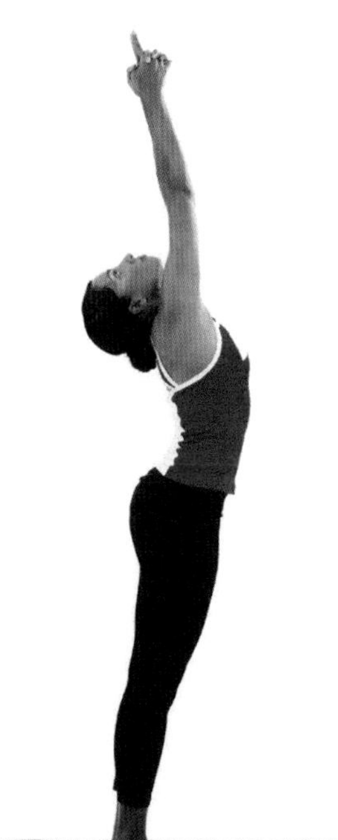

02

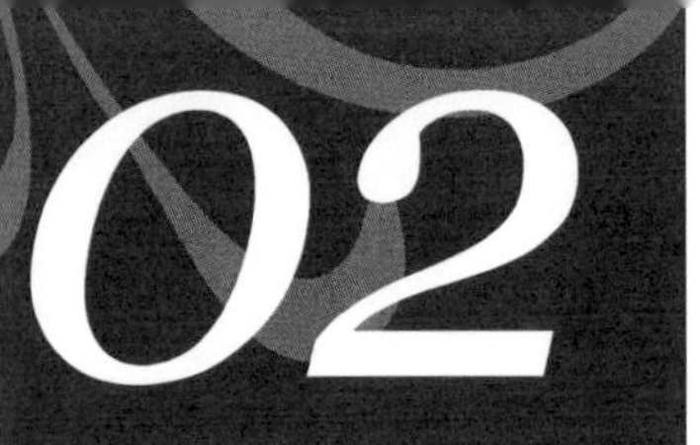

Ardha Chandrasana

Half Moon Pose

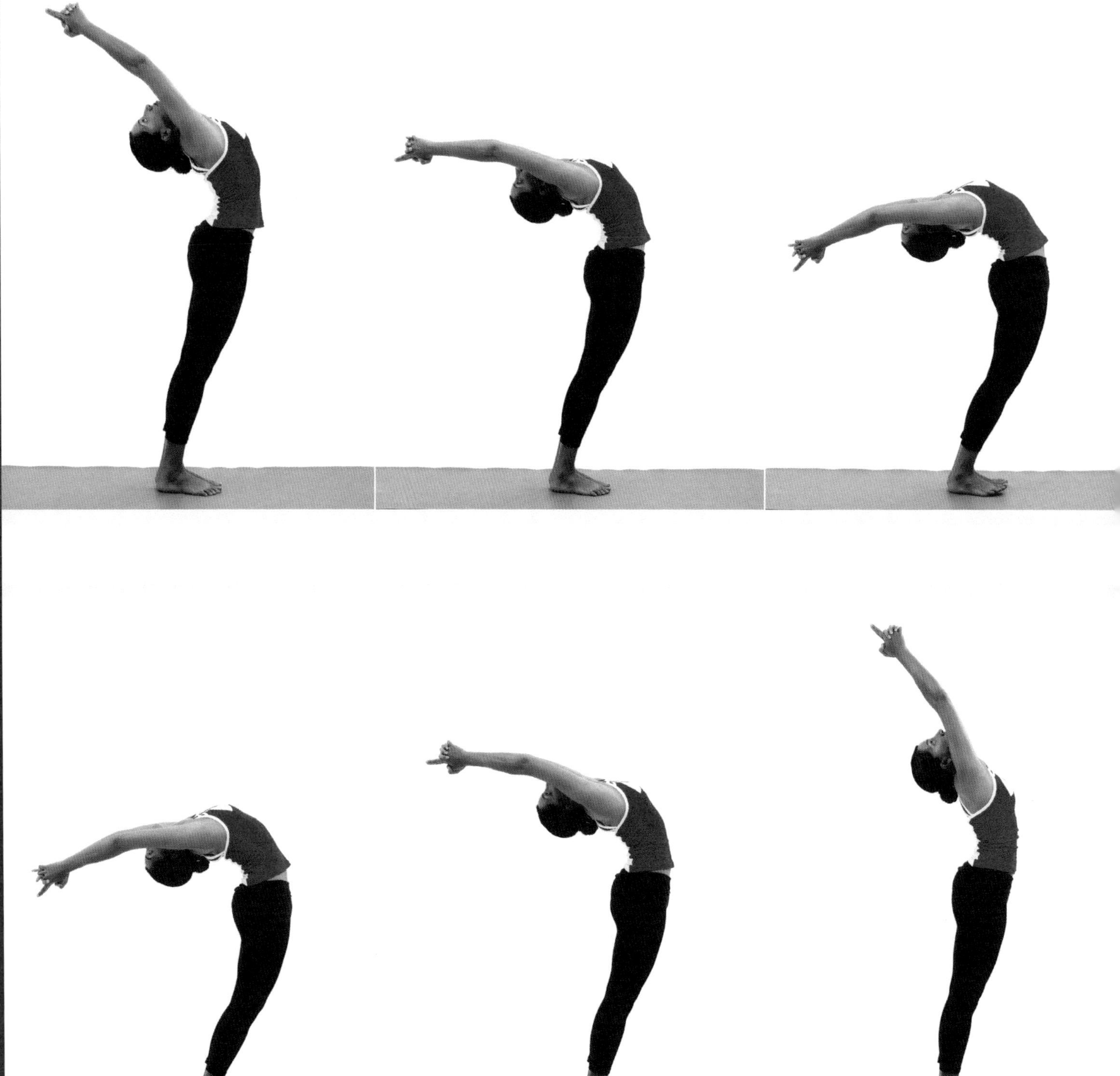

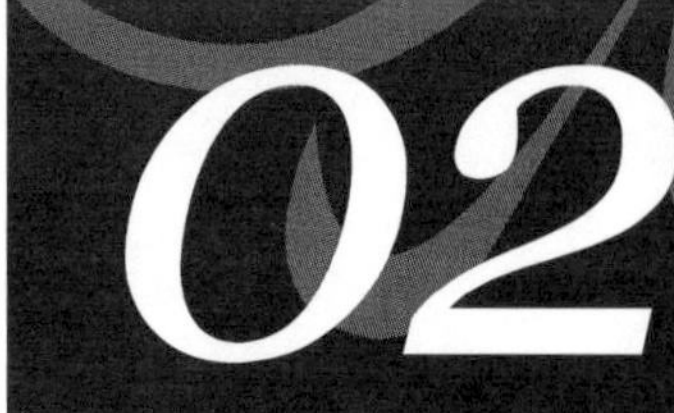

Ardha Chandrasana

HALF MOON POSE

4. **MOVE INTO YOUR BACKBEND:** As you exhale look back and move your arms back to the back wall. This will initiate the backbend. With strong legs and arms, extended spine and relaxed neck, your backbend emerges.

5. **YOUR COUNTERWEIGHT:** Your hips are actually the counterweight to your backbend. So it is vital that you push your hips forward, arcing them beyond your feet. Move strong legs and hips forward, lift the body up and back in an arch while arms approach the back wall or floor. Every other part of your body moves in the counter direction to your hips. In other words your hips move forward and everything else goes up and then back.

6. **WEIGHT IN THE HEELS:** You actually bring the weight back into your heels. This in itself would seem as if it would not work and is surely one of the finessing parts of an experienced yogi's pose. It takes courage to swing the weight there having the confidence that you will stay upright and not find yourself on the floor.

7. **LET YOUR UPPER BODY GO:** Keep the foundation very strong. The sensation in the pose is one of falling backwards letting gravity pull you back, aided by your line of sight and amazingly counterbalanced by the forward movement of your hips.

8. **YOUR KNEES:** Commonly the knees bend. Make sure that you keep them locked out. It may lessen your apparent backbend, only your ego will argue against this. Push your hips forward at the same time.

9. **YOUR THROAT:** In a backbend your throat is experiencing an intense stretch. The skin across your throat and chest is quite taut. Rather than zeroing in on the tightness, see if you can further soften the back of the neck. Your breath may need to be modulated to keep the oxygen moving into your body. Greener yoginis who generally have lesser breath resources may find it more difficult to breathe deeply. Shorter shallower breaths are fine. Just keep 'em coming.

10. **YOUR EYES:** Look back and not up. You will go where you are looking. Try to see the back wall, the floor where it joins the back wall, or even your mat.

11. **YOUR ARMS:** Recommit them and make a concerted effort to take them back to the floor.

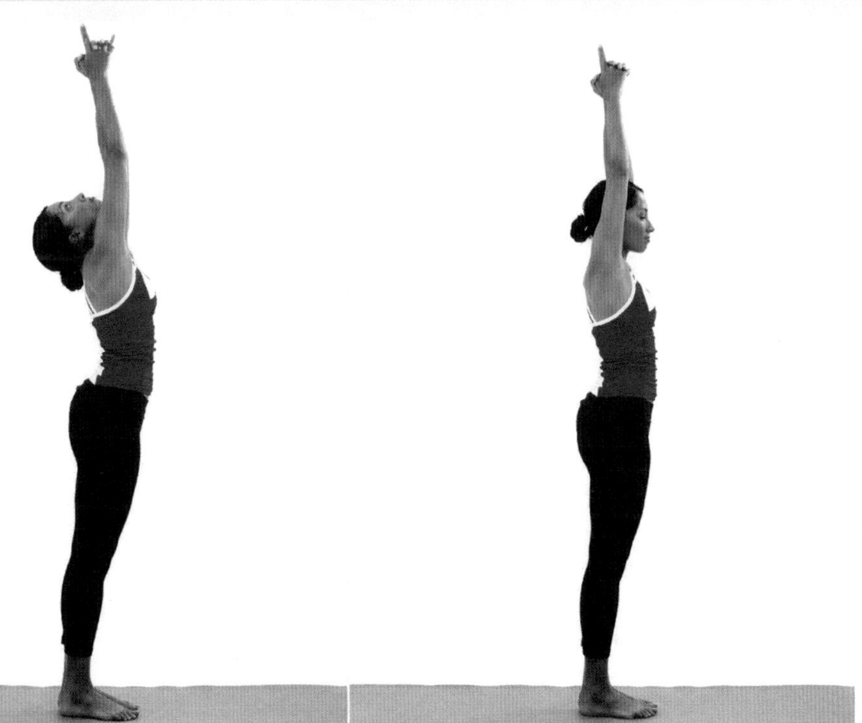

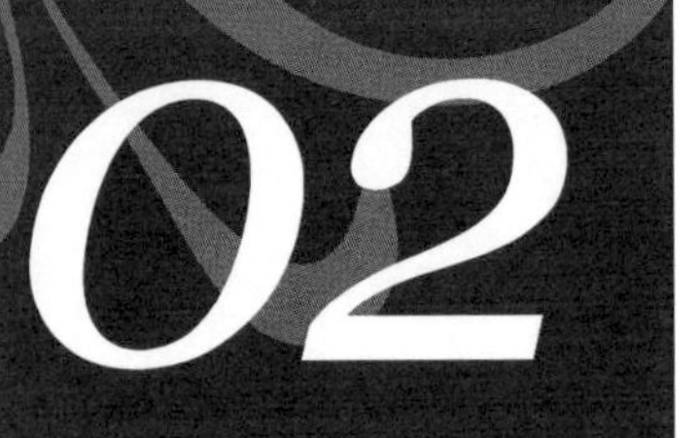

Ardha Chandrasana

HALF MOON POSE

Release

Make sure you inhale your body back to center, moving slowly to avoid dizziness. The buoyancy in your lungs will give you some assistance. Bring your chest and arms up. Keep your legs strong. Your head comes up the very last. Meet your eyes in the mirror. You are now ready to enter the 4th part of this pose – the big forward bend called Hands to Feet pose.

Common mistakes and how to fix them

Legs bend or not locked: Bending the legs gives a false sense of the extent of your backbend. It challenges your balance and instead of surrendering to the pose, your muscles will risk damage and try to stop you from falling. The bend, which starts at the feet, is founded on a very strong base of solid locked out legs. It extends upwards through the torso and shoulders, and through arms to fingertips, in a long lean arc. Intensify the backbend by pushing squeezed hips forward and bringing the weight back to the heels.

Weight in the toes: Students usually develop faith in the mechanics of this pose over a number of classes. The counterweight works perfectly to support the body. Pushing the hips forward strongly allows all your weight back in the heels and further allows the arms to go back too. Trust in the forces of nature.

Neck is tense: Not surrendering your neck to gravity is perhaps the biggest barrier to success. Holding the neck up creates tension in the neck and shoulders which is potentially damaging and painful. The fix here may be as simple as bending your elbows slightly. You may have (or think you have) very good reasons to hold your head up, including some valid ones; acute pain due to injury, certain types of cervical spine damage. However, the most common reasons are fear and unfamiliarity.

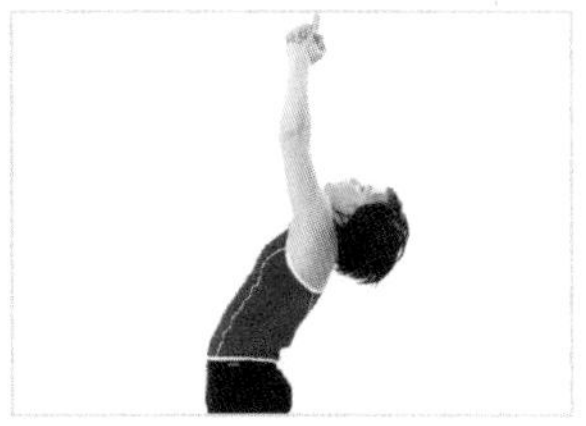

For protection from danger, all animals react adversely to exposing their underbelly (comprising heart and major organs). As yoga debutants the risk seems real: Will I fall over, what is that strong or intense reaction in my heart, my solar plexus, my throat?

Once familiar with the exercise, we know that, no matter how big the backbend is, we are safe.

Reactions in backbend are unconscious attempts to keep you on your feet. They include bending legs, slack muscles in the butt and legs, and leaving the weight in the toes.

Go with the energy, don't fight it. Allow the head to be pulled by gravity and fall weightily from your neck towards the spine. Fear eventually makes way to trust, tension to release. Tight head, neck and shoulder muscles give way to loose long and relaxed ones.

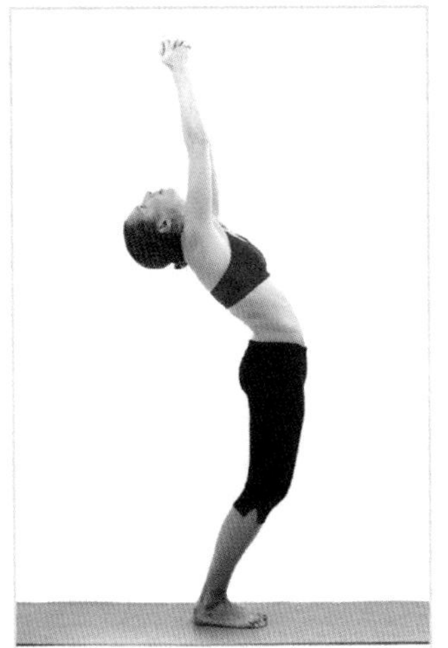

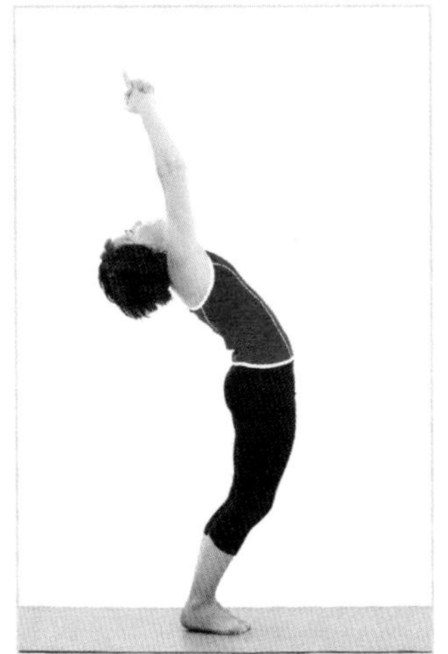

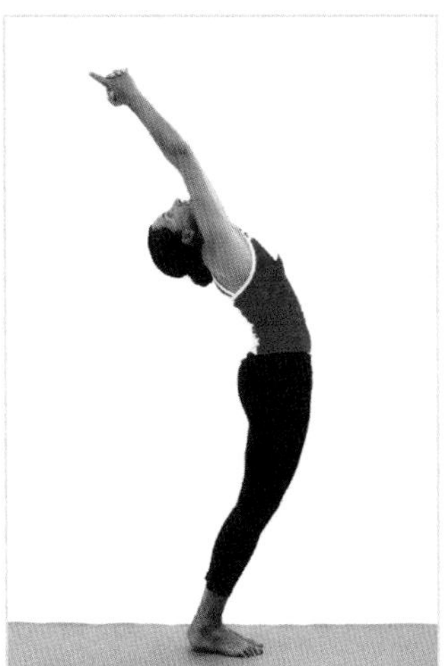

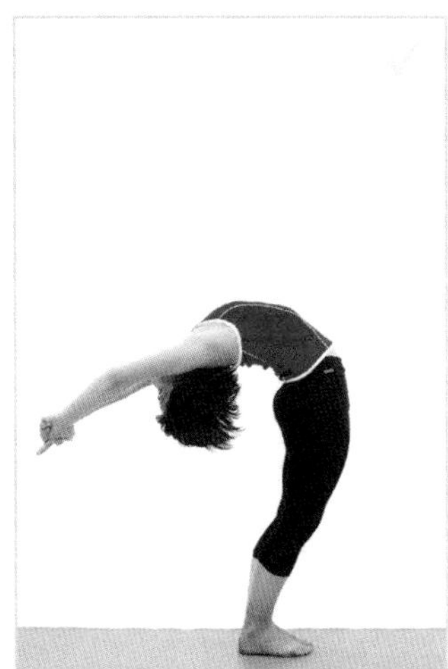

Ardha Chandrasana

Half Moon Pose

The important safety elements are:

1. When instructed to let go of the head behind you on your soft neck; do exactly that. Let go, and use your eyes to take you where you need to go: 'Where your eyes look, your body follows'.
2. Keep the legs extremely strong and push hips strongly forward.
3. Lift out of the spine before and while going back.
4. Take and then keep the weight back in the heels.
5. Your body will not fall over backwards. Your body, your shoulders, your chest, your neck and your spine will open with vast reserves of space to explore.

Not looking back: When all conditions are right your potential to create a deep backbend is greatly improved. The act of placing your visual attention (whether correctly or not) does more to determine the depth of your backbend then just about any other condition. It can greatly affect neck tension, the ease in which you allow your head to rest back, or where your weight lands.

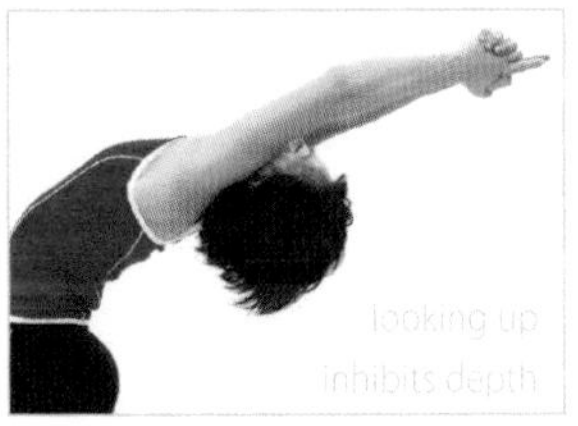

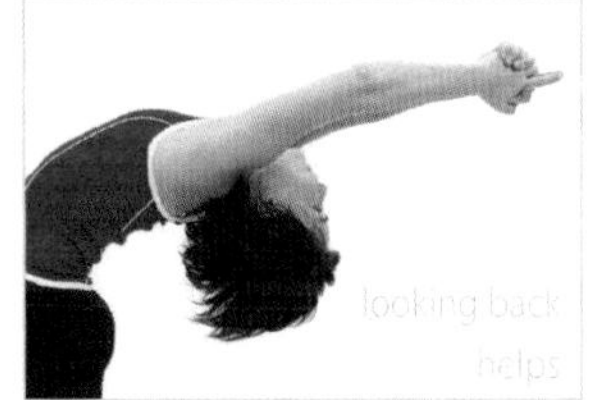

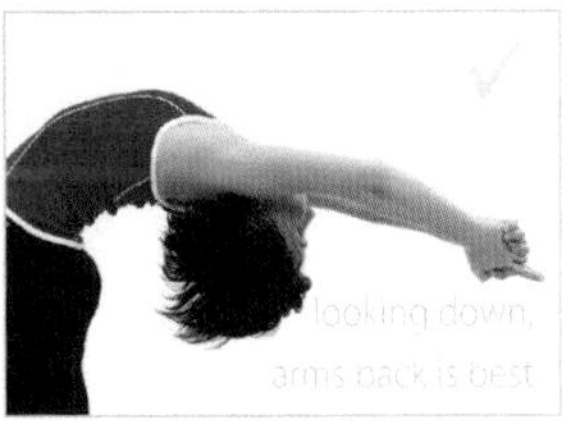

Test it out by doing a backbend while keeping your eyes locked on the ceiling. It stops even very flexible students in their tracks. This misdirected visual focus seems to connect you with your emotional body. Anything strong that you experience mid-pose will feel intensified when you drop your eyes (toward your chin) and can cause you to come out early.

For an opposing exercise for positive results enter your backbend and locate the furthest point behind you. Next set aim to move beyond it. Whatever you do, don't look up, and, don't look down your nose. Look back and down, take your arms back too.

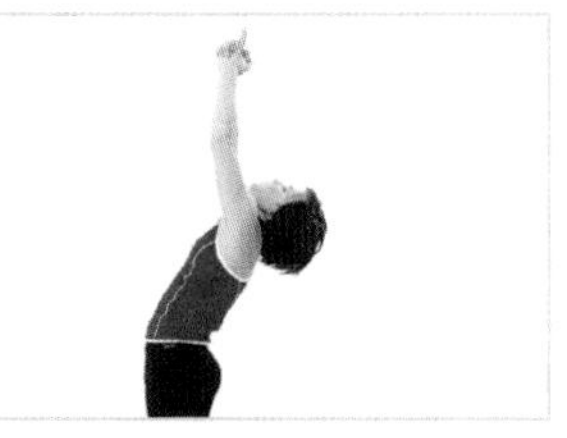

Arms reaching to ceiling: Too often students will actually keep their arms up over their heads to start, go back into their backbend but leave their arms up, fingers pointing to the ceiling. Obviously the backward movement is minimized but also the eyes tend to look up toward the fingertips. Look back, and take your arms back. Feel your chest and shoulders open as a result. A lesser mistake is not bringing your arms back as much as you can.

Gone too far?

There is really no possibility of going too far here. Some students have the most amazing backbends. Some will actually get their fingers close to or on the floor behind them. These students are most certainly using their line of sight to take them even further. For example when I go into this pose I am first looking for the back wall, then the floor, then the back of my towel and then my feet. Just keep looking beyond.

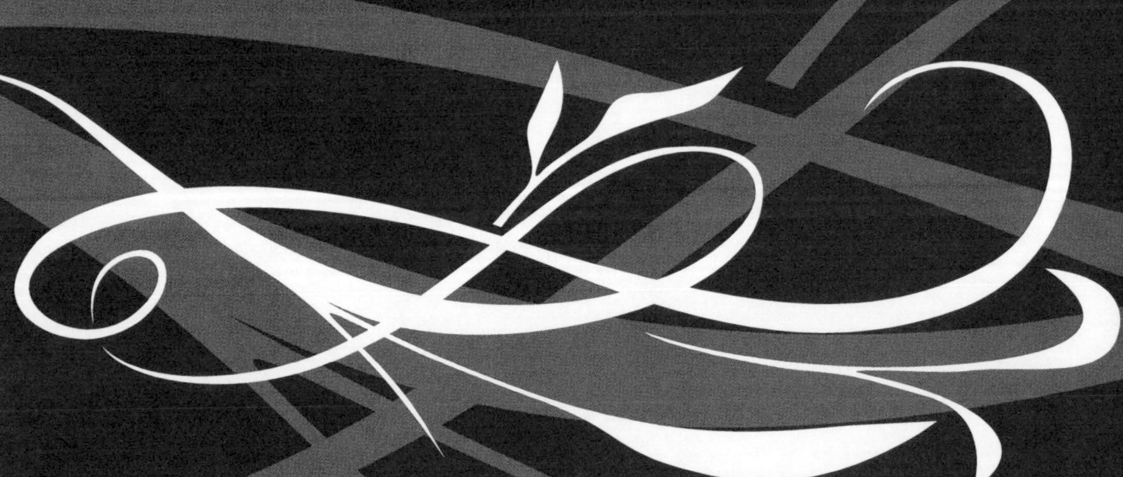

Pada Hastasana

People are always blaming their circumstances for what they are. I don't believe in circumstances. The people who get on in this world are the people who get up and look for the circumstances they want, and, if they can't find them, make them.
—George Bernard Shaw

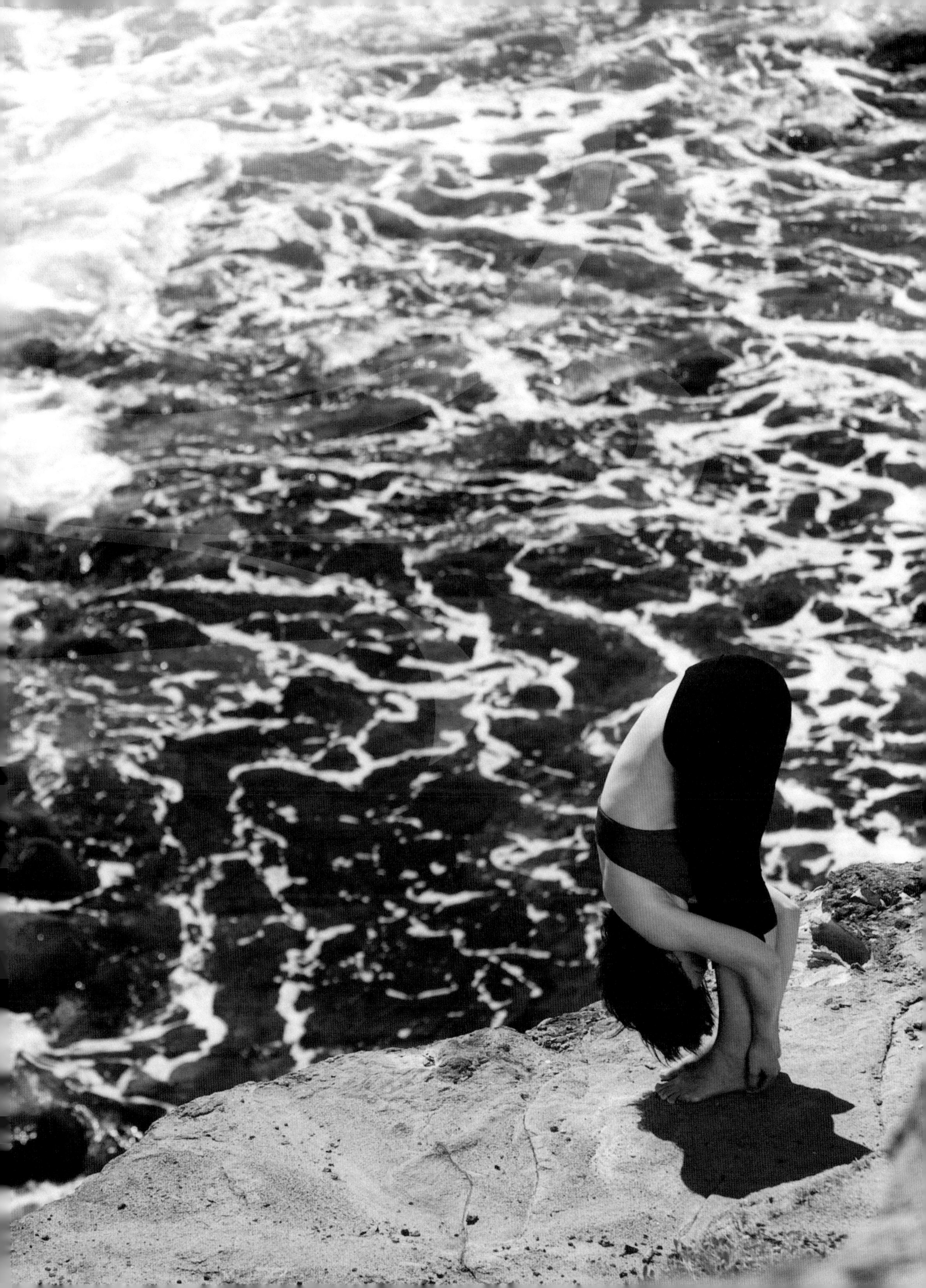

Pada Hastasana

Hands To Feet Pose

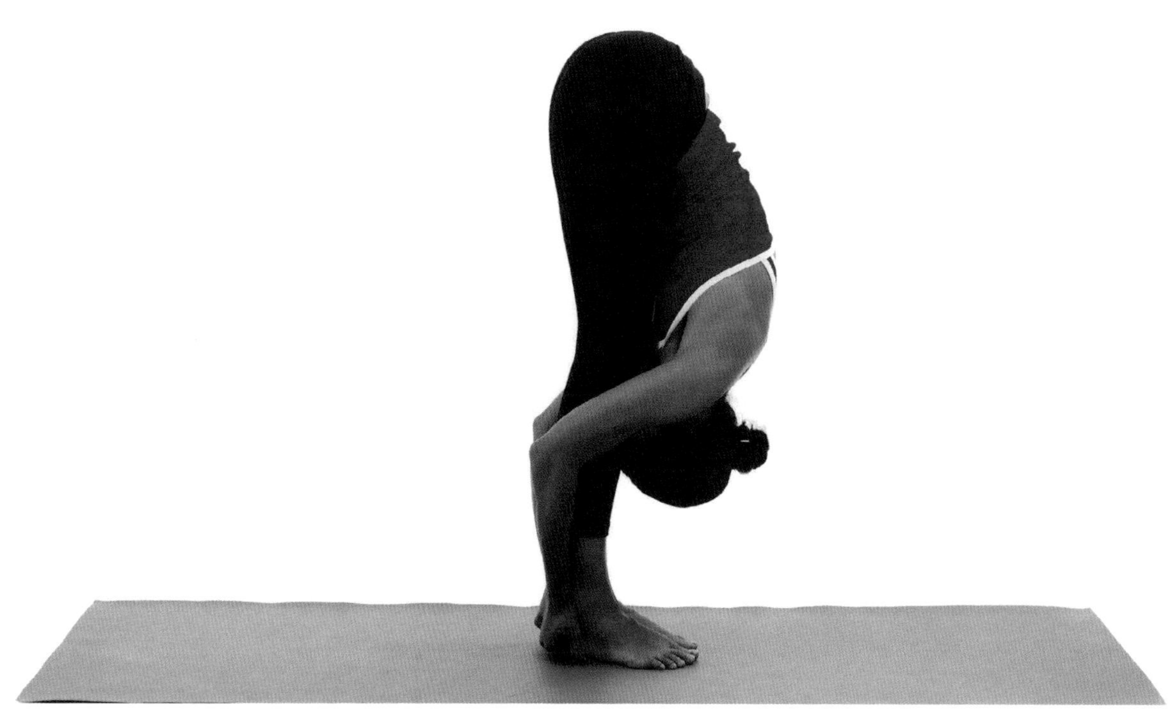

The essentials

This is an intense forward bend which will naturally give you a great stretch to the back side of your body and legs. Most students really look forward to this part, even though there are lots of groans!

This pose is incredible. To get this pose right you have to rely on precise execution. Employing the concept of reciprocal inhibition we can open up the whole backside of the body. There are some very specific mechanics to getting this to work for you.

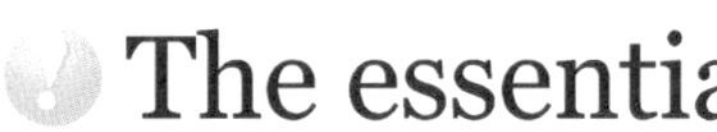

What makes this pose so difficult to get right?

Done incorrectly this pose will:

- Tighten your shoulders and neck
- Cause strain in the lower spine
- Tighten the legs and the back (the converse is what you want)
- Be very tiring

Thankfully there are some clear ways to get this to work for every single body type out there. It might not always be a textbook picture but with the proper elements present it can be achieved. This is one of the few poses where I can tell what sort of attention you have been getting at other studios. There is no excuse to get this one wrong - especially because the results can be disastrous. We will tweak this together now.

A word about forward bending

Our lives are full of forward bends, yet it is right here that we need to be careful. It is on the entry to this pose where weakness in core strength is highlighted. Bending forward puts all sorts of stresses on the body and spine. Many apparently strong looking individuals have difficulty bending forward citing disc and muscular problems.

Remember to listen to your body. It is important to use the hydraulic pressure of the organs against the spine to support you on the way down to the floor. It is also important to talk to your teacher about alternate ways to get to the floor if you are experiencing spasms in your mid or lower back.

Pada Hastasana

Hands To Feet Pose

The technique

The warm-up

You have just exited your backbend so you are standing upright with your arms over your head.

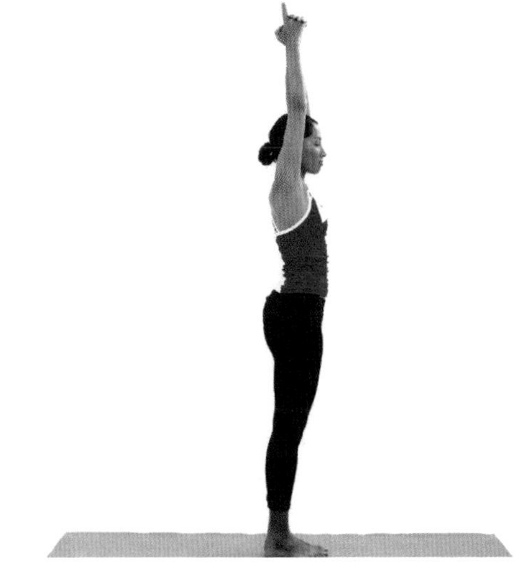

1.1 **Getting To The Floor**: Inhale the extension in your torso and arms. Draw in your abdomen to help protect your lower spine, raise your pelvic floor and as you exhale, hinge at the hips - with arms, head and back constantly aligned - to bring your hands down to the floor. The warm-up routine (which is great for opening up your legs, hips and lower back) seems simple but definitely needs clarification.

1.2 **The Warm-Up**: In an ideal world your hands will hit the ground in front of your feet, and you will warm up, shifting the weight from one leg to the other straightening and bending your legs alternately to warm and loosen the joints and stretch the legs.

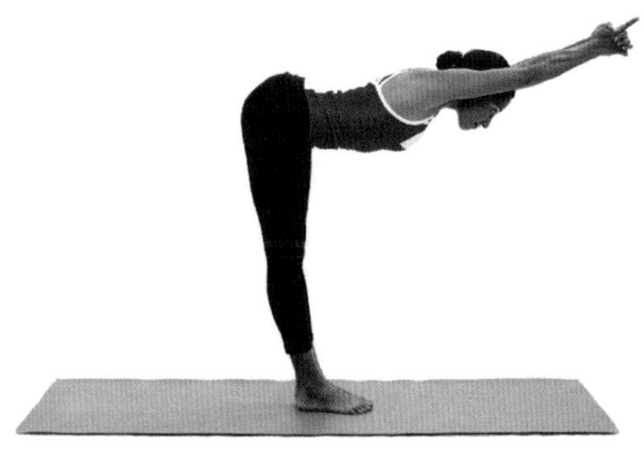

1.3 **Warm-Up For The Not-So-Flexible**: No matter how flexible you are, your warm-up position starts with palms on the floor. For the less flexible keep your back and legs straight as long as you can, then separate your hands and allow your palms to come to the floor as far out as they need to be. Your feet always stay where they are. Bend your legs if you need to, to get your hands in place. Your initial position will be with straight legs similar to a downward facing dog or 'V' shape.

Similar to a runner's warm-up, lift one heel to bend that leg, while the other heel drops to the floor. Lean heavily into the locked out leg to stretch and loosen the hips and lower back. Take 3-5 seconds on each leg for 3-5 cycles. A quick wiggle of the hips does absolutely nothing.

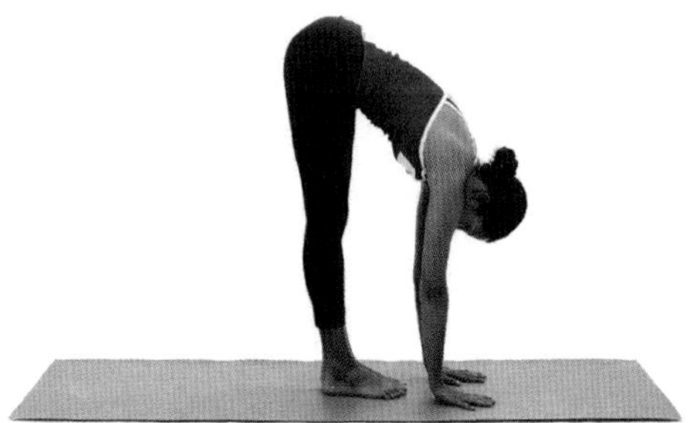

1.4 **Palms On The Floor:** The tighter your body, the further your hands are forward of your feet, and the more heavily you lean into your hands. Your palms on the floor create a crucial safety mechanism to protect your hips, hamstrings, spine and even sciatica conditions. If you can take all the weight in your hands then you can safely drop each alternate heel to the ground as you bend the other leg. As you stretch that heel down you can modulate the pressure in your hands so that the stretch becomes long, safe and effective. I recommend staying about 3-5 seconds in each stretch.

Pada Hastasana

Hands To Feet Pose

regular flexibility

warm-up

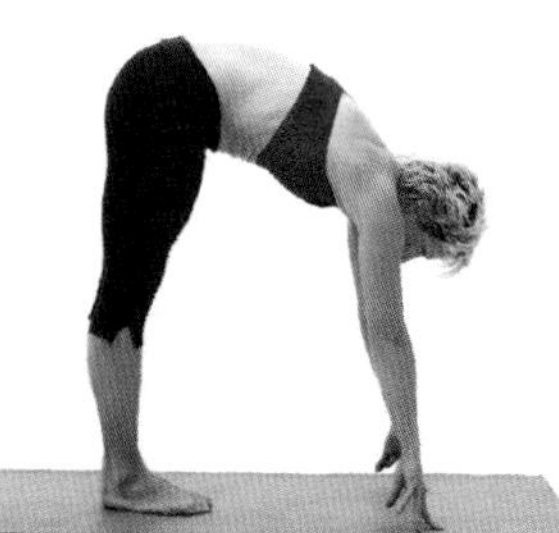

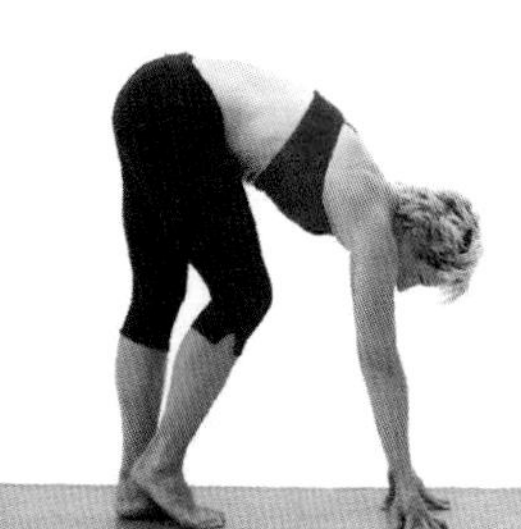

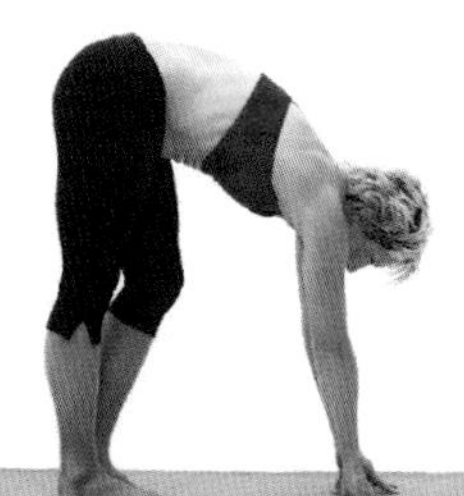

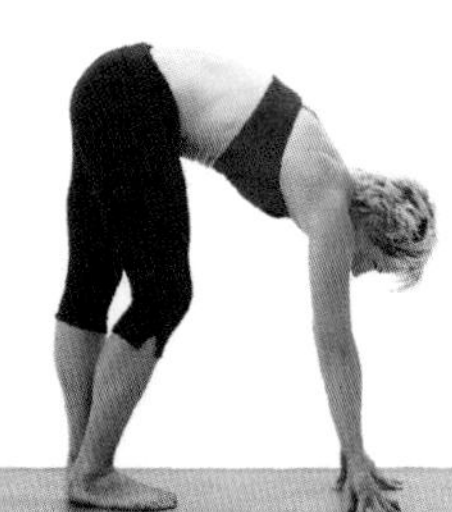

flexible warm up

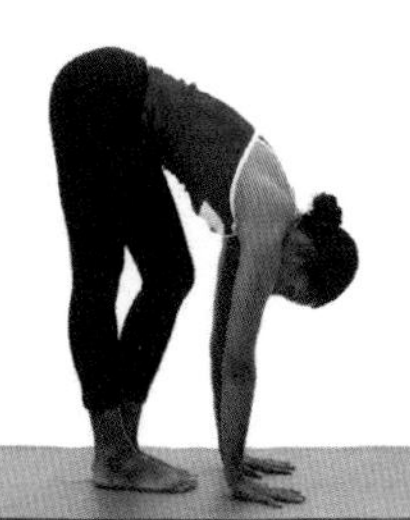

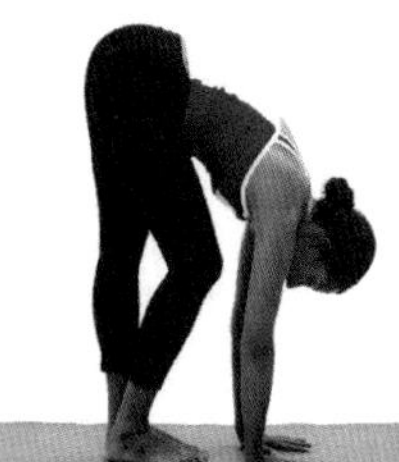

inflexible warm-up

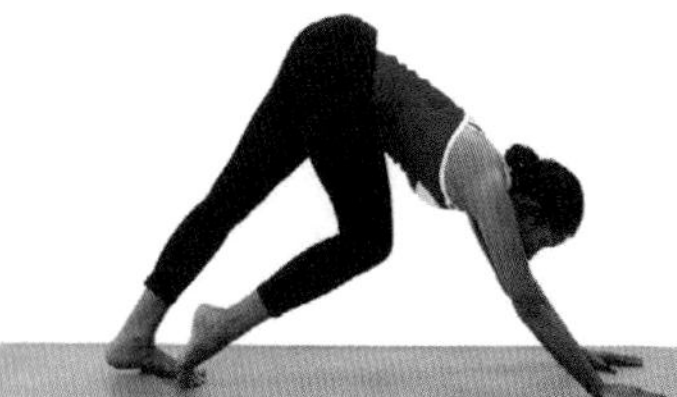

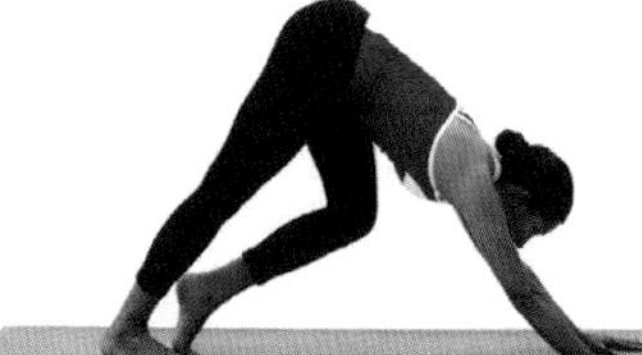

1.5 **Does Squatting Help?**: I see a lot of students squat. I have never found this to be effective. I can say however that every single student that I have helped with the technique of loosening up the hips by leaning into each one slowly while keeping the palms on the floor has found this to be the most effective stretch.

1.6 **Your Feet Stay In One Place**: Remember to keep the position of your feet the same as in your side bends. The exceptions are for pregnant or larger bodies where you place your feet at hip distance apart. As your body opens up you will find you have to walk your hands out less far until you eventually bring your hands down near your feet.

1.7 **Loosening Up For The Super-Flexible**: The more flexible you are, the closer you will position your hands to your feet. Try leaving your heels on the ground and bending and straightening your legs in turn. Lean well into each hip. Want some more? Then bring the weight way forward into the toes. The more stretch you want and get, the less pressure you put on the floor with your hands. Try different positions to place your palms or the backs of your hands; in front, to the side, behind you. I rest the back of my hands passively on the floor just to support me so that I don't fall when I take the weight forward.

Pada Hastasana

Hands To Feet Pose

03

The pose

2.1 **Walk Your Hands Back To Your Feet:** Those of you who placed your hands out for warm-up, will have to walk them back again.

2.2 **Your Legs:** Bend your legs (your feet are still in position and have not moved since the beginning of class).

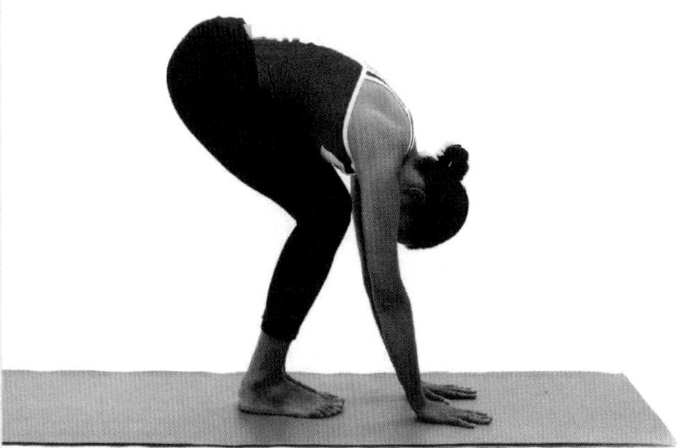

2.3 **Your Body On Your Legs:** Elongate your body and then lay your torso on the upper legs, the chest on your knees. The legs stay bent. The degree of leg bend is flexibility dependent. The tighter you are, the more you bend your legs here.

2.4 **Arms Around The Back Of Your Legs:** Bring your right arm around the back of your right leg and place your fingers under your foot and facing directly onto the mirror. Your elbow points toward the back wall. Your shoulder is relaxed away from the ear (up toward your hip). Now bring your left arm around the back of the left leg and position similarly, fingers forward under the foot.

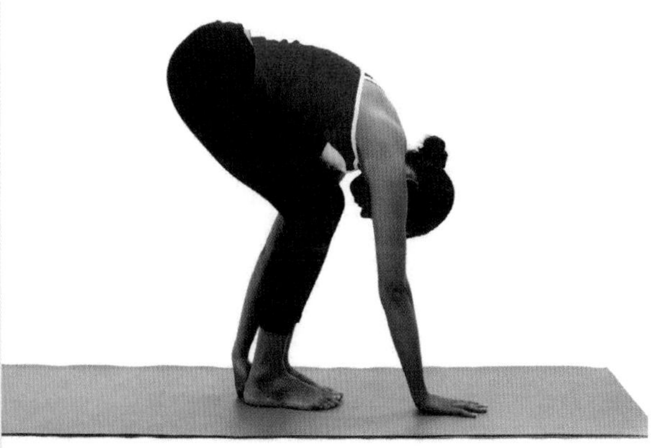

2.5 **Your Fingers:** All 10 fingers are parallel, facing forward. Line up your baby fingers together to touch. If you are very flexible you may even be able to overlap your little fingers.

2.6 **Your Head:** Let your head drop to fully loosen up your neck. You can test its relaxation by gently nodding 'yes', and shaking 'no' and then letting it hang.

2.7 **Pull, Lengthen, Press, Pull:** Inhale deeply and then on your exhale PULL upwards on your heels. Pull against your feet and lift the hips up while you pull your chest and body down onto your legs. You must execute a pull to engage the biceps muscles to draw your elbows up and behind your legs. The mere intention of trying to get your elbows to touch together will help you achieve your outcomes. The biceps' pull facilitates upward shoulder movement away from the ears (toward the ceiling).

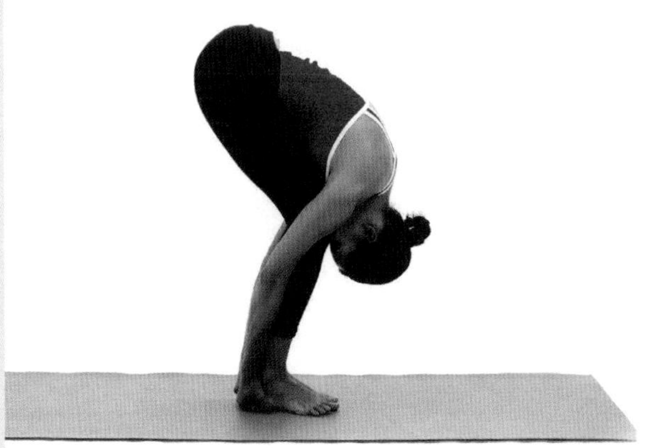

2.8 **Body On The Legs, Hinge At The Knees:** Your body MUST remain on your legs for the entire pose. To do this you pull on your feet while you simultaneously lift your hips up toward the ceiling by hinging at the knees, with the eventual aim of straightening the legs.

Pada Hastasana

Hands To Feet Pose

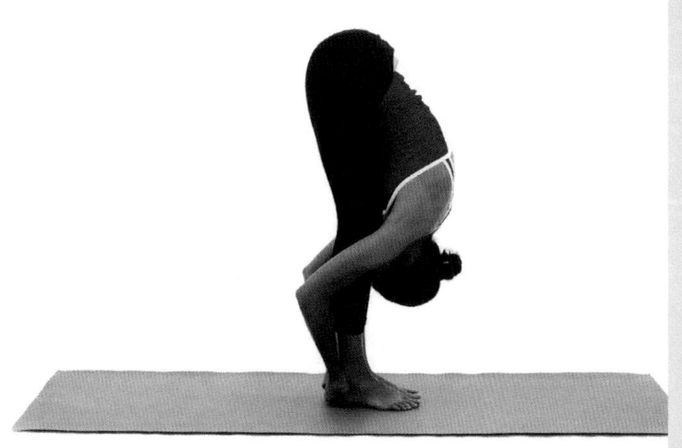

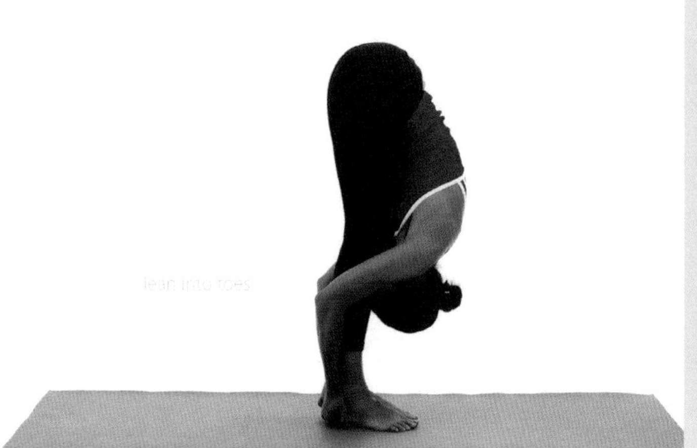

2.9 **Delicious Stretch**: The stretch that is created is amazing. If you do this pose correctly then it travels the entire back side of the body from heels through your hips and then down the whole length of the spine.

2.10 **Head to Feet**: Pull with the hands, lift the hips, relax into the stretch with big breaths and allow gravity to pull your spine down. One day the top of your head will be close to or touch the top of your feet, your legs will be straight and locked out and the stretch will be extremely satisfying.

2.11 **Even More Pull, Climb Your Body Down**: Take a big inhale and 'climb' your body down further on to your legs. Walk the top of your arms around behind you as if they are climbing up the outside of your thighs (which lifts your elbows and draws them together). On your exhale continue to re-engage the pull and lift. Surrender to the stretch and feel yourself growing long.

2.12 **Even More Stretch, Weight Into Toes**: Once you have discovered your sweet spot then it is time to roll the weight closer into the toes. No, you won't fall over because of Newton's Law – every force has an equal and opposite reaction. Pulling against your feet, your feet exert a downward force. As you lean into your toes you are perfectly counterbalanced.

Release

On your last exhale you are still pulling the body onto the legs, hips lifting up, leaning forward and feeling that stretch. Finish your exhale, let go of your grip and hang there for a moment to momentarily let the blood recirculate. Straighten your legs if they are not already straight. Bring your arms back out in front of you. Reverse out of your posture on an inhale by hinging your strong body around your hips to standing. Exhale your arms down to your side, make contact with yourself and stay as still as you can keeping the breath flowing.

Common mistakes and how to fix them

Many of the errors center around correct grip. The fingers have to be well positioned as do the hands. These and other important actions to avoid are listed below.

Fingers at an angle: Your fingers should be parallel in the grip and all facing forwards. Otherwise a totally different result is not only possible it is very likely.

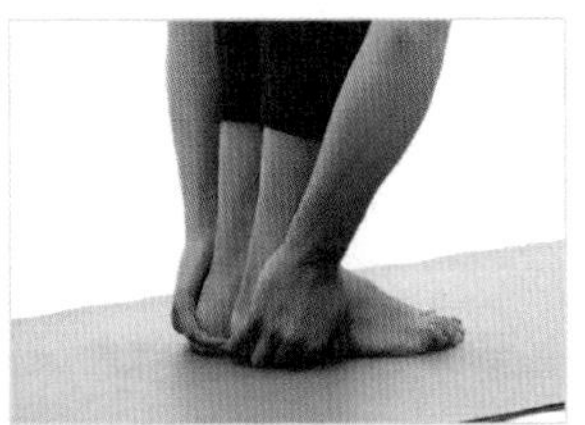

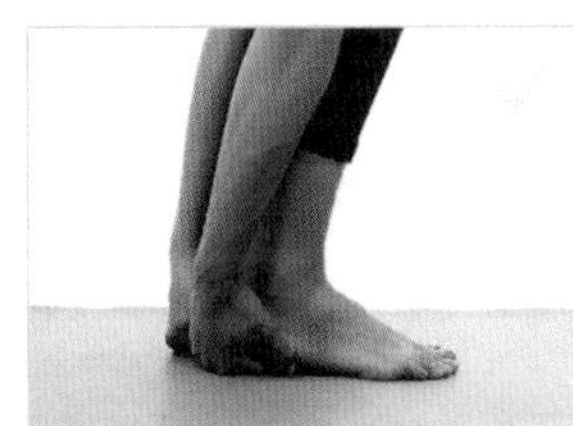

Thumbs over top: Your thumbs should never be on top of your feet. Otherwise your shoulders tend to be recruited in the pull. Grip your feet with all fingers including thumbs together.

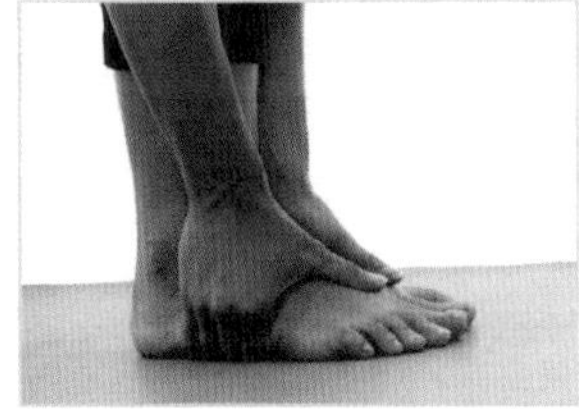

Elbows out: Don't let your elbows bend out to the side, pulling your shoulders down with them. Keep them tightly in against the legs, elbows directly behind you.

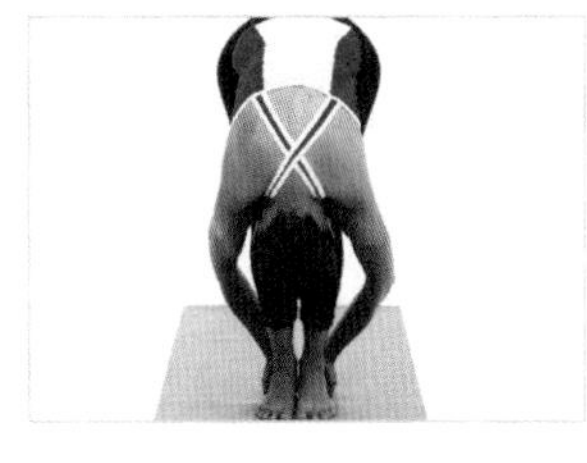

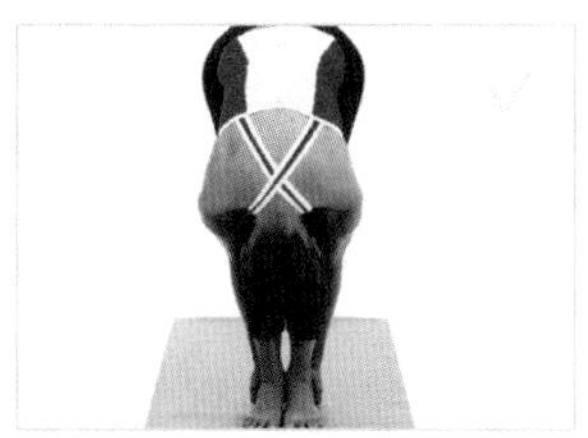

Hunched shoulders: Never shrug your shoulders. In this inverted position it means keep them away from the floor.

Space created: Ensure your body NEVER separates from your legs. A rounded spine and especially one where the body and legs separate produces undue pressure on your lower spine. Your back is nestled against your legs and therefore is straight and never rounded. This protects the back as do the hydraulic forces of the organs against the spine (as you hold your belly in).

***Hanging out, can't reach the feet**: Some students actually just hang because they can't touch their toes. You are getting absolutely nothing from this pose if you cannot bend down and least get your body and your legs together.

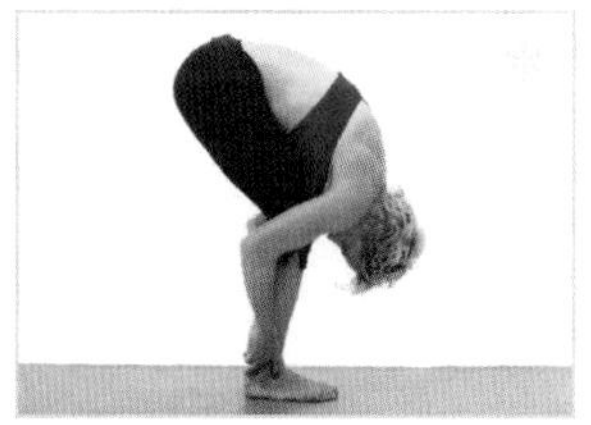

You may not be able to get your fingers under your heels in the correct orientation but some grip is better than no grip. You may have to be content with holding on at your calves or ankles. Pulling pressures will start to open your body and you will make great progress – certainly far in excess of just hanging your body in space.

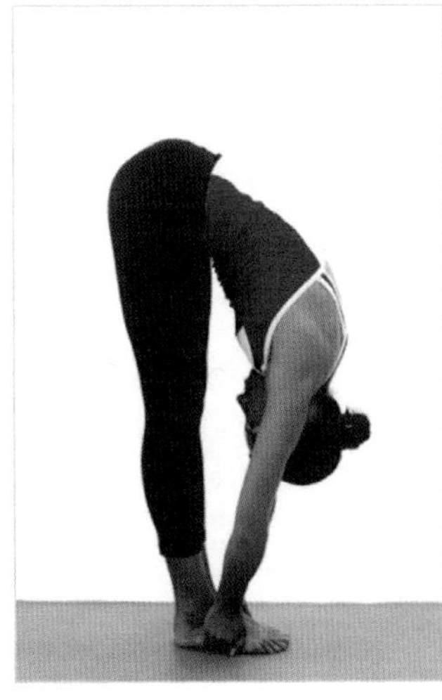

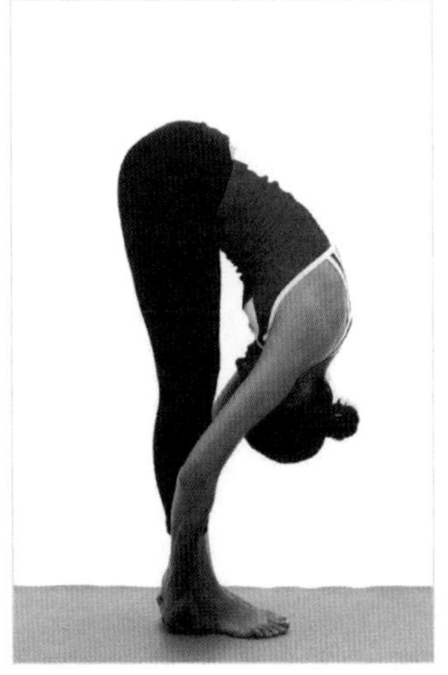

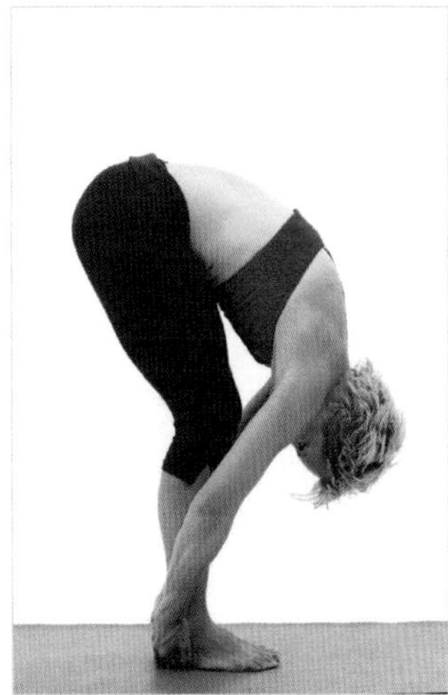

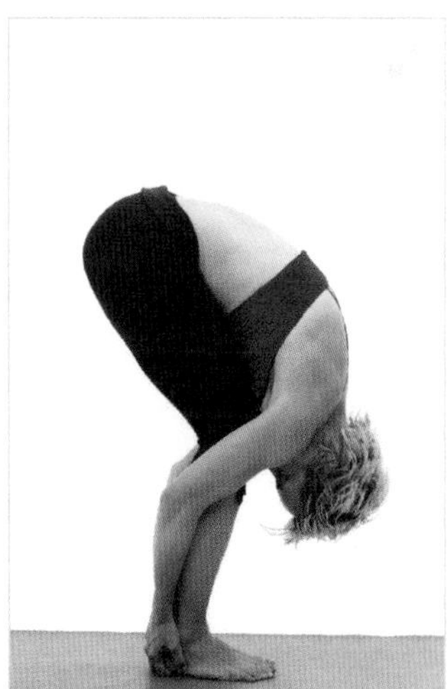

Pada Hastasana

Hands To Feet Pose

Straight legs or body on legs? Which should be priority?: There is a mistaken belief that straightening the legs is more important than the body on the legs. Never let the body separate away from the legs.

If you can't reach your feet (see above) then bend your legs as much as you need to in order to squash your body firmly on to your legs. You may need a modified grip behind the ankles. Maybe, if your body size is large, or you are pregnant you need to separate your feet up to hip distance apart. Then pull. You will feel your body open and your back will be straight. If you are not convinced, do the reverse; straighten your legs, round your spine and pull and feel the tremendous strain in your lower back.

Hinging at the hips: If you hinge at the hips allowing the body to separate then the pulling force actually creates strain in your back – your back will round and your shoulders will strain. Once your body is on the legs, you must only hinge at the knees.

Grip moves: Keep your grip constant. Don't allow it to slip to the side.

Stiff neck: Stiffening the neck creates tension in the shoulders. Loosen the muscles in the neck and let your head hang.

Crucial elements of the technique explained in detail

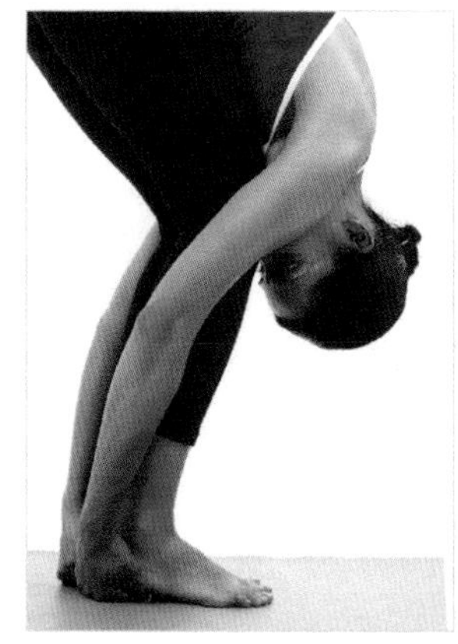

Pulling with your biceps

The body-opening power of this pose happens because of a number of body reflexes. The major one is a reflex device called 'reciprocal inhibition'. This is the simultaneous relaxation of one muscle (or group) and the contraction of its antagonist. Here you contract your biceps muscles and pull hard with your hands, and the back side of your body relaxes and opens up. This will happen even if your legs are not straight or locked out. So keep your legs bent if you have to, in order to maintain body to leg contact. You protect your spine and have greater stretch and opening.

Through your pose you are trying to get your forearms more closely aligned. If your elbows are distanced then this is a sign to recommit your arms by 'climbing' your upper arms up your legs to further wrap your elbows behind. This action further isolates the pull to the biceps.

It creates length and stretch which is felt through the whole backside of the body; from the heels through the back of the legs, up into the hips and then up through the whole spine. It aligns your forearms together and parallel and ideally they will just about touch.

Another way to think about this action is to pull on the heels and try to lift your elbows.

Don't pull with your shoulders

Drawing the strength from your biceps muscles relaxes the shoulders away from the ears so that there is no pulling component from them. This alleviates any damage from shoulder-shrugging and spine-rounding.

Protect your spine

Using your biceps creates back length. Your spine is protected because your body is cradled against the legs and the hydraulic pressure of the organs compresses against and safely cushions the spine muscles.

Hinge at the knees

Accompanying the pull is a most definite lift of the hips to accentuate the lengthening stretch. The movement is a hinge at the knees so that:

- The body stays sandwiched or glued to the thighs at all times
- The body stays in the same relationship to the legs
- The forces pull the body onto the legs.

Separating body and legs means the shoulders start to pull instead of the biceps, the elbows start to move around to the side of the legs and the grip changes (from behind to the side). Aim to keep the elbows behind the knees, pull with the biceps and lift by hinging at the knees!

The grip around the foot

The ideal grip is from behind but not all bodies can manage it. You may have to alter your grip if:

- You find it impossible to balance in the crouched position
- You cannot reach your feet.

If balance is an issue then you really should introduce a small distance between your feet. Keep them parallel. This may be necessary with larger bodied students, pregnant women, or those of you with very tight hips or shoulders. Get as much contact of your upper body against your legs as possible.

Sometimes the grip under the feet is compromised. Whatever happens aim first to get your fingers under your feet.

If unable to reach, then aim for the ankles, or the back of the calves, with thumbs on the outside. Your palms would be placed against the leg and facing the mirror. The thumbs will need to move laterally to get a positive grip on the leg with less slip. Keep the elbows moving to the back wall. Think of drawing elbow points upward.

Gripping at 90° from the side causes elbows to splay out and the pull would be more from the shoulders. Thumbs on top of the foot will not allow the shoulder relaxation. So keep the thumbs pointing in the same direction as the fingers.

If given the choice between grip on the feet and body away from the legs, or grip on the calves and body contacting the legs, CHOOSE the latter. Always keep the body on the legs even though it may introduce other challenges.

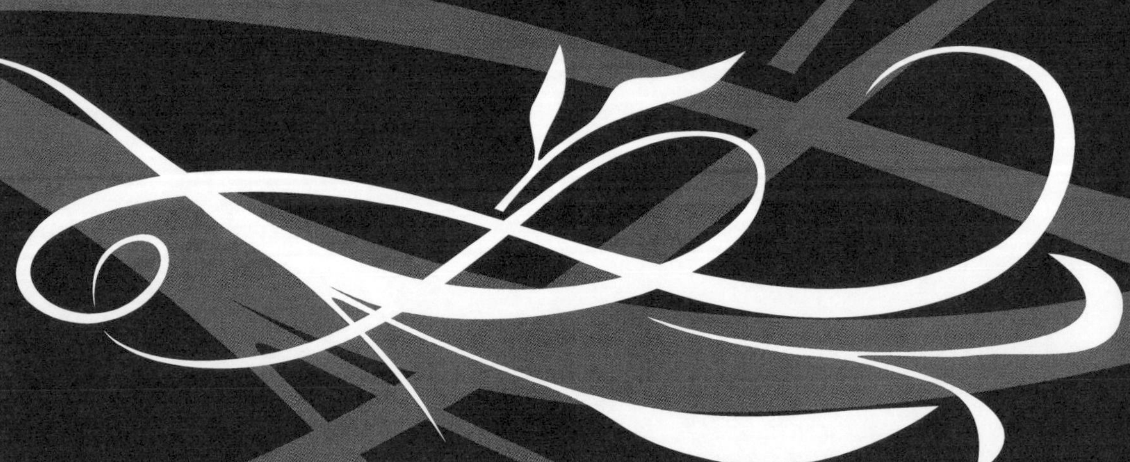

Utkatasana

Our dilemma is that we hate change and love it at the same time; what we really want is for things to remain the same but get better.
—Sydney J. Harris

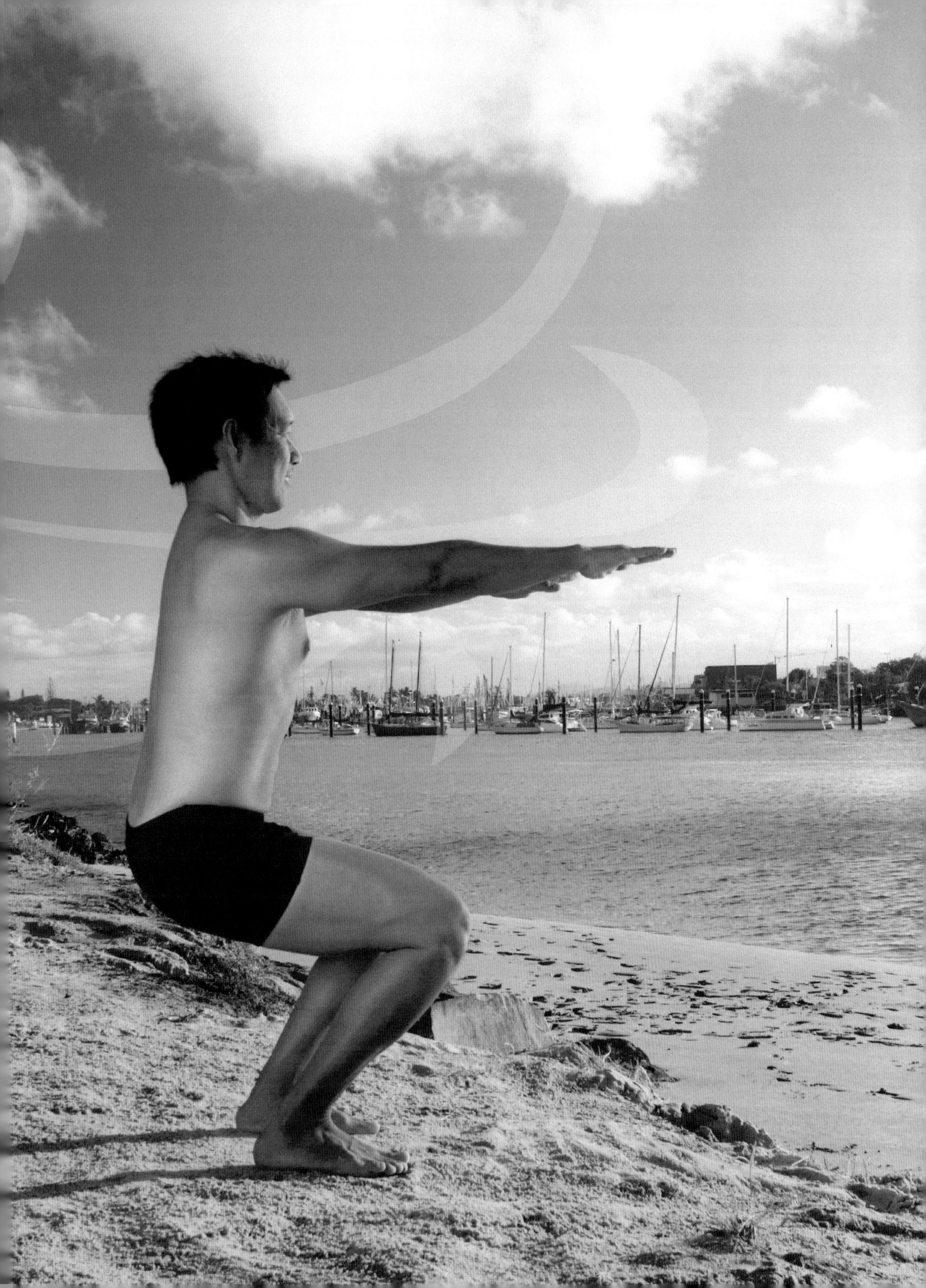

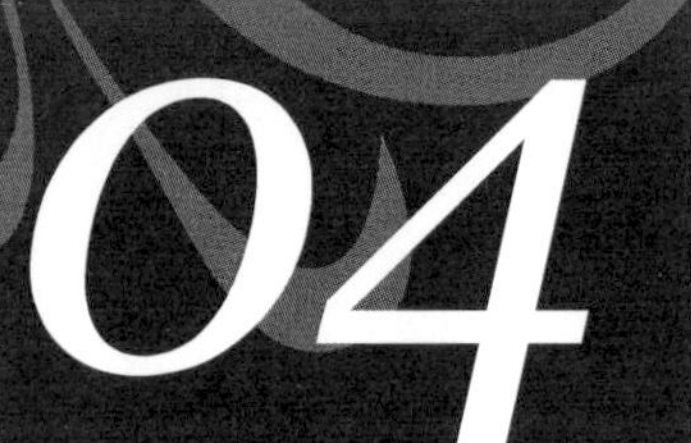

Utkatasana

AWKWARD POSE

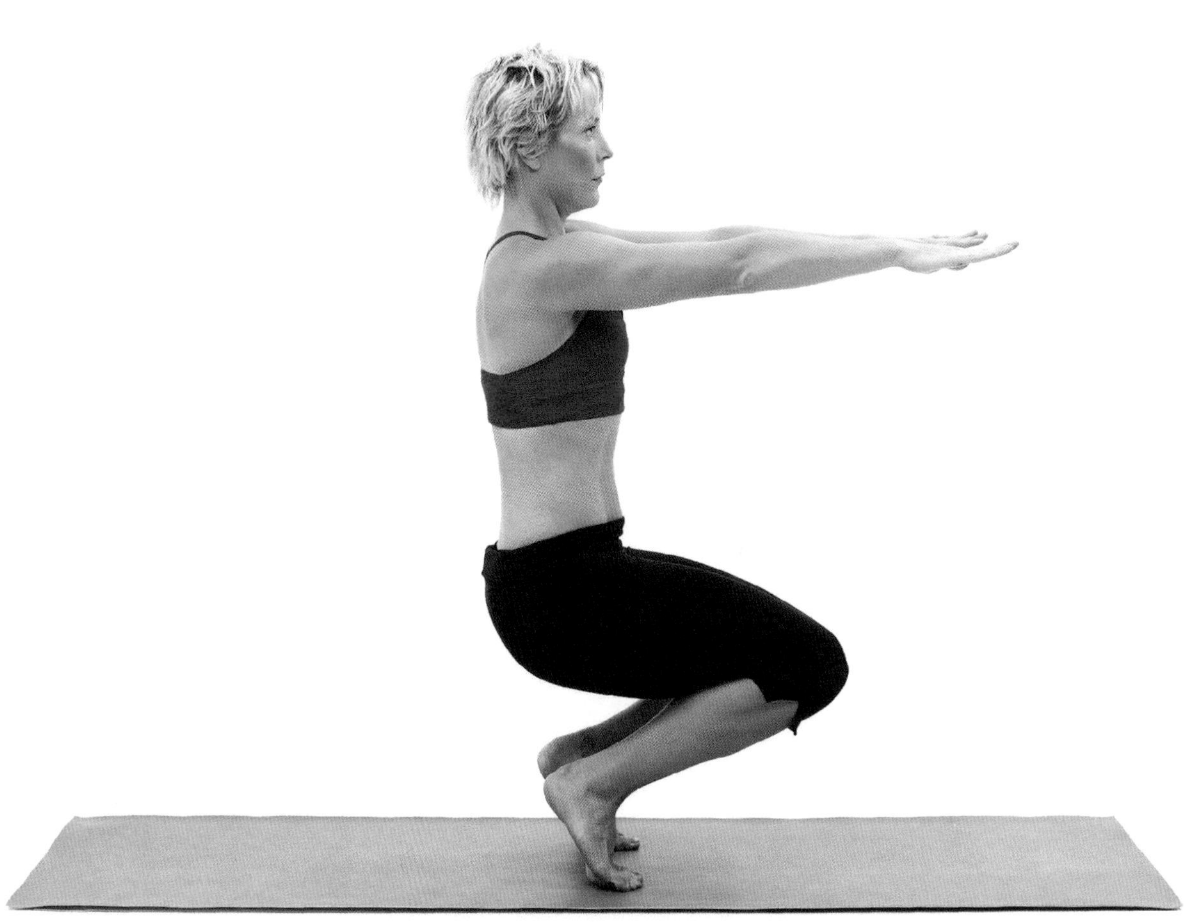

The essentials

This pose, just following Half Moon is a great hip and ankle opener. Performed in three parts it really strengthens your big muscles in the legs and arms, and calls for you to have great stamina and focus.

If you are just starting out, you will look around in Half Moon and Awkward and wonder how these amazing people could possibly keep their arms over their heads, or in this case, arms raised out in front of them for so long without faltering. Well have faith, 2-3 classes in fairly rapid succession will have you discovering that same font of energy.

What makes this pose so difficult to get right?

The hardest part about this pose is ironing out the confusion between the three parts. In Part 1 your challenge will be dropping your bottom to the right level as well as keeping your feet exactly parallel, because doing both feels completely abnormal. Part 2 it is opening up your ankles and Part 3, well, you will know how strong your leg (particularly the quadriceps) and core muscles really are and how much control you have over your movement. Students may lack stamina, strength, flexibility or have a fear of looking silly.

Utkatasana

Awkward Pose

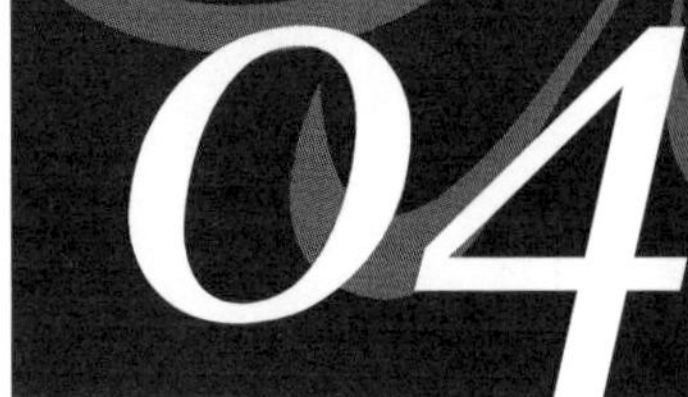

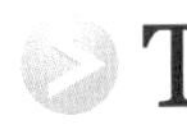

The technique

The set-up

You will only need to step out the one time to position yourself for all three parts.

1.1 **Step Out Hip Distance:** Leaving your left foot where it is, step your right foot out so that the feet are about hip or shoulder width apart. I find that when your arms are up parallel then best alignment comes from positioning the arms over the legs. Avoid having to bend forward to measure a specific distance because in essence every body is different. Besides you will get too distracted from your meditation.

1.2 **Arms Up Parallel To Floor And Each Other:** Inhale and bring your arms out in front of you, palms down. Your arms are parallel both to each other and the floor. Correctly positioned arms extend directly from the shoulders; you can see the tops of your forearms in the mirrors (as the common malposition is to bring them up too high).

1.3 **Your Arms Are Strong:** Extend your engaged arms strongly forward from the shoulders all the way to the fingertips. It is as if you were attempting to touch the mirror BUT at the same time lengthening the distance from the ears to the shoulders by squeezing the shoulder blades back and down.

1.4 **Feet Parallel:** Draw your heels slightly apart so that if you looked down, you would see 2 imaginary straight parallel lines emanating from your heels directly through your feet to the mirror. You will probably feel slightly pigeon-toed. The directions are the same for those with malformed feet, just be more calculated with your foot positions. Simply ensure that your feet are neither turning in nor out. When looking at your reflection, you won't see any part of your heels. Foot position is critical for the hip opening to occur.

1.5 **Heels Square:** The back of your heels are parallel with the mirror (ensures good square hips).

1.6 **Head Up:** Keep your chin up parallel to the floor. It need not change for the entire pose.

1.7 **You Are Ready To Begin.**

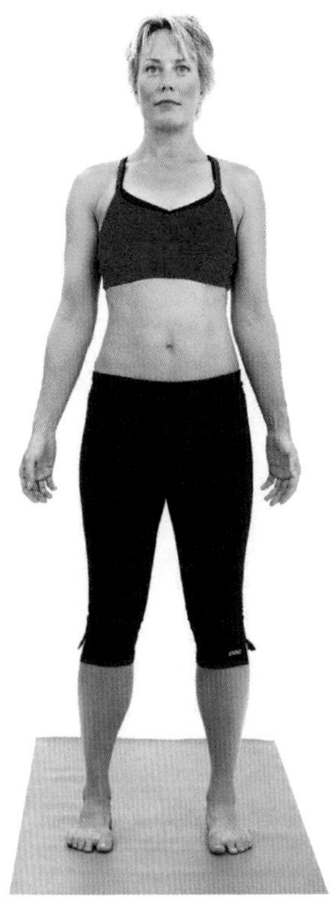

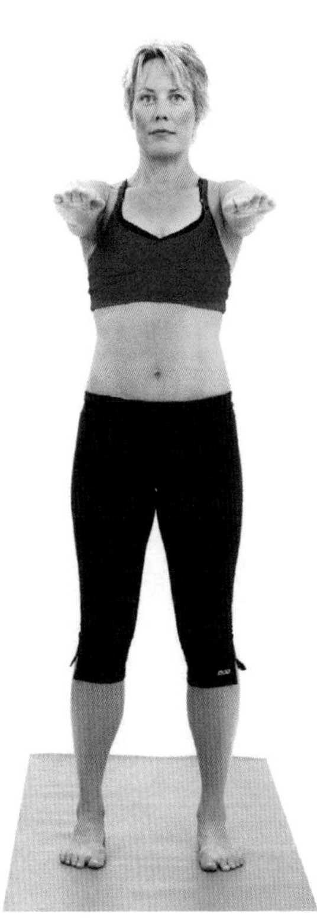

Utkatasana

Awkward Pose

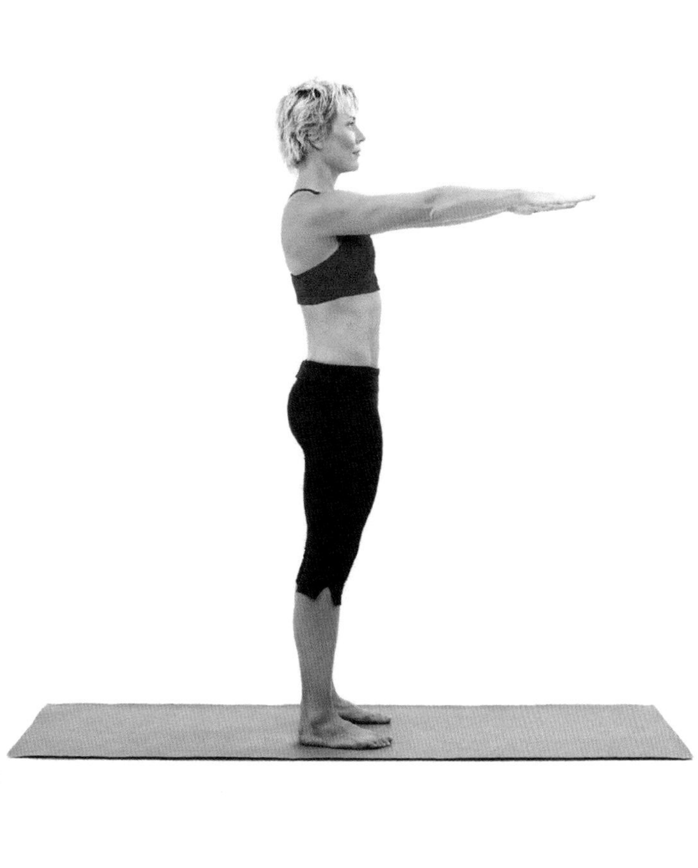

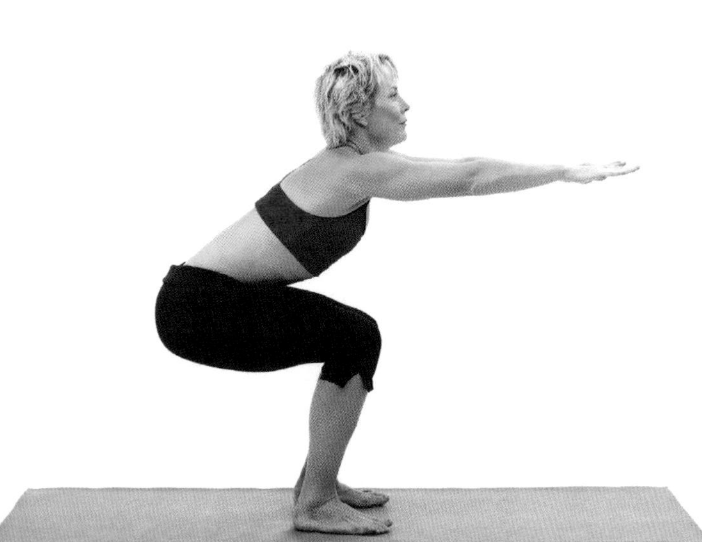

Part 1 Utkatasana

2.1 Inhale, Recommit Arms: Lengthen and strengthen the arms with shoulders back and down.

2.2 Exhale, Bottom Out: Exhale, strengthen your core and then poke your bottom out behind you and sit down.

2.3 Thighs Parallel: You must try to get your thighs down parallel to the floor.

2.4 Feet Flat: Keep your feet completely flat on the ground and take the weight back into the heels.

2.5 Keep Knees, Feet, Legs All Parallel: You must aim to keep your feet parallel and resist the movement of the feet – most commonly and naturally the heels move in and the toes move out to make it easier to get in position with less strain on the hips.

2.6 Arch The Spine: Get your upper body moving backward arching your spine, lifting it up off the legs to get your chest up. You are trying to look like you are sitting in a chair with a horizontal seat.

2.7 Chin Up, Chest Up, Bottom Down: Do this trio of actions continually to settle you down and backwards in the pose.

2.8 Lift Your Toes: Lifting your toes up off the ground brings the weight back even more. This will also help you further lift your chest up. It will feel like you can barely keep yourself from falling over. In order to resist falling you strengthen your body and arms.

2.9 Release: Inhale as you actively push up through the heels. It gives you energy and keeps your focus and body strong.

Tip for Part 1:

Here is a little 'trick' to help you lift your body up further off the legs to vertical, and increase ankle flexibility. Push your knees toward the mirror (you can feel the ankles open and the shins and calves stretching) and then bring your weight back in the heels lifting the chest. Push forward and then settle back, maybe even a couple of times.

Utkatasana

AWKWARD POSE

04

Part 2 Utkatasana

With arms still strong and feet apart begin Part 2.

3.1 **COME UP ON YOUR TOES**: Inhale and raise up on engaged, strong legs to balance on your toes. Push the weight forward into your toes as far as your ankles allow. It helps to 'lock' ankles into their furthest opening. No matter how flexible, your heels stay as high as possible.

3.2 **STRONG ARMS**: Re-engage your strong arms. They will tend to slacken as you focus hard on lifting up through your ankles and balancing on the toes so have some attention to continually keep arms activated.

3.3 **STEADY BODY WITH CHIN UP**: Maintain your focus in the mirror, at one place high on your body – eyes, third eye or throat for example. Your chin stays up parallel to the floor. Calm your breath and find your balance.

3.4 **SIT DOWN AND KEEP YOUR CHEST UP**: Inhale length; exhale, draw in your abdomen and sit down while keeping your feet in your heels-up-high position. Your chest stays high up off your legs, back parallel with the wall. Your spine will arch as you 'sit' and your pelvis tilts a little.

3.5 **LEGS PARALLEL**: Your knees face forward and your legs neither splay in nor out.

3.6 **WORK YOUR HEELS UP**: Resist your heels dropping at all. As soon as you feel your heels start to drop, stop, (you may have to slightly elevate your butt) work your heels back up and then lower your bottom again.

3.7 **PUSH INTO TOES, LEAN INTO ANKLES**: Work flexibility into your feet. Push into your toes and not the balls of your feet. For best results, the more weightily you lean into your ankles, the easier this pose will become. Eventually you will create a straight line from your (bent) toes, through your ankles, to the knees.

3.8 **THIGHS JUST HIGHER THAN KNEES**: To direct more weight into your ankles your hips should be slightly higher than your knees.

3.9 **RELEASE**: Inhale as you push up through the toes. Exhale to lower your heels back to the ground. Arms stay strong, feet stay apart; ready for Part 3.

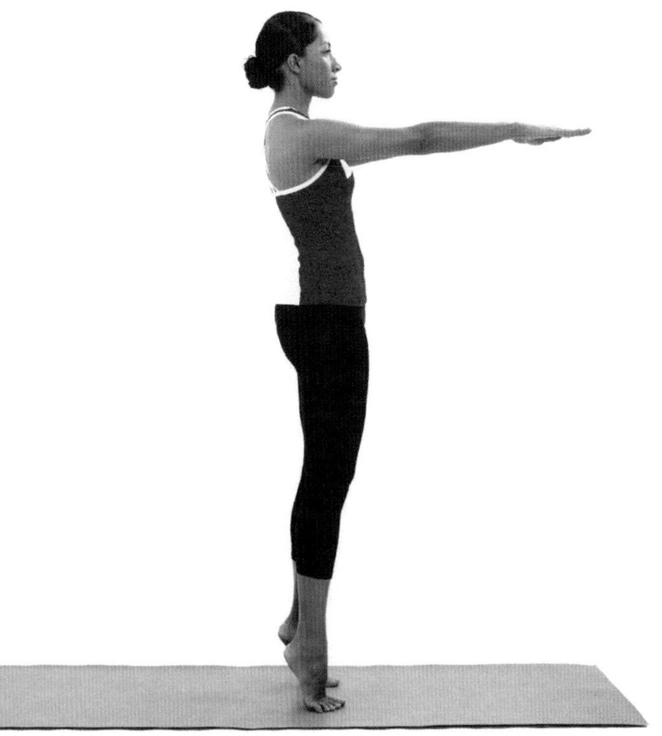

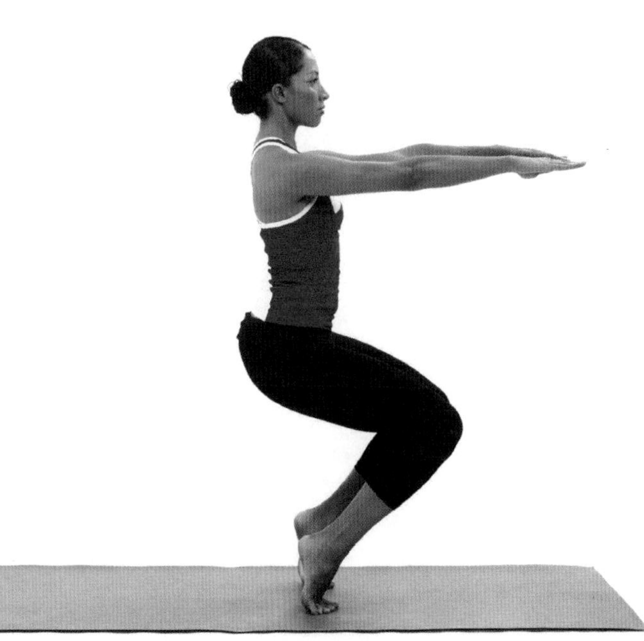

Utkatasana

Awkward Pose

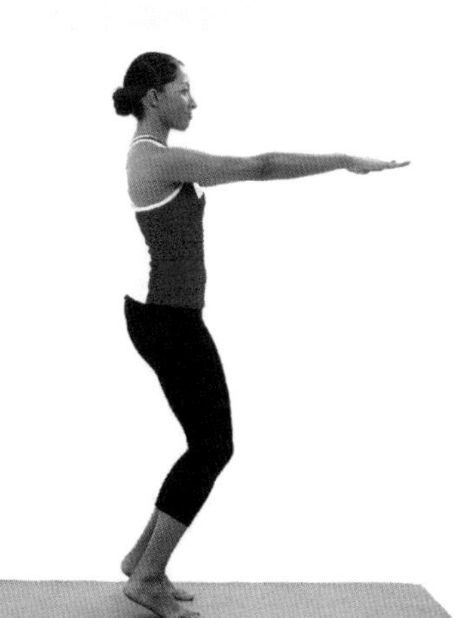

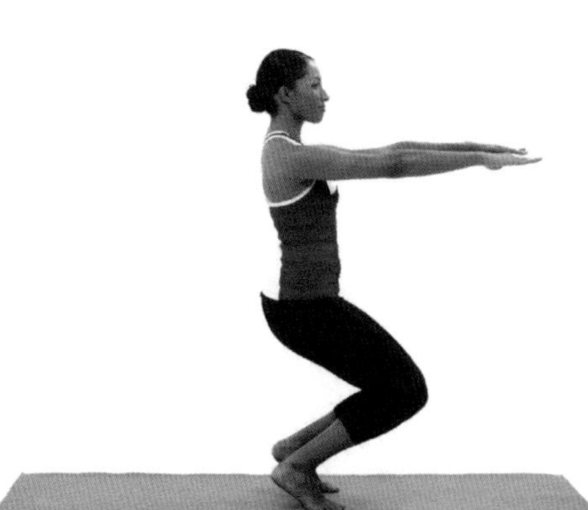

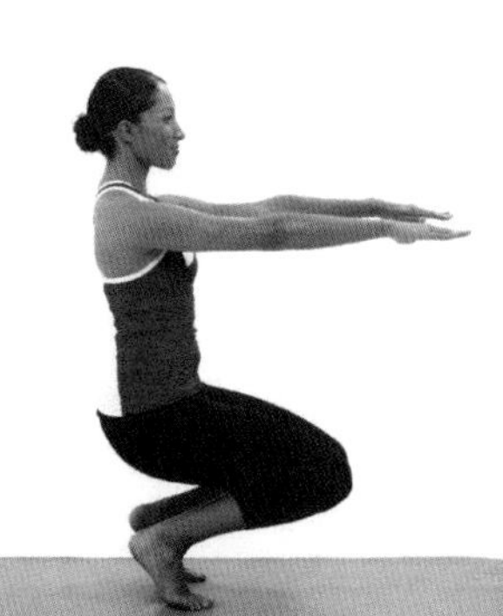

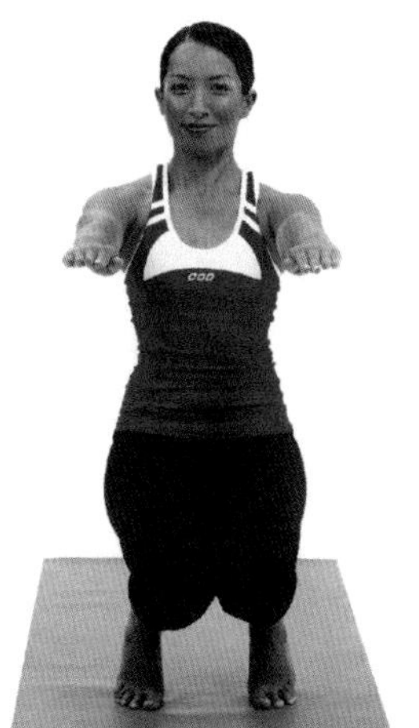

Tip for Part 2

This tip safely improves your ankle flexibility. Sit at the edge of a chair, couch or even a toilet with your toes contacting the floor. With your bottom strongly supported you can now raise your heels and strongly weight your ankles forward.

Literally lean all your weight into your toes to open up both toes and ankles. This is easy without the distraction of balance and will go a long way to improve your physical yoga practice.

Part 3 Utkatasana

4.1 **Recommit Your Arms**: Strengthen and lengthen your arms. Keep them strong from the get-go 'til you release.

4.2 **Knees Together**: Inhale length into your torso and as you exhale, bring your knees together and squeeze them very strongly. Allow your heels to come up off the floor creating a small gap the width of a finger or two.

4.3 **Slide Your Body Down**: Take another breath. Exhale, engage your core and start to lower your straight, lengthened and VERTICAL spine down as slowly as you can, so that your hips come to within an inch or two (a few cms) of your heels. You must resist the forward movement of your body to keep your spine vertical.

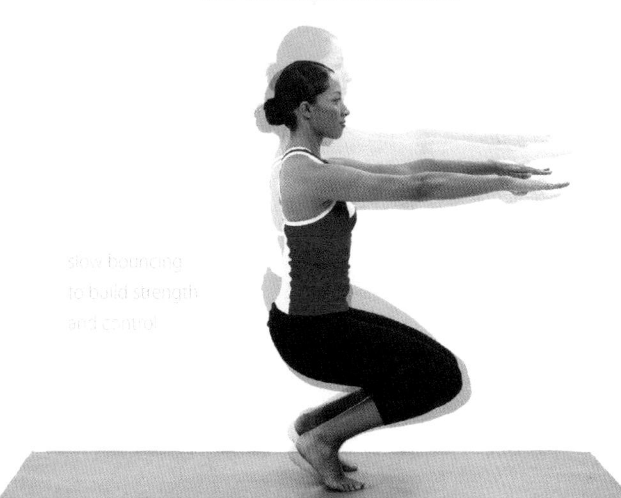

slow bouncing to build strength and control

Utkatasana

Awkward Pose

04

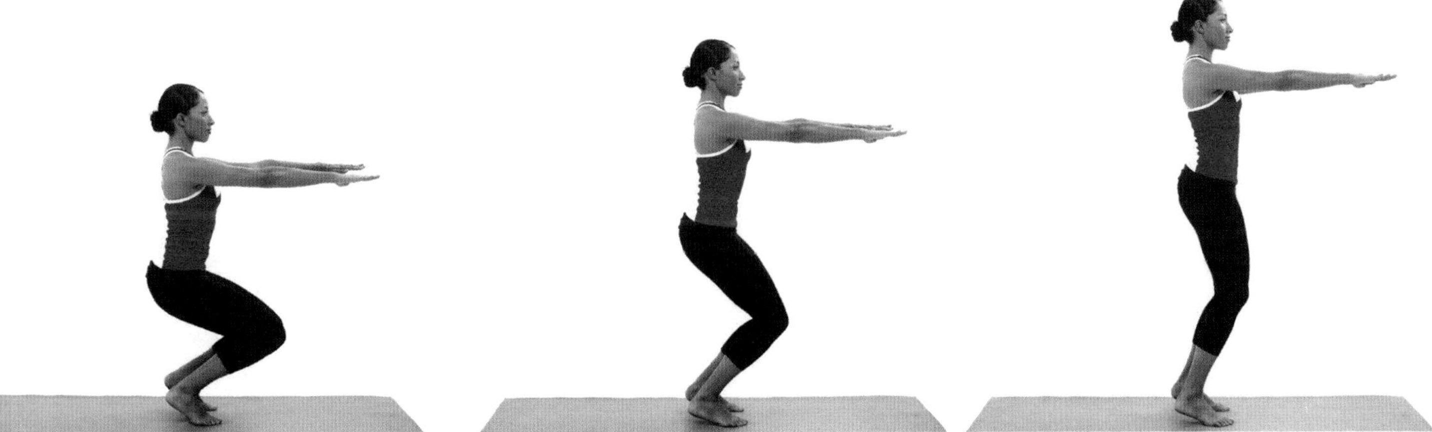

4.4 Knees And Inner Thighs Squeeze: You must keep your knees squeezing together all the time.

4.5 Heels Up: Your heels will come up off the floor. They have to, to keep your body vertical. Beginners: Always start with heels off the ground. As you become more flexible your heels may actually stay on the ground initially before descent.

4.6 Shoulders Positioned Correctly: Keep your shoulders down and back away from the ears. Position them directly above the hips – you may arch the spine.

4.7 Breathe: Keep the breath flowing. I find longer slower breaths makes the recruitment of strength in the arms and particularly the legs much easier.

4.8 All Actions Constant 'Til The End: Keep your chin up, chest up, bottom down, heels up, knees squeezed, arms strong 'til it is time to release. You are strengthening your adductor muscles in your thighs and supporting your torso on a strong foundation to build your core muscles.

4.9 Grow Your Strength: You are asked to take 10 seconds to ascend and descend or sometimes simply to take as long as possible. Don't get judgmental or fixated on how long it takes you. It can be extremely variable and depend on many prevailing physical and mental factors. Try to lengthen the time it takes to get into and out of this exercise. Building strength will continue to happen while you descend and ascend as long as the knees keep squeezing together and the arms remain strong. The stronger you become the longer you will be able to keep your back up straight and vertical.

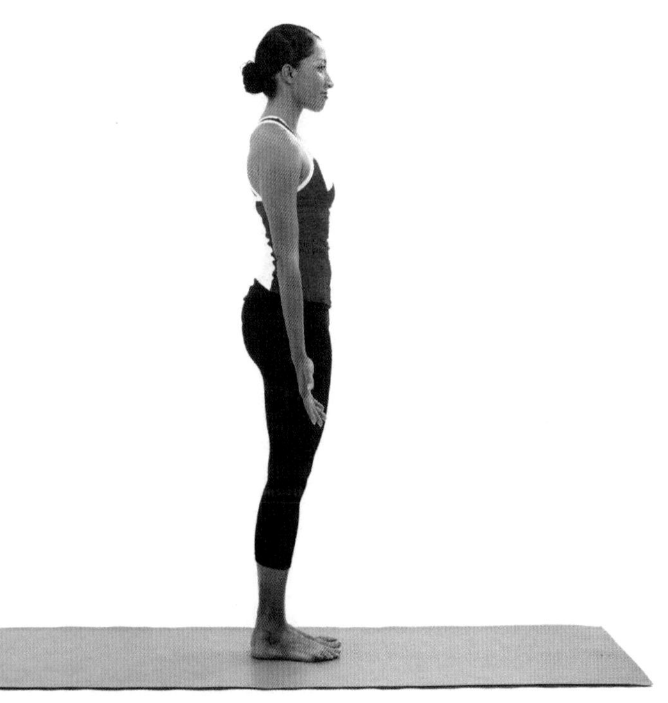

Bouncing

Scripted classes ask you to bounce before exiting Part 3. The danger is that you can risk great damage if done too fast. Only 'bounce' if you can slowly and deliberately move up and down 1-3 times (each movement takes about 1 whole second).

However I recommend this self-limiting and non-risky move: Recommit core engagement and squeezed knees, reactivate your arms and THEN raise up to a hover point above your heels. Your ability to raise up and then stay there will build that desired strength and control. You will exit from here. If your knees are weak then wait to attempt this element as building strength happens over time with practice of all poses.

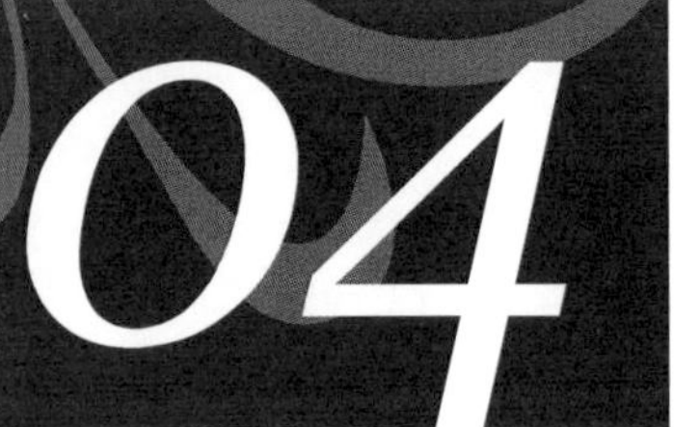

Utkatasana

AWKWARD POSE

Release

To release you need to take a big inhale, draw in your abdomen, engage your core muscles and on the exhale, start your ascent to completely reverse the movement. You absolutely must keep the arms strong, and above all keep the knees squeezing 'til you find your heels back on the floor and you are standing upright. Exhale your arms down to your side as you bring your feet back together again for your Savasana.

Common mistakes and how to fix them Part 1

Slack arms: Your ability to work this pose and balance is severely compromised with slack arms. Students commonly allow their arms to 'hang' from their shoulders, fingers dangle, with wrists barely engaged, arms slightly bent and forearms soft. This error is most commonly seen in young women who are typically quite flexible and lack upper (if not whole) body strength. They look good doing yoga but need concerted effort to build much needed body strength.

Lengthen and strengthen with a movement that starts with your correctly positioned shoulders. Activate your arms right through the elbows and wrists to the tips of your fingers.

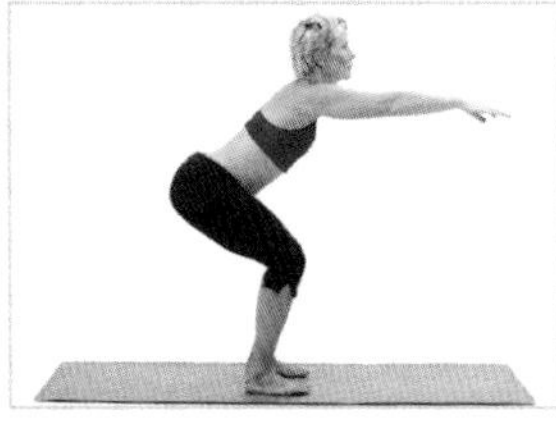

Bottom is up: When your bottom sticks up in the air, the weight quite comfortably falls evenly over the feet, even forward into the toes. The center of gravity is more over your knees and the pose becomes – dare I say – too easy! The students who are most likely to keep their bottoms high are the ones who feel a little silly looking as if they are doing flying superhero impersonations!

In order to feel your quadriceps muscles really working (to hold your body up) you need to have your thighs parallel to the floor. You are one of the minority if you look like you are sitting upright in a chair. Your lower spine flexibility is important here, but what seems to be more of a determinant in gaining depth is the flexibility of your ankles and general body strength.

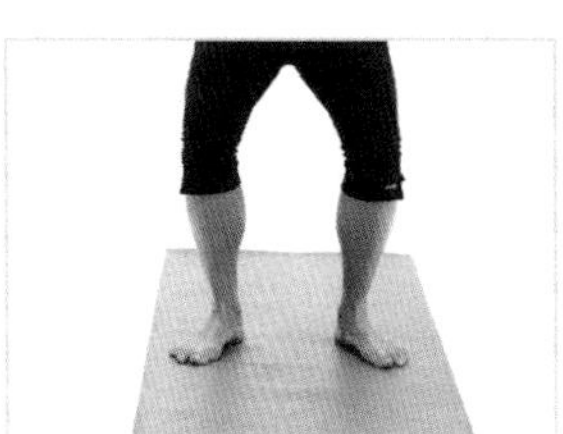

Fanning feet: When feet fan out to the side you can sit down lower and more easily but your hips will lose the opportunity to open. Resist this foot movement and keep feet parallel.

Weight in the toes, or heels up: If weight distribution is incorrect, your heels may even come up off the floor. Leave your feet flat and swing the weight backward into the heels. Try lifting your toes so that the balls of the feet stay planted.

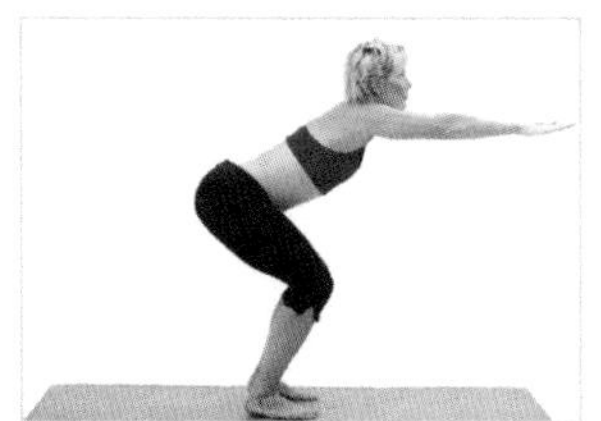

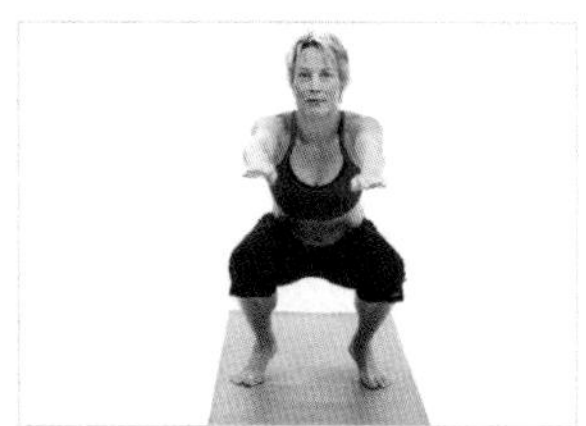

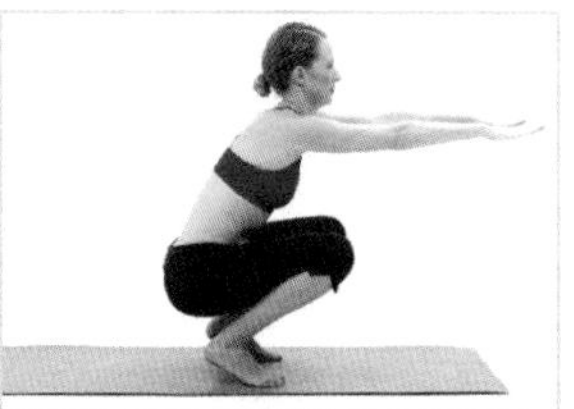

Sitting down too low: Avoid leaning on your haunches. It is possible to go too low in this pose. Some students even lift their heels up off the floor as if they are simply squatting. These two errors may be accompanied by fanning the feet outward. Both result from dropping the bottom and not lifting your chest up off your knees.

Common mistakes and how to fix them Part 2

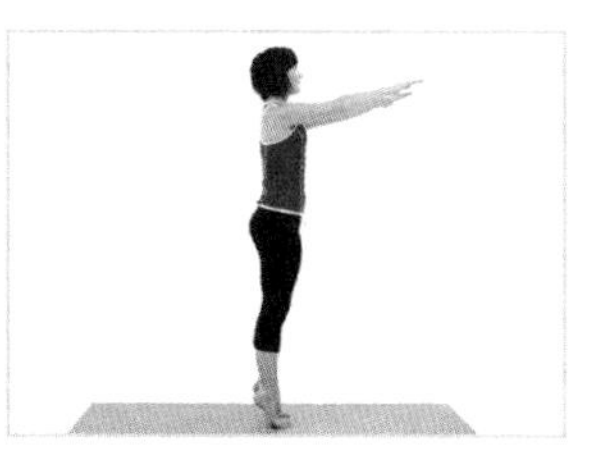

Everything goes up: Often newcomers to hot yoga will rise up onto their toes with an accompanied upward movement of their shoulders and arms. The arms slacken and come up about 10 to 20 degrees during set-up. Simply drop the arms enough to see the tops of your forearms. Keep them parallel and strong, and squeeze your shoulders down and back.

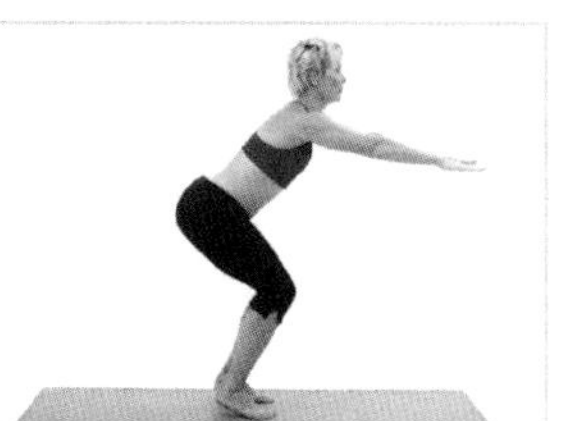

Heels drop: Often the heels drop as the bottom descends. Simple logic indicates that you should be able to keep your heels as high as you had them on your set-up. Be conscious of driving weight through the ankles the toes and not the balls of the feet. Lifting your chest will help recruit your quadriceps muscles into action. Improving leg and core strength will yield results over time.

Arms slacken: See Part 1 mistakes. Activate your arms fully to fingertips and squeeze your shoulders down and back.

Body comes forward:

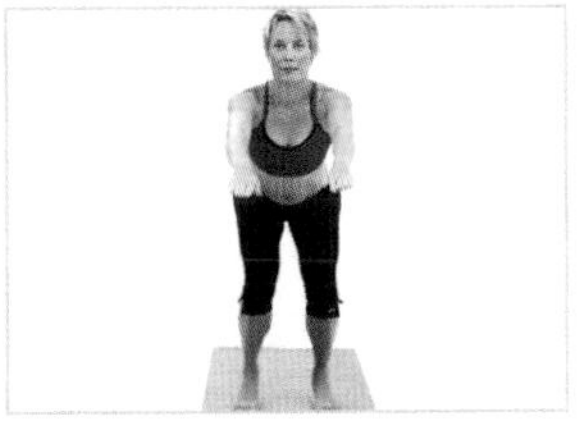

The body should remain upright, parallel to the wall. Arching your spine against activated arms will help. It counterbalances the force pushing forward through your ankles. This error is hard to fix during the pose. Better to re-work your descent.

Thighs lower than knees: The thighs are never lower than your knees. Otherwise the center of gravity shifts backwards, the heels drop and the balls of the feet get weighted.

Common mistakes and how to fix them Part 3

Knees separate: Students may find it difficult to squeeze knees together the whole time, often descending with them hovering close, but not together. It is a question of safety so please, ensure your knees not only touch, they squeeze. This is crucial for bolstering support for your spine and knees and building leg strength.

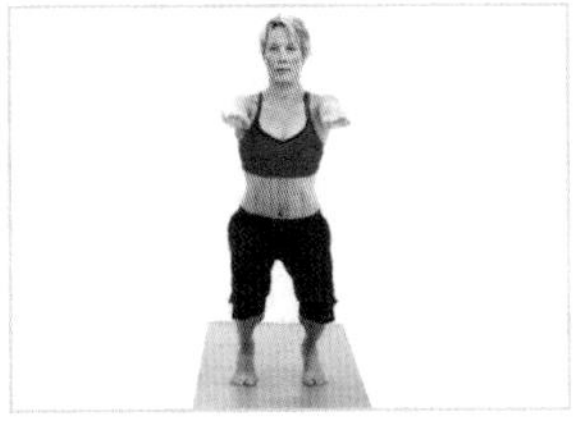

In the early stages of practice, or even after a break away from hot yoga, if your quadriceps muscles are feeling weak then modify your speed of descent to ensure contact. You may have to speed it up a little rather than experience muscle 'failure'. Or descend less far and work on regaining your strength from practicing other poses. Tomorrow is another day.

Heels stay down:

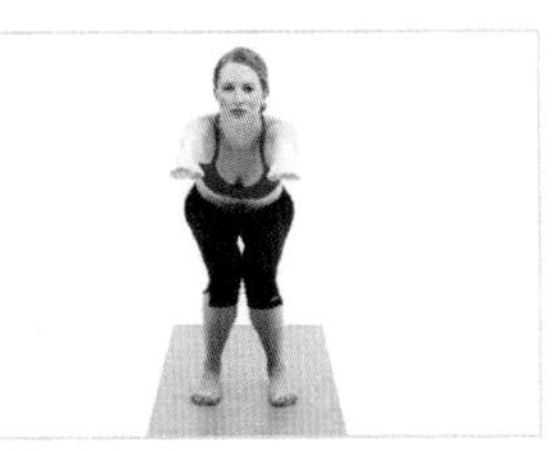

Newcomers either neglect to lift heels off the ground in set-up or lay them back down on the floor as they descend. They end up doing something like the Part 1 pose with their bottom out backward and their chest forward.

The 'trick' here is to set up with the heels just off the ground. Then, focus totally on squeezing the knees and sliding your straight back down in a completely vertical fashion (whether this translates 100% to ideal pose or not). As a result no thought will need to be given to the heels at all.

Arms slacken: It is extremely difficult to lower your body vertically if your arms lack energy.

Knees too high or you're resting on your calves:

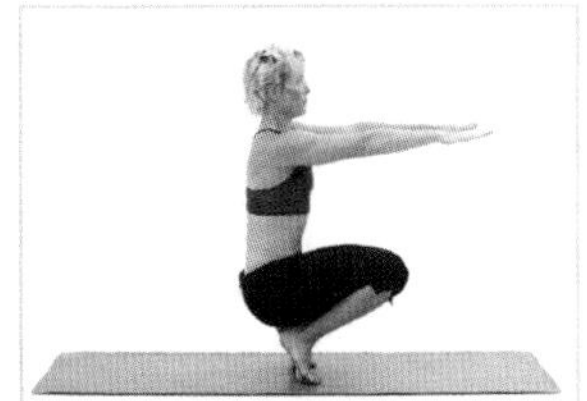

Finishing your pose with your knees higher than your hips means that your arms and legs were insufficiently activated during descent. In such cases you end up squatting with your hamstrings resting on your calves, your leg muscles unable to resist gravity. Sometimes you will find yourself here because you simply have no more energy resources.

When the knees are too high, attention may be needed in several areas. Check whether your heels started off the floor; or if you need to engage your core or arms or squeeze the knees more. Your aim is to build sufficient strength to hover with space between the upper and lower parts of your legs, your hips slightly higher than your knees. This will also greatly aid your exit.

A note about arms:

In all likelihood each set (comprising all 3 parts) takes about 2 minutes. As such it is impossible to recruit 100% of the fibers of your arms' muscles and keep them strong 100% of the time. Naturally it will require periodic commitment and recommitment. At the very least it will help you to ensure that the arms remain consciously and mindfully strong for the entry, pose and exits of each part.

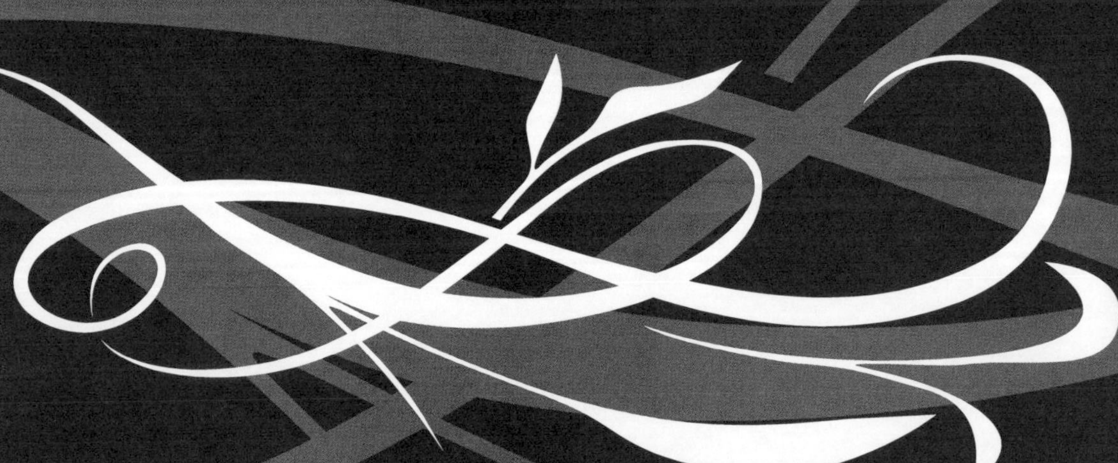

Garudasana

It takes as much courage to have tried and failed as it does to have tried and succeeded.
—Anne Morrow Lindbergh

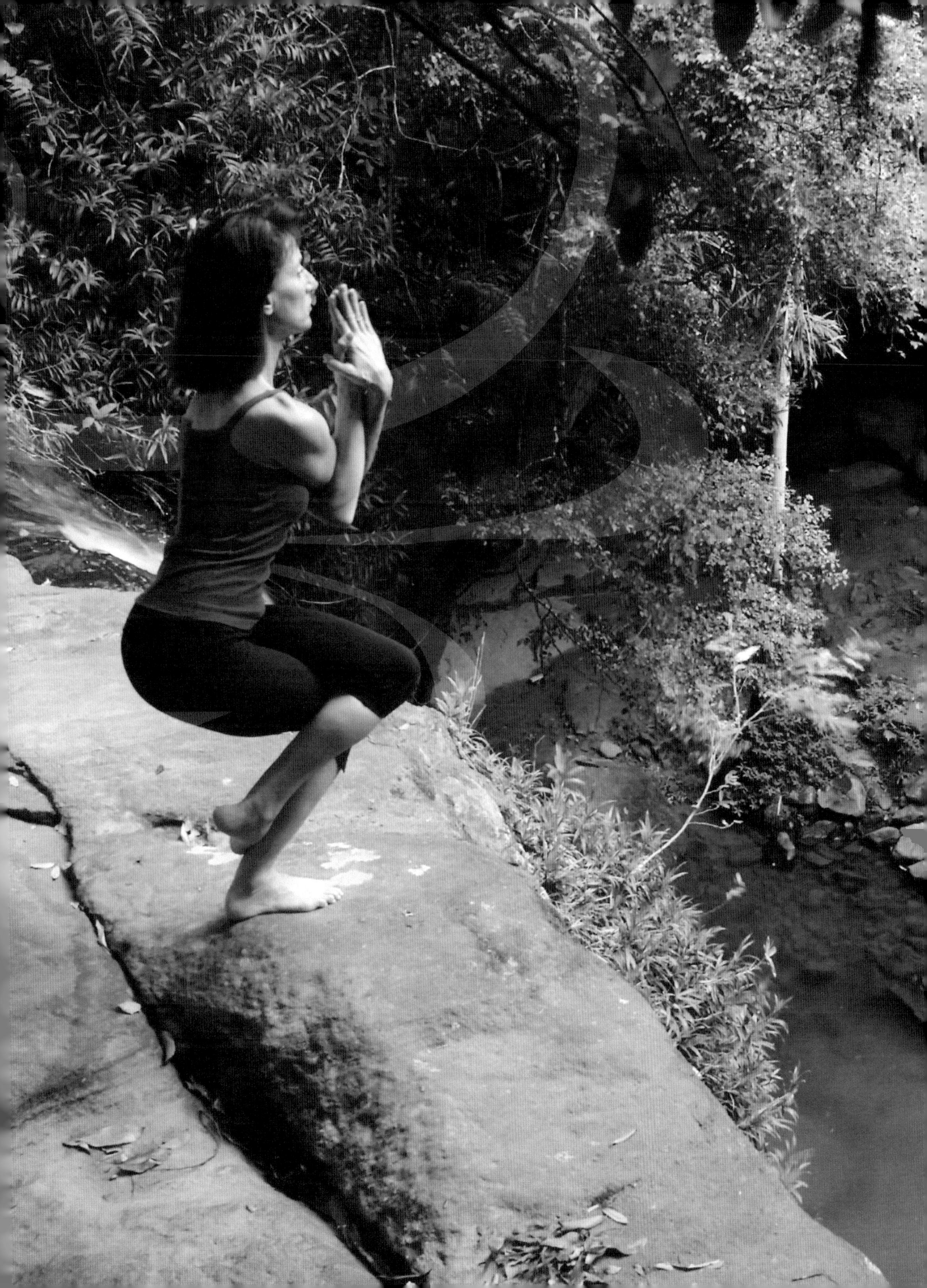

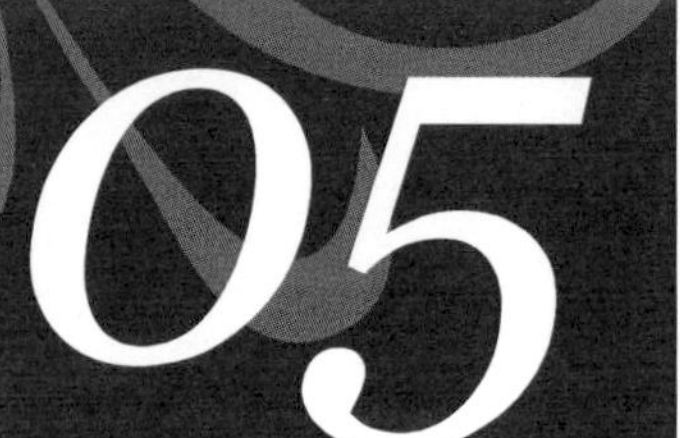

Garudasana

Eagle Pose

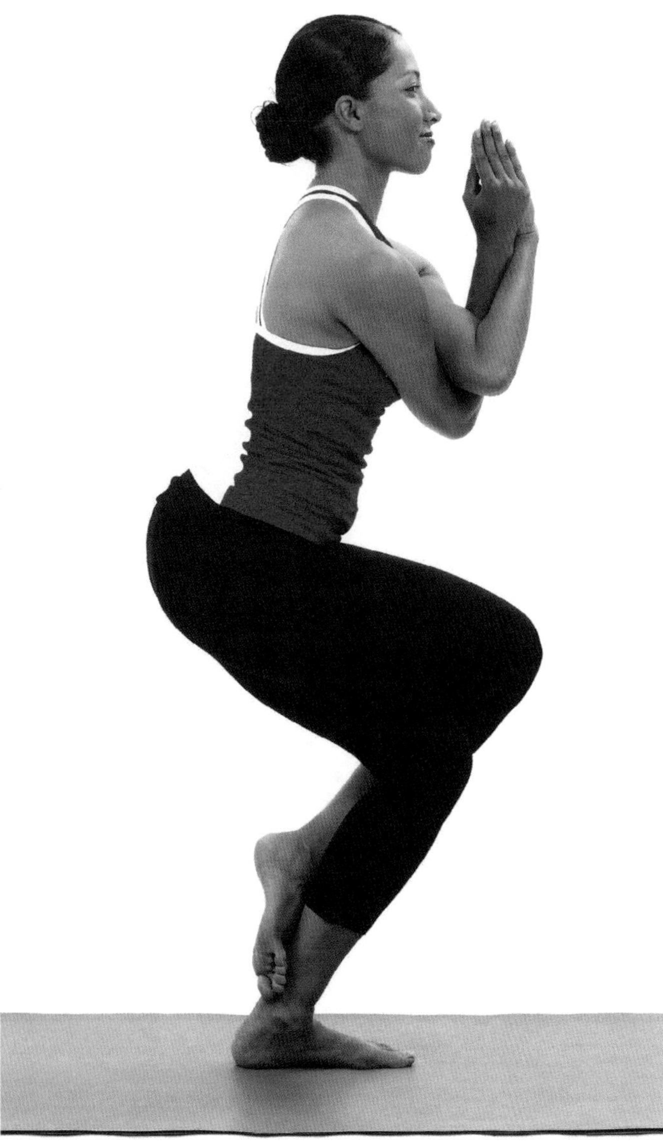

The essentials

Eagle is often jokingly referred to as a 'pretzel' type pose. It warms up the large leg and arm muscles in readiness for the rest of class. Said to improve your sex life, Garudasana limits blood flow around the sexual organs, while your legs and arms are twisting. Simultaneously there is deep stretching through the shoulders and hips creating more flexible joints. Eagle pose is particularly good for opening ankles, knees, wrists and shoulders.

What makes this pose so difficult to get right?

Got any tight parts in your body? Well, if you don't know, then Eagle will diagnose them for you! Injury, short muscles, tight joints, bulky biceps and thighs will make this one all the more challenging. The geometry of the intertwined legs and arms with the body sitting down low, while trying to keep the chest up high, makes for an interesting journey.

The set-up is crucial to this pose and will determine the depth to which you can go. Most students will sit their bodies as low as they can when they set up. Surprisingly keeping your upper body perched high while bending the knees with strong even foot weighting will paradoxically allow you to sit lower in the final pose.

Garudasana

Eagle Pose

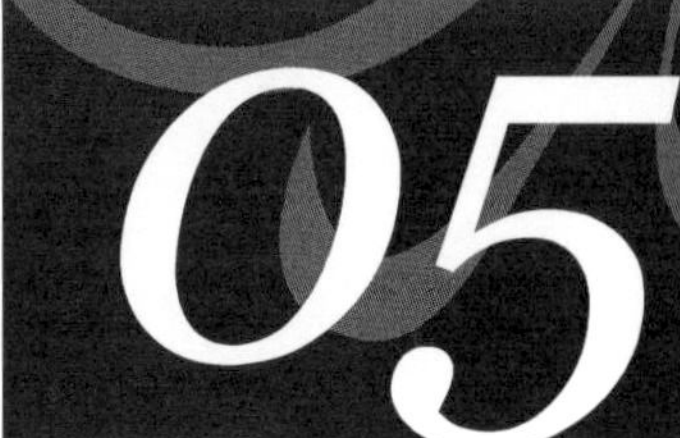

The technique

The set-up

Eagle is usually approached in 2 stages. You set up the arms and sit down. Then you set the legs in place, balancing on one foot and work the depth. Start with shoulders down and back, palms forward. The feet are together. Inhale and bring your arms up over your head.

1.1 **Exhale And Swing Your Arms**: Swing your arms down in front of you. The right arm goes under the left. Cross them above the elbows and then cross them below the wrists.

1.2 **Hands Together In Prayer Position**: The 'trick' with the hands is to always keep the palms facing inward while the arms swing and cross. They will continue to face each other when the elbows bend and the hands come together in prayer position in front of the face. If you can't manage prayer position then interlock your fingers or get at least some contact between the hands. Grabbing hold of a thumb is a common technique.

1.3 **Sit Down Low With Heels Flat**: Sit low into your hips as you arch the spine to keep the chest up as high as possible. Try to position your shoulders directly over your hips as you stick your bottom out behind you. Both feet are firmly and evenly planted because your center of gravity is along a vertical axis: Your weight is pulled down through it, and not forward.

1.4 **Pull Arms Down**: With your arms intertwined pull them down toward your abdomen. Ensure you keep the chest up and open, and the shoulders down and back. The higher the chest is kept up, the better the alignment and the less adjustments mid-pose.

1.5 **It's Awkward**: Sitting down low in the hips feels 'awkward' but it is very stable. The hips are back, body up, arms wrapped, and feet flat on the floor.

The pose

2.1 **Start Strong And Stable**: You are stable and grounded down through both hips and both feet. Pull on your elbows without letting your hands fall forward – keep them close in to the face.

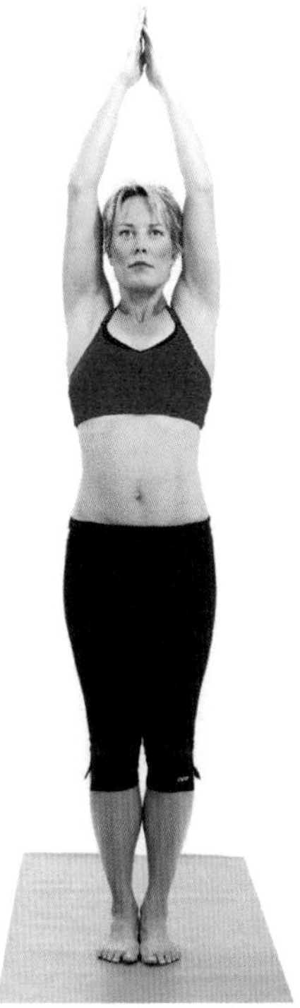

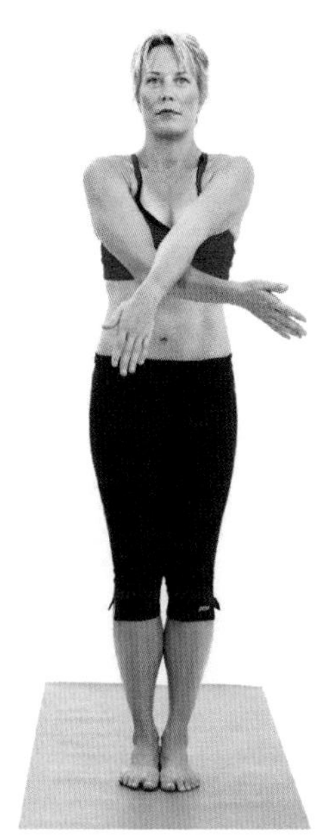

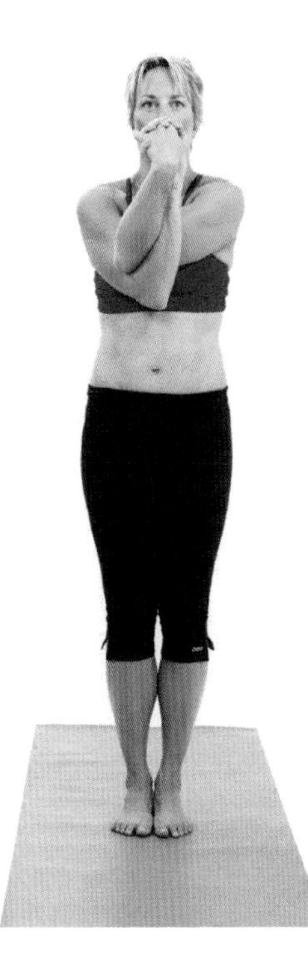

Garudasana

Eagle Pose

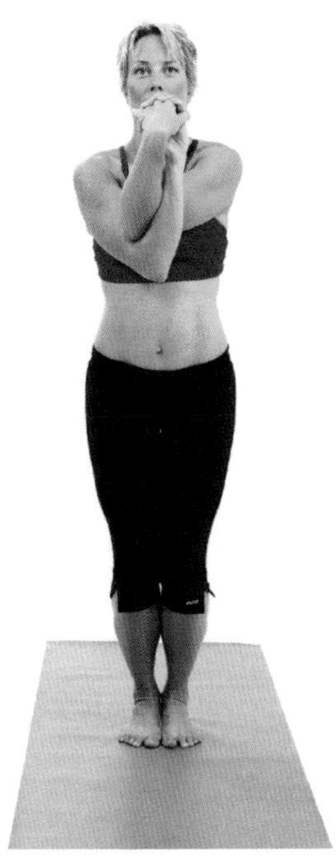

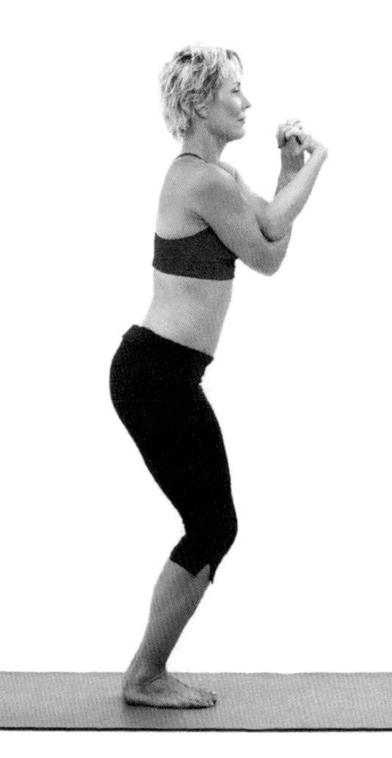

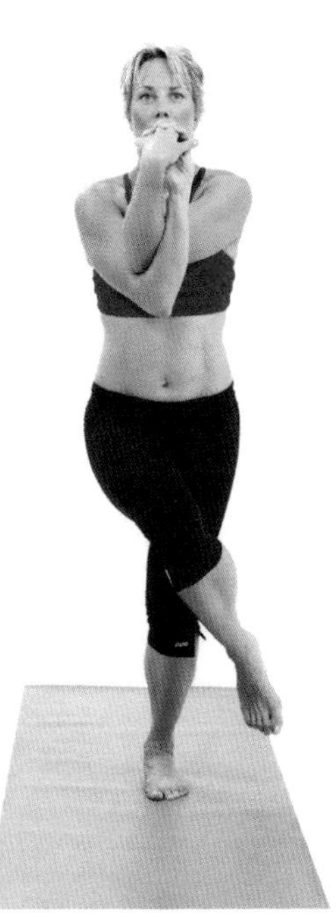

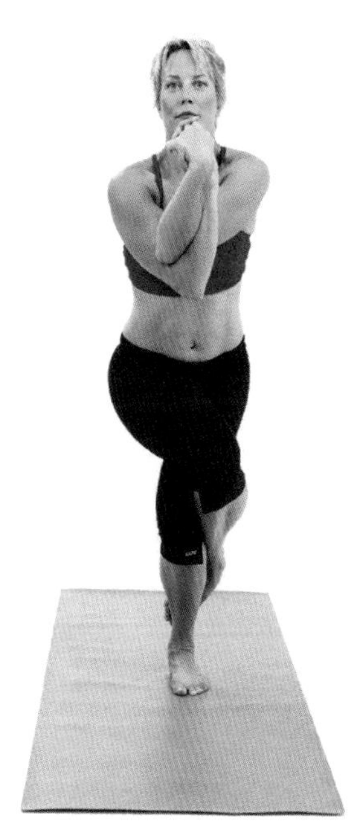

2.2 **Lift Your Leg And Wrap It Over And Around**: Only your right leg moves as you pick it up and wrap it over and around your left, bent, grounded leg. Your head and body stay still without raising even an inch. Aim to hook your toes behind your calf muscles.

2.3 **No Space Between The Legs**: Use insistent downward force to squash your upper leg onto your lower leg (which acts as a seat). Your foot slides down the back of the standing leg. Your strongest lower body compression happens when you have an airtight wrap with no gaps.

2.4 **Arms Continue To Work**: As you pull down on your elbows your shoulders work themselves back and down. This helps you center and balance yourself. Feel the tension-dissolving stretches through your neck and shoulders.

2.5 **Arch The Spine And Sit Down Low**: Imagine you are sliding your vertical spine down a wall. Keep your chin up, chest up, bottom down as you continually arch your spine. Allow the seating and pulling forces to work along with gravity. Direct the energy vertically through your supporting ankle to optimally open your hips and ankles.

2.6 **Square And Level Alignment, Stack The Joints**: Stacking your joints in a vertical line between nose and toes will align your body squarely to the mirror and floor. Some teach shifting the knees or arms in opposite directions. However, I have found the best way to describe this: Square your hips off to the mirror. Doing this creates a better outcome by also and more importantly enabling you to easily lift your chest (back) up.

2.7 **Keep The Weight Back**: Shift the balance of weight to your heel. It helps to arch the spine, which keeps the chest up.

It is no surprise that students with very flexible ankles do very well in this pose to keep their chests up and sit down low, low, low. If that is not you, then keep leaning into your lower leg to help open up your ankles and routinely bring the chest up and weight back to keep you from collapsing forward. These are very deliberate yet subtle movements.

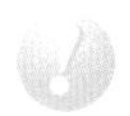 Release

As you exhale for the last time, sit down as low as you can, while pulling on your elbows and keeping the chest up. Feel that sliding sensation as you sit close to your ankle. On your inhale start to straighten up, uncross your legs, and then your arms and swing them back up over your head. Now exhale and swing the left arm under the right as you enter left side Eagle directly from your arms-up position without any break. Correspondingly, after you sit down, your left leg is lifted to position itself over the right.

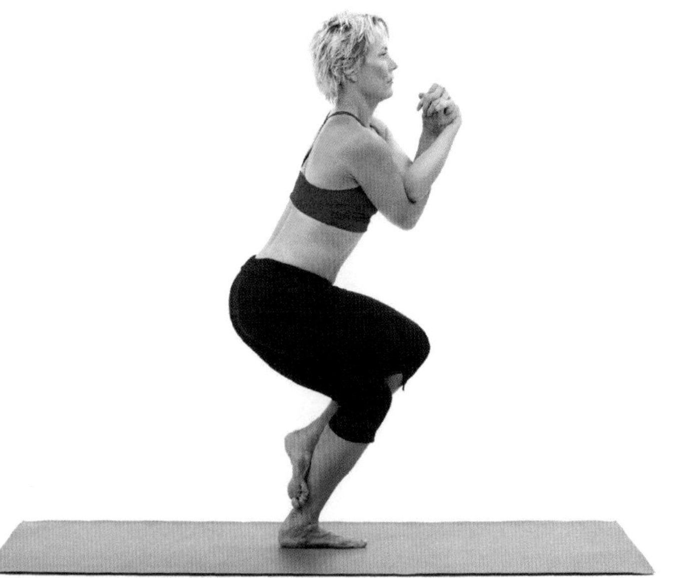

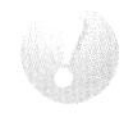 Second set

This is one pose where both sides and both sets follow on from each other. With your first set finished, you will continue directly into the first side again without rest. Cycle through 2 sets of Eagle and finish with a standing Savasana.

 To drink or not to drink?

After finishing Garudasana, most teachers offer a break to collect yourself before moving on to Standing Balancing poses. Some tell you to take a drink and others not. The important thing is that at this stage your body is warmed up. You are mindful of your yoga practice, your breath, you are connecting with yourself in the mirror, and ready to go on.

I always ask my students to be conscious of their decisions at this point. If you ritually reach for a water bottle, then resist this habit and become more mindful of your needs. Is it that you need to drink, or is it that you are using the activity as a means to distract yourself from what is really going on? Perhaps you divert your eyes and attention so that you don't have to stand there with your own company looking in the mirror. Sometimes this simple action can make us feel the most vulnerable – the inability to confront ourselves in the mirror. Just be, there is nothing else to do between the postures but breathe. Take that literally and figuratively and make tremendous spiritual, mental, physical and emotional breakthroughs.

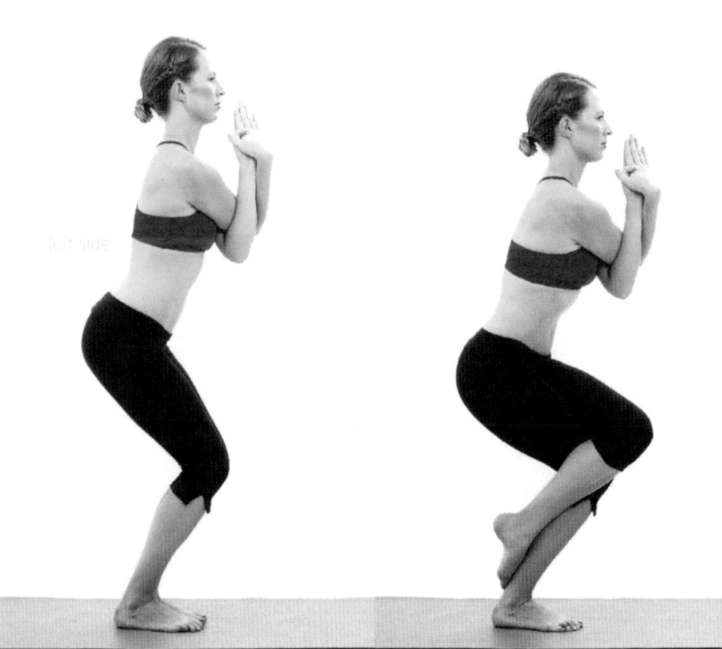
left side

Garudasana

EAGLE POSE

Common mistakes and how to fix them

Can't get the arms wrapped: Capabilities vary enormously when trying to get the wrap. While some barely manage to cross the arms above the elbows, the most common difficulty is getting the hands to come together, even to touch. Maybe bulk is getting in your way, or muscle or joint tightness.

Do what you can to approach your hands and eventually your palms together. Try to get some purchase on the arms to pull the elbows down towards your belly. You may have to grab a thumb, a finger or maybe even use a small towel to provide the purchase and pull.

many acceptable hand positions

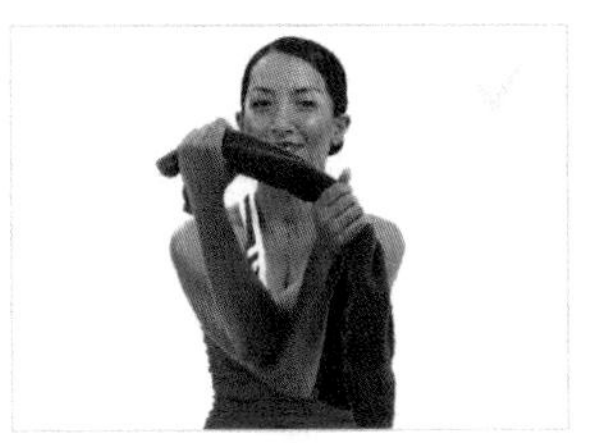

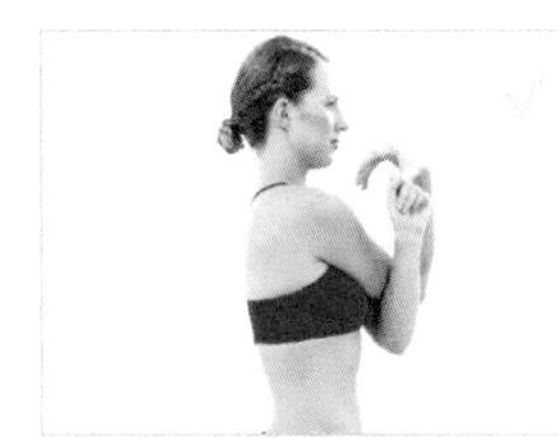

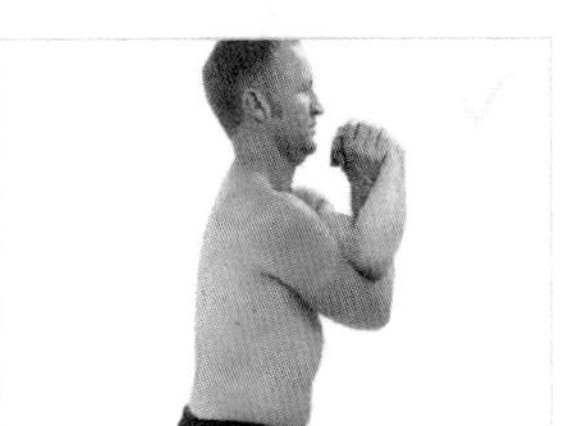

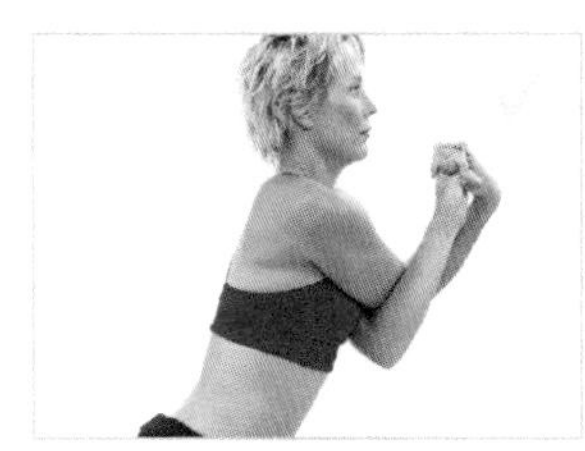

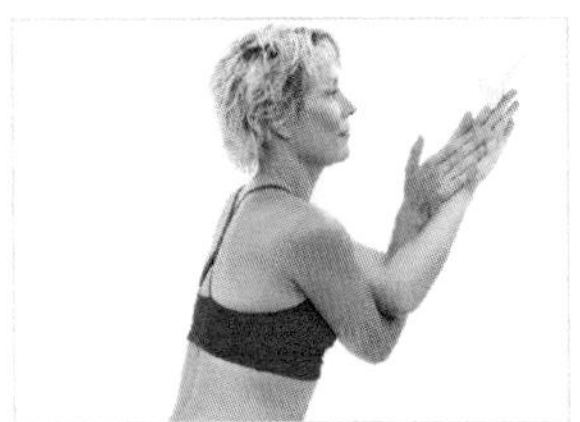

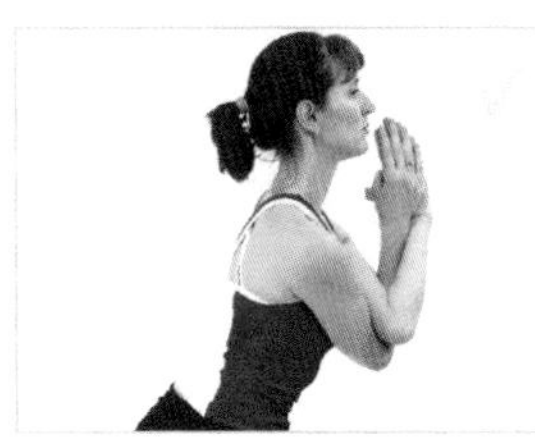

Can't grip your hands together in prayer position: No problem, just try to get some grip between the 2 hands. Perhaps only the index finger will just barely reach the thumb. Or the lower hand only reaches half way up on the palm. If you can interlock your fingers at all, then try to 'wrestle' your arms down into a more secure position. You may find yourself now able to reach prayer position. If not, just keep your fingers interlocked.

Can't get the legs wrapped: Join the club! Most people can't get the full wrap. It doesn't matter. Have the right intention, alignment and do the work!

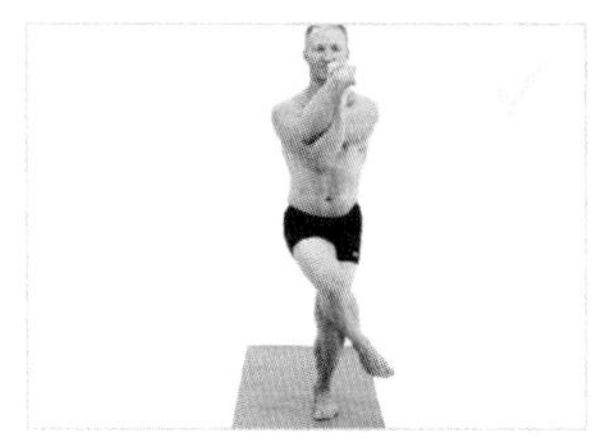

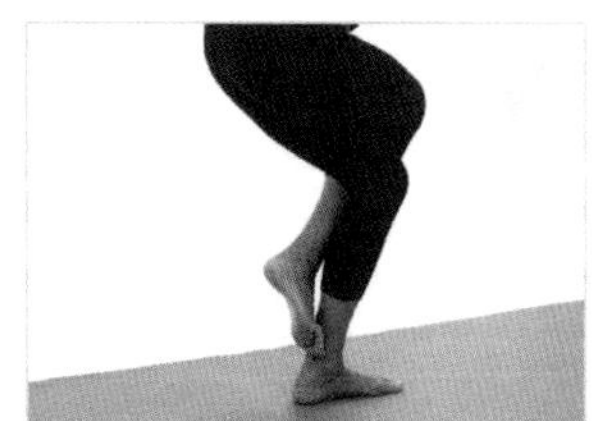

The wrap ranges from:

- Knees barely crossed with a leg waving in the air
- to a kind of squat, body forward, crossed knees and the leg pointing down
- To a toe hooked around the back near the Achilles tendon, not quite poking around
- To a full wrap with no space between the legs (good compression) and the foot behind the ankle and toes visible in the mirror.

Standing leg doesn't bend: Many new inflexible students straighten the standing leg when trying to hook their toes around behind. Set up by keeping the chest high and sit low and keep it there. Don't let your head bob up when you lift and wrap your leg.

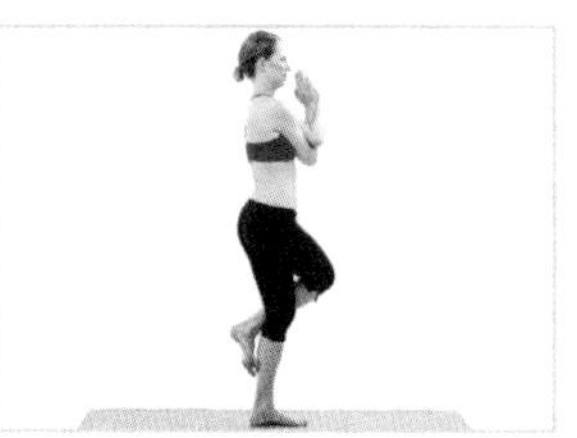

What if you are super-flexible?: The very flexible just work harder at sitting as low as they possibly can. Keep shoulders over hips, solid central alignment and a tight wrap, no gaps.

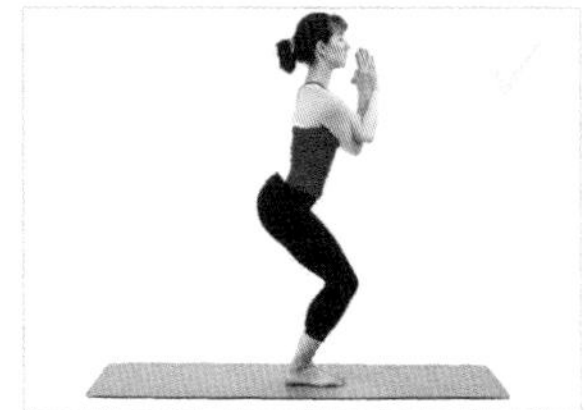

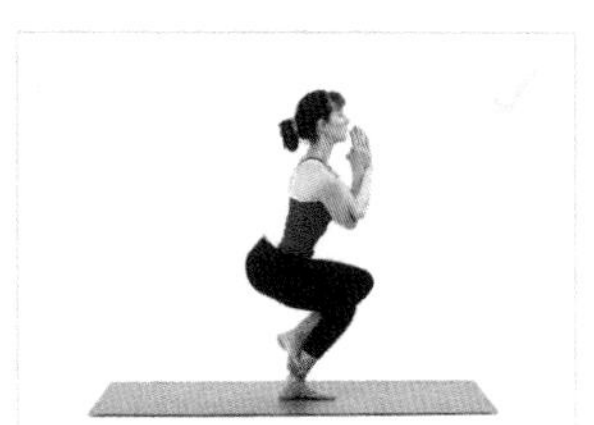

Shifting weight: Many students lift one leg off the ground and consciously place their weight on what will be the balancing leg, for even a moment before starting the leg wrap. Never take the extra step of shifting your weight. It makes your hips uneven and may unnecessarily cause alignment and balance problems that require mid-pose corrections.

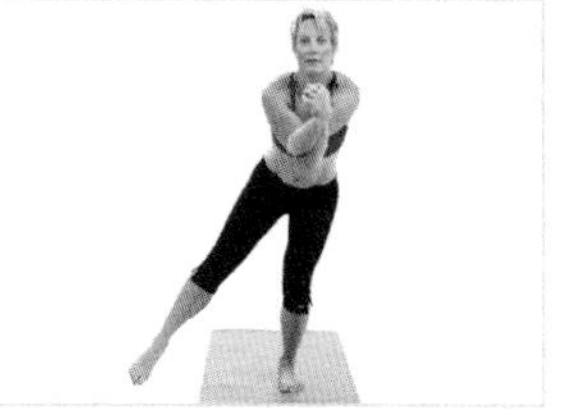

Garudasana

Eagle Pose

05

Ask yourself this if you need convincing: Do you really need to consciously shift your weight when you are lifting one leg up off the ground? One such leg-lifting movement is walking. Get up and place a thumb on top of each hip to take note of their relative positions. Take a few steps and notice how your hips stay even to the ground (barring some physical problem). Do it again, but consciously lean heavily into your hip as you place each foot down. It will remind you of an over exaggerated feminine-model-type jaunt.

Your skeletal structure is not the only system that holds your body up in space. Your muscles and your connective tissues are vital to scaffold the body into balance. This is a recurring issue in all one-legged poses.

Next time in class observe your hip positions and keep them stable. Your unconscious mind will take care of your balance. Sit down low, keep the chest up high and find your balance, on both feet. When entering the pose simply pick up your leg and wrap it over. You will balance more easily and have less corrections. Allow your body's own intelligence to guide you through.

Sitting down the wrong way: Many students set up with their hips too low hinging the body forward at the hips and hovering over their thighs. They believe sitting low will make it easier to go deeper in the final pose. It doesn't seem like a big mistake. However renegotiating good alignment is practically impossible from here. It involves getting the body back up again, before being able to lower your bottom closer to the heels.

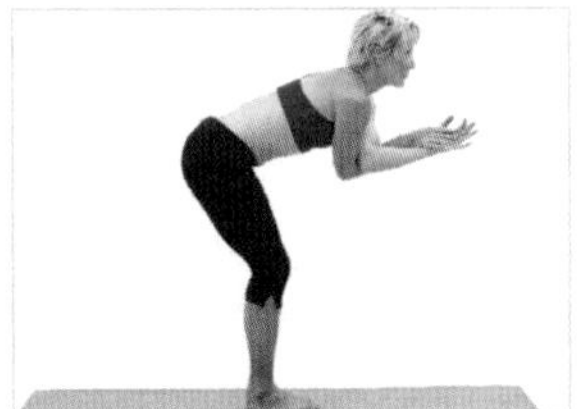

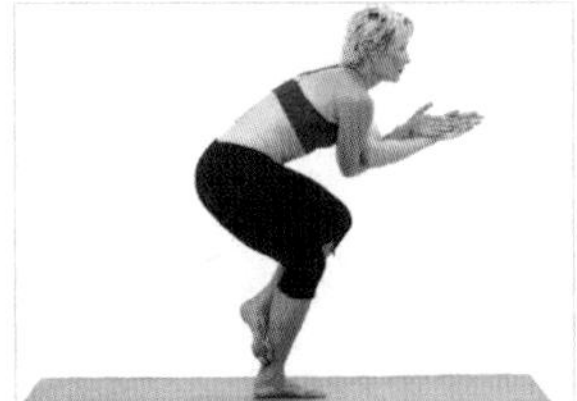

Avoiding the problem is easy: 'Measure twice, cut once.' Keep the weight evenly distributed over both feet as you sit down as low as you can into your hips. You must leave your chest up high and resist any forward body movement. Pull on your elbows and preserve correct shoulder position. Feel your spine arch, stick your bottom out backwards.

Set up your alignment and then work the depth. You won't be able to sit down as low as before, but I guarantee that you will find it far easier to sit down much further after the wrap. Your body literally slides down vertically, holding its correct alignment.

Any injuries or muscle tightness may make it impossible to enter the pose unless you bend forward. This happens. Do what you can keeping the above points a priority. Hips down, chest up, wrap. Don't force the knees.

Rounded spine, pulling the shoulders and elbows forward: Rounding your spine can be a result of incorrect set-up or pulling on the elbows incorrectly. The shoulders will be pulled down and forward:

1) If the upper arms come away from the chest
2) If the forearms come away from the upper arms and
3) If there is incorrect scapular movement. To position your shoulder blades down and back, arch the spine and pull your elbows down and in toward your abdomen.

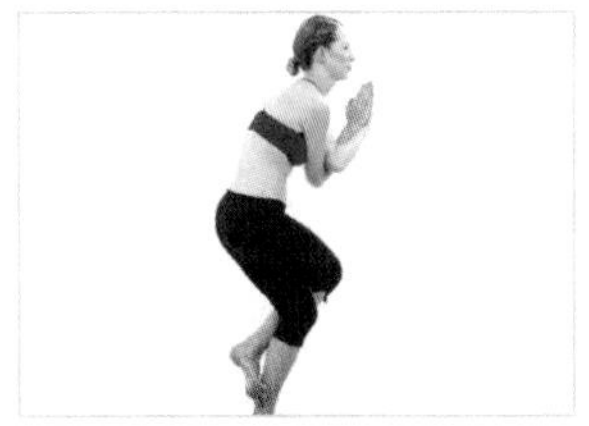

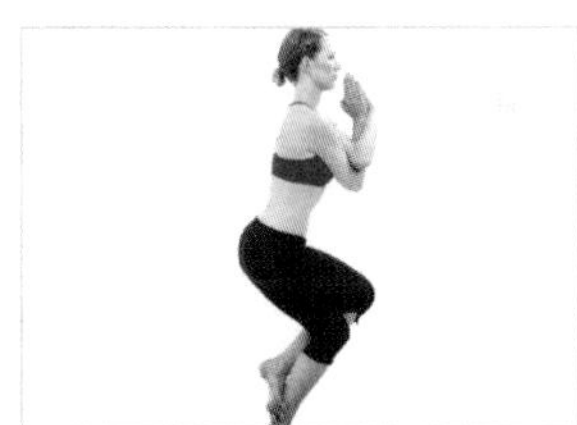

Body collapses forward, hips misaligned: Tight or injured bodies that can't go deep, often collapse forward and in their effort to deepen the pose, allow their hips to go off asymmetrically. The forces on the body become imbalanced. The only way is to retreat, move the chest up and square off!

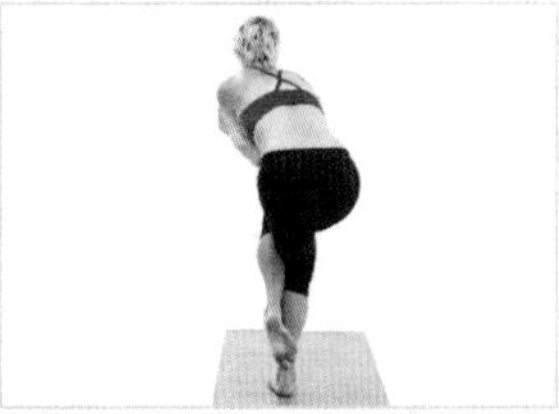

Legs and arms shift to opposite sides: Centrally stacking the joints can be a challenge. When wrapping the right leg over top, the knees tend to point left. Your body tries to balance out by moving your arms to the right. To fix: Focus on squaring the hips. You will avoid the confusion of moving legs and arms in opposite directions. Your body's own intelligence will create the gross correction and restore balance. Making the final refinements in stacking the joints will now happen more easily.

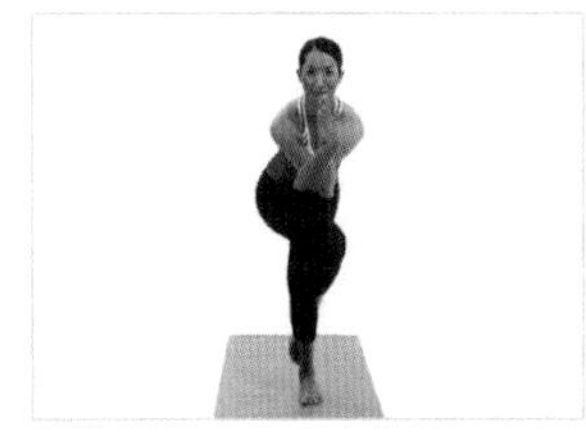

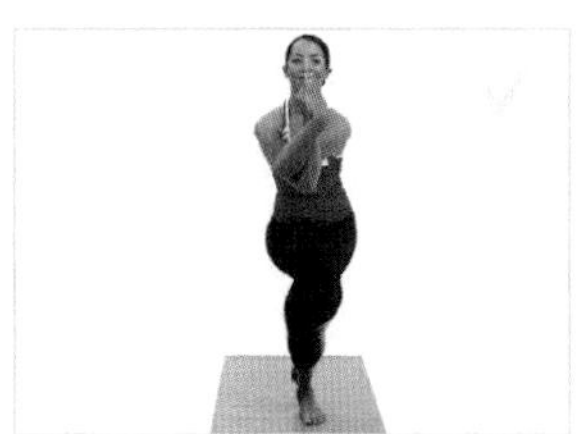

Shifting weight into the toes: Often tight bodies hinge at the hips with the body forward instead of upright. The toes take more of the weight, the chest drops and the hips actually start to lift, straightening the lower leg. Move the chest up, square off and sit down as you weight the foot evenly.

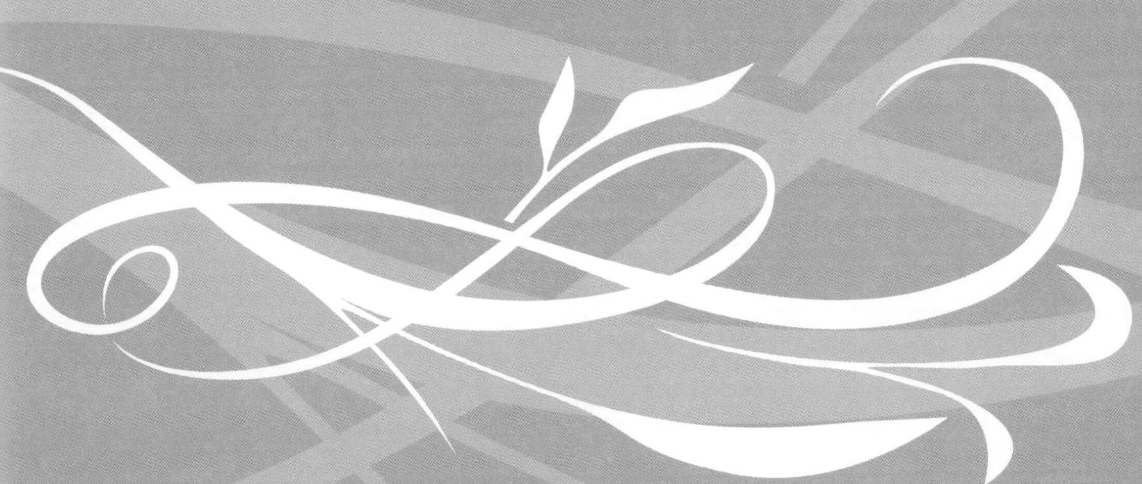

Dandayamana Janushirasana

Excellence is an art won by training and habituation. We do not act rightly because we have virtue or excellence, but we rather have those because we have acted rightly. We are what we repeatedly do. Excellence, then, is not an act but a habit.
—Aristotle

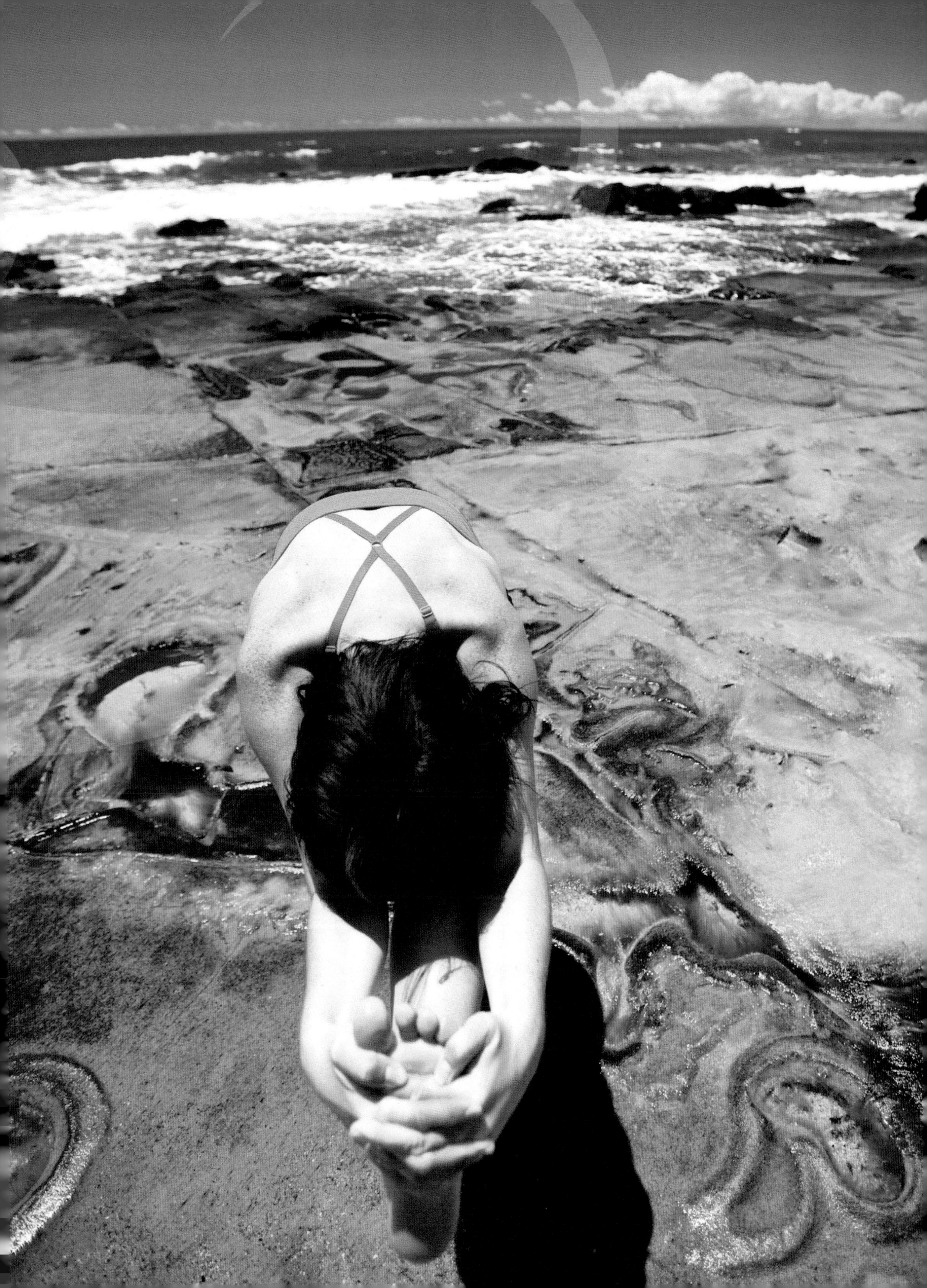

06 Dandayamana Janushirasana

Standing Head to Knee

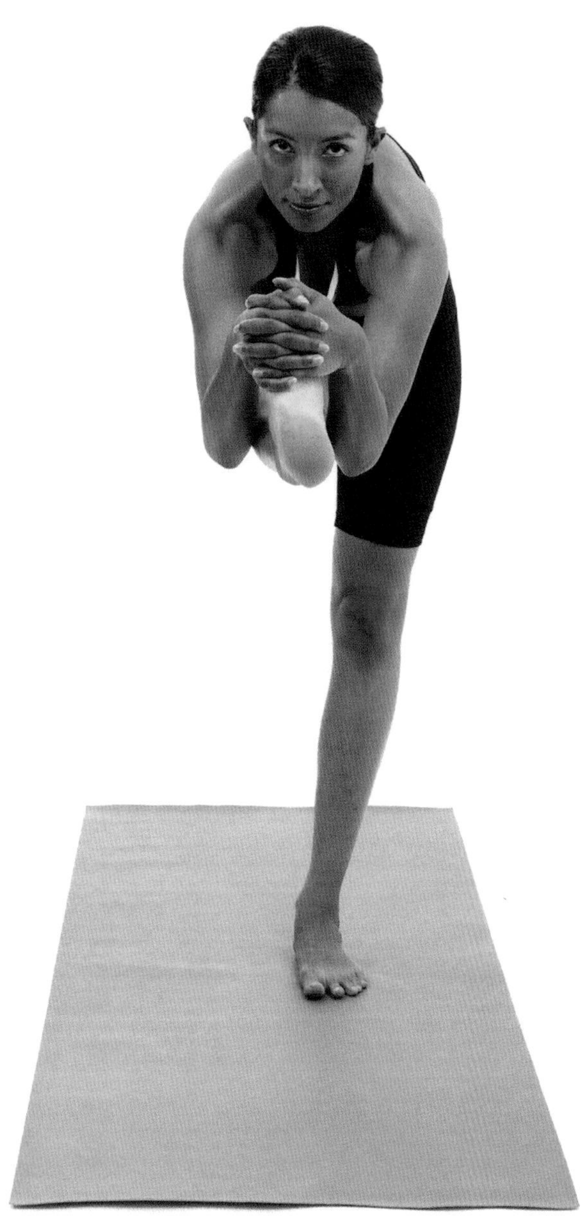

The essentials

Although we have worked hard up to now (and let's face it – it's hard *not* to work hard in a hot yoga class!) it isn't usually until this point – after your mini-break – that somehow we feel that the work is just beginning. The strong cardiovascular poses are just around the corner. All that stamina, focus and concentration and standing on one leg. Until you have done a hot yoga class it is hard to believe that yoga could possibly raise your heart rate sufficiently to be classed as cardiovascular exercise. How could this be – while you are standing still? We, the hot yoga cognoscenti know better!

This pose requires tremendous commitment and recommitment. It is, after all, difficult to stand in a single position for a whole minute and completely lock out the big muscles in one leg, while simultaneously rounded over with the other foot in your hands. It requires a controlled steady breath, calm and still body and therefore a calm and still mind, persistence and stamina, a strong core, and a steady gaze.

What makes this pose so difficult to get right?

Split into 4 distinct 'Parts' (which lead you to the position indicated by its name) Standing Head to Knee challenges you to be extremely mindful of your abilities so that you appropriately push yourself to the next stage and, at the same time remove your ego from the equation. Otherwise you will find yourself striving to get past a point where you can no longer maintain all the foundational and strength-giving aspects of this pose. Most students will not have the physical ability to get past stages 1 and 2. Most students will at some time, neglect or disregard the signs and progress beyond where they ought to be, or worse skip a stage altogether. Let's take a look at this very important process.

Dandayamana Janushirasana

Standing Head to Knee

The technique

At the end of your break, stand with your feet together, knees facing forward, hips square, arms externally rotated, shoulders down and back. If you have bunions, please adjust your feet to stop them fanning outward. Your breath is calm.

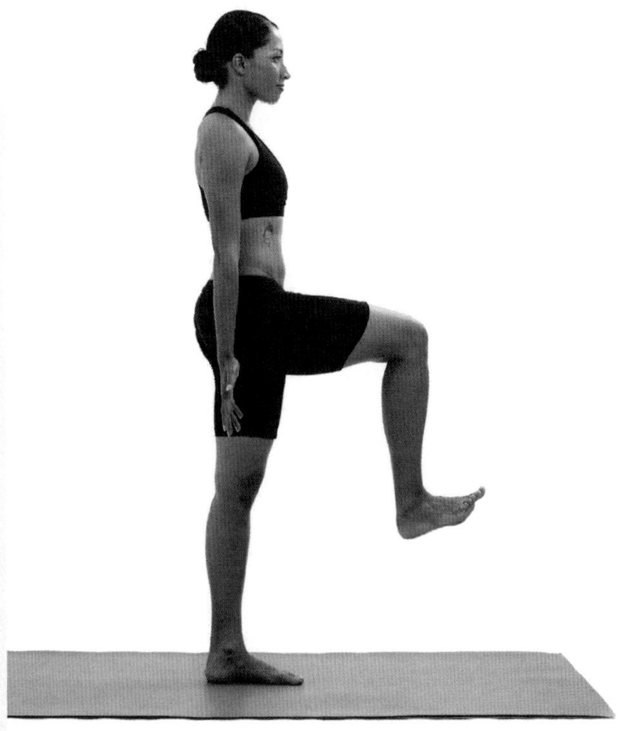

Part 1

Your leg positions

1.1 **Even Hips, Lock The Knee**: Your hips are even and square to the mirror and level to the floor. Lock your left leg, fully activating your quadriceps muscle. Your kneecap lifts and your leg cannot bend.

1.2 **Lift Your Other Leg**: With hips stable in position, lift your right leg up so that your thigh is parallel to the floor, knee at the same level as your hip.

1.3 **Leg At Right Angle, Flex Foot**: Your leg is bent at right angles so that your heel is directly under your knee in a vertical line. Flex your foot strongly.

1.4 **Stamina**: The position of both legs stays constant for a whole minute. Read on for exceptions to this rule.

Your arms and upper body position

1.5 **Round Over**: Inhale length. Exhale, engage the core and with your chin parallel to the floor (looking forward) round over and interlock your fingers under the ball of the foot.

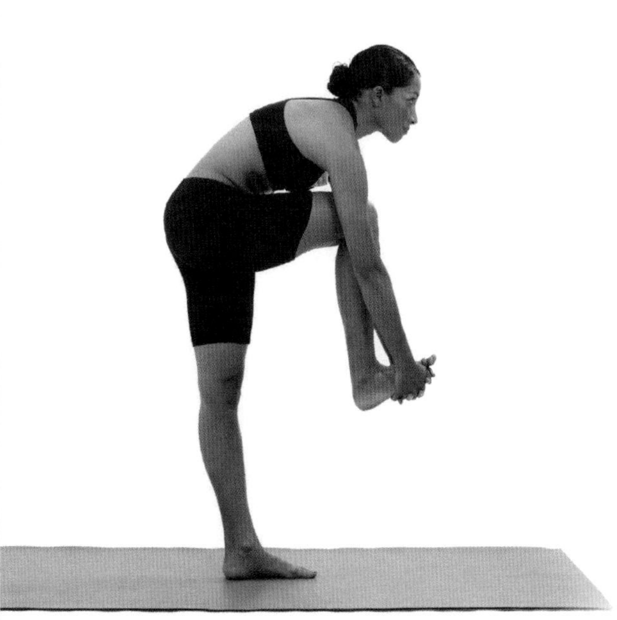

1.6 **Relax Arms, Support Foot With Interlocked Fingers**: Your arms are relaxed. Your 8 fingers interlock fully, thumbs stay with the fingers but don't necessarily interlock. Together they form a cradle for your flexed foot. Incorrectly crossing the thumbs to draw the palms together or placing them on top of the foot are both big mistakes. See later.

1.7 **Support The Foot, Hip Flexors Work**: The strength of the hands, arms and shoulders does not lift or hold up the leg. There is minimal weight in your hands. Holding the leg in position requires primarily solid hip flexor work, backed up by simple hand support.

Dandayamana Janushirasana

STANDING HEAD TO KNEE

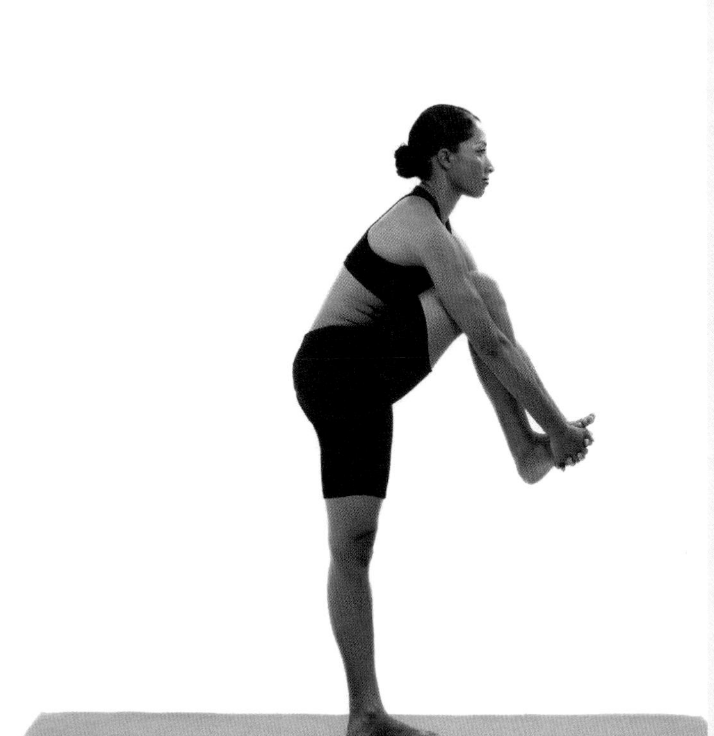

Part 2

The majority of students find their limit exploring Part 2 and never manage full extension. Once there however, this part may be your easiest. You could literally spend minutes balancing with both legs locked, the upper parallel to the floor.

You must be able to lock your standing leg for 60 seconds before you are ready to go beyond Part 1. Your first attempts are always in the 2nd set, never the first. The spine straightens to lift the chest and create the leg extension. Moving the leg forward from a rounded spine is very risky. Don't rush, make considered movements. Lock your left leg and inhale, draw in your abdomen to protect your lower spine and as you exhale do the next 6 listed actions at the very same time:

2.1 **HANDS PULL BACK THROUGH THE BALL OF YOUR FOOT**: Pull back on the ball of your strongly flexed foot. The heel resists the hands' pull by pushing strongly toward the mirror. The traction in your extended relaxed arms gives you something solid against which to push. As long as your foot stays flexed, the back of the extended leg feels a deepening stretch no matter how fully you extend.

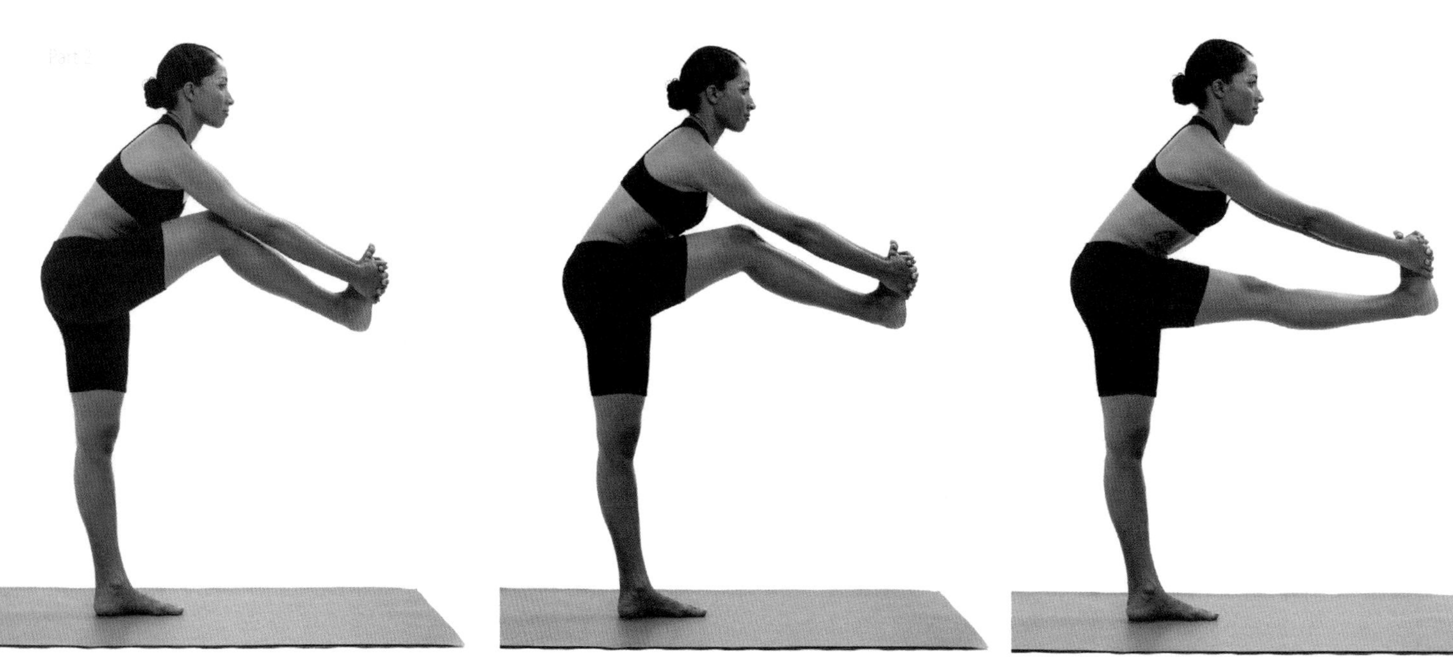

2.2 **Lift Chest, Straighten Spine, Push Heel**: Simultaneously lift your chest as you push your leg out. You transform your rounded spine to a long straight one. Shoulder blades squeeze back and down.

2.3 **Knee High**: Lift your knee up as you move your heel forward, almost as if you are lifting your knee to your chest to raise your heel.

2.4 **Heel At Hip Level, Protect Your Spine**: With your knee high your heel does not drop below the level of your hip as you 'kick' out. Ideally raise your knee and heel against extended arms so that your heel reaches the same level as your hip immediately. This is your inbuilt safety mechanism so that you never ever have undue strain on your lower back, even if the upper leg is not completely extended or locked out.

2.5 **Ensure Your Standing Leg Is Locked**: Recommit to locking your standing leg for a solid foundation.

2.6 **Head Up**: Keep your head up with chin parallel to floor. It will allow you to balance, and stop you falling forward. Your eyes should be looking forward at eyes, throat or third eye. Consider it a rule that, when you can't look at your own face, that you should never let your gaze settle below the standing locked knee.

2.7 **Full Extension**: Arms are relaxed, extended and in traction, both locked legs are at right angles to each other with the raised foot as strongly flexed back as possible.

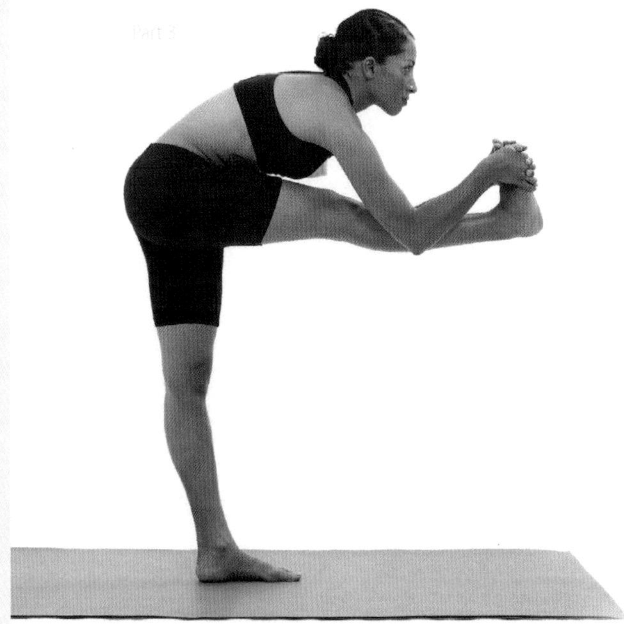

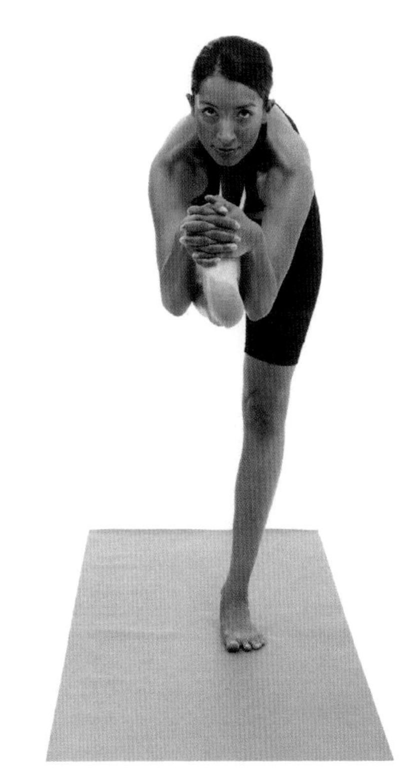

A tip for Part 2

While your ego wants you to move on to the next step, I encourage you to stay in Part 2 for a fair number of classes before progressing to Part 3. The traction forces collectively created by your body, legs and arms is the perfect vehicle for learning balance, easily. So while the leg is fully extended, body upright and focus steady, move the leg around from side to side and up and down (quite randomly). Learn how to save yourself from falling over due to destabilizing forces. Parts 3 and 4 pose even bigger balance challenges. Part 4 you will have to balance while your eyes have a moving visual focus. Solid Part 2 practice will help you get your head on your knee because you will already know how to recover.

Dandayamana Janushirasana

STANDING HEAD TO KNEE

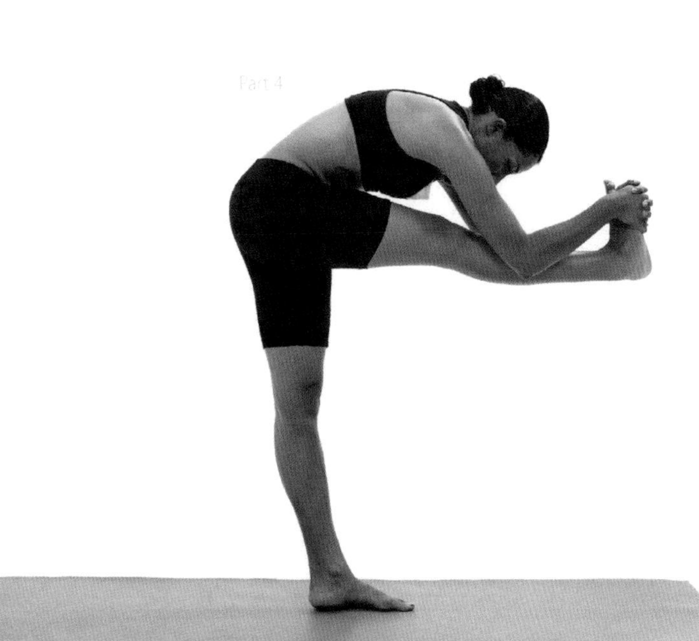

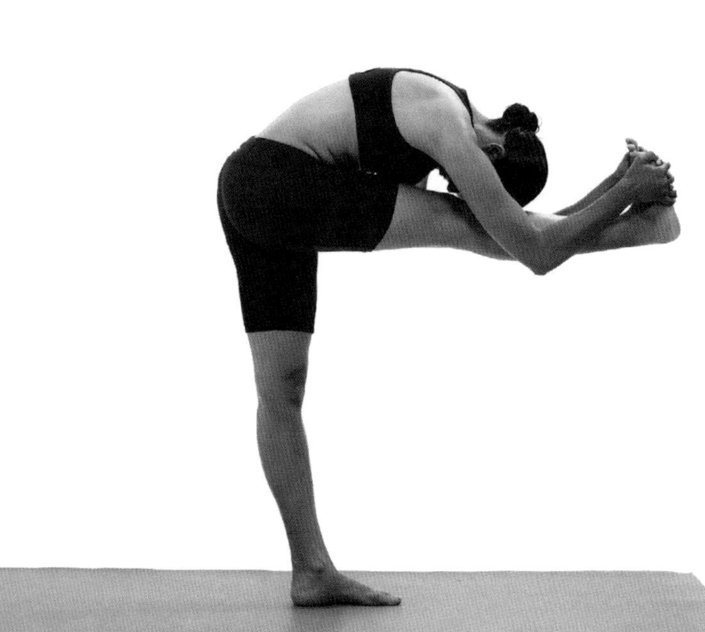

Part 3

Your locked legs are at right angles. Keep your eyes focusing forward. Inhale, and as you exhale:

3.1 **BEND YOUR ARMS**: Draw in your abdomen, keep the same pull and push forces of your hands and feet, and now bend your arms.

3.2 **RELAX YOUR WRISTS**: Your wrists need to be relaxed to maintain the hand pull yet allow your elbows to move down below your extended leg.

3.3 **YOUR SPINE ROUNDS**: The spine will automatically transform from straight to round as your elbows bend.

3.4 **ELBOWS HUG YOUR CALVES**: Aim the points of your elbows in as if they could touch below your legs and under your calf muscles. In a nutshell that is it.

The difficulty lies in your ability to maintain the position of your locked legs as an unwavering constant, and simply bend your elbows. You are learning how to balance while changing your center of gravity without dropping your heel. Pay particular attention to flexing your toes backwards and feeling the heel extend. Breathe! These are all vital lessons for getting your forehead on your knee.

Part 4

This is where you bring your forehead onto your knee. Transiting your visual focus from the mirror to your abdomen will challenge your balance and concentration. It must constantly shift until you reach your destination – for example –down your leg, through your knee and then to your belly button.

Most will start by putting their nose on their shin. This is not head to knee, but it is a valiant start. Move smoothly as you shift your focus. Slowly round down and tuck your chin to land your forehead on your knee.

To stay in position for the eventual 45 seconds that I hope you aim for, you will need to have a fixed place to rest your eyes. I may end up looking below and through the space between my legs settling my visual focus on the floor. In times of great focus I will look at my stomach. Finding a fixed target is a great starting point and easier to maintain when spending 45 seconds balancing on one leg and upside down!

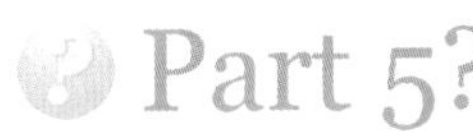

Part 5?

Yes, I did say there are only 4 parts. However there are some who can take this pose one step further. Once the head is on your knee, reach your strong arms, parallel to your leg, toward the mirror. This is a huge challenge for your balance, strength and focus. Attempt it firstly in the second set.

The 75% rule

Moving through to Parts 2, 3 and 4

Most people get much less than they should from this pose. The scripted approach to classes has them move slowly through Parts 1, 2 and 3 to finally put their head on the knee for a second (where most fall out). This does not maximize one's efforts. Typically a student moves to the next phase when they can no longer tolerate being still. It is far easier to constantly move the body than to stay motionless in one position.

In my lessons, the first 60 second set IS the first part of the pose; read on for the exceptions. Over ninety per cent of yogis find that their biggest challenge in this pose is when simply rounded over supporting their bent leg. To stay still for an entire minute takes great stamina, focus, patience, persistence and concentration. Until you can lock the leg for the entire 60 seconds, don't even attempt to kick out either in the first or second set.

Second set gives you 30 seconds to extend the leg for the first time, or work on the new wherever you are at. If you are consistently getting and holding your head on your knee then I have a rule by which you can work...

Spend 75% of the time in the final part of the pose.

Yes, 75% or a whopping 45 seconds of the time with your head on your knee. Anyone who can put their head on their knee can (perhaps too easily) spend 15 seconds, moving slowly from part to part, cycling through at their leisure.

As soon as your legs are in position, hands are interlocked and everything is stable, don't procrastinate! Lift your body and extend your leg. Once settled, bend your elbows. Then bring your forehead to your knee. Don't waste any time. Get there and deepen your experience. Your humility and sense of humor will be required as you work on your stamina and persistence.

When should I extend into Part 2?

If you can lock the leg for 60 seconds then your first attempts at Part 2 happen only in the second set. Once Part 2 is mastered, your efforts to attempt Parts 3 and 4 also take place in the second set. Your challenge is to push your envelope without involving your ego.

I'm not yet at Part 4. Can I still use the 75% rule?

Yes, you can. If you are 'stuck' in Part 1, then I encourage you to hold your rounded body over your lifted leg for the full first 60 second set. Then attempt progress toward full Part 2 extension only in the 2nd set. Work toward spending 3/4 of second set in full extension. Once both legs are fully locked out for the whole 25 seconds, upgrade your challenge to holding your legs in position for 45 seconds in the first set.

The same goes for exploring Part 3. First try bringing your elbows down in the second set only. Aim for a 25 second hold. Only once this is achieved, should you even attempt to bend your elbows down in the first set. No matter where you are at, second set is for spending 22-25 seconds in your fullest expression of Standing Head to Knee.

Important safety elements for Part 2

- Your spine is straight, your arms long and in traction
- Your well interlocked fingers hold the ball of the foot for maximum leverage and definitely NOT the arch.
- Keep your ankle flexed and toes pointed back.
- Pull against your foot, push against your hands, heel extends.
- Keep your ankle at the same level as your hip as you extend; initially lift your knee and ankle to the correct position.
- Controlled steady breath.

Never, ever

- extend your leg before your standing leg is locked out.
- let your heel drop below your hip on your extension.
- let your extended foot relax, keep it flexed.

Second set

Second set is only 30 seconds long. Most students will stay in Part 1 for set 1, and move to their fullest extent in set 2 for at least 22-25 seconds. See my 75% rule above for more details.

Release

As with most poses, you are called on to exit in the reverse fashion to your entry. This is so that you don't just 'wait' for the end and flop out. Be mindful and use control of your muscles to scaffold your spine.

Dandayamana Janushirasana

STANDING HEAD TO KNEE

Common mistakes and how to fix them

Part 1

The mistakes that occur are often a result of flagging energy or lessened attention to the basics.

The leg unlocks: A leg can 'lock' to different degrees. The final stage firmly secures the knee. To keep it strongly locked you will cycle between 90-100% for most of the time. Watch your knee in the mirror, see the quadriceps muscle draw the knee cap up. See it lock into position. That in itself is a good beginners' meditative focus and will often stop them 'thinking' about too many other distracting and destabilizing things.

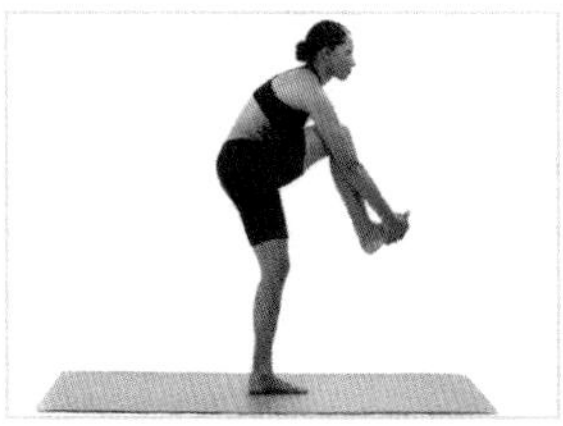

Eyes down: Looking down to the floor or in front of the mat, drastically increases the tendency to fall forward. General rule of thumb: Never drop your eyes lower than the reflection of your standing locked knee. Ideally you will work on eye contact but look where you can on your body. Remember the phrase: 'Where the eyes go the body follows'. Looking in the mirror not only keeps your body up, your balance will improve and knee-locking will be easier.

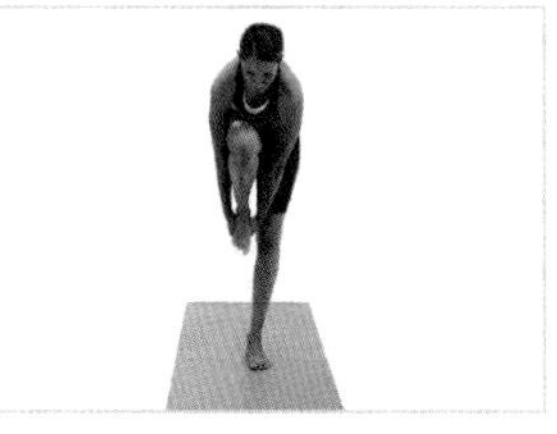

Leg angles back: The lower leg often folds backward (from 30°-60°). The eyes tend to look down. The thigh either stays parallel to the floor or it moves up toward the chest. The foot no longer flexed, usually wraps down over the hands. Falling forward is more likely especially as students often bend the standing leg to stop themselves falling.

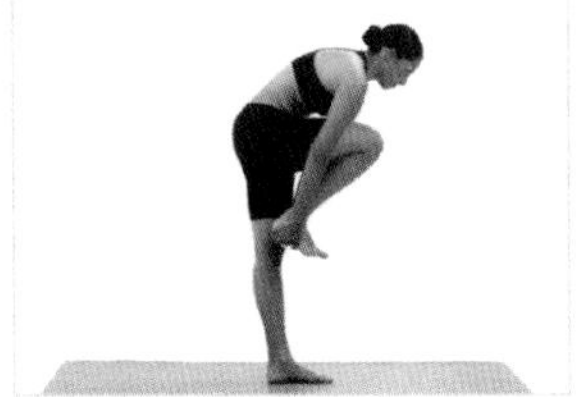

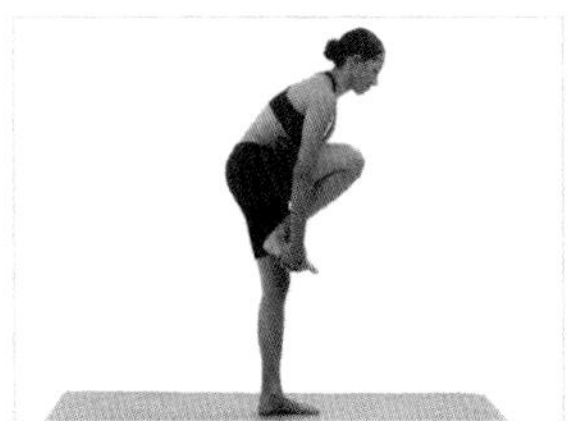

This is fairly easy to correct. Shift your visual focus. Look forward no lower than the reflection of your standing knee, grip correctly at the ball of the flexed foot, with the heel extending vertically to the floor, and of course, lock your knee.

Leg angles forward: Angling the lower leg toward the mirror puts great strain on and can be dangerous for the lower spine, especially if the thigh drops below parallel. The more the heel moves forward the more strain on the lower spine. The shoulders start to strain, the foot relaxes and pushes down into the hands. Basic to understanding this pose is that moving the foot forward in this fashion is NOT the way Part 2 is accomplished. Keep Parts 1 and 2 totally separate.

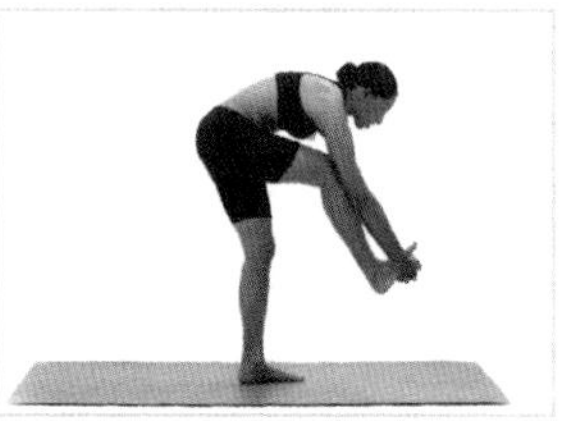

Thumbs on top: In this mistake, the thumbs either start on top, or shift from underneath. This seems harmless, but it recruits different muscles in the arms and shoulders causing tension. It leads to a cocktail of some or all of the following:

- Foot loses strong flexion;
- Toes relax down and point to the floor;
- Foot leans on the hands;
- Hands then arms, and shoulders, and lower back take the strain to actually hold up the foot;
- The biceps contract and shoulders get pulled down;
- Body falls forward;
- At some stage the eyes drop to the floor;
- The whole body tries to stop itself falling over;
- The standing leg unlocks and bends.

All these forces are destabilizing and cause stress on the lower back. Put your thumbs underneath!

Leaning into hands: The problems caused by this mistake and "Thumbs on top" are very similar. They occur in a different order. Here the cascade is set off by leaning the weight of the foot into the hands even if thumbs are correctly placed. Next you will probably feel the downward pull of your shoulders, and back and neck strain. Review 'Thumbs on top' again to cross-check. Shift your attention to relaxing your arms; flex your foot and ensure your thumbs are underneath; bring your knee to hip height using your hip flexors to maintain the lift. You should be able to take your hands away and have nothing change. Get your chin up and look forward.

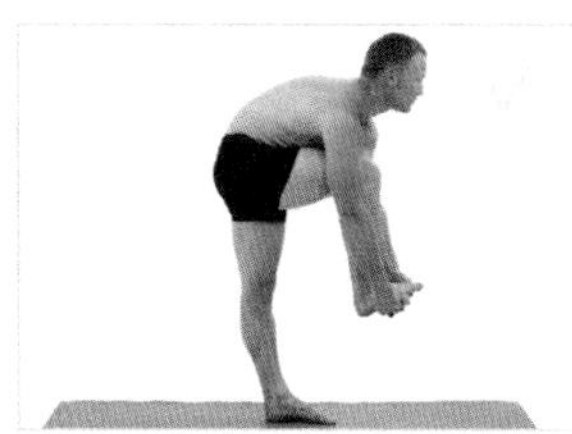

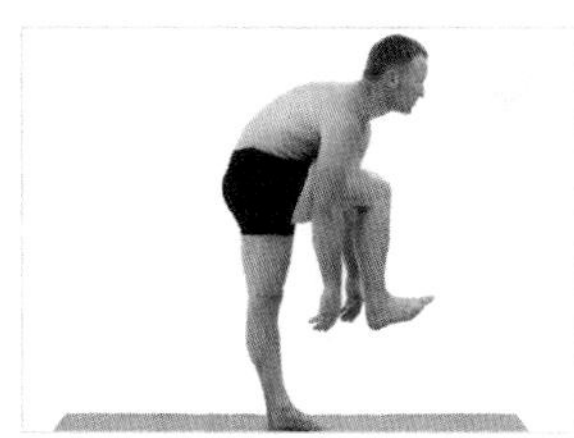

Holding at the arch: The mechanism of this position is lost with a mid-foot grip. It causes the toes to move down (wrap over the hands) and the heel to move up. Without exception you must hold at the ball of the flexed foot for Parts 1, 2, 3 and 4.

incorrect grips

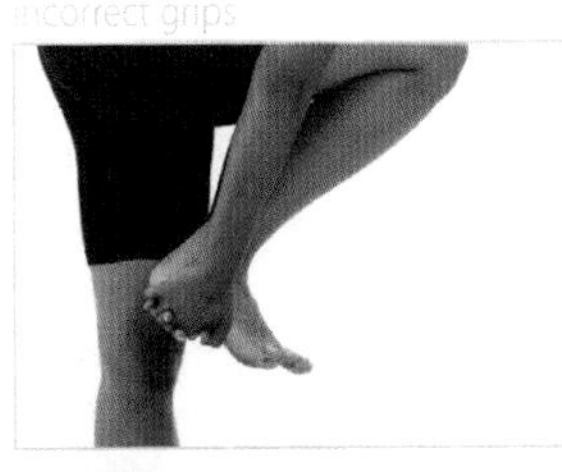

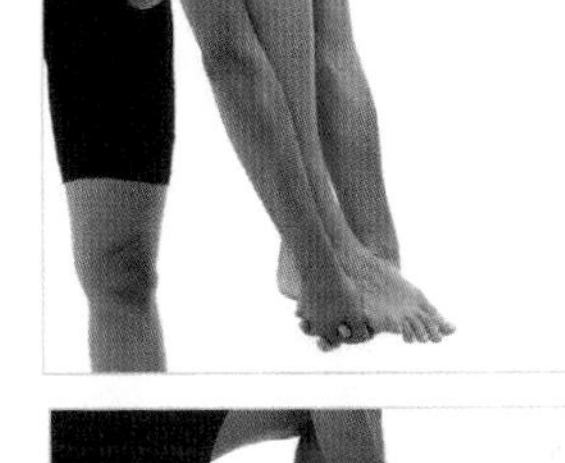

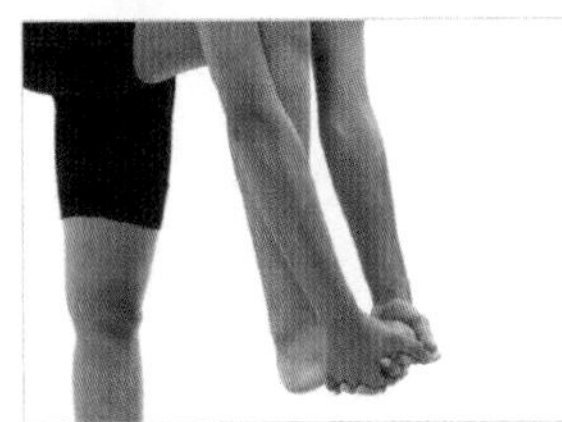

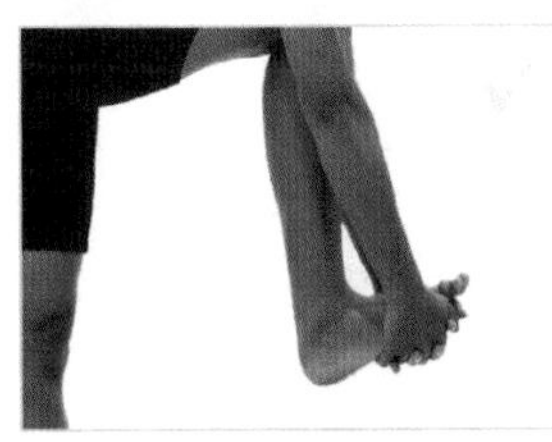

Chin drops: A drop of the chin usually accompanies a drop of the eyes. Always keep the chin parallel to the floor for Parts 1, 2 and 3.

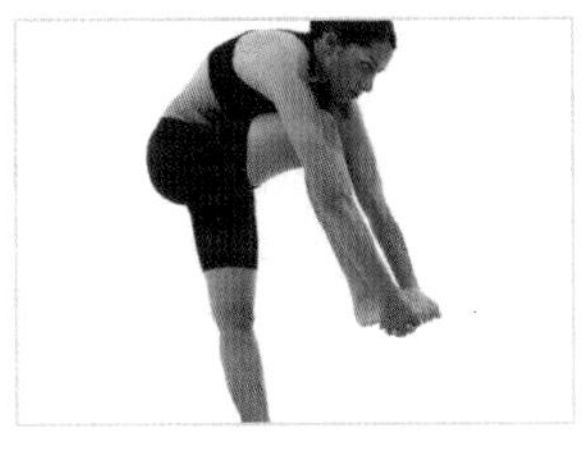

Stiff arms: The arms and shoulders stiffen up causing the weight of the leg to push down into the hands. Relax the arms and only use the clasped fingers to pull back against the flexed foot. Support your foot, don't hold it up.

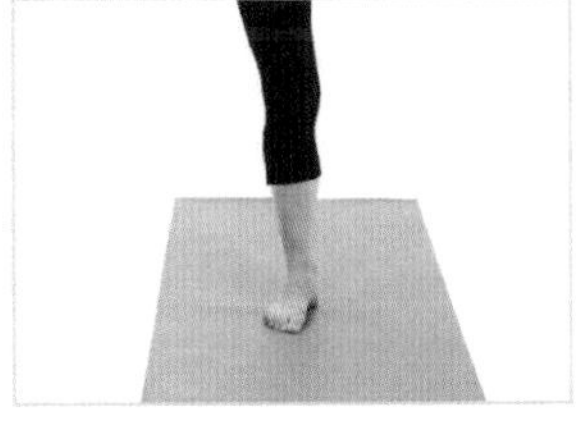

Foot is at an angle to the mirror: Most students will at some time – and usually unconsciously – shift the direction of their standing foot to an angle that creates easier one-legged balance by fanning their toes out to the side. Conscious awareness is all it takes to keep your toes directly on to the mirror. It may cause your ankle to wobble more, but you will learn balance, improve your core strength and it will be easier to lock your leg.

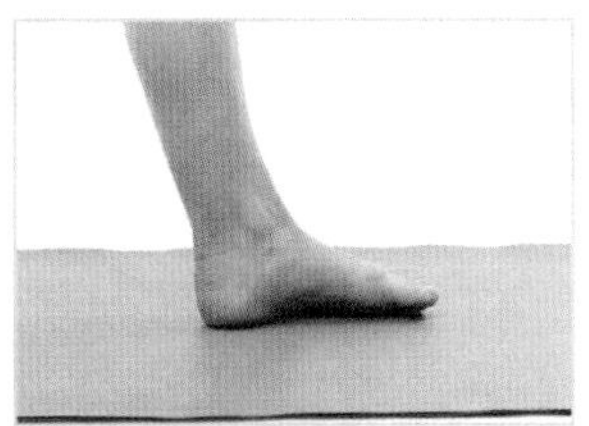

Foot lifts: When balancing on one leg the inside of the foot often lifts transferring the weight to the outside. Push the ball of your big toe back onto the floor. Your center of gravity shifts forward and centrally and make for easier balance.

Shifting the weight to your standing leg: Many teachers tell their students to shift their weight to the standing leg. Just like me telling you when to blink, this is an unnecessary instruction. When was the last time you fell over because you lifted up a leg to walk or climb a step? (See 'Mistakes' in Eagle pose.) Lifting a leg automatically shifts sufficient weight for you to balance, without having to think. Consciously shifting the weight exaggerates the movement and causes a change in hip orientation. The unweighted hip now slumps lower than the other and your spine curves laterally. Ultimately when asked to shift your weight, you will spend time correcting all the ill-effects.

When I simply ask my students to lock one leg then lift the other, their hips stay square both to the floor and to the mirror. Remember 'measure twice, cut once' and you will know intuitively that correct prior set-up will pay enormous dividends.

Try this; with or without a mirror. Press the heel of your palms down on the top of your hips. Shift the weight, lock that leg and bend up the other leg for Part 1 position. Notice the slumped hip and what it takes to get your hips and leg back to alignment. Start again but do not shift the weight. Encode the sensation of maintaining even hips before and after lifting your leg into position.

Picking up the foot instead of meeting the foot: Asked to simply lock out a leg and then round down to pick up the other, is potentially a dangerous movement for those with weak backs, weak core muscles, and tight bodies. Those unfamiliar with this pose risk damage, often because they are simply overwhelmed with new instructions. So try this move yourself: Place your hands on your hips and then set up your legs as described in 'the technique'. Round over to meet your foot (which is already in position) rather than pick it up. Once you understand how to separate the elements, the risk is removed and you will not need to place your hands on your hips.

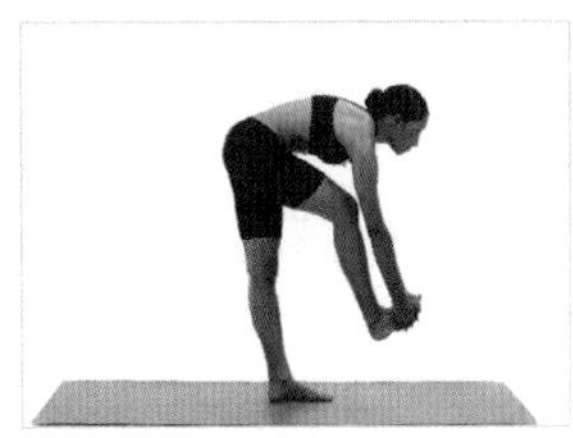

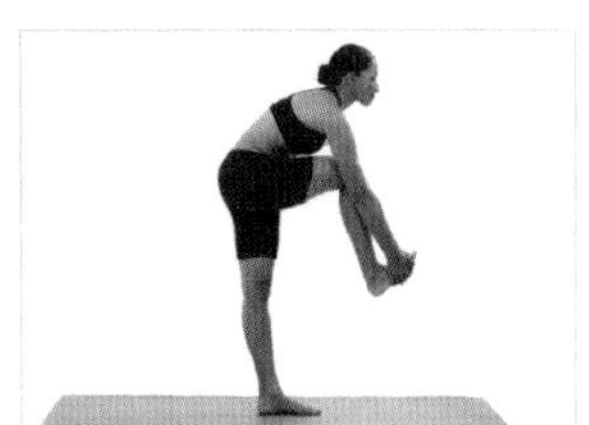

Dandayamana Janushirasana

Standing Head to Knee

I can't even get my hands under my foot, what do I do?

This is more common than you think. Some students will have to clasp just below their knee with fully interlocked fingers.

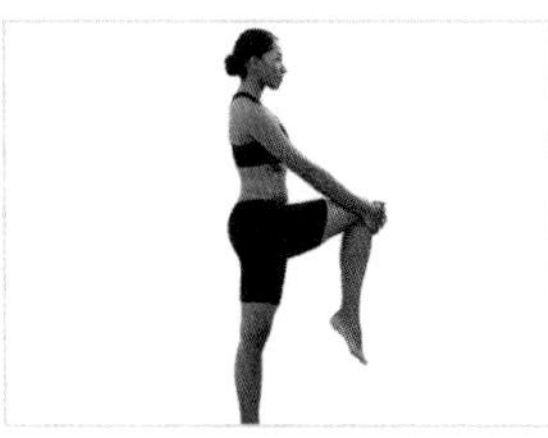

- The lifted leg is completely relaxed.
- The foot is not at all flexed.
- Gravity is pulling the leg down against straight relaxed arms. The leg 'falls' into the clasp of the hands creating an active stretch which opens up the hip.
- The back is upright and straight.
- The locked leg is the primary focus and takes precedence over all other actions.
- The aim is to allow the flexion to open the hip area, create strength in the back, quadriceps muscles and ankles, and of course, balance.

Some students need to use a wall for support. This is fine. As long as your priority is to build strength and balance through locking your standing leg, then you are making progress.

Part 2

A revision of the section detailing Part 1 mistakes is advised. In addition there are these mistakes which can have serious outcomes:

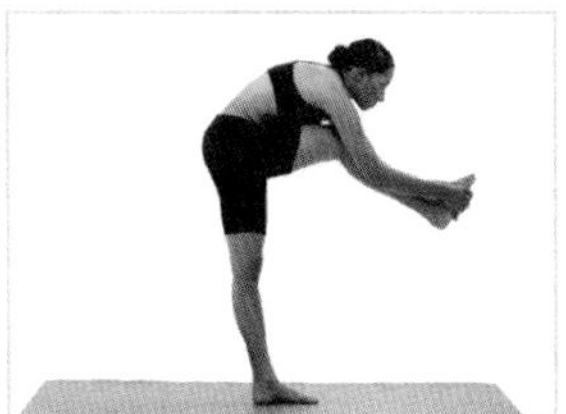

Chest down: Sometimes the spine is straightened slightly but the body hinges at the hips. The arms bend as the leg and body come forward in this mistake. There can be some confusion regarding the similarities between Parts 2 and 3. As this is Part 2, arch the spine and lift the chest to correct. Arms stay in traction as the leg extends.

Flexed foot flags: Often the foot loses the flexion due to any number of errors, when the body is fighting falling over. Students often simply forget to keep up the flexion and accidentally point the toes forward in an unconscious attempt to lengthen the leg. Lift the chest, pull on the ball of the foot and really focus on extending the heel away from you.

Keeping a rounded back, or extending by hinging at the knee: Holding a round spine not only makes extension dangerous and difficult but you have to really work to keep yourself from falling over. Your pose will be all about TRYING to balance instead of CREATING balance with correct stance. The arms cannot straighten, the foot won't stay flexed and the leg drops and causes back strain.

The extension is not a simple straightening of the leg or a forward movement of your foot to meet the height of your thigh.

Moving from Part 1 to 2, the spine needs to lift and straighten. Your straight arms and heel move up in an arc as you extend your leg. The knee moves upward and must be higher than hip height while the foot travels to full extension at hip level to remove the risk of back damage.

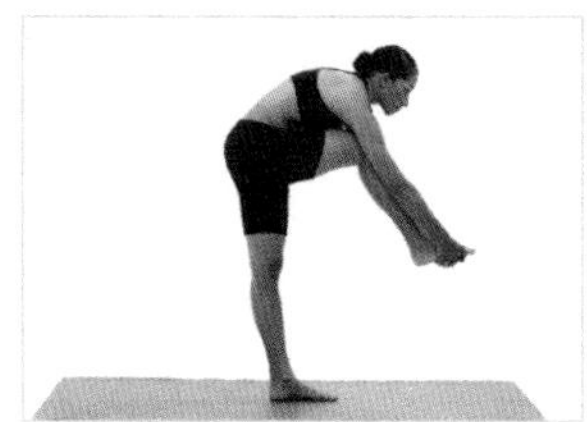

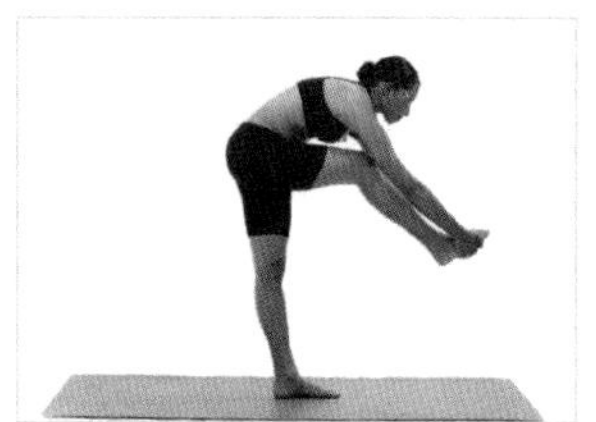

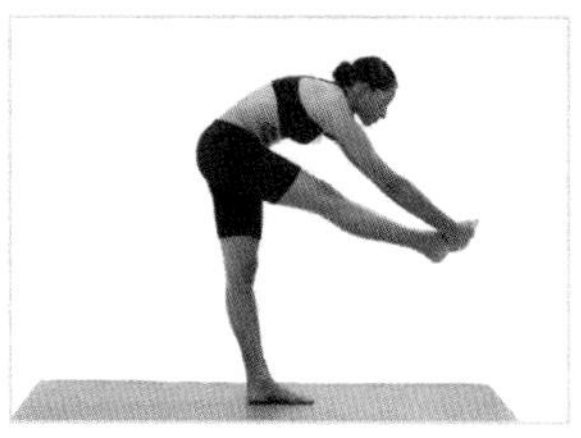

Knee drops: The knee drops if the spine is rounded when the foot starts to extend. Your leg will more likely end up angling down to the floor. In an attempt to stop you falling the arms fight back by bending and pulling. You will point your toes to the floor, put all the weight into your hands, and hey presto, you will fall over.

Just as in the previous mistake the fix is similar. You will have to lift your chest, straighten your arms and spine, and raise your knee.

Arms bent, elbows out or down: Bending the arms will obviously involve the biceps and shoulders. The body will come forward. It will be very hard to keep the balance and hard to keep the foot flexed. The leg extends by creating traction against lengthened arms. See above!

blending Parts 2 and 3

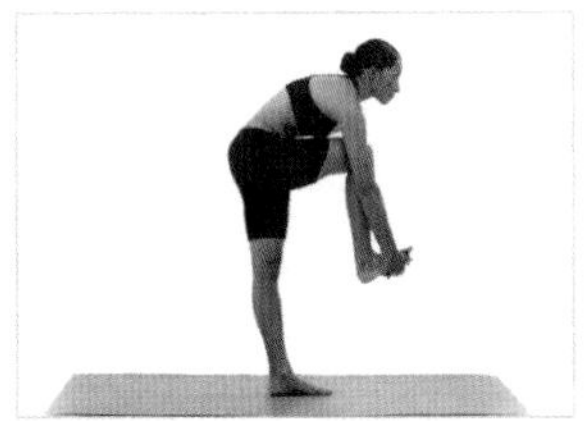
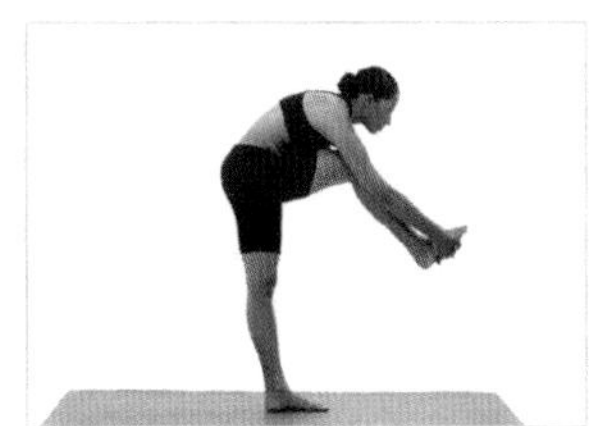
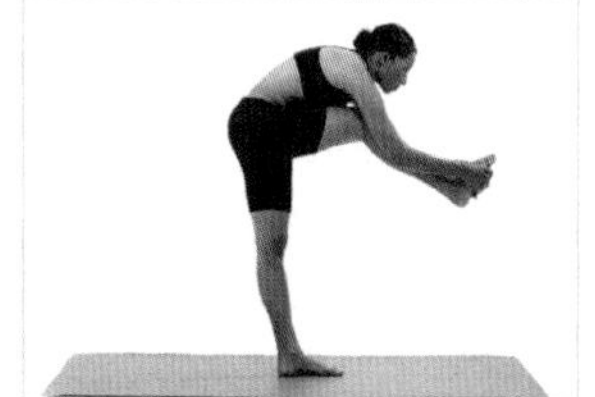
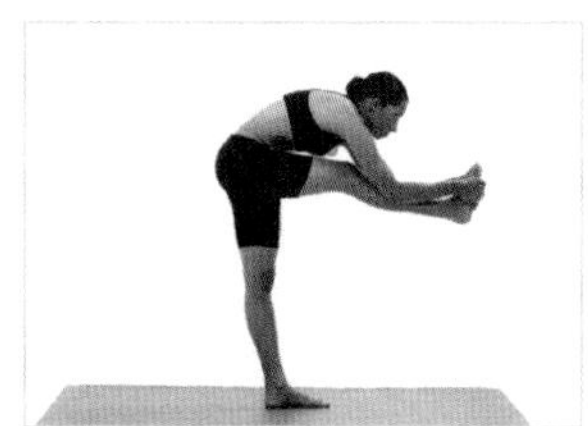

Part 3

Allowing the foot to relax: When the foot relaxes the back of the leg shortens and toes point to the mirror. The grip slips toward the heel. You have to try to stop yourself falling forward. See mistakes in Parts 1 and 2. This usually happens as the elbows start to bend down and is as a result of conscious mind overwhelm; too many things to think about! Allow yourself a steady learning curve which includes making mistakes. Next time as you bend your arms down, keep the pull strong on the ball of the foot.

Elbows are out: Tuck them in and down towards the calf muscles.

Blending Parts 2 and 3: The most common mistake is moving from Part 1 to a hybrid of Parts 2 and 3. With the back already rounded over the leg in Part 1 it is a common misconception that the body remains down as the foot lifts, and the elbows stay below the leg. Make all 3 parts distinctly separate.

Part 4

Forehead to shin: You are almost there. The aim is forehead to knee and students usually place their head progressively up their leg as they continually stretch themselves to learn new balance over time.

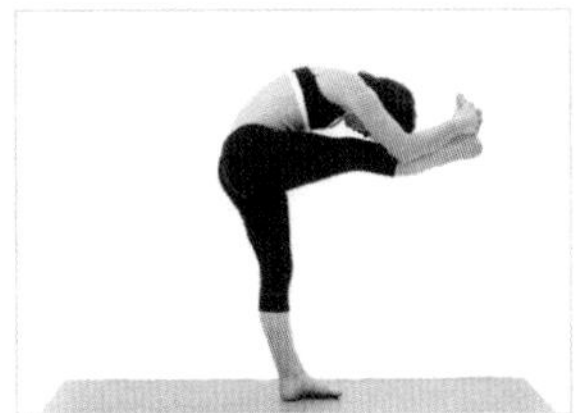
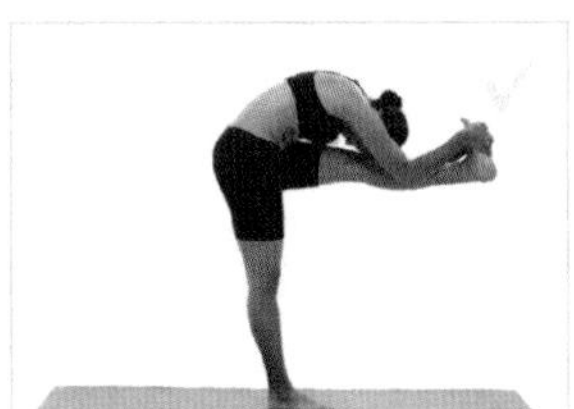

A backbend between sets

Some studios invite students to put their hands on their lower backs and do a backbend. I DO NOT support doing any backbend between the sets or right and left sides. This is totally counterproductive and unnecessary. If this has been your routine then it may feel strange not to do it the first time. Be patient. Wait for your back bend. It is coming next in Standing Bow pose.

If you want theory, then here it is. Take a look at the chapter on the tourniquet effect for more detail. You stretch, compress, and twist, limiting flow to different areas of the body. Everything works to, on release of the pose, create a burst of blood through those areas flushing and cleansing.

A forward bend after Camel before Savasana is ill-advised because it doesn't allow the full tourniquet effect to work its magic, the flushing is less effective. Extend this reasoning to Head to Knee and get better benefit. If your studio teaches this, it is OK to just stand there while others choose to do a backbend. It is not mandatory and certainly not part of the pose itself.

Dandayamana Dhanurasana

Our greatest glory is not in never falling but in rising every time we fall.
—Confucius

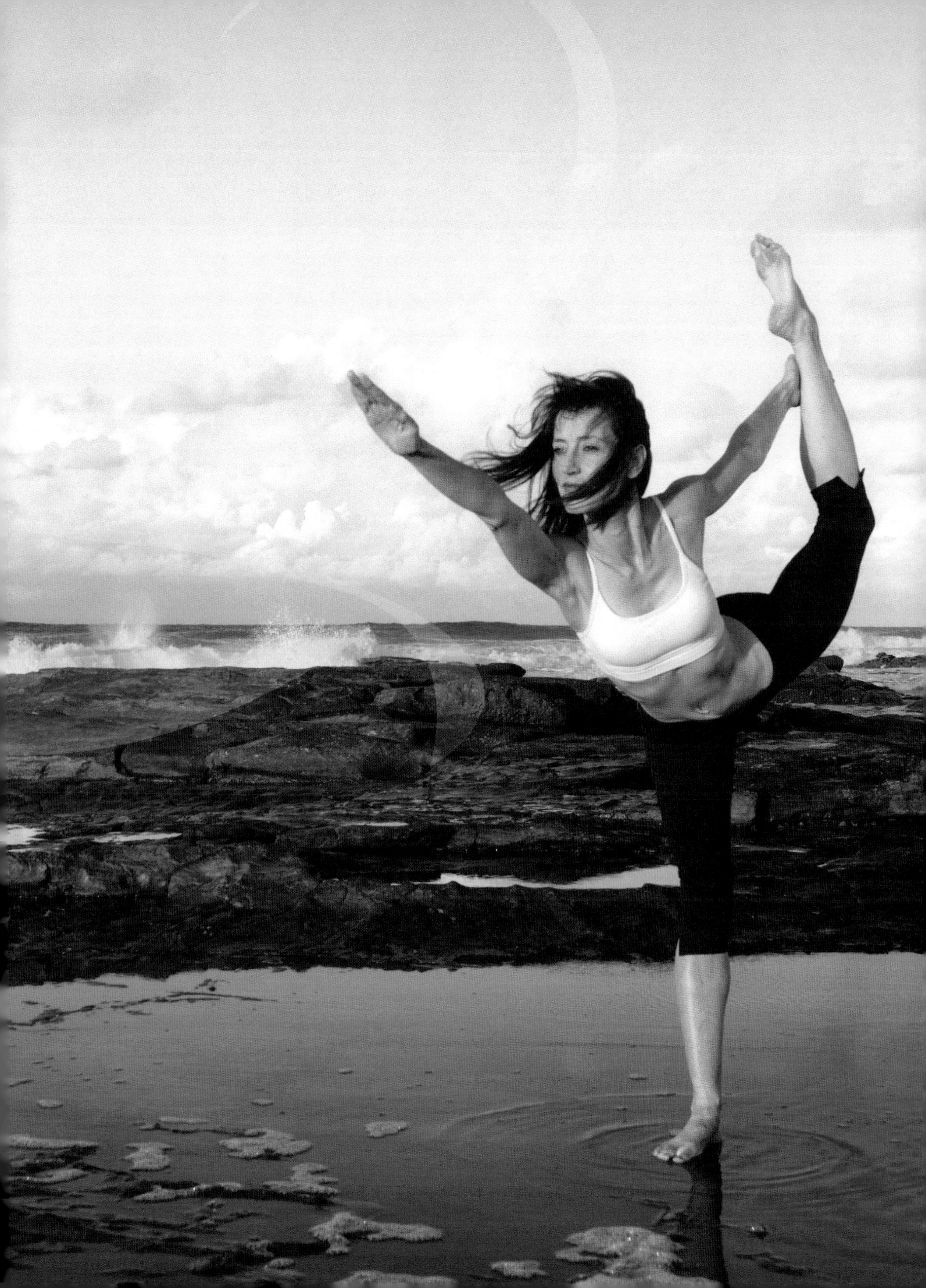

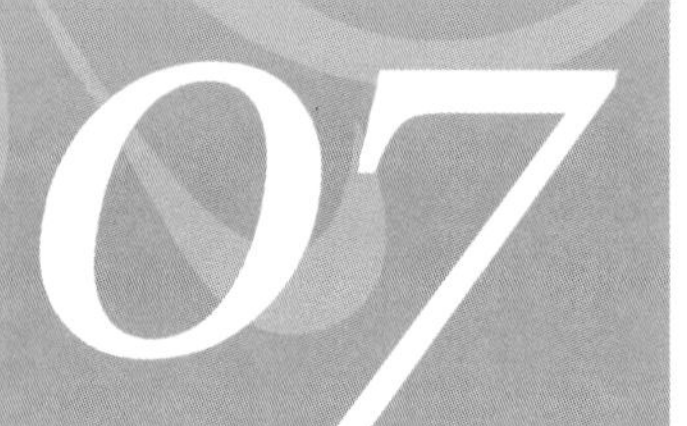

07 Dandayamana Dhanurasana

Standing Bow

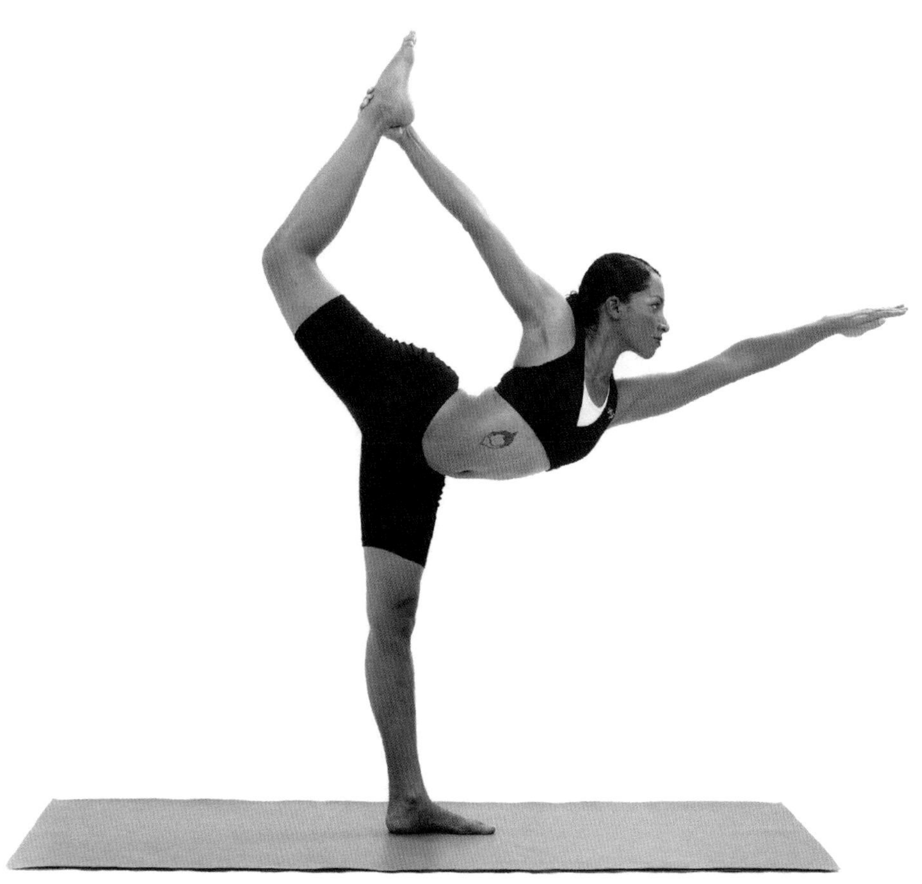

The essentials

Who doesn't like Standing Bow? A strong proud pose, there are not many who cannot grab their foot and kick to feel that awesome stretch through the chest and arms, and the strength in the leg. Once you discover the key to this great position then you can't help but do good solid work. With some precise instructions, everyone eventually has their own 'light bulb moment' and finally 'gets' what they need to do.

What makes this pose so difficult to get right?

When you are a new student in the room, you could be forgiven for thinking that this pose requires you to throw your body down toward the floor to raise the leg up toward the ceiling. Positioned behind more advanced yogis you see only a back and front view, which distorts your real understanding of the intention of this pose. What you don't see is the side view, the way the body opens up into a flourishing backbend supported on a single leg.

Immediately following this pose is one called Balancing Stick where the body comes down parallel to the floor. In a strange misapprehension, most approach Dandayamana Dhanurasana as if it were a combination of the 2 poses. Let's break the components down and find out how to make these 2 poses completely separate.

Here we move from a strong standing balancing forward bend (Standing Head to Knee) into a strong backbend, also balancing on one leg. The prime experience is an opening of the hips, the abdomen, the shoulders, the chest, the arms, the lungs, and the throat. This is a very liberating pose – great for the spirit. What we need to do now is work out what beliefs or misunderstandings that we need to leave behind.

Dandayamana Dhanurasana

07

Standing Bow

The technique

The set-up

You find yourself now standing in Savasana looking in the mirror. Your shoulders are down and back, because your arms are externally rotated. Your palms should naturally be oriented forward toward the mirror to some degree. This opens your chest. If you are someone that finds deep conscious breathing difficult, then 'force' this arm position until your muscles comply without complaint, and practice your relaxed stance.

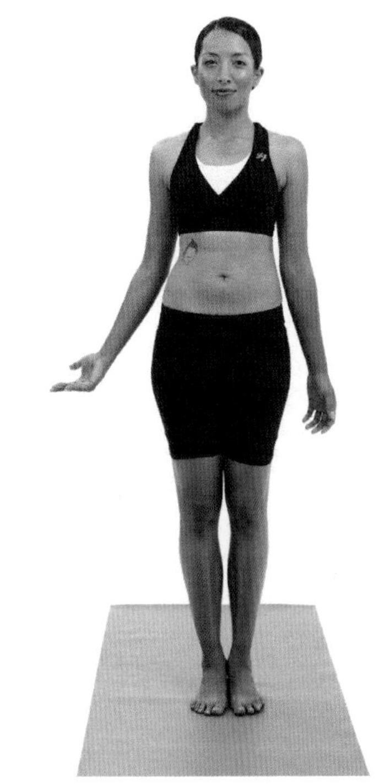

1.1 **Feet Square And Leg Locked**: Make sure your feet do not fan out to the side, keep your hips square to the mirror. Lock your left leg strong and long.

1.2 **Initial Hand Position**: Start with palms forward and arms gently relaxed down. Open, or externally rotate your entire right arm more, so that your right palm opens out to the right wall and falls a little behind you at the level of your bottom. There is a slight comfortable bend in your elbow which is in close to your waist.

1.3 **Holding The Foot**: Bend your right leg up and grab the inside of your right foot just below the toes. Your hand is already in position. Keep the 5 fingers on the inside of the foot – not gripping around it. The weight of your leg on your outstretched arm will straighten your arm and be supported by your hand. Your right shoulder will naturally be pulled a little behind you beginning a slight upper torso twist.

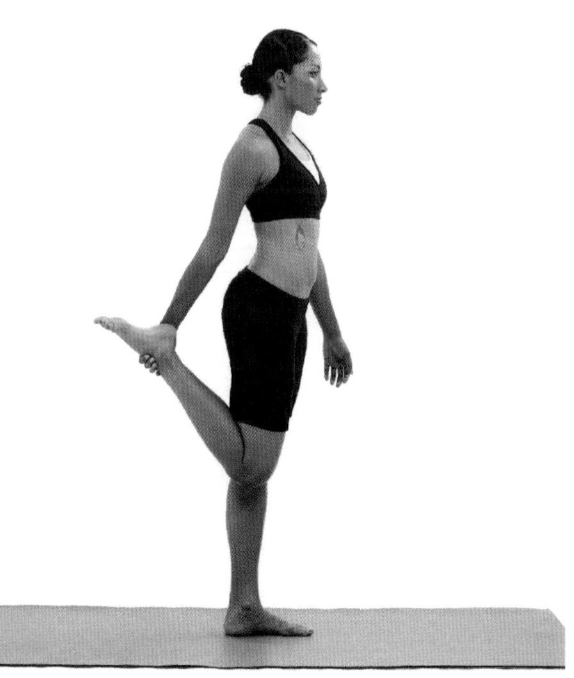

1.4 **Hips Square And Level**: Allow your knees to line up from the side, squaring your hips to the mirror and floor. You should feel some stability here facing the mirror with your foot in your hand, while balancing on one locked leg.

1.5 **Raise Your Other Arm**: Inhale your left arm up over your head, bringing it into a vertical position ending with your palm facing the mirror. Try to draw the arm back so that it is behind the ear, keeping your chin up parallel to the floor. Aim to keep your arm here as long as possible through the pose (yes it will move, but try). The extension is activated from the shoulder to the fingertips, with no shrugging.

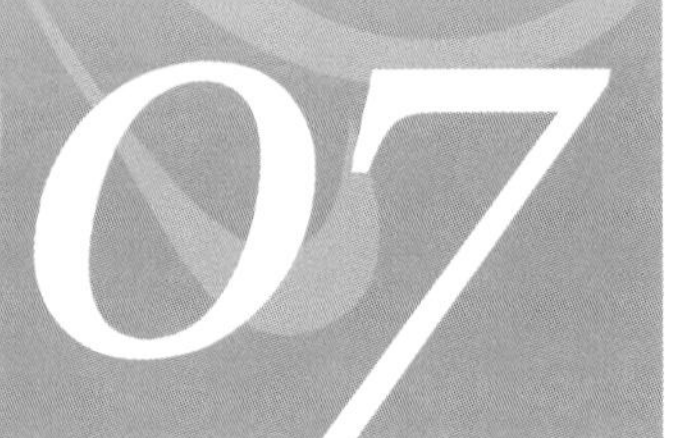

Dandayamana Dhanurasana

Standing Bow

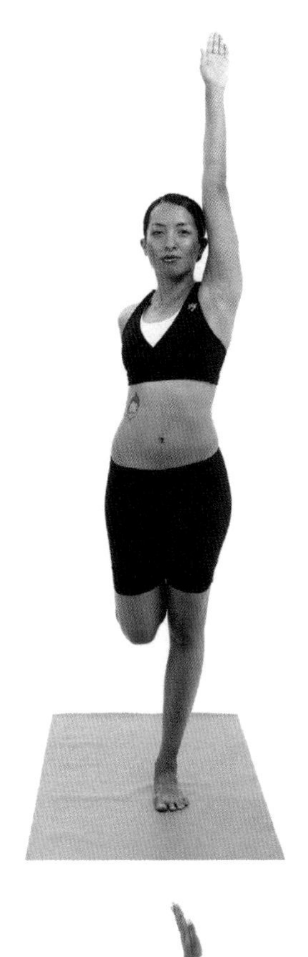

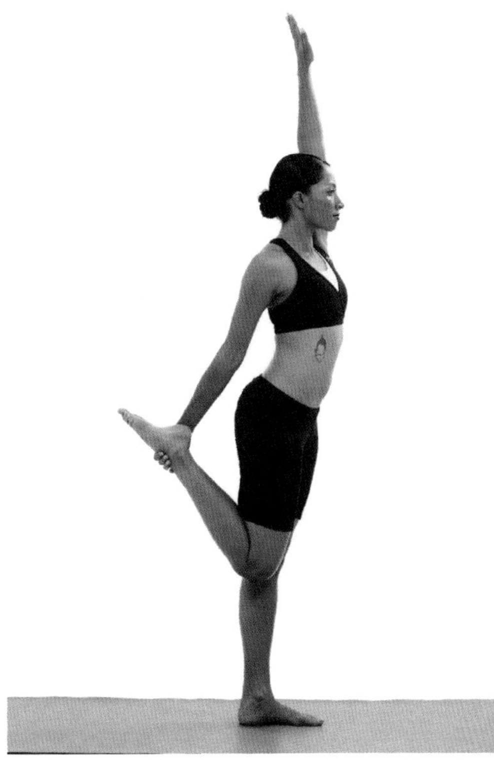

The pose

You are now standing very tall and strong from your left standing leg all the way to your extended left fingers. The imagery of trying to be as tall as possible will help you keep extended. There are a few distinct elements spread through the whole pose. Let's look at what happens now. Regardless of the extent to which your kick takes you, you will still be doing the same thing.

2.1. **Inhale Length, Exhale And Press The Foot Back**: Inhale length from heel to fingertips, and as you exhale press your foot into the hand and your knee up to the ceiling. Most students get the backward kick but need some coaching in how to carry through their kick of the thigh up to the ceiling.

2.2 **Chin Up, Keep Breathing**: The chin stays up parallel to the floor. It stays in the same position the whole time. Longer slower breaths will help you focus and balance.

2.3 **Press Back And Up Squarely**: To create the pose, the knee comes back behind you in line with your hip rather than flaring out to the side or turning out the hip like a dancer. No matter how flexible you are, when viewed from the side the knee of your upper leg must be, at the very least, behind your standing locked leg (even if it's just a little) in order to create the right traction and open the body. That's when you can check in to that lovely stretch along your right quadriceps muscle.

2.4 **Continue To Press The Leg Back, Knee Up**: Apply this driving force right until the end. This is a concerted, continuous action which creates the magic of this pose.

2.5 **Keep The Arm High – Always**: You must keep your left arm up as high as possible THE WHOLE TIME. Have the intention to keep it behind the ear just as you started even though it will drop. The tighter your shoulders are, the harder it is to open your shoulders (and the harder it is to keep your arm raised).

2.6 **Kick Your Body Into A Parabolic Curve**: In this pose your backbend is not just your back. It is the parabolic shape that your arm, back and leg create in unison. In other words, the bottom of your parabola is your lower spine. You have to create the biggest and tightest parabola that you can while you are standing.

Dandayamana Dhanurasana

Standing Bow

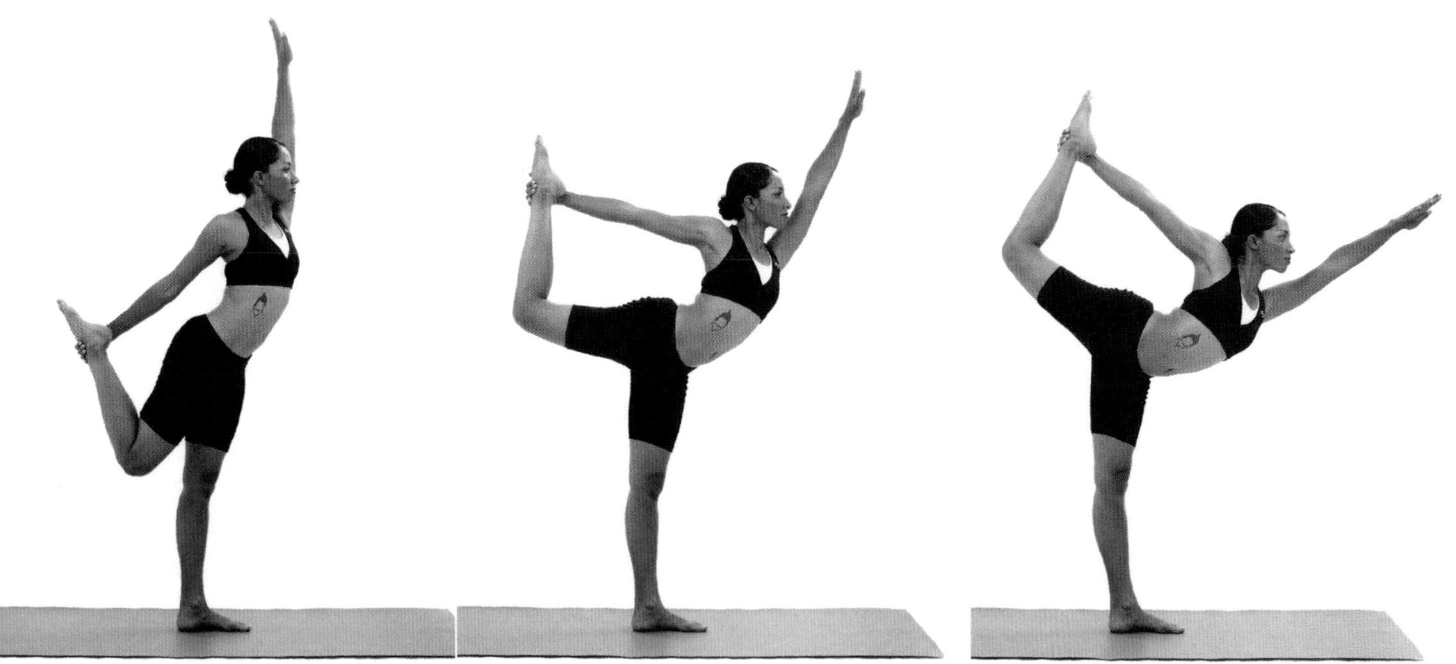

2.7 Belly Down Parallel To Floor: Once your curve is created, set it in concrete and then rotate around your standing hip to bring your belly more in parallel with the floor. As you press back harder, your body comes down BECAUSE you are creating a bigger back bend and a MUCH BIGGER KICK! Press the leg back while you lift the chest and try to touch the ceiling against the forward movement of your body. In effect, you are deepening your backbend and creating a tighter upward facing curve.

2.8 Rotate At The Hip, Don't Bend Forward: The success of this pose relies on a strong ROTATION of the parabola around the hip. It is NOT A HINGING movement of the torso at the hip. Continue to resist the forward and downward movement of the chest to keep it up high.

2.9 Create Traction Through Kicking And Stretching, Line Up Your Shoulders: The more you press the leg back, the more the shoulder gets pulled behind you by the force of the kicking leg. The more you 'kick', the more you can stretch your other arm forward and upward. Create this liberating stretch by consciously relaxing the shoulders so they can align themselves one behind the other. Try to face your chest to the side wall.

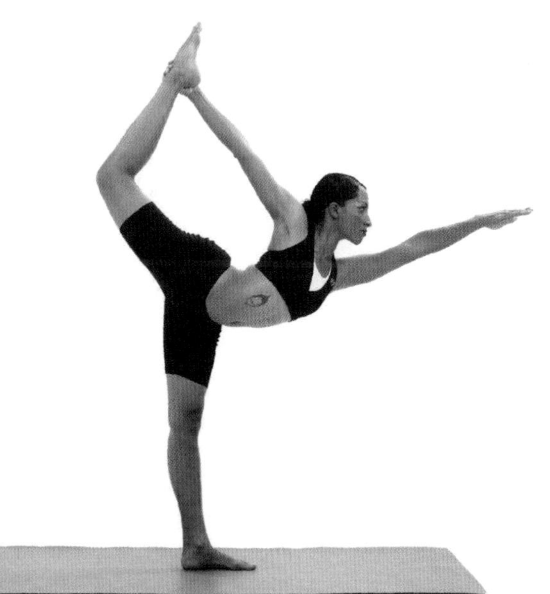

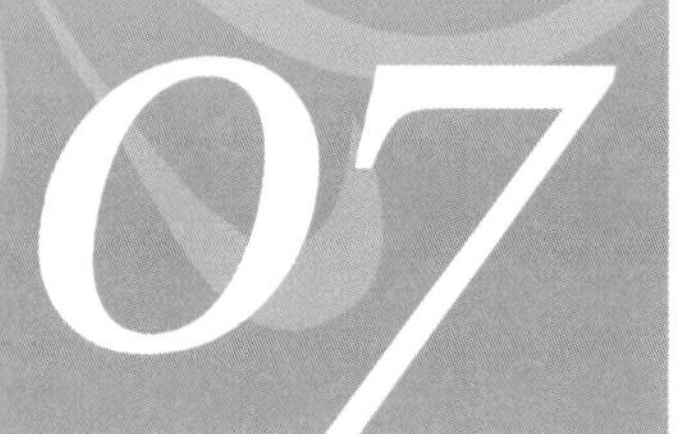

07 Dandayamana Dhanurasana

Standing Bow

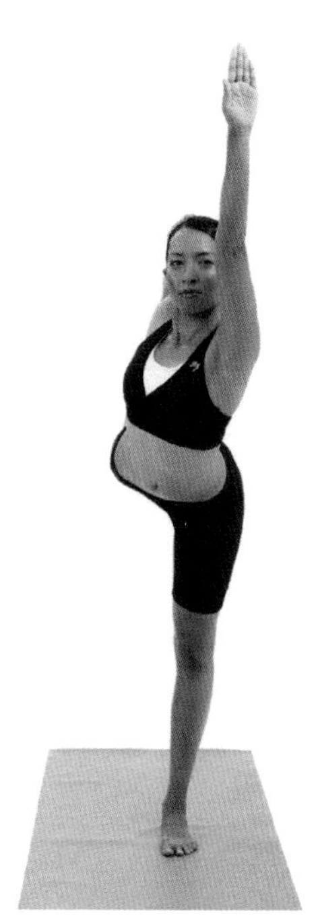

2.10 Feel The Powerful Stretches: Feel the stretch from the palm of your extended hand through your arm, through your shoulders and down your other arm to the hold on your kicking leg. Your shoulders are literally pulling in opposite directions. Observe the stretch in your kicking leg from the front of your foot, ankle and shin, through your quadriceps across your hips and up through your chest, in your throat and under your chin. Continually revisit the basics.

2.11 Aim To Do The Standing Splits: Try imagining that when you kick your leg, you are trying to straighten it out behind you. The only thing stopping you is your hand which is holding your foot. The forces therefore translate into a backward kick of the foot and an upward kick of the knee which with time may take you into the standing splits.

In summary, here is what you do

Press back your leg against a stable upright body. When you have moved your upright body and leg into their maximum parabolic expression, start to pivot that parabola forward around the standing leg hip. Preserve that backbend while lowering the body. Continue to press the leg back, to stretch and reach with your arms. These actions. which stay constant for 60 seconds, all conspire to improve your backbend.

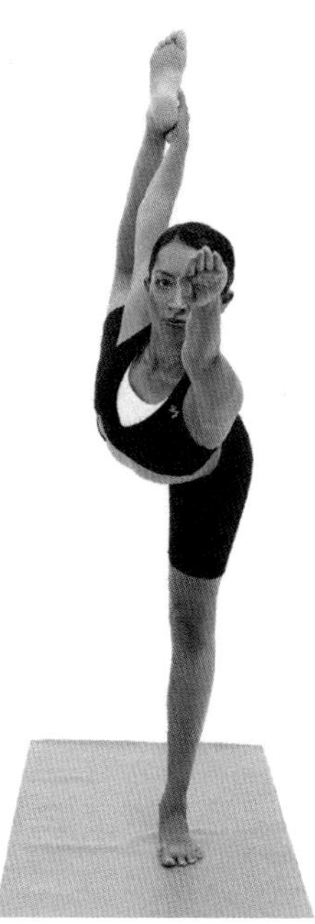

What if you are super-flexible?

If you are very flexible then chances are you find this pose very easy to get into. You look good in it, that's for sure. However, just as a very muscular person needs to balance their body by building flexibility, the highly flexible need to attain balance by building strength. This requires work. If your arm is extended in front in a relaxed fashion – somewhat resting in the air, or if you kick easily into the splits (or almost into them) then you still have a lot of work to do.

Your job is to really re-visit the basics. Challenge yourself to lift your chest right up so it is parallel to the mirror. Anyone can have their whole upper body parallel to the floor – but then your backbend will all but completely disappear. Drop your abdomen parallel to the floor, keep your chin from dropping so it too remains parallel. Keep pressing your leg not just back, but up, up, up. And lift your arm up, up, up against those strong forces of gravity. For extra challenge and strength-building only ever hold at the foot.

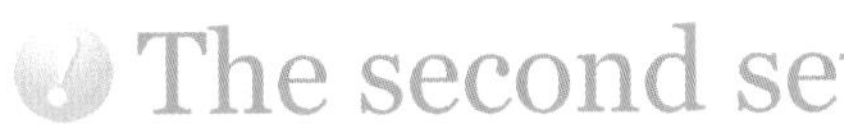

The second set

There is really no difference between the sets except for the timing. With only 30 seconds in the second set there is less stamina involved so most will feel a renewed sense of ability to really go for an even bigger kick and higher stretch, in an effort to deepen the pose. As I like to say, press a little higher, stretch a little further and remember to breathe deeply into your belly.

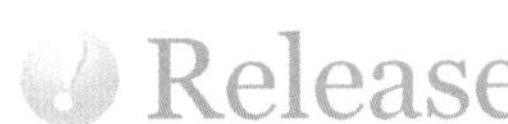

Release

Remember the parabolic shape you are trying to tighten and the leg that you are trying to straighten behind you (but can't because of your hand grip)? When you get to the end of your 60 or 30 seconds, you will release your hand from your foot and as you do it will straighten behind you down to the ground. At the same time you will bring your body to upright.

In trying to reverse the pose to get to standing you should finish upright with your forward extended arm up by your ear, then exhale it down by your side. Often you are kicking so hard at the end that you may even fall or stumble forward. However if you can, meter yourself out of the pose, pressing less and less so that you still feel those forces of traction while reversing back to Savasana.

Common mistakes and how to fix them

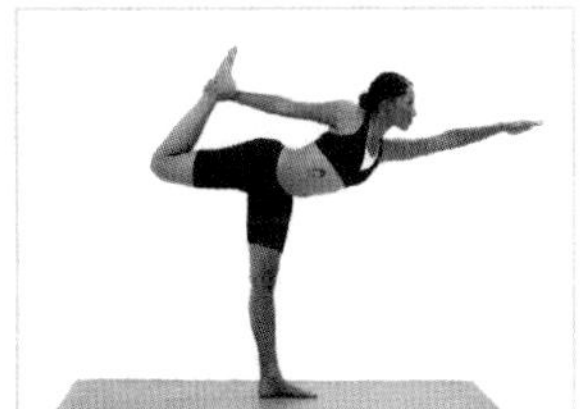

The biggest and most common error: Without a doubt the most obvious error is consciously dropping the body down before experiencing your fullest kick. It is only an illusion that the body has to come forward to create this pose. What you must do instead is work an arch into your chest and raise your arm.

The trick is to actually resist the downward movement of the chest and arm. Work solely on the creation of the biggest backbend that you can manage by keeping the parabolic form tight. Lift the chest and have the intention of touching the ceiling against the forward movement of your body.

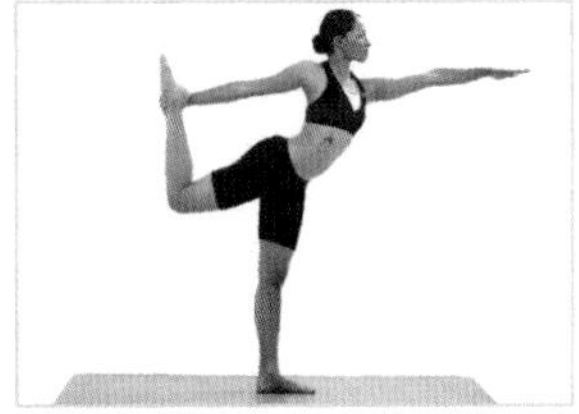

Dropping the arm: The next most common error is committed by beginners who drop the arm down to a position parallel to the floor, or level with the eyes. It arises out of taking a visual position-cue from the flexible or advanced students. The command is a retrospectively created one and comes from observing the final arm position of those who have their leg kicked high behind them or are approaching the full standing splits position.

The instruction to bring the arm down unfortunately does not delivery the body-opening results and in no way helps you to deepen your pose. If you drop your arm prematurely you are no longer allowing the kick to drive the posture and you cannot push your body down against your upward lifting arm. You lose the very important traction forces that allow you to effortlessly balance in Standing Bow.

Little wonder that students who drop their arms parallel to the floor also drop their bodies and can't seem to get their leg up high behind them. They can't balance easily and this graceful pose becomes a struggle. Set up the pose correctly, and regardless of foot height, always keep your arm up high while you kick back and up. It may help to occasionally have someone help you hold your arm up to stop it dropping down toward the floor. Over my time as a teacher I have had to change what we say at my studio to accurately reflect the actions required. Focus on the actions that yield results.

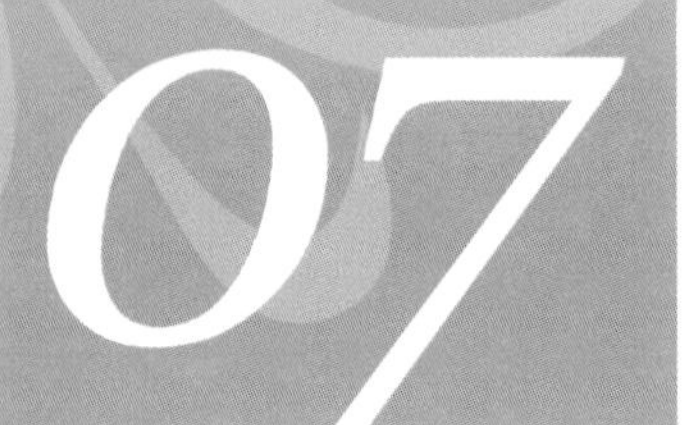

Dandayamana Dhanurasana

Standing Bow

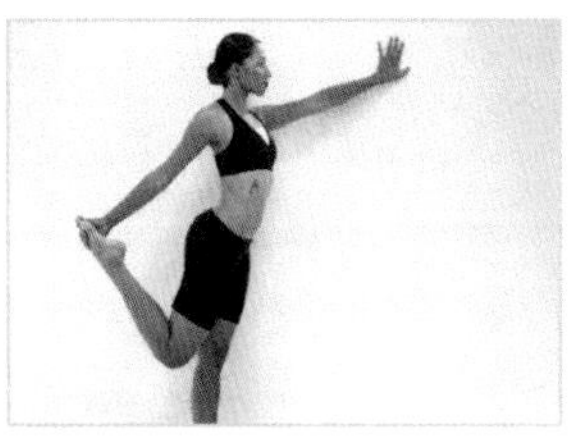

Balance difficulties, or you can only do one of the 2 basics: Many students, at least initially, find it difficult to balance on one leg. Oftentimes a new or inflexible student can hold the leg and not lift the arm, or extend the arm but not hold the foot at the same time. Sometimes it is a question of strength in the locked out leg. Try standing next to a wall and use it for support when necessary.

Difficulties may arise from a number of sources. These include injury, illness and tightness. Tight or frozen shoulders, inflexible ankles, wrists or knees, all complicate, but thankfully benefit from, Standing Bow. Typically men who have strong muscular torsos are generally more inflexible and have tight latissimus dorsi. This hampers the cross body stretch and opening the chest. This pose is renowned for improving or healing frozen shoulders and is excellent for encouraging post-operative healing in shoulder reconstructions.

Can't lock the knee: Locking the knee is often a work in progress. If your problem is just standing on one leg and you cannot yet grip your foot then I recommend standing next to a wall (if you need help with balance) or simply stand on your mat, and focus on locking your knee for 60 seconds (even without lifting your foot). You can focus on keeping your hips square so that there is no leaning and just lock the knee.

Thinking too much: Don't think about balance! You have to let go. If you are thinking about balancing then you will most likely sabotage your own efforts. What you have to do is CREATE the balance. You do this by following the correct pose actions: Simultaneously press the leg back and up and stretch your arm forward and up, all on a solid locked leg foundation.

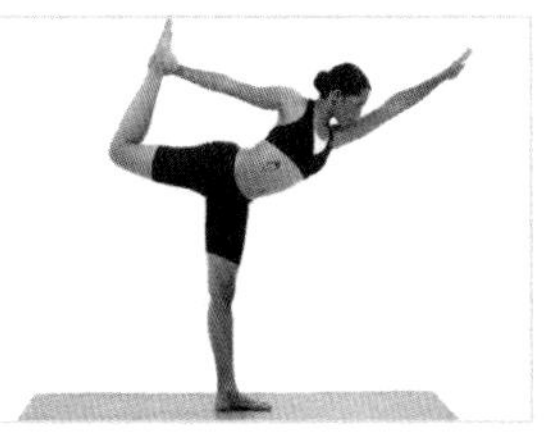

Chin drops: Dropping the chin is a sign of thinking too much. If you look down you may have lost mindful breath control, you are likely to have lost the upward movement of your upper body and the strength of your kick will be hampered. You are most likely to fall out. Look up, and revisit the basics.

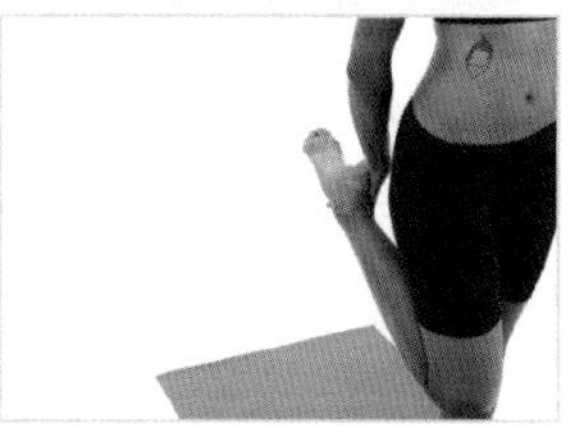

Basic grip error 1 – the inward rotation (or reverse hand) grip: There are basically 2 wrong ways to grip the foot. The first most common way is the inward rotation grip. This completely sabotages the pose and complicates the pose beyond belief. Students turn their palm backward, bend their elbow out and end up grabbing under their foot with their fingers and their elbow pointing to the wall.

If it feels strange, or too uncomfortable you are probably doing it wrongly. Let go, turn your palm forward to the mirror. Bend the arm a little and keep the elbow in contact with the waist and your palm facing up. Drop your hand in its stationary position and lift your foot onto your outstretched fingers. Simple!

The problems with a reverse hand grip: It is uncomfortable! It creates a twisting rotation which not only strains the wrist but rolls the shoulder forward and down. This in turn, counter-twists the torso making the mechanics of Standing Bow not only seem difficult but actually makes it impossible. How can you roll the shoulder forward and down (with the wrong grip) and take it behind you in a stretch?

The problem therefore is not only in back shoulder but in its relationship with the front one. The shoulder of the outstretched arm will move a little backward. So you see that it completely defies the principles when you have the wrong grip. It will close the chest. It will take each shoulder opposite to their intended direction, hamper your backbend and all the accompanying stretches. Get the grip right! Enough said.

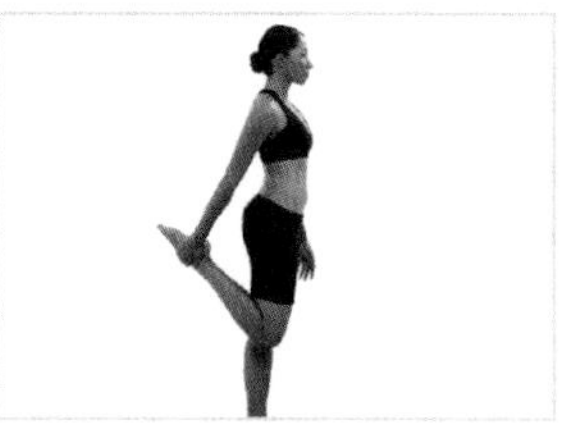

Basic grip error 2 – the outer foot grip: This second error is not nearly as serious. It involves the student extending their arm down by the side with the palm facing the thigh and simply lifting the leg to grab the foot from the outside. Although the shoulder will not have its backward position, it will not significantly hamper the stretch of the front shoulder. This foot hold is not as potentially damaging as grip error 1.

In fact I recommend this grip to students who have limited shoulder movement and for whom the correct grip is acutely painful. In this way they get much needed space and circulation in the joint. Their shoulders get restored, and can often recover from injury, shoulder reconstruction and frozen shoulder conditions. It does not take very much time for them to get enough healing that they eventually can grip correctly.

Kicking back but not up: The upward component of the kick is the hardest to accomplish. If there is no force driving your leg up through the power of the thigh then the body is more likely to move down towards the floor. You will look as if you are doing Balancing Stick, with your leg sticking up at right angles behind you. In doing so your arm will probably also drop in line with the body.

Sometimes a little assistance can give you a taste of the sensations to look out for when doing the pose correctly. I occasionally stand behind a student (mid-pose) and grab onto their ankle. At the same time I place a steadying hand on their lumbar spine I instruct them to kick further. I help provide the upward force through the ankle and intensify the backbend with my hand. From that class forward the student learns to deepen the pose, kicking higher.

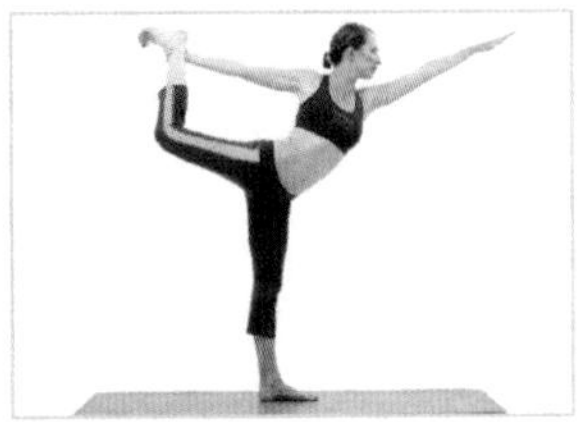

Kicking with a flexed foot: This usually happens if the grip is at the articulation of the ankle and foot. The foot flexes and the foot can kick back, but the knee tends to move down. The leg generally moves in the same direction that the toes are pointing. Hold at the foot and your ankle and foot flexibility will improve. Your pose will be more challenging. Your strength will improve.

Frozen shoulders

Students with frozen shoulders deeply benefit from Standing Bow pose. The stretch and traction across the shoulders create space and better circulation, not to mention movement of impurities out of the joint space. I have had a number of students who have also had shoulder reconstructions. It is very gratifying for them (and me) to facilitate a return to a full range of movement in the shoulder and arm, often within a small number of classes.

Practicing at home?

Then sometimes mix it up a bit, maybe lift your arm first before picking up your foot. It may bring a different dimension to your balance and take you out of ritualization of your practice.

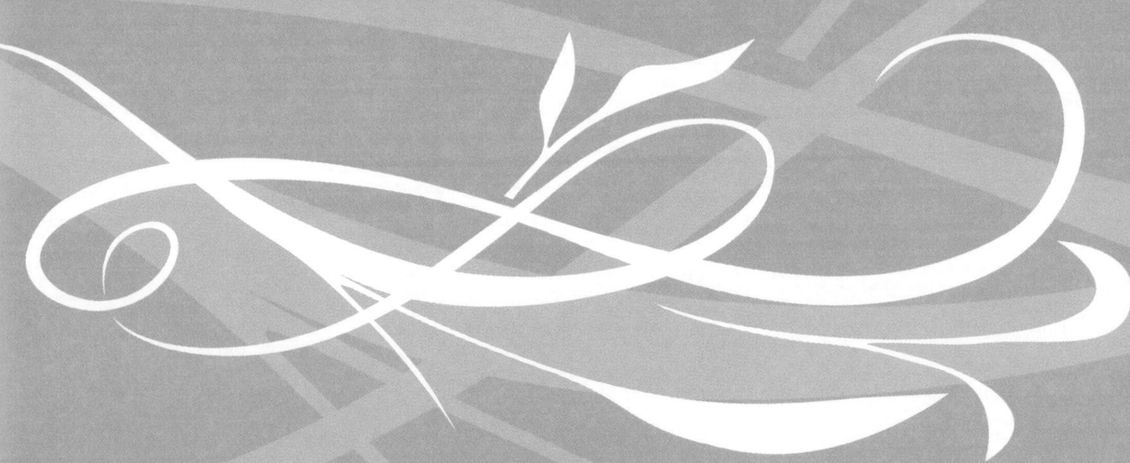

Tuladandasana

Opportunity is missed by most people because it is dressed in overalls and looks like work.
—Thomas Edison

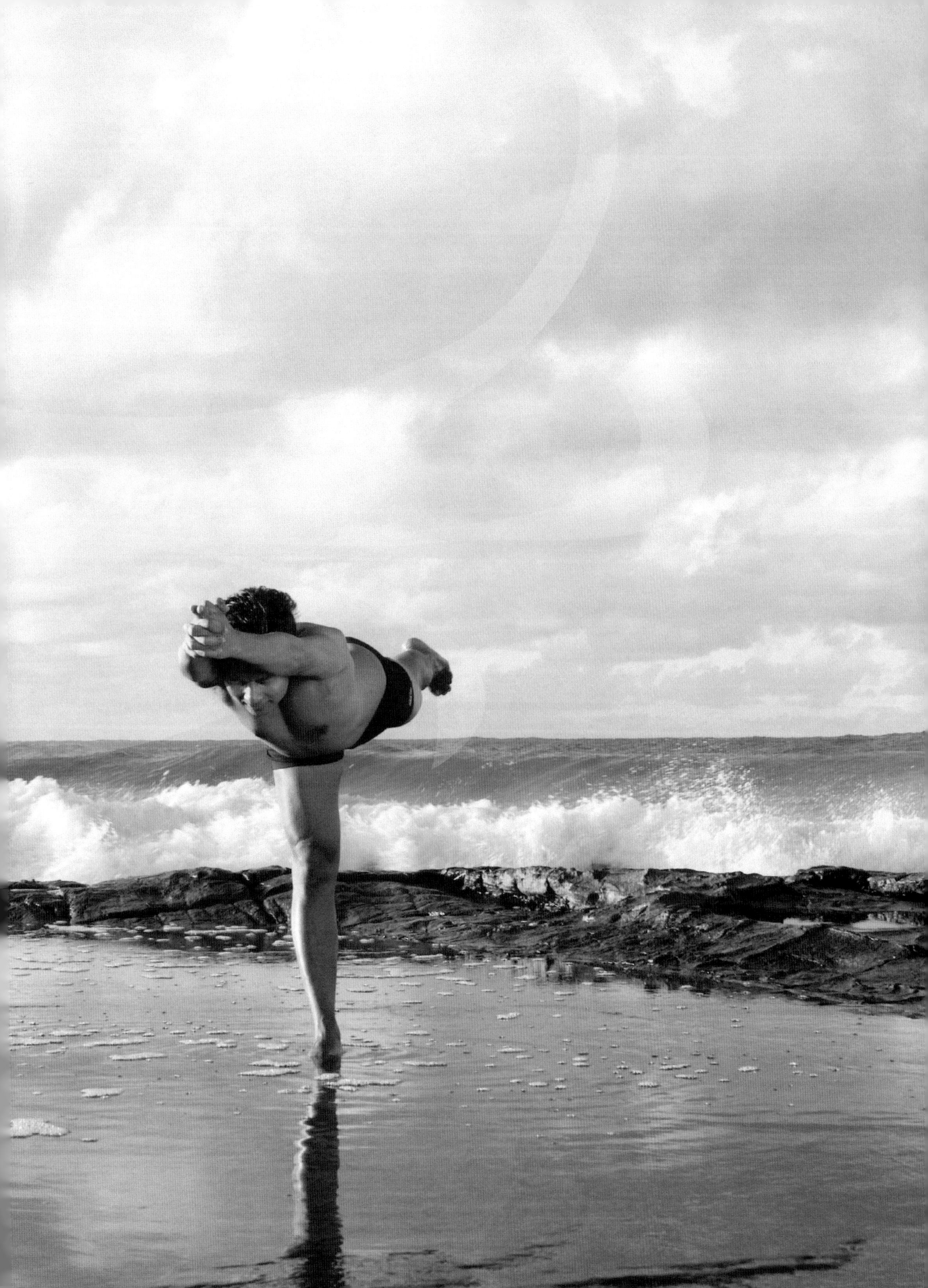

08 Tuladandasana

Balancing Stick

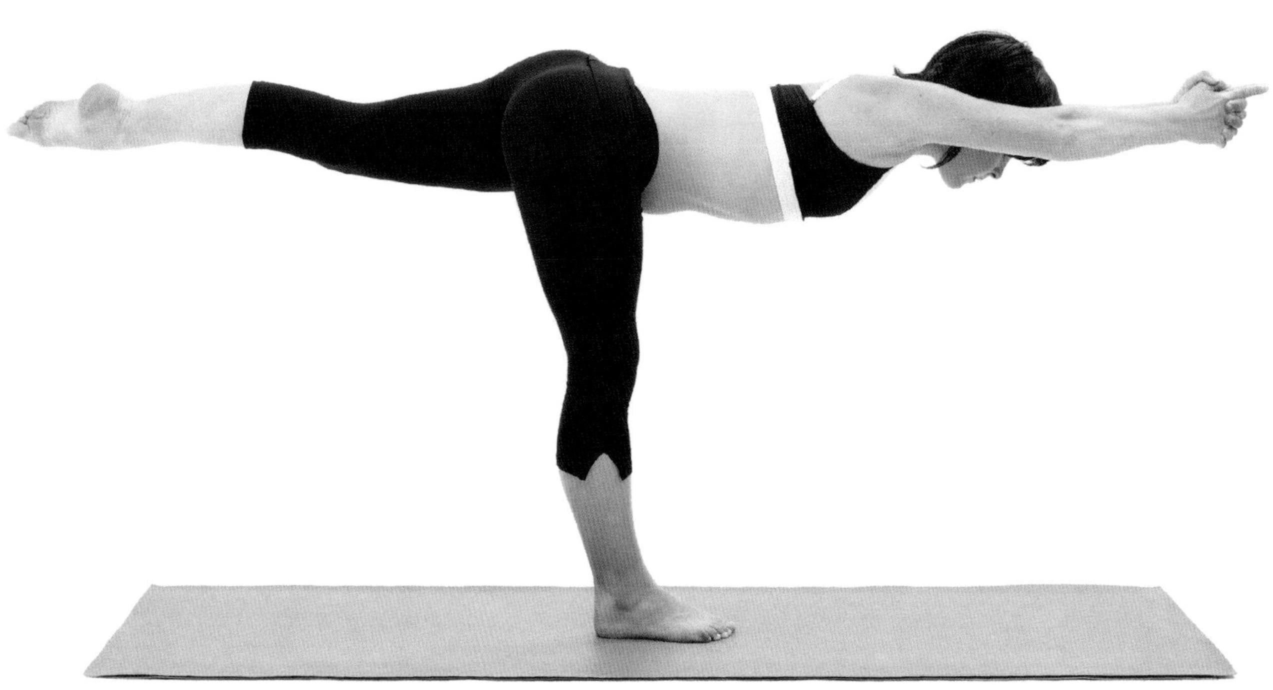

The essentials

This pose is about traction. You will learn how to stretch your entire body from your pointed fingers to pointed toes and elongating everything in between. It is very strong too, your legs are locked out, your arms are strong and the balance on one leg all multiply out to challenge you – all in one seemingly simple 10 second pose.

Balancing Stick also has a reputation for helping asthmatics. The chest opens and the lungs and heart physically stretch. It is hard to believe that the heart can work so hard in such a small time. This is great cardiovascular work and creates flushing of your coronary vessels. Face up to the challenge head on. You can do anything for 10 seconds.

What makes this pose so difficult to get right?

It is quite deceptive really. A 10 second pose should be easy, right? Balancing Stick wants to prove you wrong. Your ability to manage will depend on your strength and flexibility in equal proportions. To lengthen your body especially requires open hips, shoulders and sufficiently lengthy latissimus dorsi and a healthy core. When in the pose, you need to be strong to hold your body up off the ground like a balanced see-saw. Any single element missing will create great areas of focus for you.

This pose patently highlights the difference in your hips. Uneven hips will see you struggle to lift your leg. Maybe your latissimus dorsi are tight. Maybe you carry tension in your shoulders. Together these conditions will have you working hard not to create the classic 'broken umbrella' so often referred to. You may be surprised to discover how much this pose has to offer.

Tuladandasana

Balancing Stick

The technique

Shift yourself, if necessary, to the back of your mat or towel. You want enough room to be able to take one step forward to place that foot on the towel. Stand in Savasana with shoulders down and back.

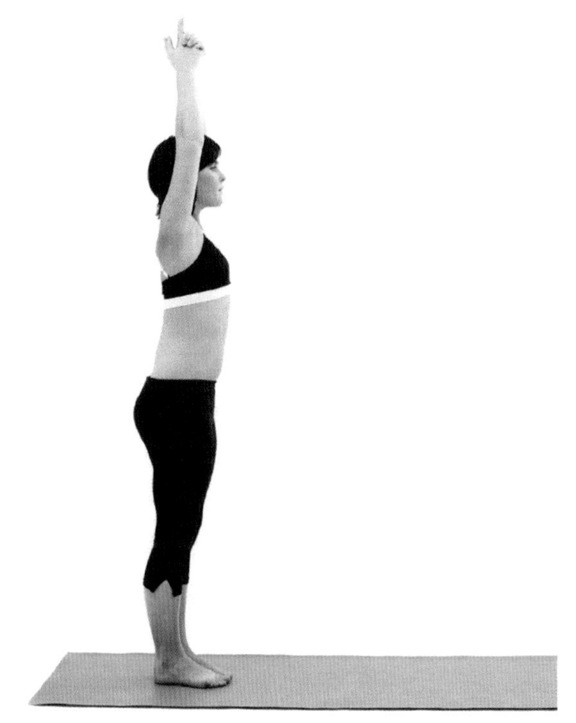

1. **Arms Up And Back**: Inhale your arms up over your head and interlock your fingers, index fingers released. Arms are only as straight, strong and long as you can manage with shoulders down and back, neck relaxed, no shrugging. A micro-bend is always preferable to tension (which will hamper your outcome).

2. **Head Up**: Chin stays up parallel to the floor. Arms are back, no shrugging.

3. **Step Forward**: On an exhale take a step forward on your right foot. Your right leg is locked and strong, supporting your whole body. Your toes (footprint) are square to the mirror.

4. **Leg Behind Strong, Hips Level**: Lift the left foot off the floor as if to take another step then leave that foot behind you, toes pointed. The toes may touch the floor behind you. Importantly, lifting the foot allows the front leg to take the weight. Square the hips to the mirror and floor regardless of position of your back foot.

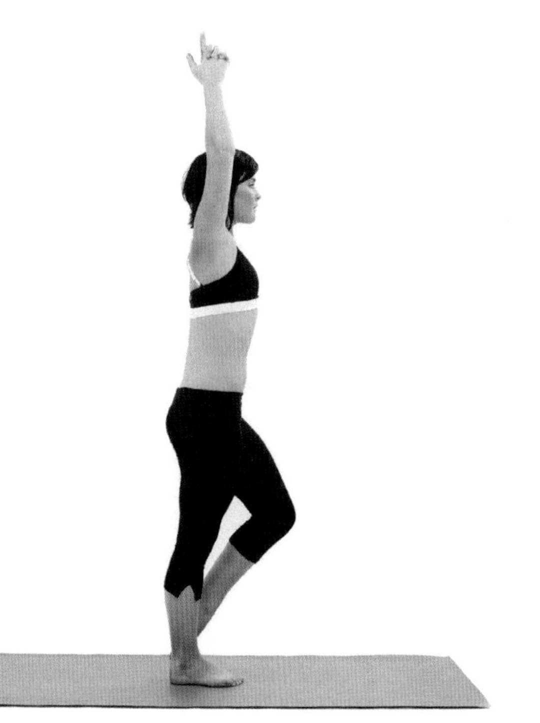

5. **Stand Tall**: With hips square and level lift your chest up and feel the extension through the front of your body right up through your fingertips as if you are trying to reach the ceiling. Lock both the standing and lifted legs strongly. In effect you are standing upright, strong and stretched, in an ever so slight backbend or arc.

6. **Inhale Length And Hinge**: Inhale length into your torso and strength in your legs and, as you exhale hinge your stationary body, arms and legs around your standing leg hip. It is crucial to try to maintain the static relationship of your arms, body, legs, chin and hips to each other. As you move simply allow your leg to come up, as you simultaneously bring your body and arms down, in an attempt to bring yourself parallel to the floor.

7. **Hip Down**: Keep the extended leg hip down parallel to the floor (not easy at all!).

08 Tuladandasana

Balancing Stick

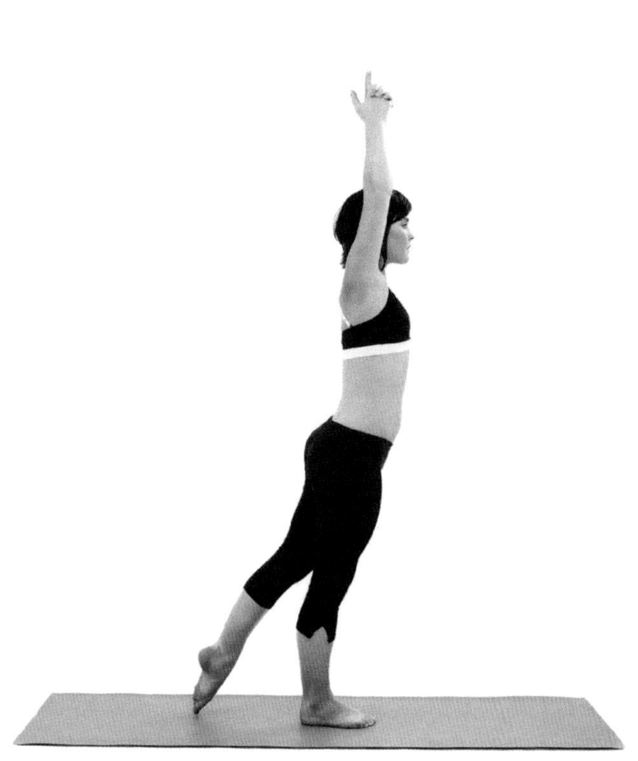

8. **Stretch Yourself And Look Forward**: With shoulders down and back you can elongate and stretch further. Ideally, if shoulders do not hunch, try to squeeze the head, with the arms by or behind the ears. But keep the chin away from the throat. If the eyes or chin drop the pose collapses. So look on the floor at least a yard (a meter) ahead, even at the reflection of your toes in the mirror.

9. **Pull Yourself Apart**: Create and feel a powerful stretch through immense traction. Use imagery and effort to enhance the extension from the fingertips to toes, through the whole body. Imagine a pulling sensation on your hands and feet.

10. **Work Hard, Continually Self-Correct**: You are aiming to maintain the same conditions in your arms, body and leg that existed before you lowered your body. Any changes in this relationship can be corrected mid-pose. Haul yourself out just enough to recreate the correct body position and reapply yourself. Although being parallel to the floor is ideal, be content if you are at your edge, with a firm straight stretched out body at any angle less than 90°.

This is surprisingly challenging. Taking the body down parallel to the floor is easy. Simultaneously keeping the arms up over the head and leg extended back at exactly parallel to the floor is where just about every student I have ever met finds they always have something to work on.

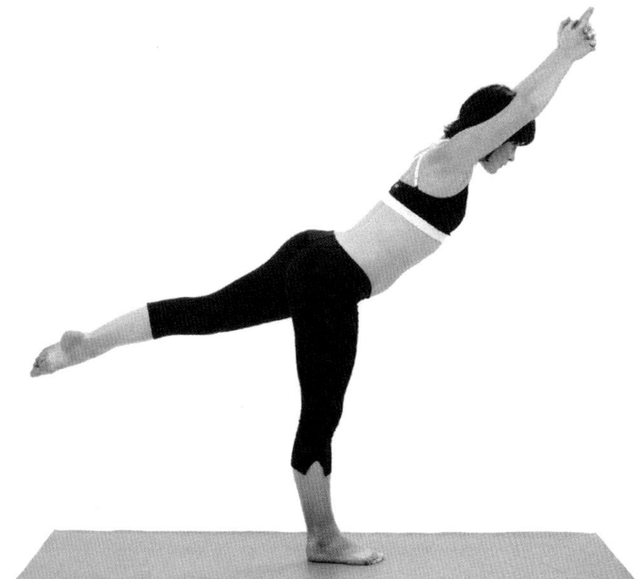

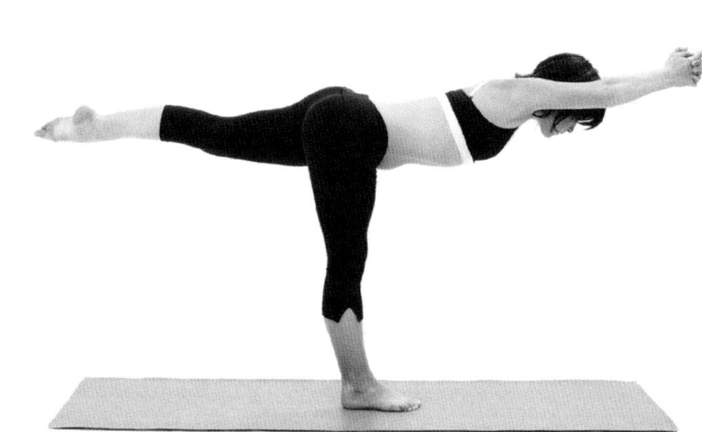

Release

Lift out of your pose on an inhale, allowing the extending leg to lower, stepping it back to your starting position at the end of the mat. Now step your grounded leg back so that both legs stand together, with your arms still extended over your head.

Keep your arms up over your head in readiness for the left side. There is a small Savasana between the sets where you will exhale and bring your arms down by your sides again. Keep your arms still and shoulders down and back. Your limbs and major joints need the renewed circulation, and rest from the hard work.

In your Savasanas your heart may be racing. Make contact in the mirror, breathe deeply with your chest open and feel your heart rate calm.

Common mistakes and how to fix them

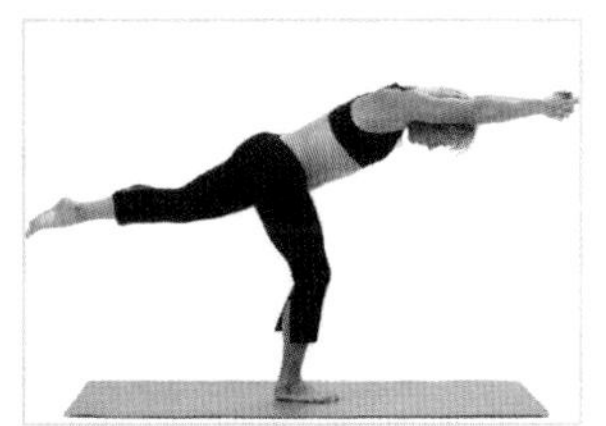

Bent legs: If your standing leg bends then balance is almost impossible. A see-saw needs a strong connection through to the earth. Your strong locked out lifted leg creates the perfect counterbalance to the forces from the torso and arms.

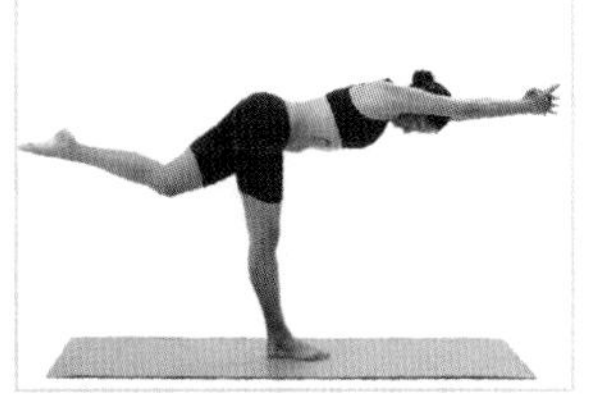

Chin drops due to body tightness: The chin tends to drop when you have tight lats or shoulders. The tighter your body the harder the extension. Keeping the arms squeezed close to the head will drop the chin and cause the arms to point down toward the floor. Work against tightness by focusing on stretching, lengthening and lifting the arms and body. Allow the chin to lift again by unclamping the head and arms and slightly bending the arms. Retreat to a point where you can sustain a straight-line form. The next error may be related.

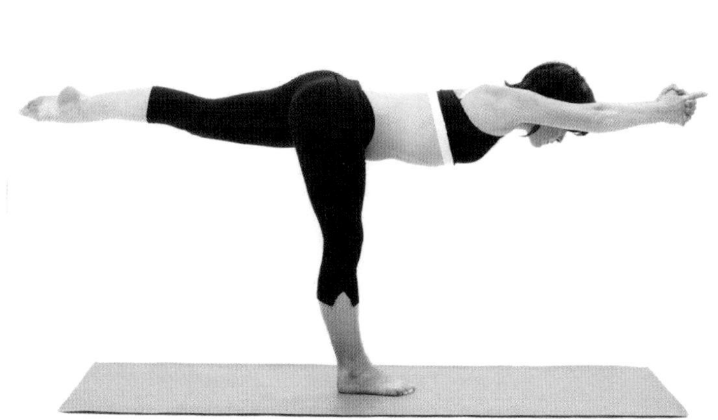

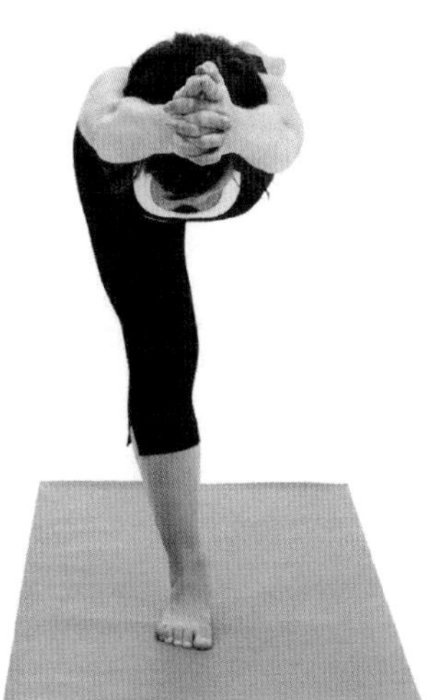

08 Tuladandasana

Balancing Stick

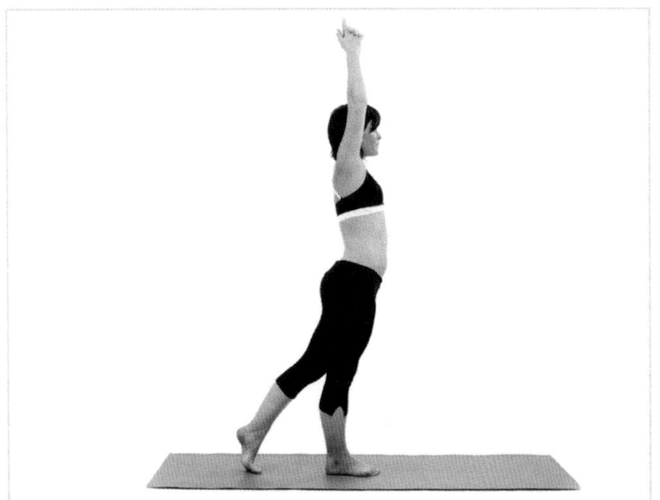

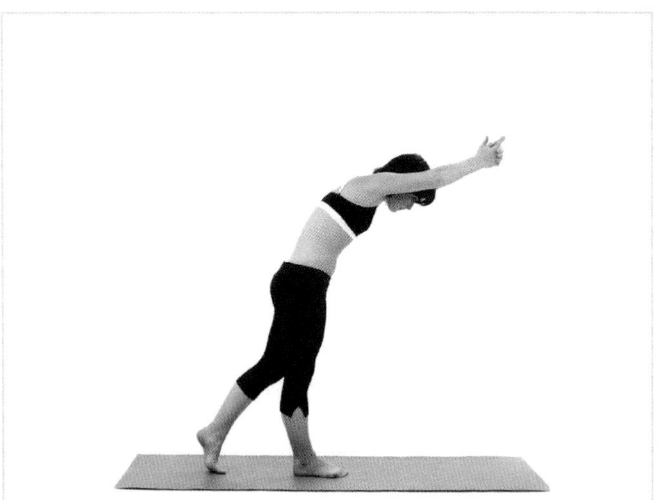

Eyes down cause chin to drop: A drop in the chin usually causes your eyes to look down. It may also cause your arms and even your legs to fall. Balance is lost and so is your ability to keep an actively strong and long body. Rule out upper body tightness, see above. This pose relies on strong forward visual focus, beyond the mat.

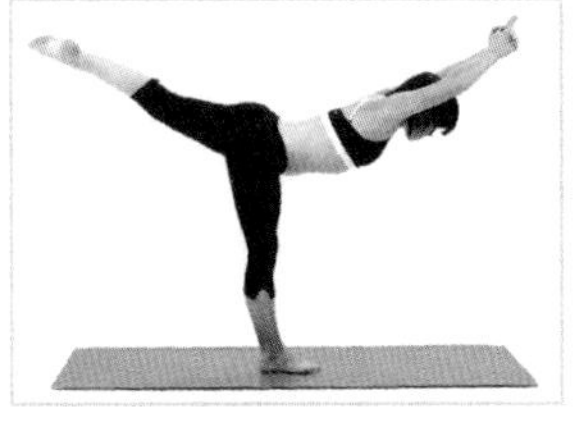

Leg too high: This usually happens when a student is close to the final pose. No matter where you are it is impossible to see how you look. It is therefore hard to finesse the pose without an observer. Commonly, in an effort to extend fully, the back leg lifts too high by about 5-10 degrees. If you are a dancer or very flexible it is very common to end up with your body taking the shape of a banana. The other fine adjustment is to drop the chest while extending the arms.

The leg doesn't lift until the body almost gets into position: Often I see students who start the upper body moving down and wait until the body is at least at 45° before they start to lift the leg. See the series of images above.

Remember to lock your arms and body and legs in that straight position and pivot around the hip. This means that everything will occur at the same time: As the body drops, the leg lifts.

This error happens mostly because the student has simply stepped forward while keeping weight in both legs. The front leg must support the weight and the back foot must come up off the floor even if just for a moment. Otherwise the body starts to dive as the weight shifts to the front leg on entry.

So remember, back leg lifts off the floor momentarily during set-up. Your body proportions determine whether your pointed toes will rest at or just above the floor. Stand tall and extended with a slightly arched spine. This will force your body to be totally supported on your front leg. Your pose will involve pivoting your form around the hip without weight redistribution.

Broken umbrella: This describes the shape of one's whole form when the body cannot sustain itself in a straight line parallel to the floor – both sides sag around the standing leg. Keep the relationship of your strong long body constant. Enter into the pose. Stay vigilant for the smallest signs of your arms or legs bending, or your chin starting to drop. As soon as they do, back out an inch or so until everything lengthens and strengthens again and rework it.

A straight body at only 30° from vertical that is strong and stretching is a far superior result to one that is 'parallel' to the floor but with flagging arms and legs. Maybe you will have only moved several inches off vertical, but you will have the traction forces to benefit from and improve upon.

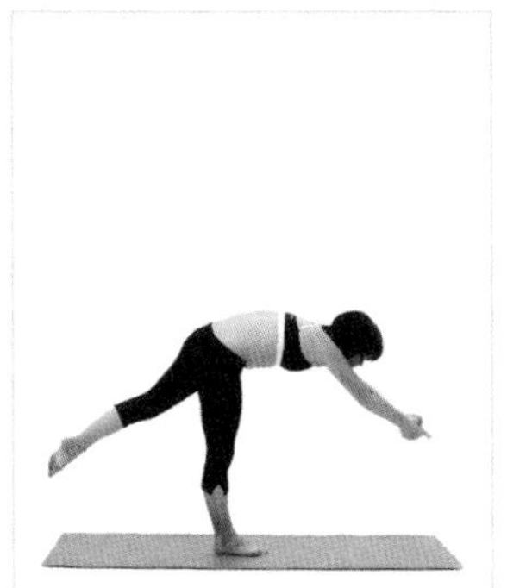

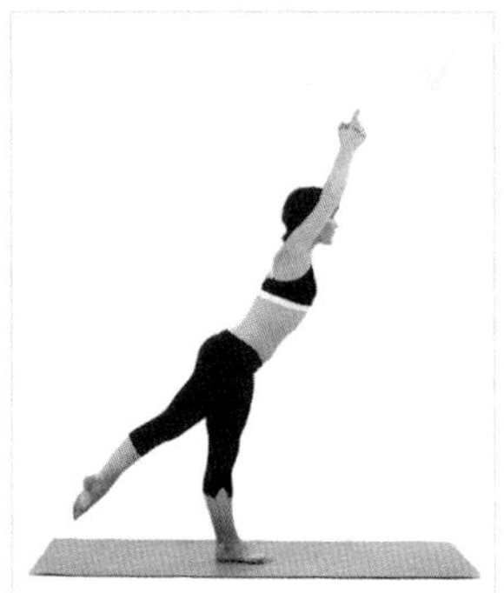

Tuladandasana

Balancing Stick

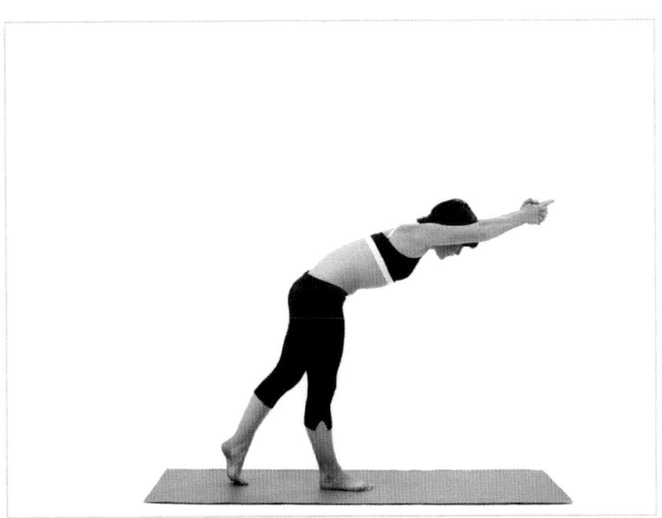

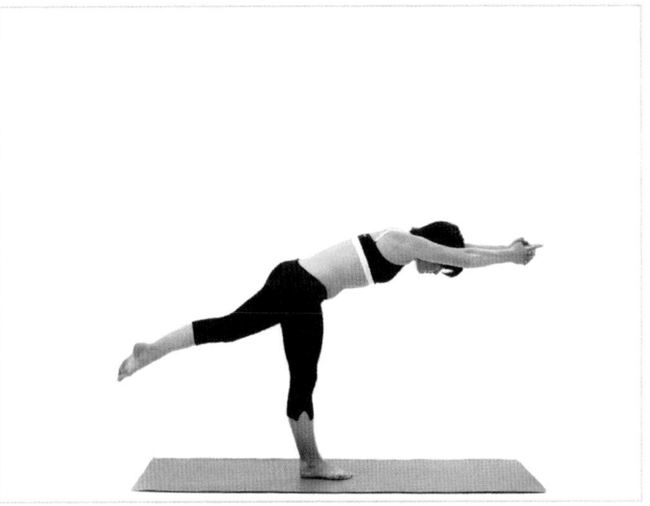

Bent arms: If your arms are slack then most likely your lifted leg is too. Strengthen and lengthen them as if to touch the mirror in front and feel the stretching sensation against the backward pull of the leg. Remember Newton's law – forces need an equal and opposite force against which to work.

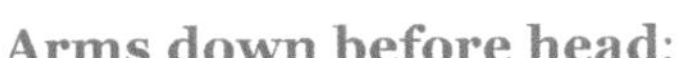

Arms down before head: If you can do so without shrugging or hunching your shoulders, keep the head clamped between both arms. The forces created increase your chances of creating a strong long body through relaxed shoulders. If properly positioning shoulders is difficult introduce a micro-bend in the arms.

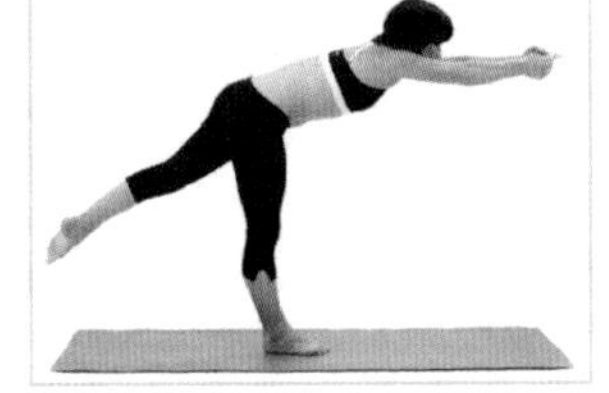

Shoulders shrug: Shoulder shrugging moves the blades wholly in a vertical direction and creates stress in the head, neck and shoulders. Drop the scapulae down and back and preserve the extension through to your fingertips. If you are tight or injured in this area you may need to bend the arms a little to decompress the tense muscles. It seems paradoxical that the lengthening of the arms and body means dropping the inside of the shoulders back and down, away from your ears. The chapter on arms and shoulders explains this very clearly and in simple terms.

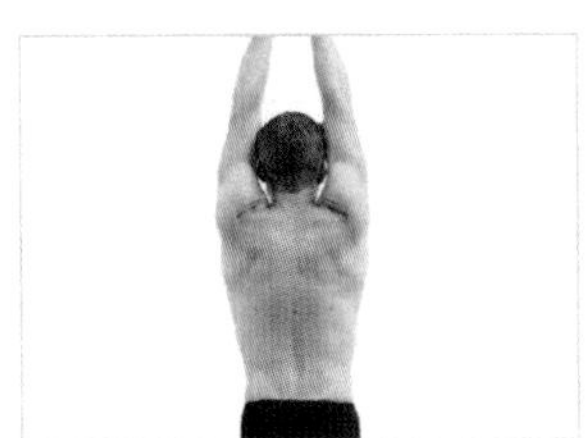

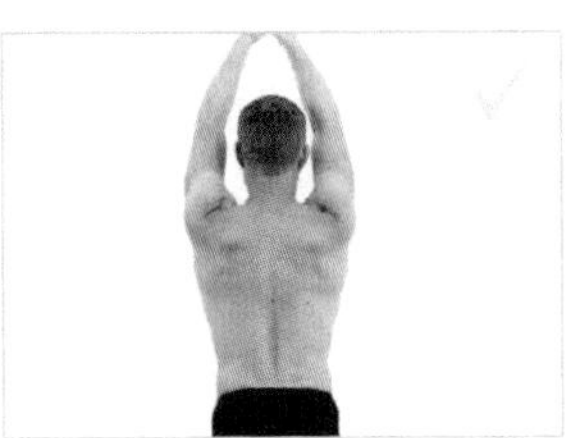

Too slow. Observe the 75% rule: Don't go slowly into this pose. Otherwise you will find yourself wasting up to 6 or 7 seconds in a leisurely transition. Just as in any pose, you are aiming to get to your fullest expression of it efficiently. The challenge is to get there as fast as you can without losing your balance. Then stay there because for the most part that is where the work happens.

Too fast: A common error (even if your set-up was correct) is to dive forward as if into a pool. The upper body goes forward toward the floor at a faster rate than the back leg lifts. The result is a 'broken umbrella' shape, or balance is lost and you fall and have to start again. Be deliberate and graceful and get there in a timely manner preserving the necessary strong straight form. Then if you find yourself bending you can straighten out and stop at that point.

Dandayamana Bibhaktapada Paschimottanasana

Laziness may appear attractive, but work gives satisfaction.
—Anne Frank

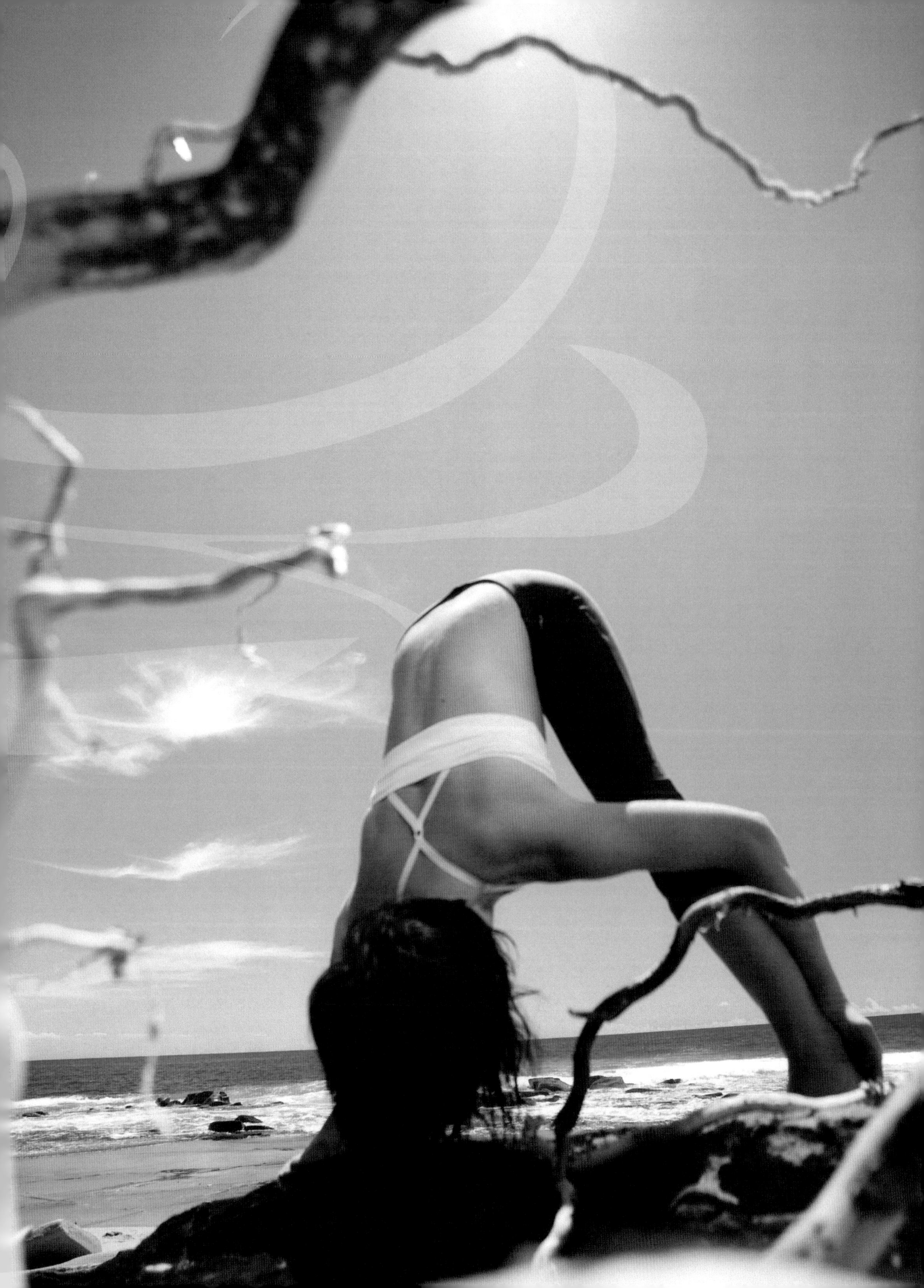

Dandayamana Bibhaktapada Paschimottanasana

Separate Leg Intense Stretch

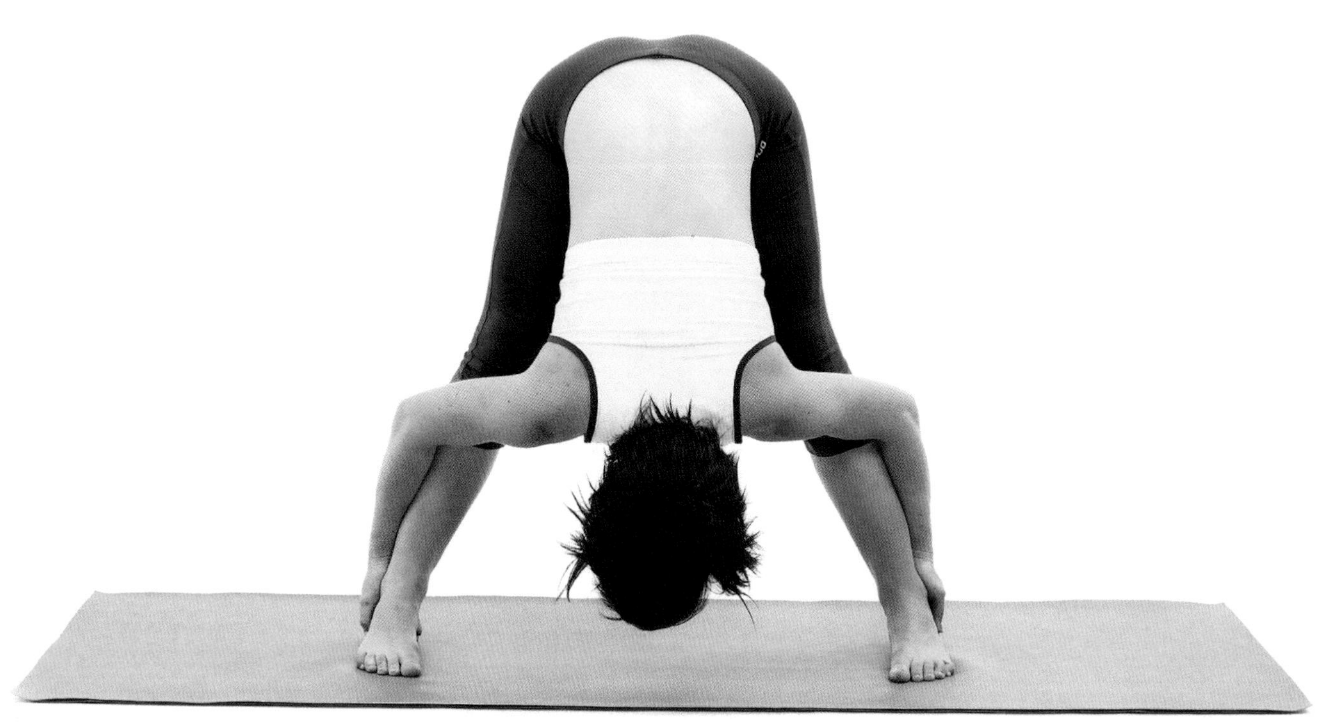

The essentials

Separate Leg Intense Stretch is a strong warrior pose. Yet its primary aim is to facilitate an incredible stretch through the spine, hips and legs thanks to the magic of several of the body's muscle reflexes. The main (or best known) reflex is that of reciprocal inhibition (the automatic relaxing response to the contraction of opposing muscles). When you understand and apply the correct use of the legs, arms and the grip you will feel the whole backside of the body stretching out blissfully – and not without some significant effort or reward!

The 45 second sets are spent bending, pulling and lifting in a very specific way. When done correctly space is created in skeletal and soft tissue systems and certain hamstring injuries can be ironed out; you should feel freedom and relief in your lumbar spine and sacroiliac joints. The chest actually feels as if it is being propelled through the shoulders. Your body will become toned and strong and the stress in your shoulders and neck will disappear.

What makes this pose so difficult to get right?

The pose must be approached correctly or you risk damage. The method I teach is totally in tune with the body's natural reflexes. If you are familiar with Bikram or hot yoga classes led by script-recital teachers then you will find this physiologically more holistic approach slightly different. I invite you to keep an open mind. Your body will thank you. This is not a rounded back posture. Years of experience shows that the power in this pose is to always, and at all costs, keep the back straight – otherwise it wouldn't be called Paschimottanasana (Intense Stretching).

If your back is round when legs are straight then you must bend the legs, especially if the body is tight. Surprisingly you'll feel a better stretch discovering hidden length in your hamstrings and lower back and possibly iron out hamstring injuries (rather than cause them).

I hope that you see by the end of this chapter that to do it in this way will serve to resolve pain in the upper body and stretch out the lower spine. A straight back is the aim. Straight legs are a bonus.

Dandayamana Bibhaktapada Paschimottanasana

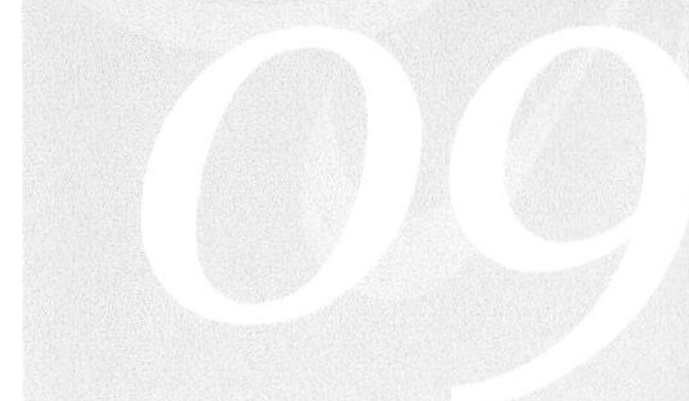

Separate Leg Intense Stretch

The technique

Find yourself to the left side of your mat. You are going to step out to the side about 3 foot (about a meter) and straddle your mat. Stand in contact with yourself in the mirror. If you are at home you may either have to change the direction of your mat or step out on the length of it.

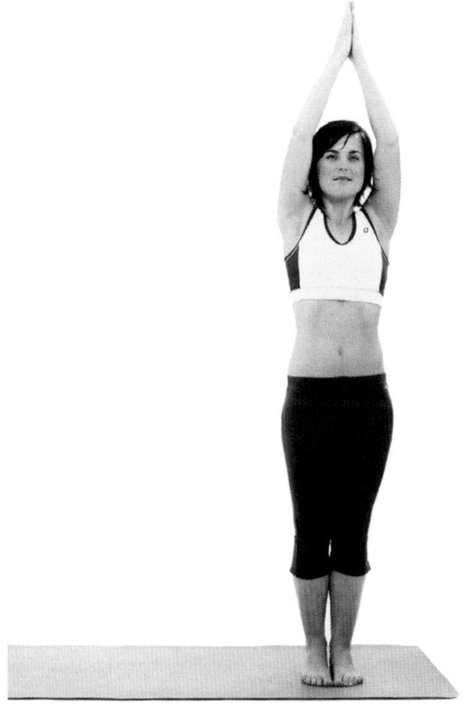

1. **Arms Up And Step Out**: Inhale your arms up over your head and on your exhale do two things simultaneously: Step out to the right to about the 3 foot (1 meter) mark and, lower your arms down so they are parallel with the floor.

2. **Arms Out**: Your arms are now outstretched as if there were one line from fingertip to fingertip right through your shoulders.

3. **Toes In**: Your feet having started out together, are now apart and parallel. If you have sciatica or acute lower back pain then you will need to keep them parallel. If you have neither of these complaints then you will bring your toes in slightly so that they are pigeon-toed. This will intensify the stretch through your hips and hamstrings.

4. **Warrior**: Stand tall and strong as a warrior. Make sure your shoulders are down and back.

A quick tip: If you feel tension in your shoulders here, with your arms outstretched, turn your palms up to the ceiling for a moment and then rotate them back down again. Feel and actually see how this draws them down and back and lengthens your neck. This is the activation of your lower Trapezius. For more detail on arms and shoulders, see pages 38-43.

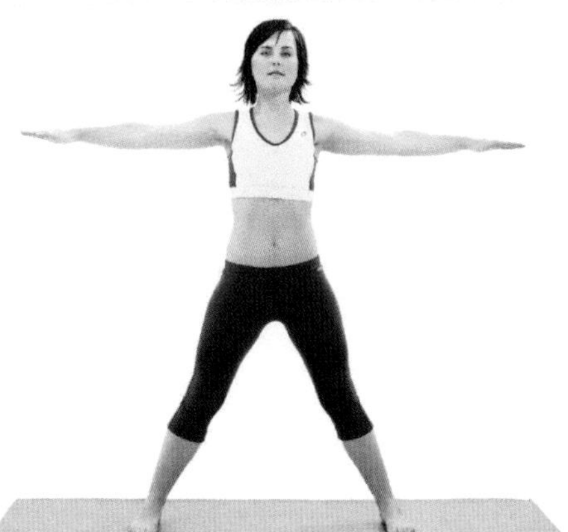

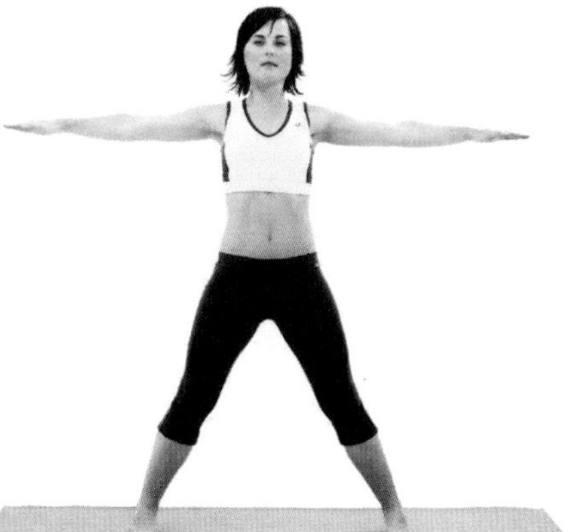

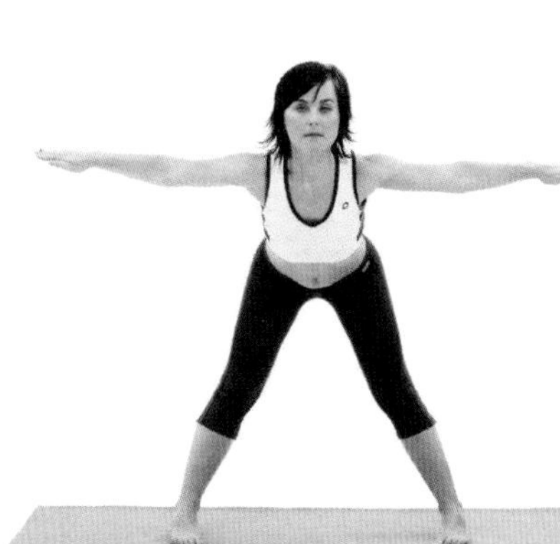

Dandayamana Bibhaktapada Paschimottanasana

SEPARATE LEG INTENSE STRETCH

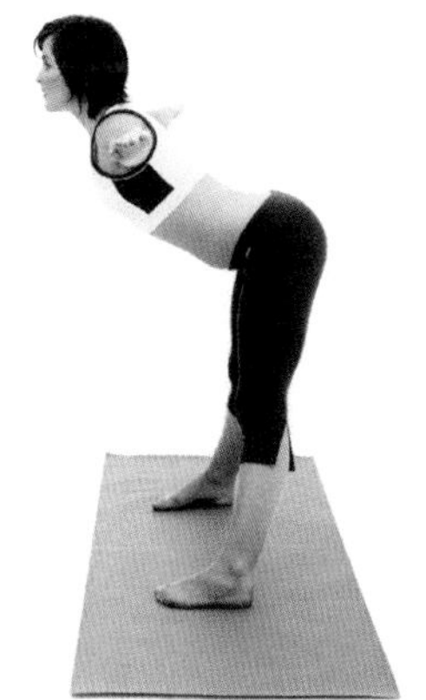

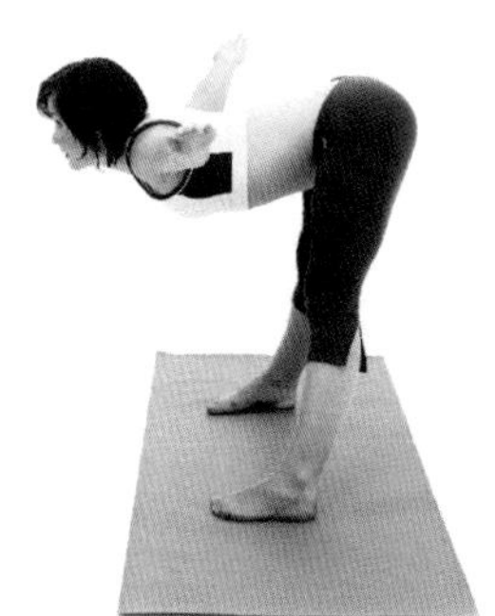

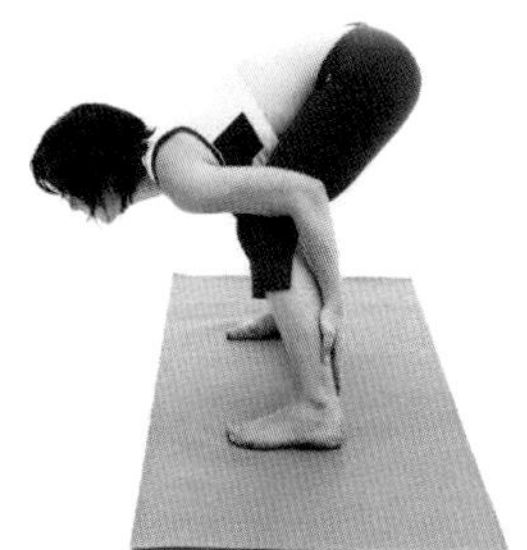

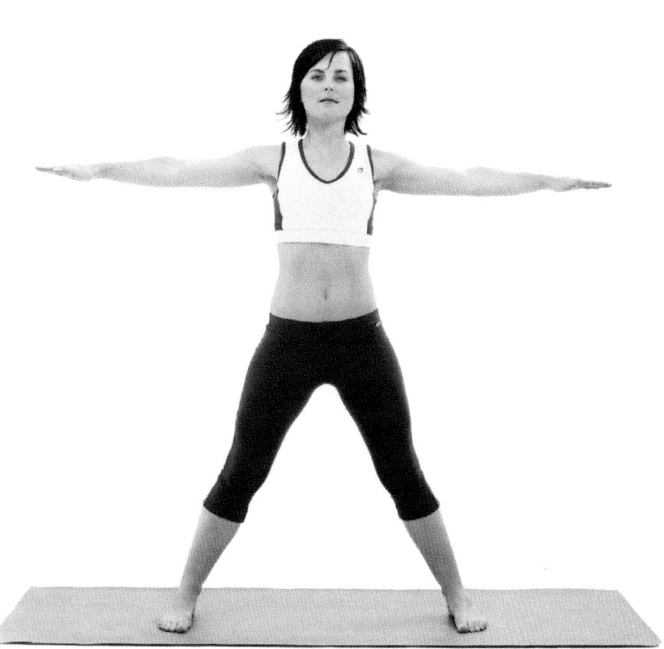

5. **HINGE YOUR BODY DOWN**: Lengthen your torso on an inhale and on an exhale draw in your core, and with arms out, hinge at the hips to bring your body down toward the floor with spine straight. To facilitate the continued ironing out of your spine keep your chin away from the chest in an effort to maintain eye contact. It is when you can no longer do this that you perform the next part of the pose.

6. **GRIP THE FEET**: Bend your legs (only place hands on the floor if necessary). Slide the hands down the back of your calf muscles and lift each heel in turn to slide your fingers under to face forward, toward the mirror. Your thumbs are on the outside of your foot and ideally your elbows are pointing up and back behind you.

7. **LOOK FORWARD, STRAIGHTEN THE SPINE FIRST**: Keep your chin away from your chest, eyes forward. In this way you work on lengthening your straightening spine from your coccyx right through to your cervical spine (your neck). Draw your chin forward like a turtle's head out of its shell and imagine touching your forehead to the floor between your feet.

8. **PULL WITH BICEPS, LIFT HIPS, STRAIGHT BACK**: Take an inhale and on your exhale PULL on your feet with your hands. Consciously LIFT your hips up to the ceiling. The action of the PULL with your biceps is crucial. Your elbows or forearms should be touching your shins. When you pull, don't think of pulling your body down, rather imagine your elbows and shoulders moving up (away from your ears towards your hips). This engages reciprocal inhibition to open up the back of the body.

9. **LIFTING HIPS STRAIGHTENS LEGS**: Lifting the hips up lengthens the legs. Most importantly the back must stay straight whether legs lock or not.

10. **WHEN THE BACK ROUNDS**: As soon as your back starts to round, back off by re-bending the legs a little and then re-engaging the pull. Always aim for a straight back. Keep pulling with your arms and lifting your hips, extending your chest forward between your shoulders. This is an energetic pose.

11. **FOREHEAD TO THE FLOOR**: As your legs start to straighten, your forehead will approach and may even touch the floor. Because the pose is all about extension you never want to rest the head on the floor and cause any spinal compression.

    The moment your forehead contacts the floor you must make a mid-pose adjustment. Walk your feet closer together an inch (few cms). Revisit the basics and start the work again. The more advanced you get, the closer your feet will be: You may only have to step out 2-3 feet (60-90cm) in your set-up.

12. **BACK STRAIGHT, LIFT HIPS, WEIGHT IN TOES**: The ultimate ideal is to have legs completely straight and locked out. The spine protrudes straight down from upward facing hips. The shoulders and elbows are drawn up. You can feel the biceps working. The chin away from the chest, as you look forward, face parallel to the floor creates an even greater spinal extension. Roll your weight forward into the toes and feel the stretch deepen. Pull, lift, roll forward.

    Even though your body is moving down to the floor, it is less about trying to get your body down there, but more about facilitation of this movement by virtue of the:

a. Pull on your heels using your biceps muscles;
b. Lifting of the hips up, up, up;
c. Position of the chin away from the chest;
d. Working of the stretch through the legs and back with or without straight legs;
e. Eventual straightening and locking of the legs.

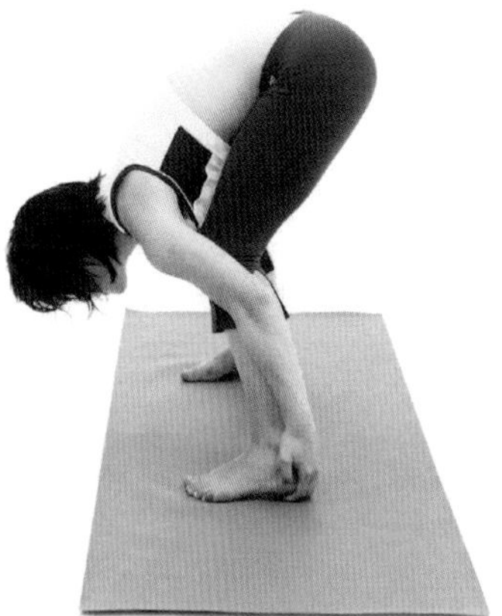

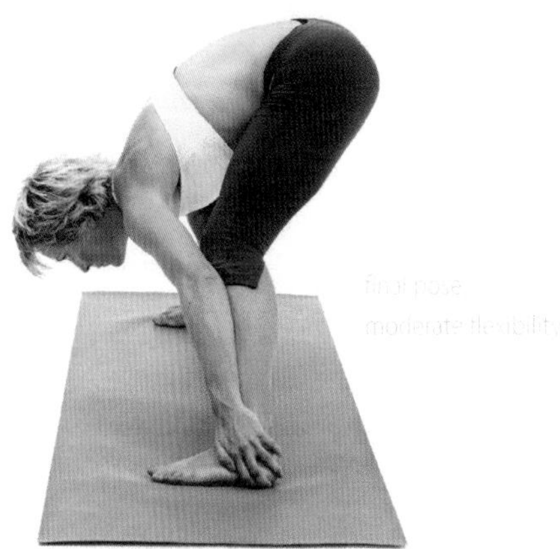

final pose
moderate flexibility

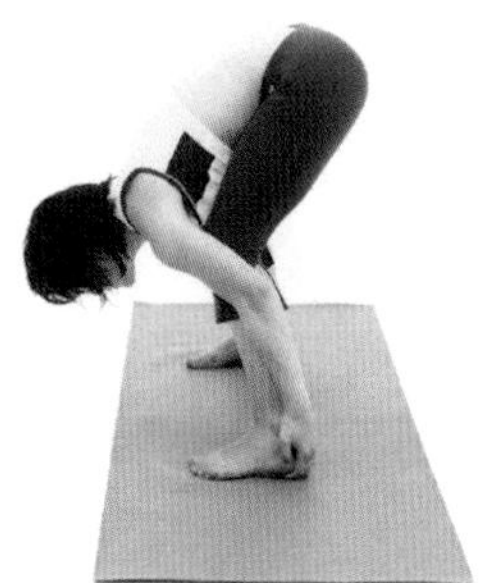

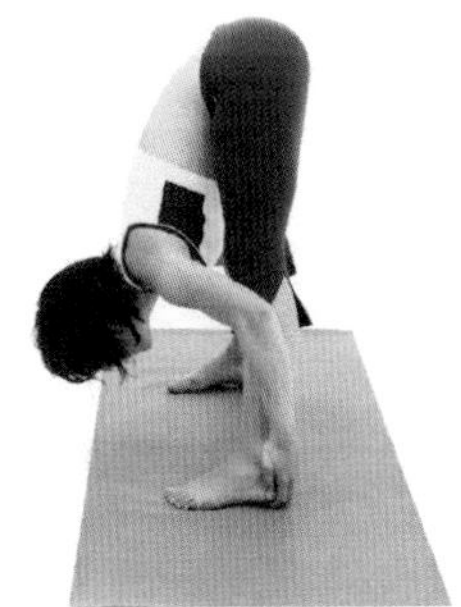

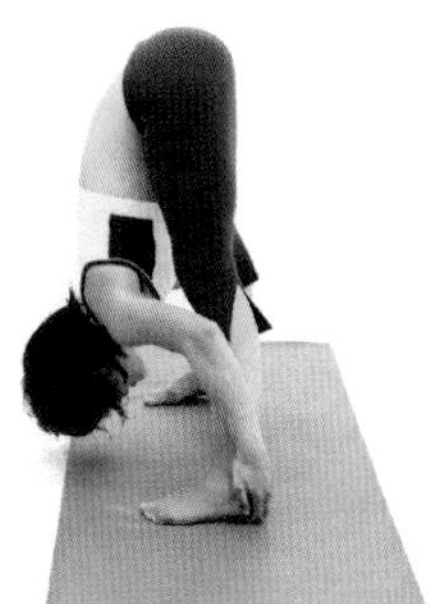

Dandayamana Bibhaktapada Paschimottanasana

Separate Leg Intense Stretch

Straighten the legs or straighten the back? That is the question.

We need yoga. And as part of our yoga routine, we need backbends. Without them nothing would counter the ill-effects of the excessively numbered forward bends that we perform everyday from the moment we get out of bed 'til the moment we get back into it. We do forward bends to get up, sit down, get into and out of our cars, to reach for something to set it back down, to pick something up. You name it, and you probably did a forward bend to get it done.

That in and of itself creates the reason for my (increasingly popular) approach to Separate Leg Intense Stretch pose. The emphasis is on creating and nurturing the intense stretch everywhere, and not just in the legs.

The second set

Many teachers say that your aim is to get your forehead to the floor. This is wrong and shortchanges your benefits. If the forehead ever touches then adjust your feet inwards an inch (a few cms) to create more leverage to continue engaging and deepening the stretch. If, in the first set you did not get your forehead to the floor, then set your feet further apart. If you did manage it, then set your feet closer together.

What if you are super-flexible?

If, in the first set, your straight legs are about 2 feet (60cm) apart, your back is straight and you feel you cannot further deepen this pose then try this. Enter second set in the same way and this time, after establishing your pull, draw your elbows away from the shins. Maintain the upward pull to keep the shoulders away from the ears. In this adaptation the shoulder blades tend to move together and muscles across the upper back strengthen.

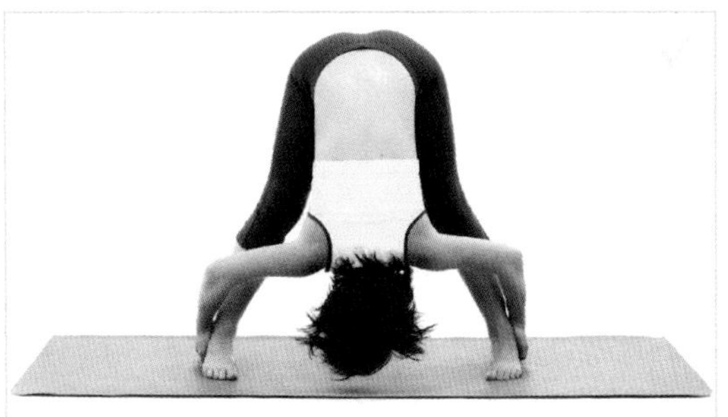

Release

Maintain the pull right 'til the last moment while leaning into your toes. Firstly let go of your hands. Then draw in your core muscles, lengthen your torso and bring your arms out to the side. Reverse out of the pose with your chin extended and spine straight. Straighten and strengthen the legs as you stand up into your warrior position.

Inhale your arms up over your head and simultaneously step your right leg back to your left. Exhale and bring your arms to your side. Contact in the mirror. Stillness.

Occasional dizziness may be a result of releasing your grip at the same time as raising your body off the floor. It can particularly effect those with low blood pressure. Provide a second or two after grip release for the circulation to re-establish itself and then come up.

Common mistakes and how to fix them

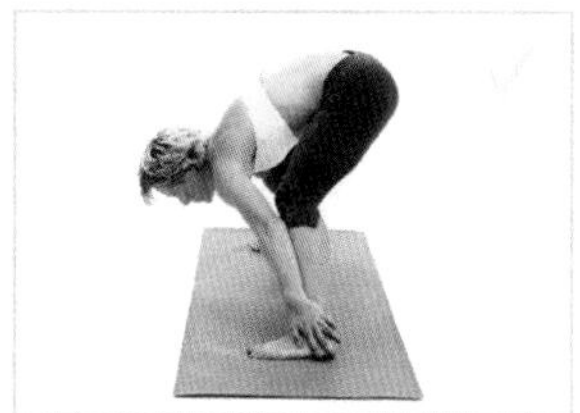

Can't reach your feet: This is a very common issue. This is just one of the reasons to bend the legs. Remember you are trying to elongate the spine so rounding it to reach the floor is counterproductive. Bend the legs and try to get the hands under each foot from behind. See 'grip' notes below.

Can't get the grip: Bend your legs. If you cannot slide fingers under the foot from behind, aim for the side of the heel. If not, hold as far back behind the arch as possible. Holding the foot at 90° from the side with fingers under the arch is the least effective grip. It recruits the shoulders which shrug. Draw the elbows inward so that the fingers point forward and in toward the center and elbows point more to the back corners of the room.

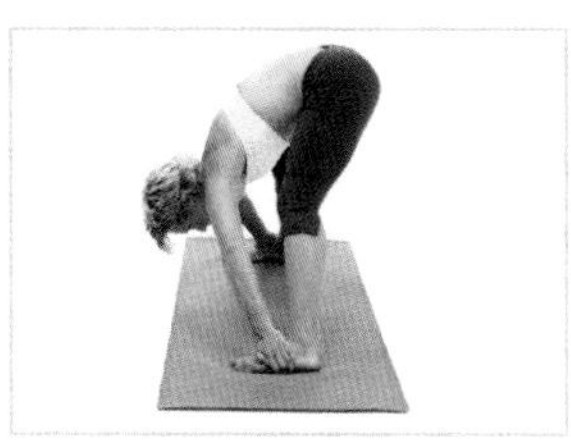

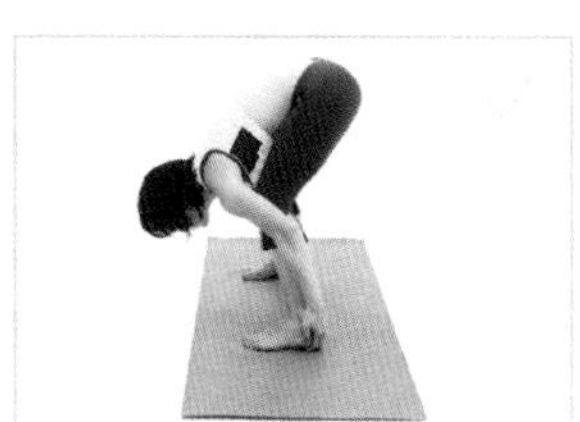

Thumbs on top of the foot: Whatever you do, ensure that your thumbs are on the OUTSIDE of your feet in order to draw your elbows out and back, and your shoulders up.

Toes point to corners: Feet fanning out can be very unstable. When toes point out (or in) stretches through the bottom, lower back and legs will be intensified, and you could risk worsening a sciatic or acute lower back condition. So, simply step out and leave feet parallel for a neutral position. If you have no such issues then pigeon-toe your feet.

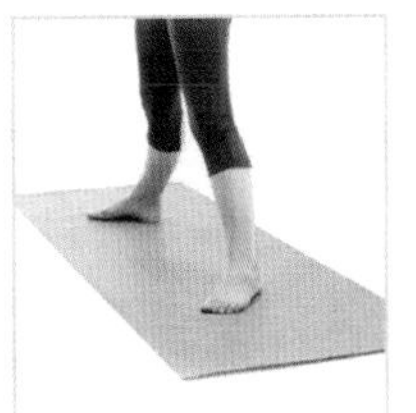

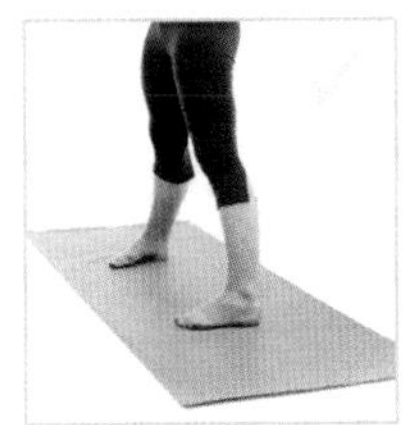

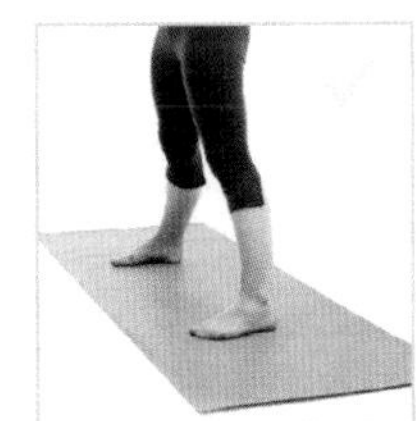

Hanging out: Some students are tempted to just hang when they can't reach their feet; back rounded, straight legs and arms dangling. This pose is not simply about the effects of gravity. Your body will not open and lengthen without the proper grip and pull. Follow correct technique: Protrude the chin to lengthen the spine, bend your knees to reach your fingers under your feet, then pull.

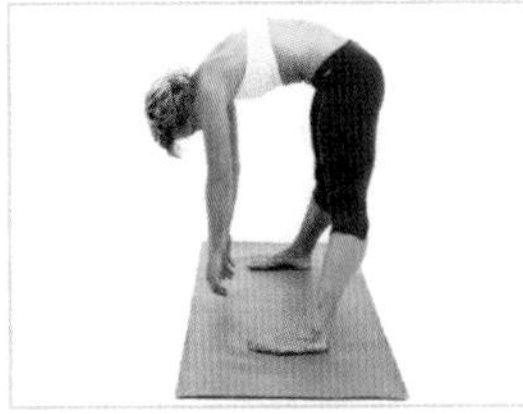

Hands at the ankles: Placing the hands under the feet will give you the best leverage and stretch. This is impossible for some students due to inflexibility, injury or larger body size. Instead place the palms on the back of the bent legs as low down as you can. The thumbs may need to envelope the outside of the leg to get the pull. Apart from this grip, the technique is the same: Bent legs, straight back and pull with bent elbows pointing behind you rather than out to the side.

Feet too close: Many new students assume the reach is easier when feet are closer. They place them at about 2' (60cm). Mostly the stance is equal to or wider than 3' (1 meter) if the mechanics are to work. Bend the legs to grab the feet; work on straightening your back rather than your legs. As your flexibility improves, foot distance narrows.

Hunching and pulling with shoulders: Use your biceps to pull, not your shoulders. Let them move up away from the ears and towards the hips.

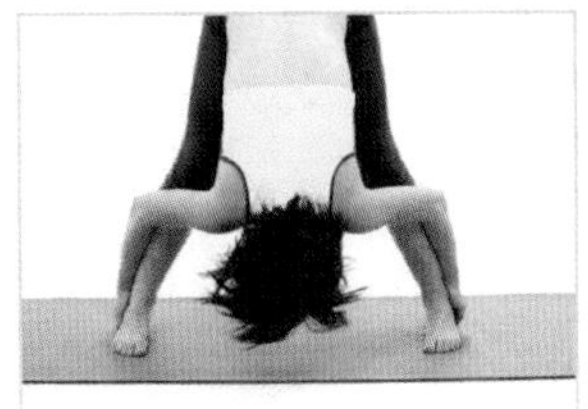

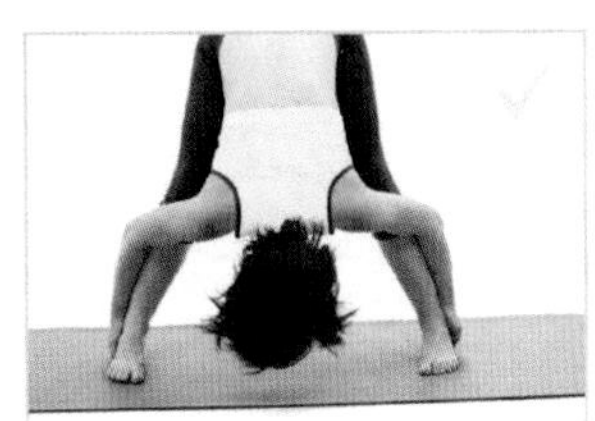

Feet too far apart: Your feet are positioned too widely if; your arms have to be straight to reach your feet; and your legs are straight and cannot bend; and your spine is rounded.

The common command to step out 4' (1.2 meters) is for most just too far. Most students need to step out somewhere between 2.5' and 3.5' (0.75-1m). Bend the legs, pull with bent arms. Feel the difference.

Looking at the back wall: Many students, even flexible ones, often look at the back wall while pulling on their feet, causing the spine to round. Extend your spine long and straight by pulling your chest through your shoulders. For your whole spine to benefit the chin has to be away from the chest; the face has to be parallel to the floor; eyes look down to the floor between the feet; and shoulders move up away from the floor.

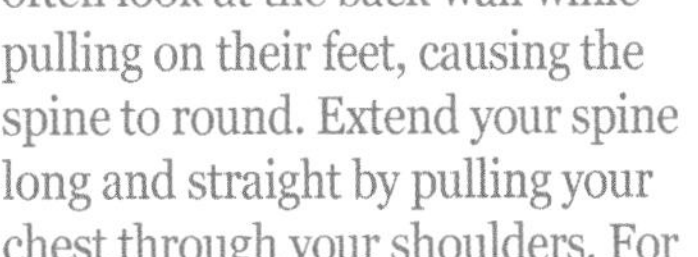

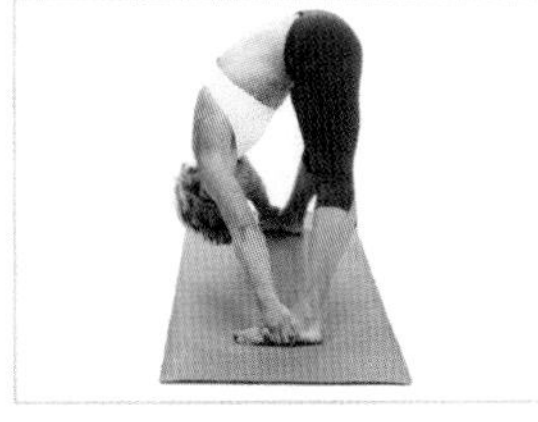

***Acute back problems can change the entry**: Lumbar or thoracic spine conditions may be worsened by the standard straight-back entry. Here's how to avoid engaging muscles and causing spasms that could cause you grief in these cases.

Once in your warrior position, keep your feet parallel, and not pigeon-toed to minimize aggravation. Tuck the chin, walk your hands down your legs, and curl the spine until you get to the floor. Now engage the pose in the regular way because it is great for ironing out such problems. Your damaged muscles will get some rest and length.

At the end of the pose, release your grip, and walk your hands back up your legs, follow your hands with your eyes, chin up last.

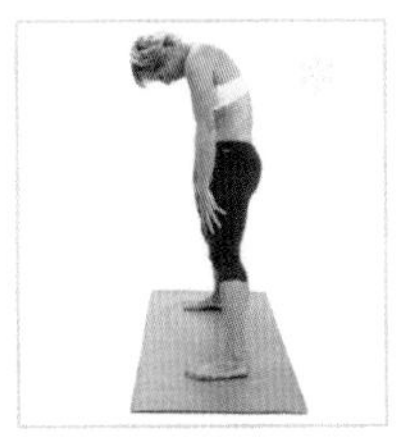

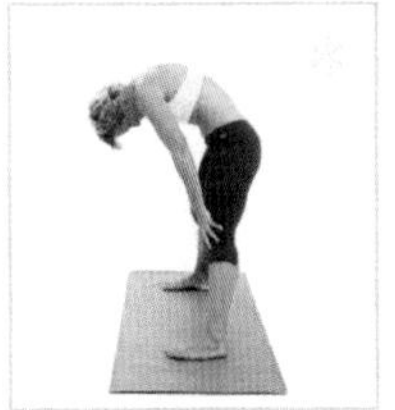

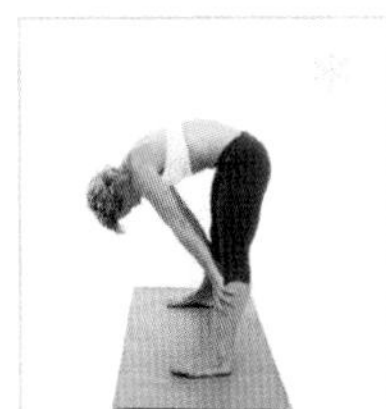

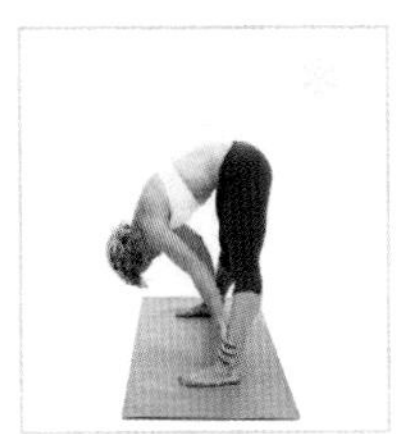

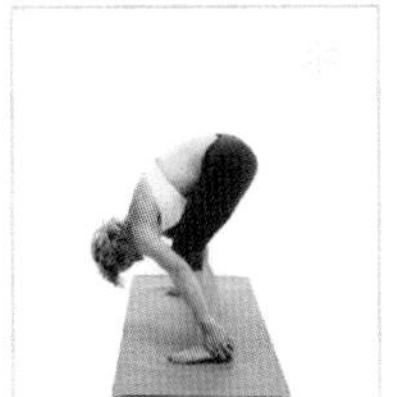

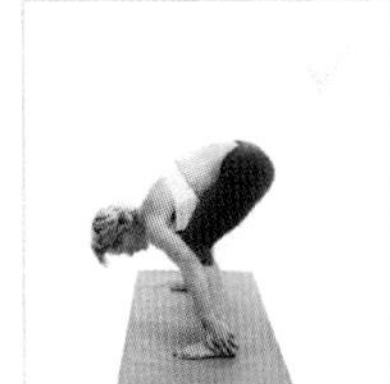

Trikonasana

You've got to go out on a limb sometimes because that's where the fruit is.
—Will Rogers

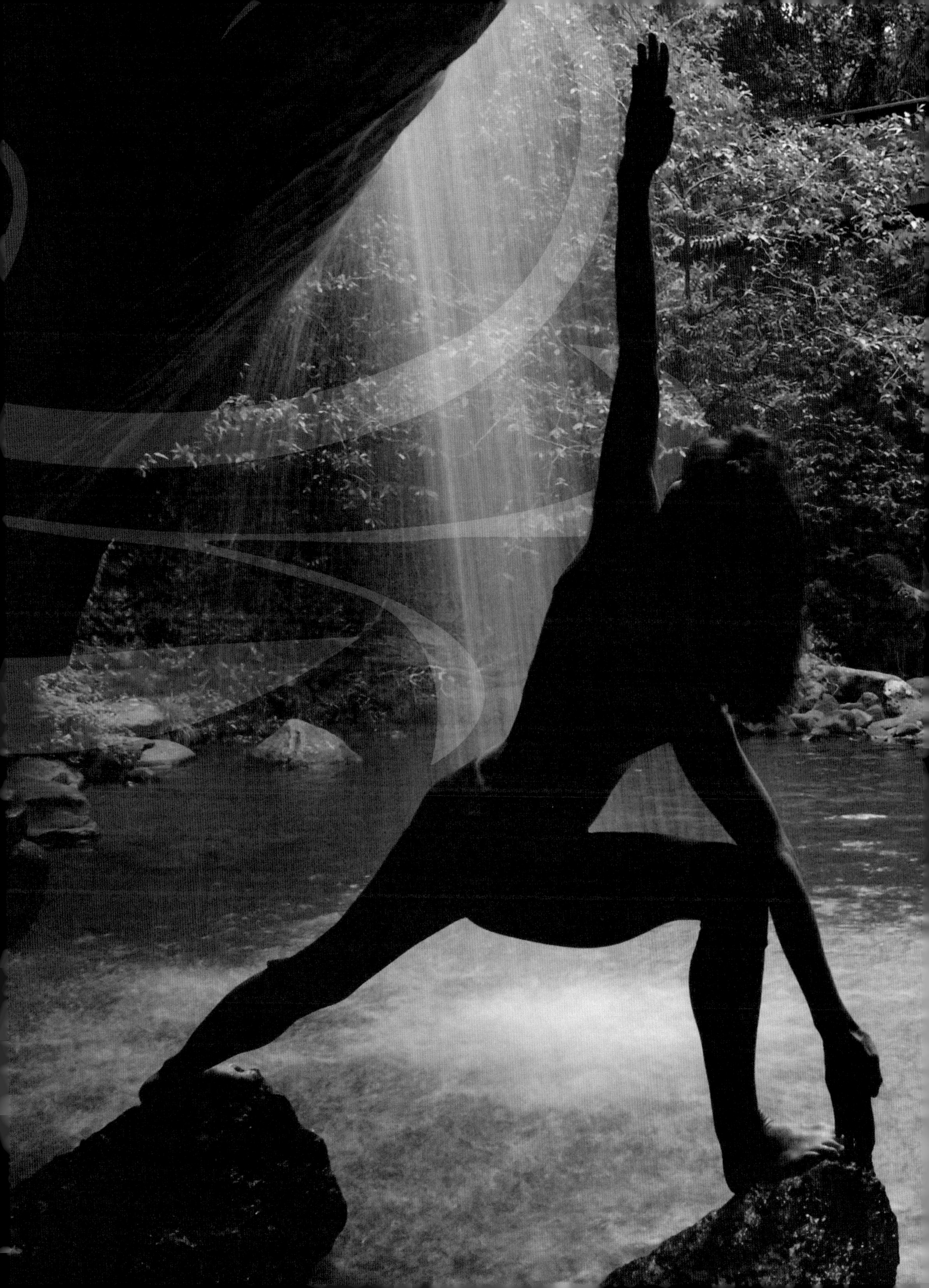

10 Trikonasana

Triangle Pose

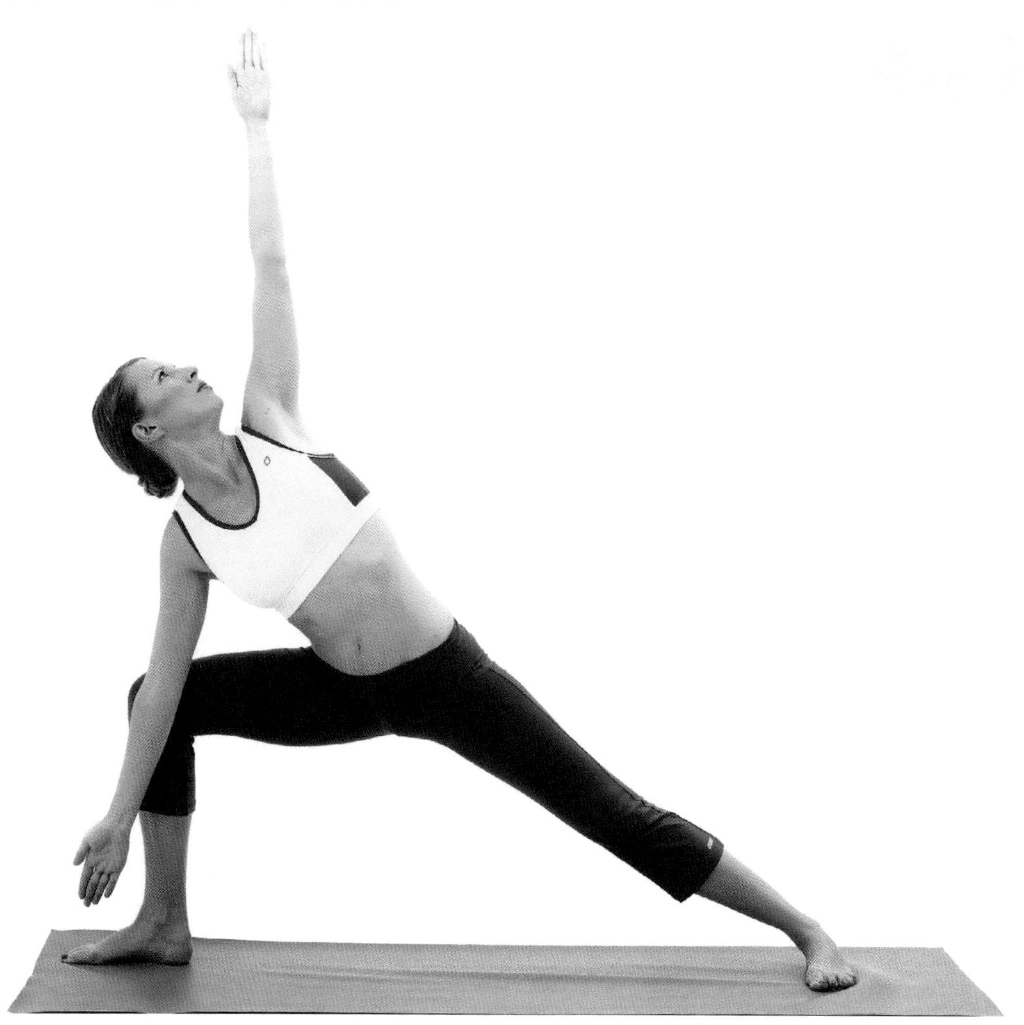

The essentials

Often referred to as a power pose, Triangle is strong and energetic providing a good challenge. You may be quite tired by the time you get to this warrior pose. The work is demanding, involving all major muscles groups. Plus, you have to try to hold your body up against gravity whilst in an asymmetrical position. It all comes down to engineering the body geometry well to take the struggle out and bring the balance and strength in.

This pose is a wonderful hip opener. The tractions deliver great shoulder stretches and body length. Your ability to hold your body up off your leg for what can seem like ages, proves your stamina, focus and ability to breathe through adversity.

What makes this pose so difficult to get right?

The challenge is to combine the right degree of strength, stretch and effort with the correct relationship of the legs, arms and body. Have your legs or arms an inch from their correct position and you can feel tired, overcome and falling to the floor. Move them back and feel energized and just about invincible!

With so many elements on which to concentrate it is little wonder that some things occasionally fall by the wayside. Even practiced yogis will sometimes find their goal elusive but other days it seems so easy. Once you discover the keys however, this pose can be your friend and consistently improve your strength.

Trikonasana

Triangle Pose

The technique

After finishing Standing Separate Leg Stretching you find yourself to the left (or at one end) of your mat. For this pose you will once again step out to about 4 foot (1.2 meters).

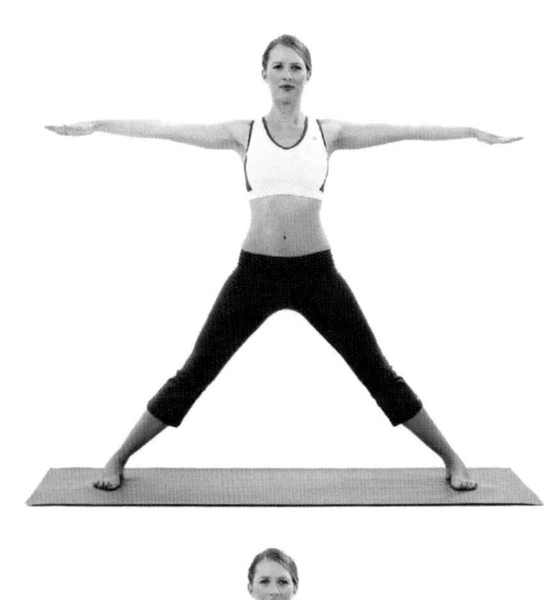

1. **Arms Up**: Inhale your arms up over your head and as you exhale you will do two things.

2. **Step Out, Arms Out Palms Down**: You will bring your arms down parallel to the floor, palms down, and you will step strongly out to the right about 4 foot (1.2 meters). There is a straight line that travels from fingertip to fingertip through your strong straight arms and shoulders. Drop the shoulders down and back to resolve any shoulder tension (see tip on page 141).

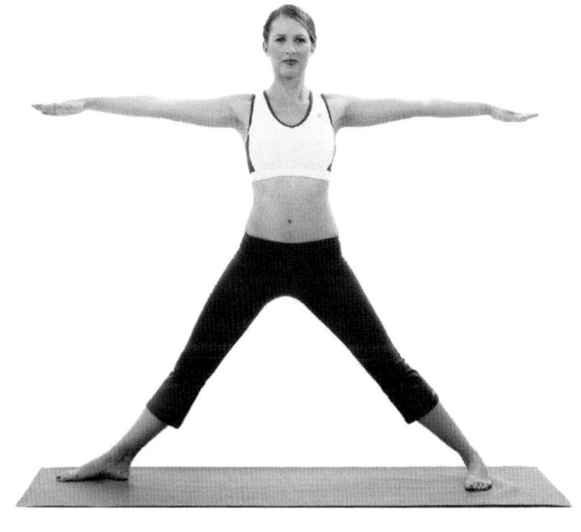

3. **Angle Your Feet, Heels In One Line**: Pivot your right foot on the heel through 90 degrees. Bring your left toes in about 5-10° to the right. This position assists hip stability and safety in the adductor stretches. The line through your heels is parallel to the mirror.

4. **Level And Square Hips**: Try to maintain your hips square to the front and level to the floor (easier too, with heel to heel placement).

5. **The Lunge**: Inhale length in your torso, lock your left leg knee completely and lunge deeply into your right knee. Your leg position is crucial here. It will not only determine your ability to balance and support yourself, but also the safety of your knee. Bring your right thigh down, parallel to the floor to make a 90° angle. Your shin is vertical. Your knee tracks directly over your ankle and should never be past your toes. Nor should it be back behind your ankle, even though this is possibly the lesser of 2 evils.

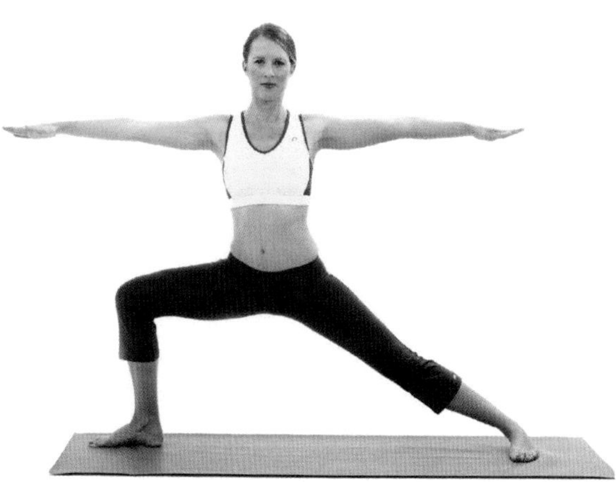

6. **Bounce Once, Settle Into Position**: You can settle in to your lunge by (optionally) bouncing once gently to tease open your hips and stretch your adductors. You feel balanced and strong. Your feet are pressing wholly and strongly into the floor and each takes the load equally. Your heels drive downwards for a powerful connection so there is stability and no hint of sliding. Your hips are square. Your palms face down, shoulders relaxed. This is your warrior.

10 Trikonasana

Triangle Pose

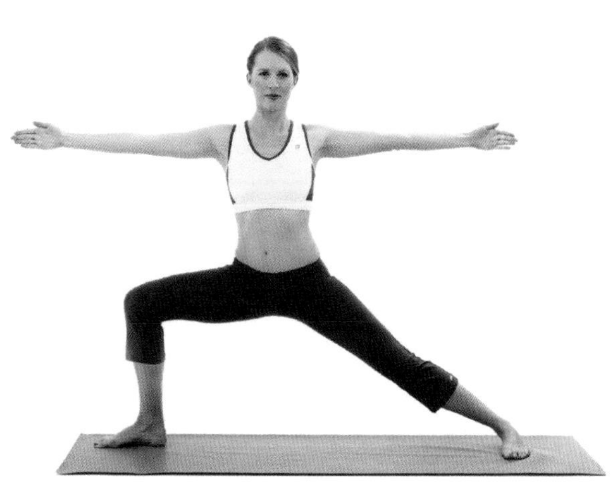

7. **Palms Forward, Arms Back, Move Into Triangle**: Take an inhale, externally rotate your arms to turn the palms forward while holding your arms back. Exhale and move your energized arms and body into position so that the elbow comes in contact with the bent knee (never below it). Be sure to continue the straight relationship of arms from fingers through your shoulders. Turn the head so the chin is over (not resting on) the shoulder and look up through your thumb and fingers stretching up to the ceiling.

8. **Press Elbow Against Knee**: Push the elbow against the inside of your right knee with a constant backward force so that the shin is vertical. The fingers of your straight arm point down toward the outside toes (and not the big toes). This creates healthy knee alignment and a wonderful active stretch from your locked leg to your bent leg opening your hips, pelvis and adductors.

   Keep your body as upright as possible. It will come down at an angle creating one of many triangular relationships obvious to you if you were to look in the mirror.

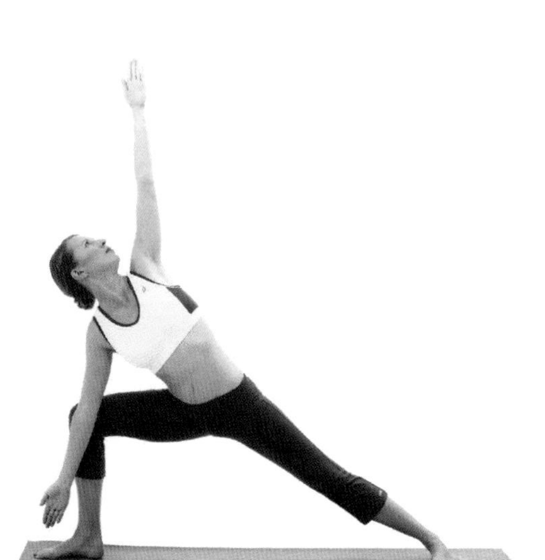

9. **Stretch Up, Reach Down**: Once in the pose literally try to reach your fingertips up to the ceiling. This creates the lift in the body and the upward movement of the energy off the floor and out of the hips. It provides the stretch across the shoulders as your other fingers reach down toward, but not touching the floor. Energy emanates from shoulders through to the fingertips of each arm.

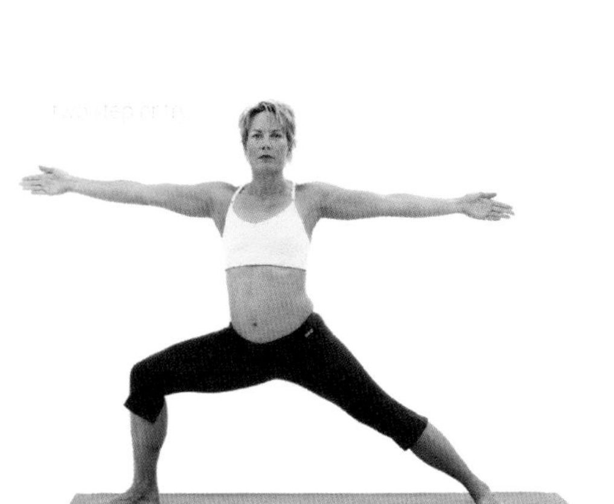

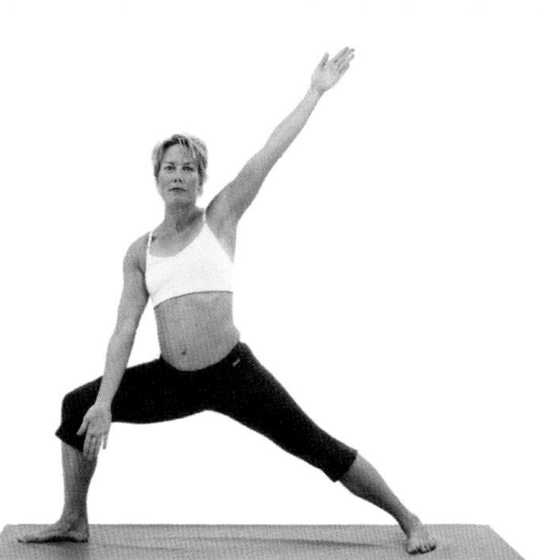

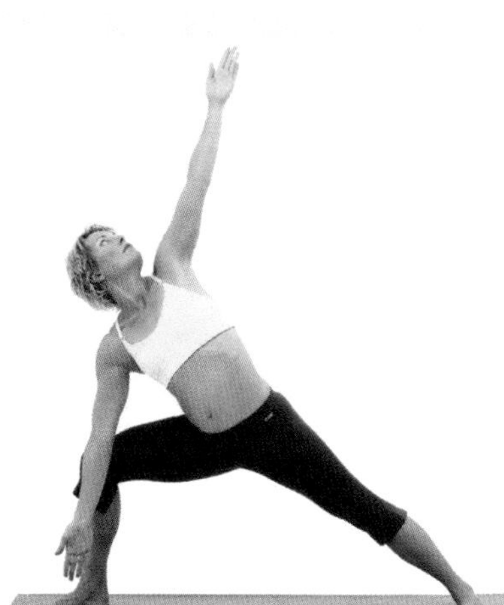

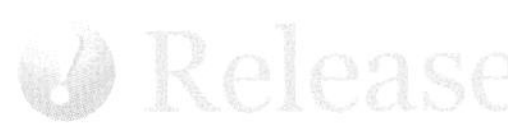

Release

Come out of the pose in the reverse fashion by releasing the arms and body, then releasing the lunge. However, most will find it so demanding that the release is somewhat less controlled. Do what you can. Maintain good focus and breath and use active feet to push away from the floor.

The second side is the exact mirror image. There are no special instructions here. Most students notice that one side is easier than the other due to natural asymmetries in flexibility.

Common mistakes and how to fix them

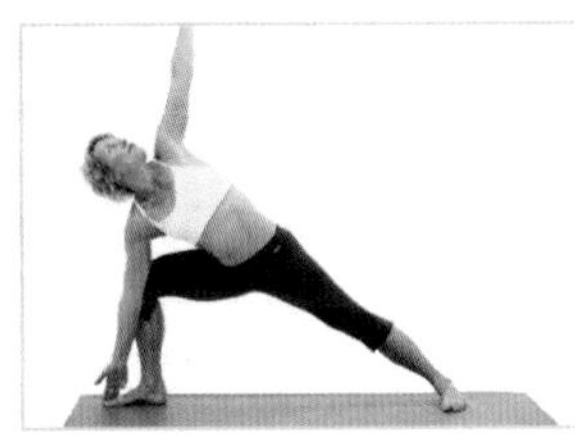

Resting fingertips on the floor between toes: The most common error is to place the fingers on the floor between the big and second toe. There are two reasons for this mistake. One is the misinterpretation of scripted instructions and the other is a confusion between this hot yoga Triangle with that of the Iyengar style where yogis actually rest the palm on the ankle, foot or floor.

Never let your fingers exert any pressure on the floor. The rule for everyone regardless of differing body geometry is that the distance of the fingers from the floor is always and only determined by precise elbow and knee contact. See following mistakes. Allow the line through your shoulders, arms and fingers to point down towards the small toes of the foot and not to the first and second toes. This is a far healthier knee position and you will get much better hip-opening.

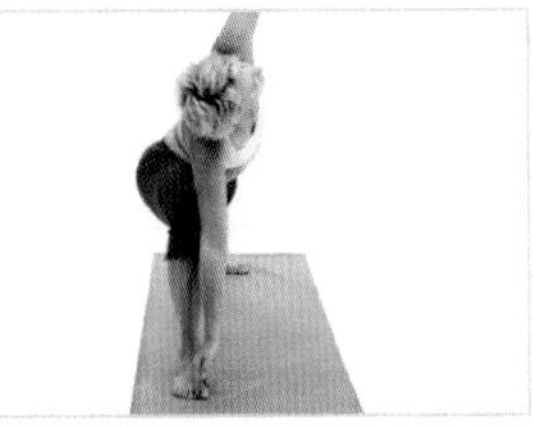

Incorrect elbow placement: More important than the finger position is where the elbow contacts the leg. There are 2 bones in the forearm. The radius which is broader at the wrist, and the ulna which is broader at the elbow. The ulna is the one you feel at the elbow point and is part of your forearm. Push backward on your knee from the ulna down (not with the upper arm). Lose ulna contact, lose balance. Bend the elbow, lose stability. Slacken the upper arm, fall forward. Contact with the upper arm against the knee will bring the body down too low. See below.

Body too low: Many students feel heavy in the pose: The body comes down too low because the upper arm contacts the knee, the arm may bend and they often lean on the knee. The only way out is lifting the body further, straightening the arm and bringing the ulna to contact; and drawing the energy out through the upper fingertips.

To counter this all-too-common problem try breaking the entry down further: Windmill your arms toward the knee and then move your elbow to your knee and no lower. The movement is thus determined by the arms, and the body comes with it into correct placement. Once mastered the entry happens seamlessly. *See photos of two step entry; page 150.

Elbow bends: An elbow bend is a sure sign that the upper arm is contacting the knee instead of the ulna. You are likely to feel heavy, lacking energy and as if you have to hold yourself up from the floor. The biceps tend to muscle the leg back and the body sways forward to try to balance. Your feet may start to slide apart, no longer being evenly anchored.

By contrast, pushing the knee back with a correctly placed elbow actually energizes your entire arm. This in turn activates the traction through the chest to the upper arm and lightens the load on your legs. This is crucial to understanding the mechanics of this pose.

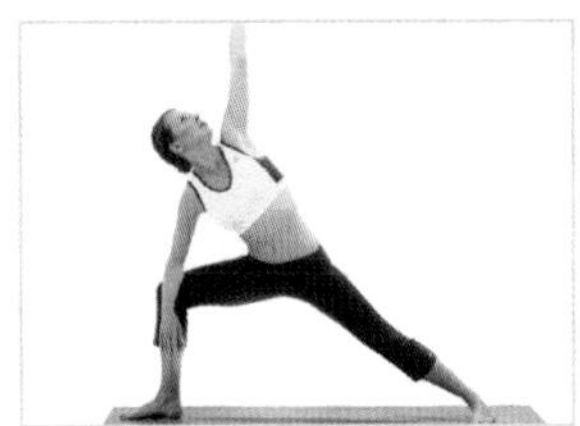

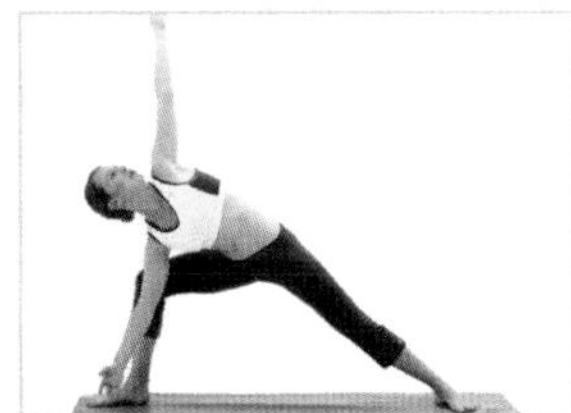

Pose collapses due to tightness or injury: For some students, after the initial lunge, the entry seems to imbalance everything. The body falls forward, the outside hip rises, the chest faces the floor, the lower arm reaches for the floor, and the upper arm floats forward.

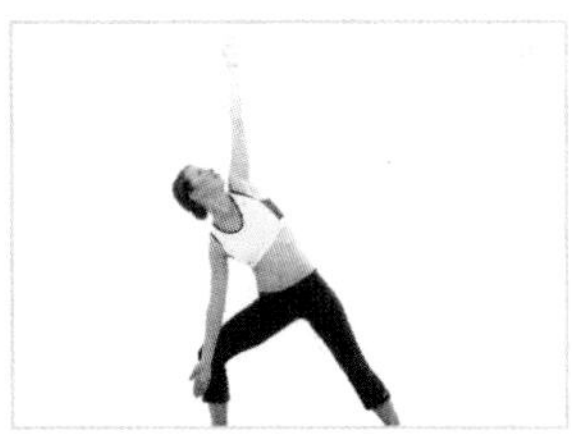

Because this problem is likely the result of injured hips or shoulders it is not fixed by elbow-to-knee placement (which can worsen the issue). This solution works: Step out less far. The lunge is less deep, the knee must be vertical and the thigh is at an angle and not parallel to the floor. Keep the body as upright as you can. The wrist or forearm pushes back against the knee. The arm is activated through to fingertips.* See photo.

10

Trikonasana

Triangle Pose

shin is angled and not vertical

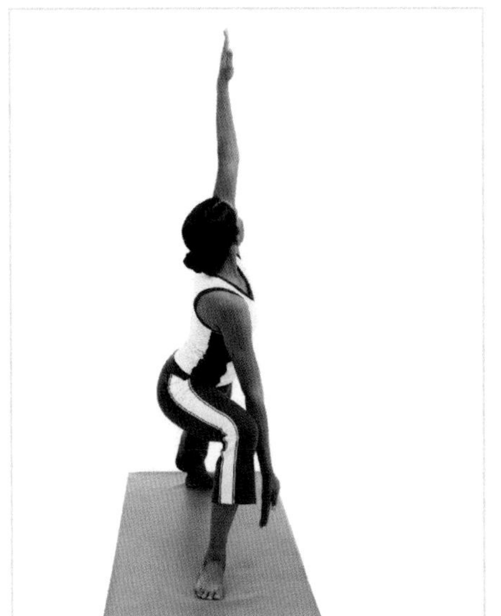
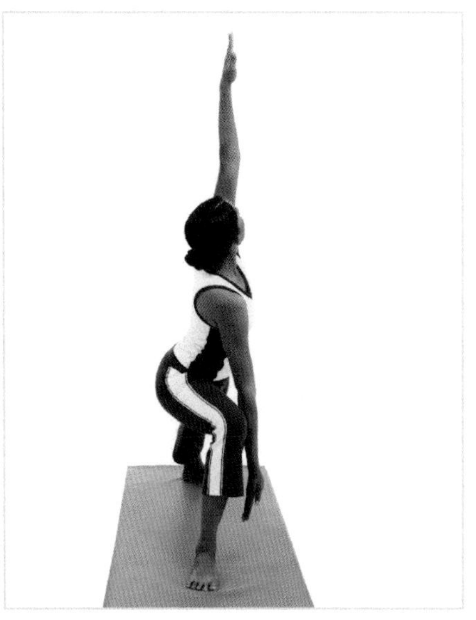
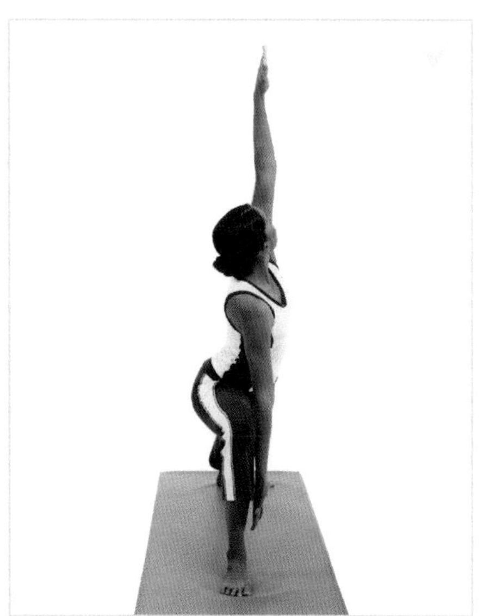

Injured and rehabilitating students have experienced consistently excellent results with my technique. It is a logical approach to create a struggle-free Triangle. Students tell me they find more balance; less struggle to keep the body up yet much more ability to push the knee back and therefore safely tease open the hips. They no longer fall forward and can create the tractions fundamental to this pose. Over time the distance between the feet widens to improve the lunge. Most graduate to the full pose, able to lunge deeply and push strongly with newly opened and flexible shoulders, knees and hips.

Shin is angled and not vertical: The shin has to be vertical in 2 planes. Not just with respect to the side wall (as a vertical line seen in the mirror) but with the front wall too (not leaning back or forth).

The foot tends to pronate when you lunge down in triangle, forcing the body forward. When the elbow pushes back on the knee with the fingers pointing to the small toes of the foot, the pronation corrects into an uplifting of the ankle. This simple action lifts the body up in good alignment. Coupled with your long and straight locked leg anchoring fully through your foot, you can feel your hips open.

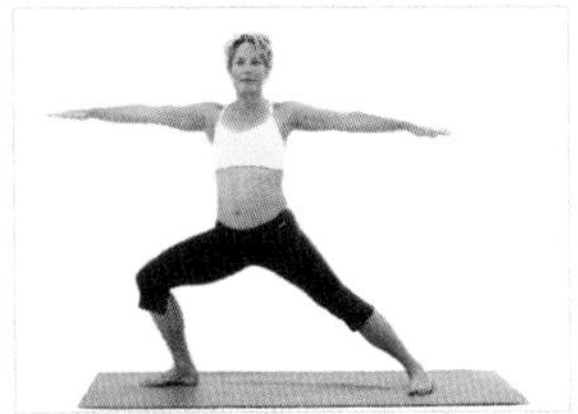
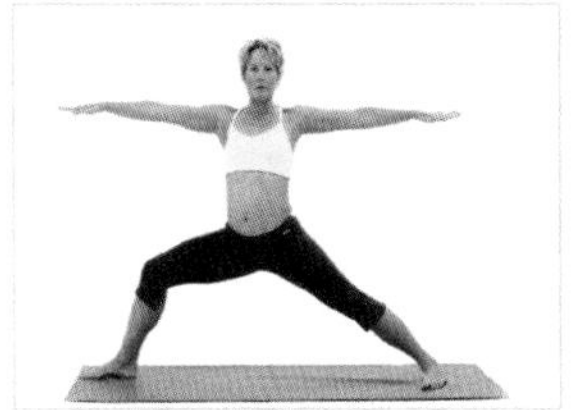

Leg bends or foot lifts: The outstretched leg needs to stay strong. Try pushing the outside of the foot into the floor, while also anchoring the big toe. In time your ankles will become more laterally flexible.

Feet slide: Join the club! However, contrary to hot yoga lore, it's not simply a sign of weak inner thighs. It may also indicate a) a need for more precise foot placement b) insufficiently pressing the knee with the elbow c) poor core strength d) inflexible hips. Drive the heels and feet downward. Continue working this pose as an integral part of your practice to holistically improve strength, stamina and flexibility.

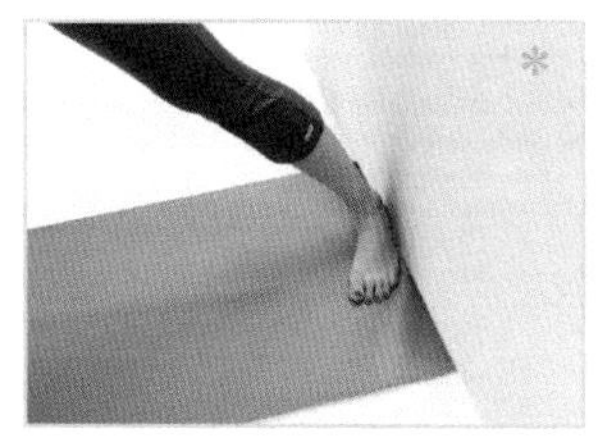

***Fear and/or pain holding you back**: If you have hip or knee problems it can be hard to settle into the lunge: Your feet slip or you feel strain at the groin, worried you may tear something. Use this temporary approach to quickly build extra physical strength and confidence. It allows you to safely hold for the pose's duration. For the first side: Stand with your left heel against a wall, your foot angled in at 30-45°. While the wall prevents one arm from being fully extended for set-up it allows you to step your right foot out to the side at the required distance.

When you lunge down you will feel stable and protected. The left heel pushes into the wall which provides a strong foundation, allowing your hip and upper body to maintain a solid position. Your confidence and strength build and you get results very quickly. You are unlikely to need the wall for more than 4 or 5 classes.

feet incorrectly aligned

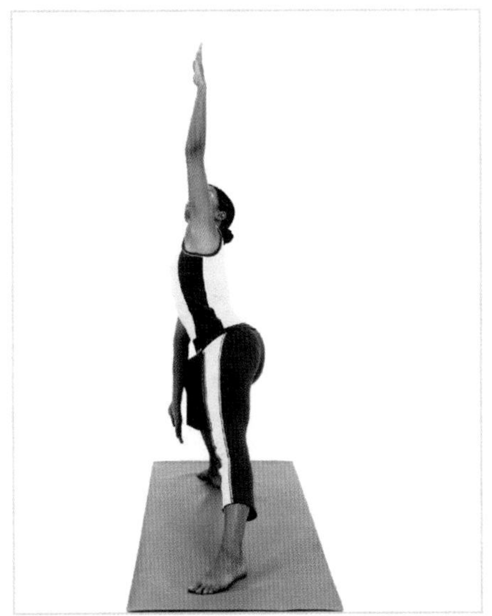

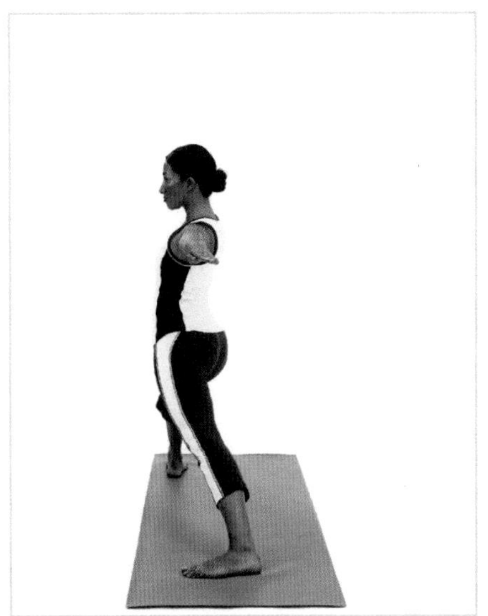

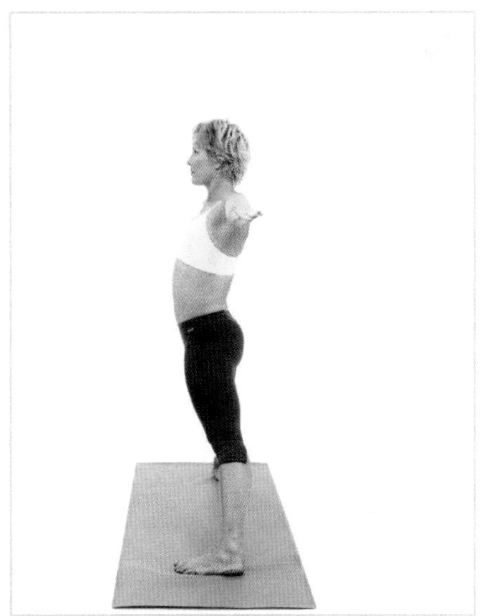

Feet incorrectly aligned: Heel to arch placement between the feet belongs to different yoga styles. Ensure heels are in one line parallel to the mirror.

Feet incorrectly angled: The outstretched foot needs to be slightly pigeon-toed in to help protect the hip. If sliding is your main problem, make sure the shin of your bent leg is vertical and you DRIVE your foot downward. An advanced distinction is to lift your toes of your bent leg up off the floor. This will draw your center of gravity back to your hips for stability and charge the feet evenly.

Feet incorrectly weighted: If not attentive most of the weight goes into the front toes, sometimes even causing the heel to lift. This puts tremendous pressure on the bent leg knee, foot and toes. This can force the body weight to sway forward and to this side. When this happens you could just about pick up your straight leg off the floor and balance on your bent leg. The pose then moves from 'warrior' to 'vulnerable'.

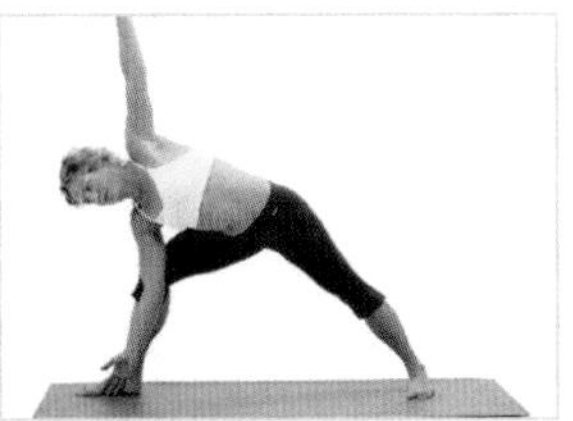

Hips ride up: When you set up, square the hips to the front and level them to the floor. The shin has to be vertical and you should feel a weightiness in the hips. Solidify the hips into position before pose entry. When the arms move, be very careful to keep the hips still, without allowing the extended leg hip to rise. Re-correction mid-pose requires a) bending the knee to regain the lunge and b) pushing the bent knee back with the elbow. The hips will again feel more settled and open.

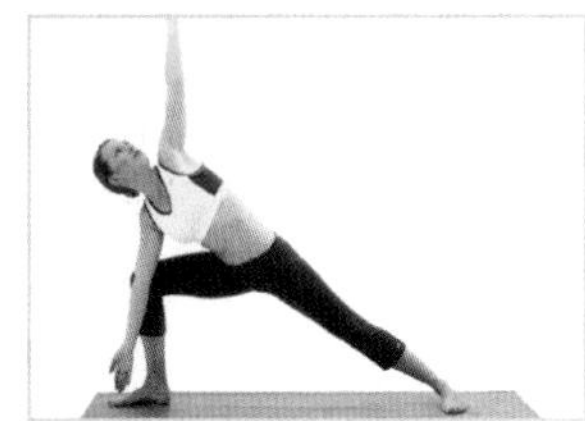

Hip of extended leg rolls down: Make no mistake, the hips should open to the front in this pose. Any instruction to roll the long leg down and forward is wrong. It makes the hips face to the side, removes the twist and transfers weight to the bent leg. If you have inflexible hips rolling the hip down seems easier: It is a stepping stone to opening hips square to the front. For those with flexible hips: The weight will be more evenly distributed. You will more easily maintain the upright squareness and alignment allowing greater traction and strength work without the struggle.

Shoulders hunch up: Your shoulders should never shrug toward your ears. Be careful when stretching the arm up. Relax your neck. Turn the head to bring the chin over your shoulder, they don't touch, the shoulder is down and back. See the chapter on arm movement and shoulder anatomy.

Sitting pretty, feeling heavy: It seems as if, when you look at yourself, that you have all the basic elements nailed. But you are feeling heavy. This happens to the more advanced students when they lose mindfulness for a time. They sit heavily into the hips without creating traction in the upper body. Activate your legs and feel your quadriceps muscles work. Push your feet into the floor and balance the leg and foot work with a strong extension through the spine to lift your torso out of your hips. I find it helps to flex the toes of my bent leg. Activate both your arms, stretching them through to the fingertips, and reach for the sky.

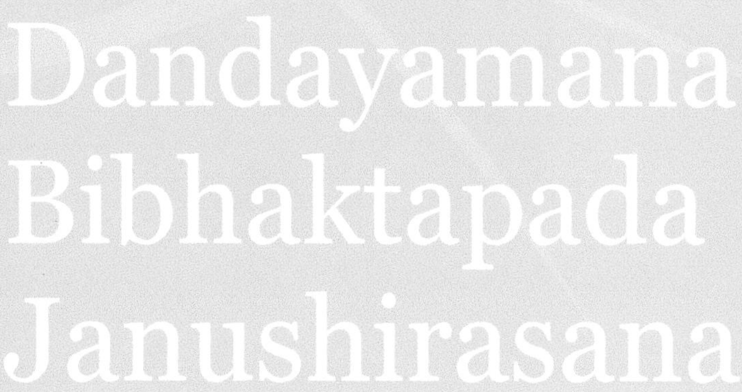

Dandayamana Bibhaktapada Janushirasana

Your vision will become clear only when you can look into your own heart. Who looks outside, dreams; who looks inside, awakens.
—Carl Jung

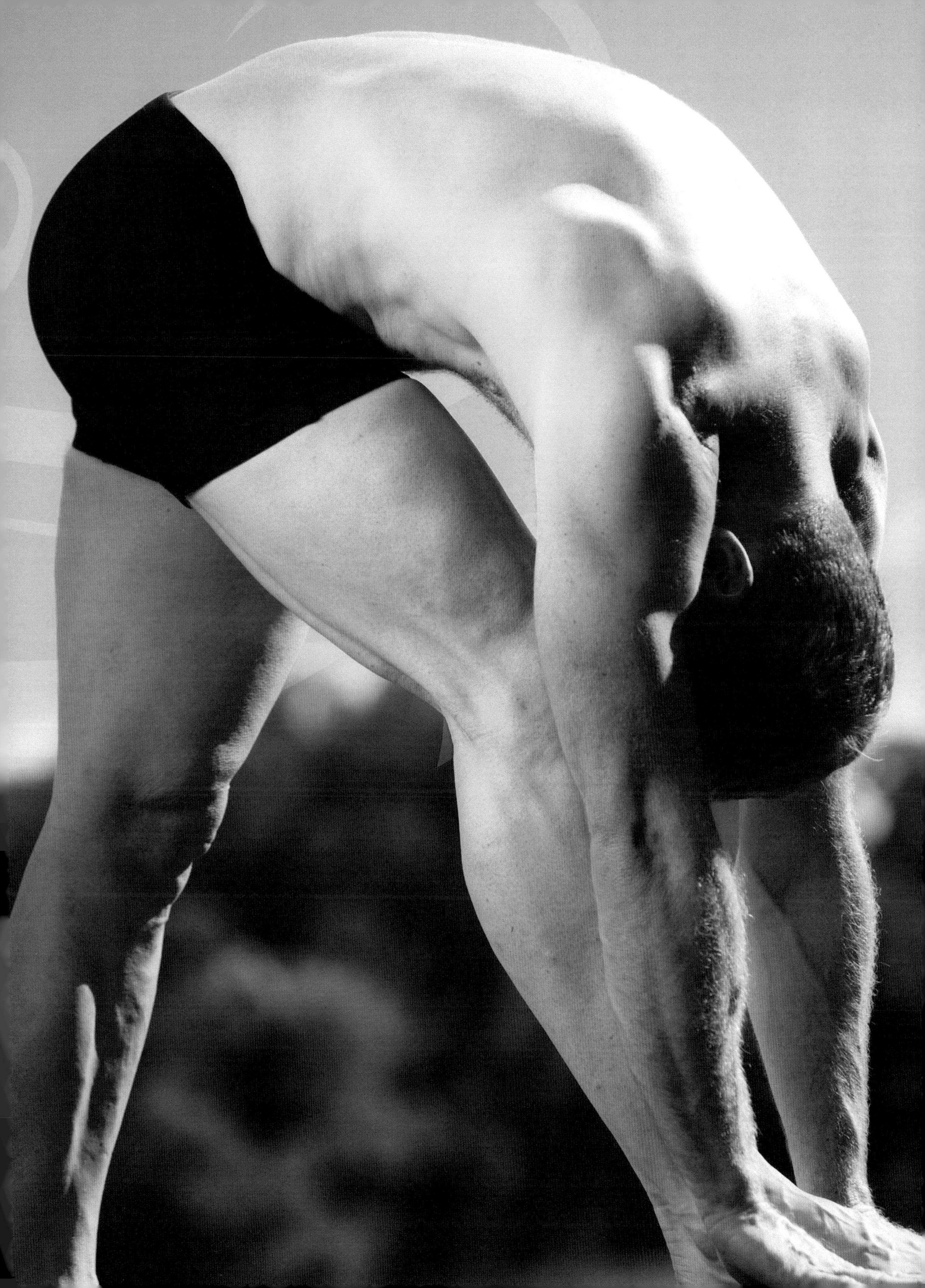

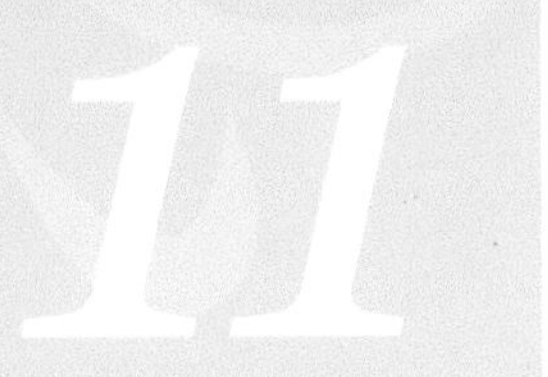

Dandayamana Bibhaktapada Janushirasana

Separate Leg Head to Knee

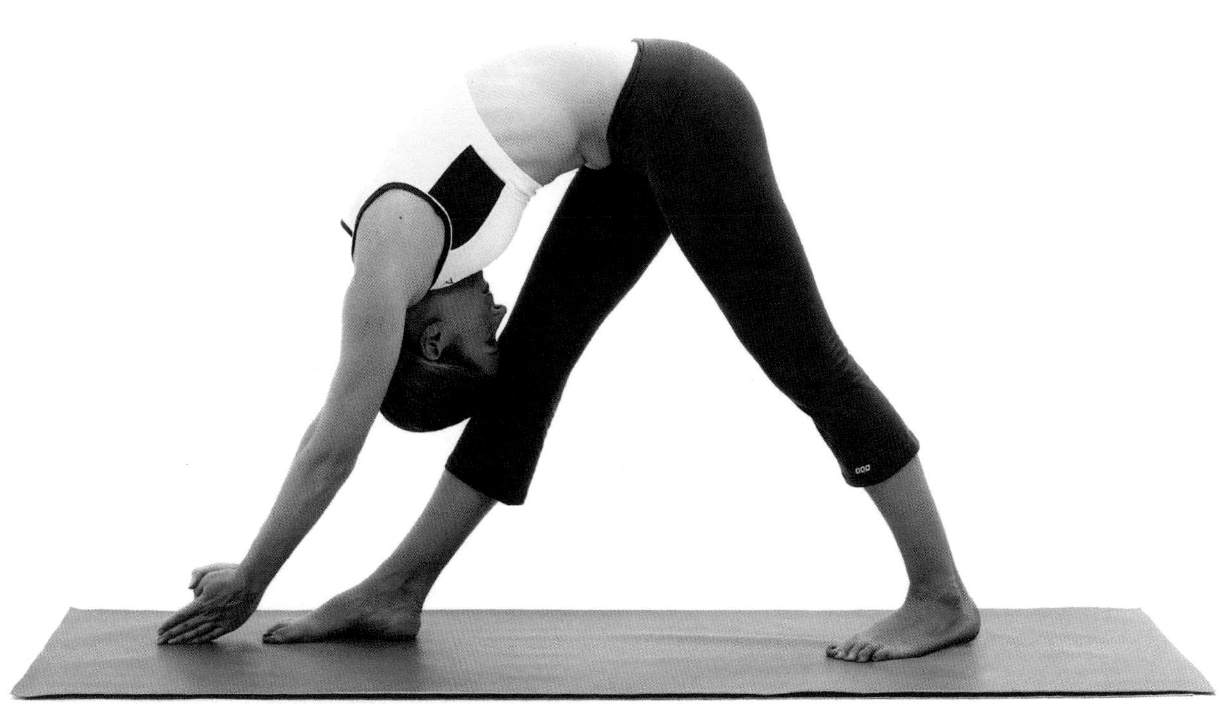

The essentials

Providing yet another opportunity to open your hips, Standing Separate Leg Head to Knee pose is a powerful forward bend with a great rounding element to particularly open the lower spine. This is a very therapeutic pose because the action of entering and exiting actually resolves muscle spasms in the mid and upper spine. Unlike the first Janushirasana pose where only advanced yogis manage to get their head to knee, the requirement here is to ensure that, wherever possible, there is forehead contact.

The eventual aim of this pose is to remain in a semi-inverted pose in perfect balance with your arms extended out in prayer position. As is usually the case, there are differences due to varied abilities in the class but we all aim to get the forehead on the knee.

What makes this pose so difficult to get right?

Primarily those with tight shoulders, hips and hamstrings can find it more challenging to create the right geometry. There is a squareness of the hips along with hand and arm placement that will take a lot of your attention.

Dandayamana Bibhaktapada Janushirasana

11

Separate Leg Head to Knee

The technique

This pose requires you to step out to the side. Stand to the left in readiness.

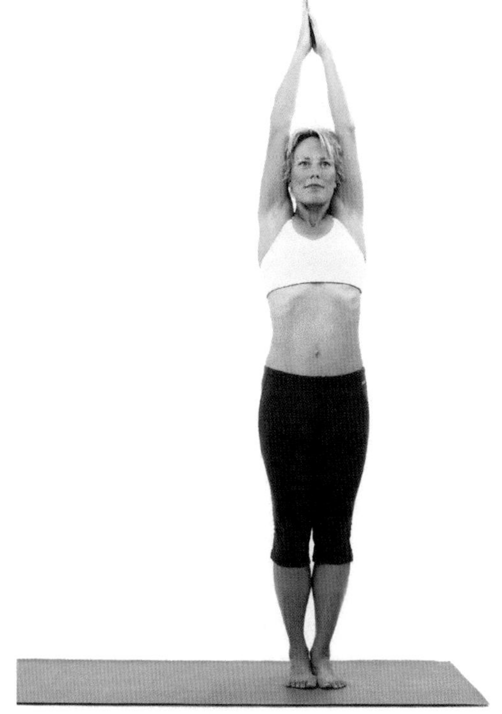

1. **Arms Up, Palms Together**: Inhale and move your arms up over your head and aim to bring your hands together in full contact from your wrists right up to your fingertips. Cross your thumbs to strengthen the grip. Shoulders relaxed, arms extended and strong. Ideally arms are straight and by or behind the ears. Introduce a micro-bend if your shoulders shrug. Your chin is up parallel to the floor for now.

2. **Step Out To The Right**: As you exhale, step your right foot out about 2½ foot (75cm). If you are straddling the mat, your feet are close to each side. Feet are parallel. The taller you are, the greater the distance. Activate your legs.

3. **Orient Your Feet**: Pick up your toes, pivot on your heels to face the right wall for this first side. The front toes are square to the wall and parallel to the mirror. The back foot is positioned at a 45 degree angle. Throughout the pose, keep both feet flat on the floor and evenly weighted.

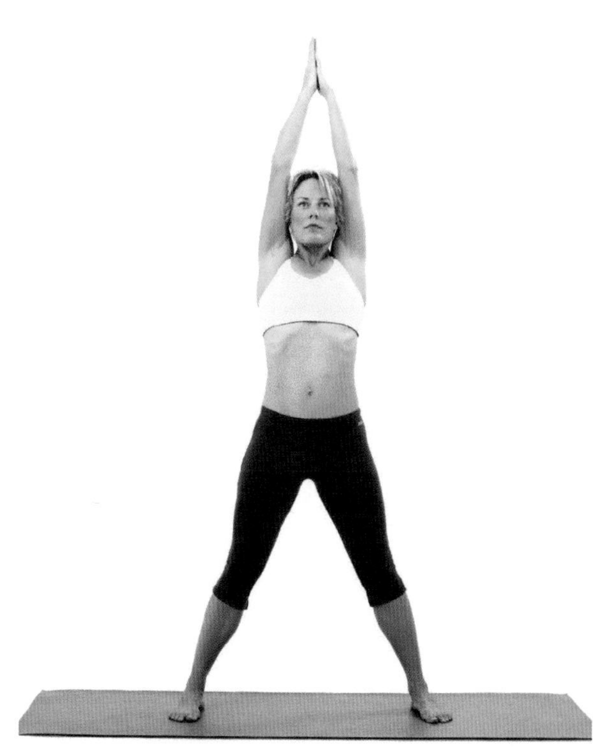

4. **Align Your Heels**: Keep your heels in one line. They are neither crossed nor separated. Take a glance down if you need to, and imagine a straight line through your toes and heel of your front foot extending right through the heel of your back one.

5. **Level And Square Your Hips**: Typically, as a result of moving your body to face the side wall, the front hip swivels down and back unevenly weighting the back leg. Square your hips to the floor and the wall to which you face by pivoting your hips. As you transfer weight back into your front foot your hip will rise up back into alignment. Lock both of your legs.

6. **Round Your Spine**: Inhale length in your torso keeping your arms back, strong and straight. As you exhale, draw in your abdomen, tuck your chin to contact your chest. This tucking action begins the rounding of the spine which continues 'til you stand tall again after release. Start to curl down from the head, looking as high up on your chest as you can while you enter.

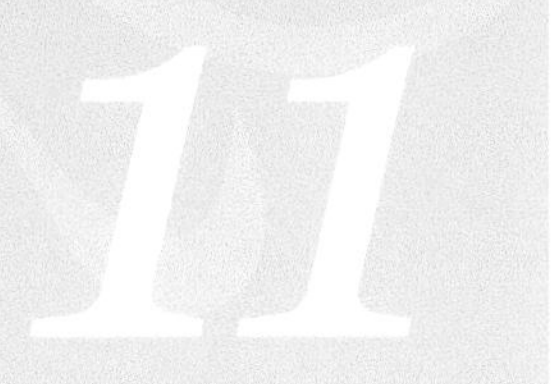

Dandayamana Bibhaktapada Janushirasana

Separate Leg Head to Knee

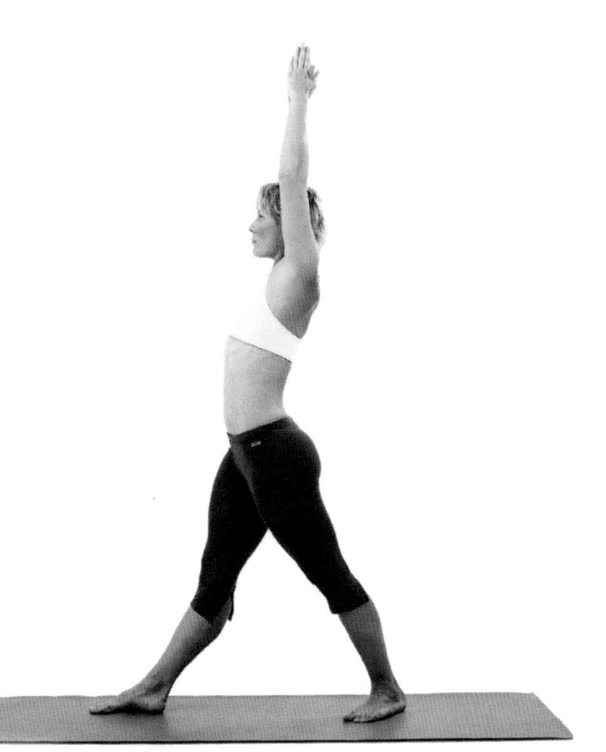

7. **Traveling To The Floor**: As you round, keep your arms in the same relative position; they stay by the head. Arms are held back even while your chin is tucked and you roll forward. As you curl down, keep the back hip forward to maintain good hip alignment. Without exception you must try to get your forehead on your knee. Keep both legs locked. At some point, however, you may need to bend your front leg to reach the floor in balance and get head to knee contact. A rule to remember: ALWAYS keep your back leg locked out with your foot flat on the floor.

8. **Hands Flat By Feet, Push Floor**: Normally hands will reach the floor and then the forehead will make contact with the knee. Palms should be flat on either side of, and close to, your front foot. For many it will provide much needed balance.

9. **With Forehead On Knee, Push Everything Away From Floor**: Most work this pose with a bent front leg. Your aim is to straighten (and eventually lock) your bent leg, constantly pushing the forehead on the knee. Actively push the floor away from you to accentuate rounding through your spine. Energized hands and arms push away from the floor and give you the leverage you need to push the knee back. Never lose the head to knee connection.

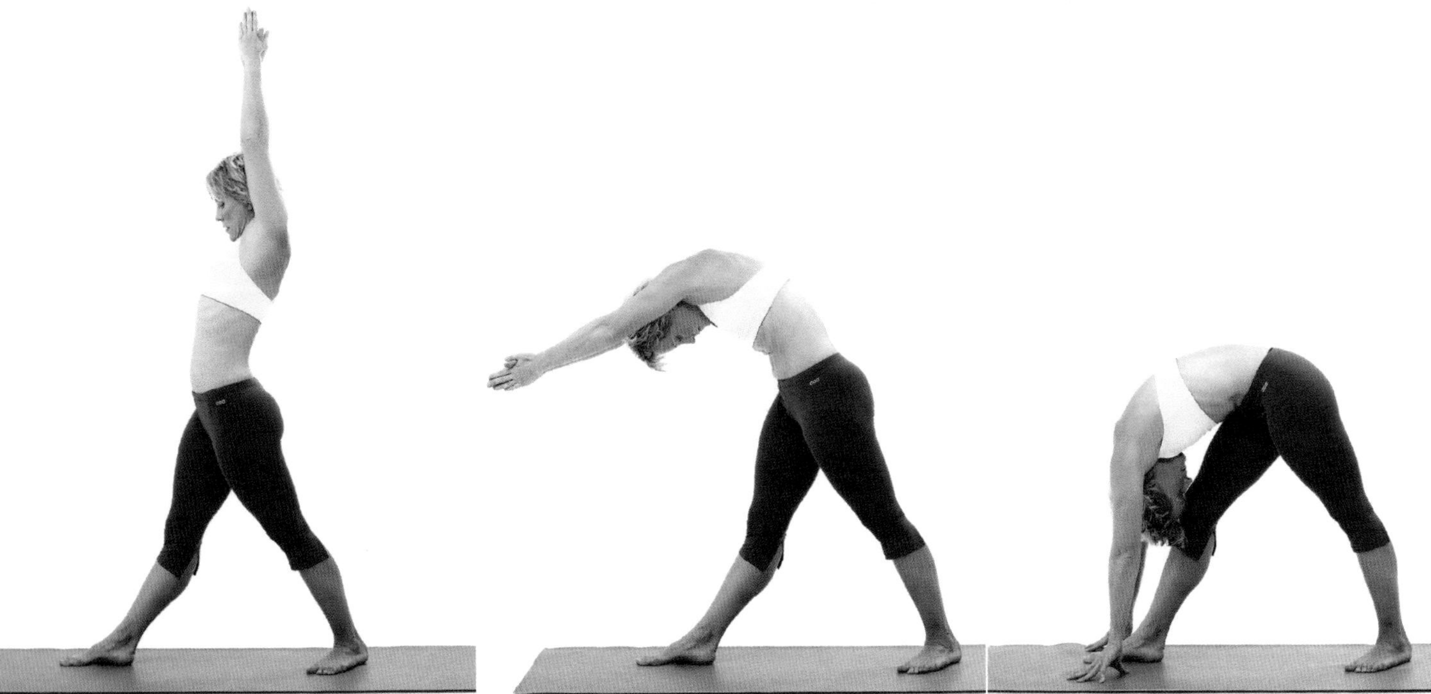

10. **LEG WEIGHT EVEN**: The way you round down, usually causes a backward transfer of weight that makes the hip of the front leg slump and shift forward. This is why teachers tell you to shift your weight into your front foot. It swivels your hips to make them square and even again, by bringing 50/50 weight distribution back to the feet. The back hip moves forward and space is created between your legs with the lift. Be careful to keep driving your back heel down and both feet flat on the ground.

11. **HANDS IN PRAYER POSITION**: I have 2 rules of thumb. 1: Only ever put hands into prayer position if your head is on your knee AND hips are perfectly aligned. 2: For best results only extend arms in 2nd set. Even if you easily get your hands in prayer realize that you get amazing spine-rounding leverage with hands on the floor in the first set, so don't waste any opportunity. Your second set will be stronger and rounder.

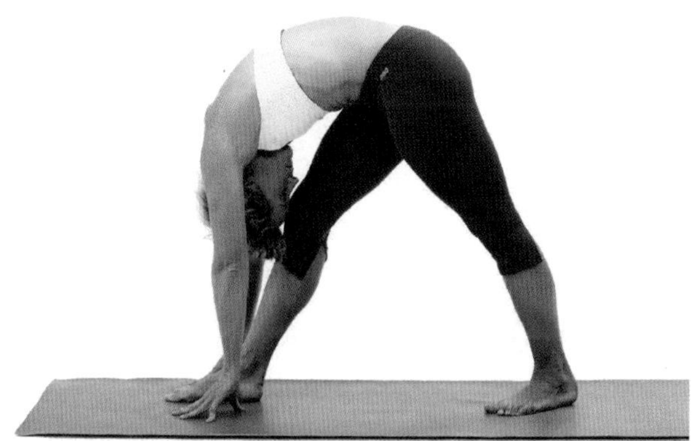

A therapeutic pose: One of the great advantages of the rounded back entry/exit is its therapeutic power. The mid to upper thoracic areas are common places for muscle spasms. Forward bends with an extended straight back, can bring on these spasms and create painful conditions. Tucking the chin and rolling forward does NOT engage the muscles that could potentially cause this damage. It helps iron out the spasms into a deep stretch. Be mindful of the position of the hips on the way in and out of this pose to ensure greater restorative effect.

You are creating maximal compression down the front side of your body while opening up the vertebral column and stretching deeply through the muscles. Many benefits arise: From intense abdominal organ compression, in your stomach, liver, intestines, pancreas and kidneys; and it is said that the head to knee contact helps optimize many vital functions through hormonal regulation.

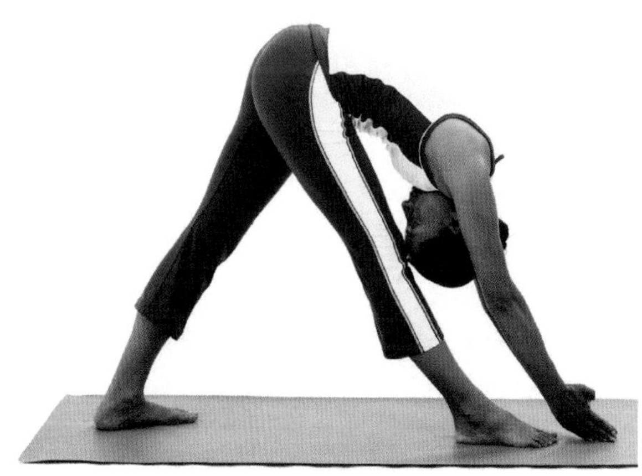

A technique tip for perfect entry: Start by tucking the chin, squaring the hips to the wall and floor, then curl. Regardless of flexibility the hips always need your constant focus. Try the mantra: 'Back hip forward, back hip forward, back hip forward'. Mindful attention to hips on entry and exit means a greater chance of creating the ideal hip position with minimal mid-pose adjustment. I guarantee better results and benefits because you will be working the pose intelligently. The outcome is mind-blowing. Students cease to struggle with balance and alignment, even those who used to find it difficult to simply place head to knee. 'Measure twice, cut once' and you will more easily form that solid platform parallel to the ceiling.

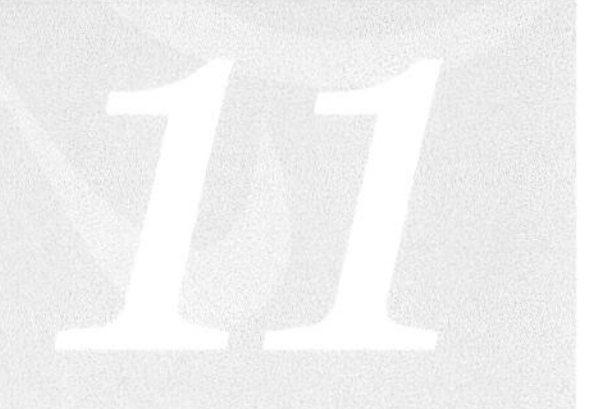

Dandayamana Bibhaktapada Janushirasana

Separate Leg Head to Knee

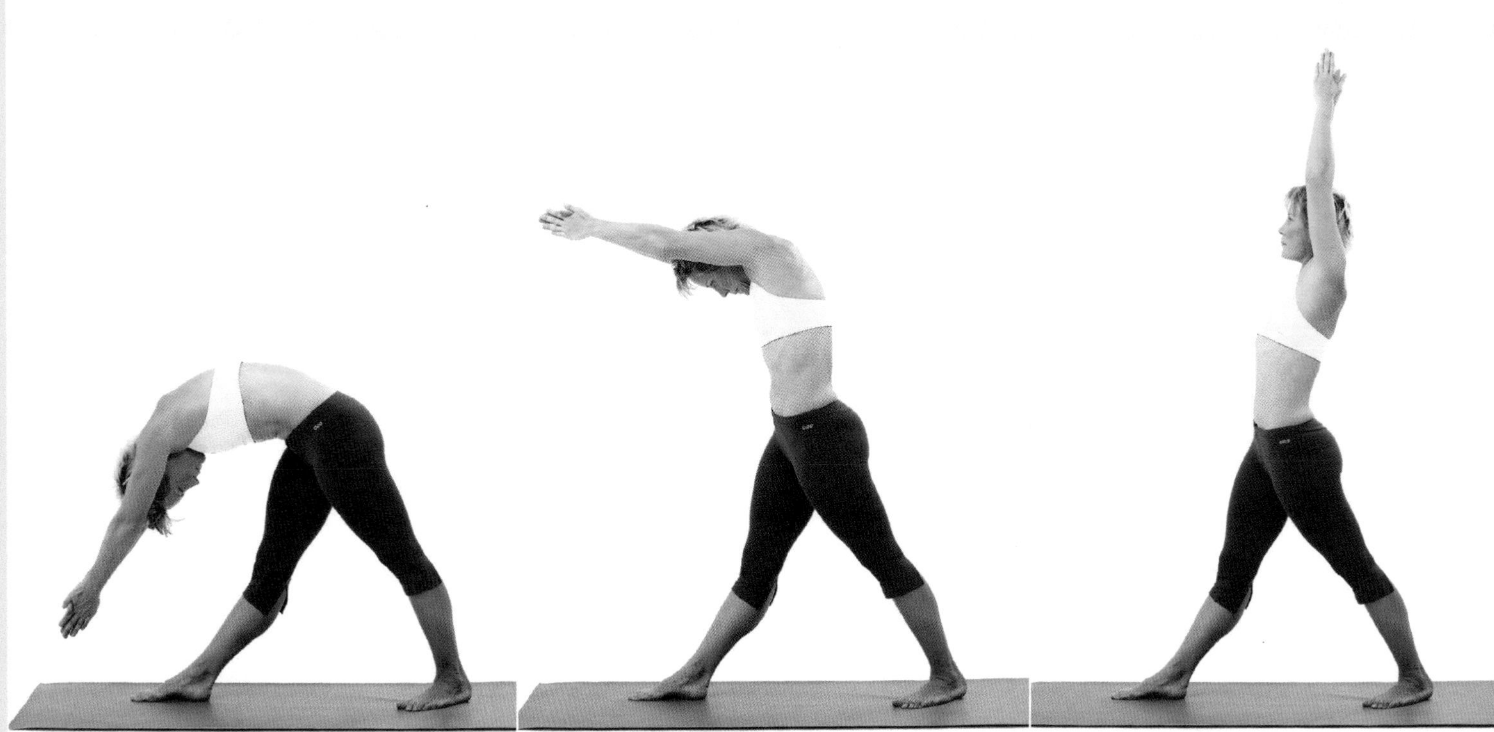

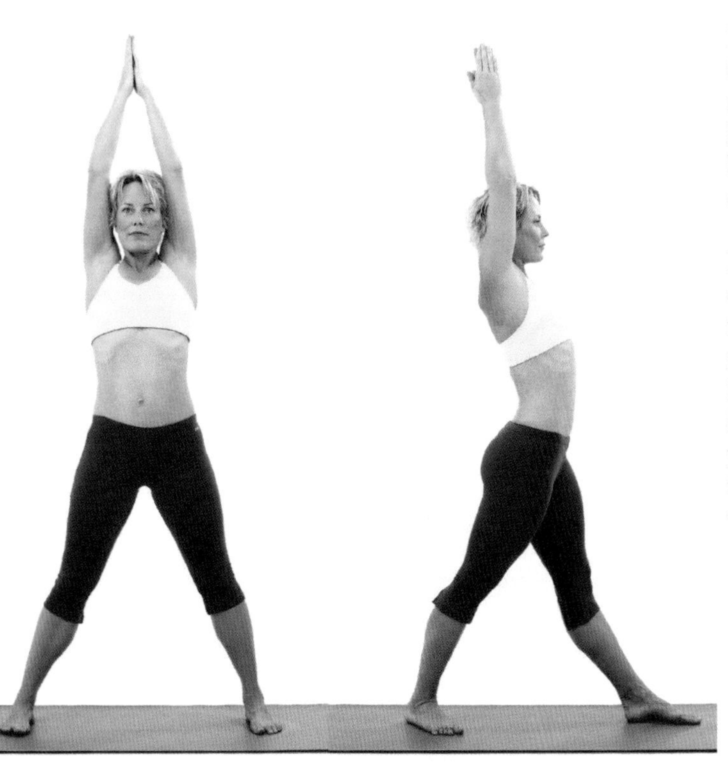

Release

Remember the mantra in the 'technique tip for perfect entry' I introduced you to? Keep your hip position uppermost in your mind on exit repeating 'back hip forward'. Keep the roundness in the spine, the chin tucked, arms with your head and your hips square to that side wall. Press the rewind button and lift out with strength and focus in an exact reversal of the entry.

Plant the heels to pivot to the front. Then pivot again to correctly orient your hips, body and feet to the left wall for the second side. Each side of each set commonly lasts 20-30 seconds once the hands reach the floor. There is a brief Savasana between the 2 sets. Work maximum spine rounding in the first set with your hands on the floor, no matter what your experience. Only bring your hands in prayer position in the second set, if, and only if you can get your legs locked out with optimal hip alignment.

Common mistakes and how to fix them

Can't get the head to knee: Flexibility may be your issue. Some have to bend the leg on the descent just to get hands on the floor. Working on hip alignment, and spine rounding through leverage from floor contact, is the most crucial activity. Always keep your back leg locked. You may bend the front leg. There will be some people despite best efforts who cannot get their head to knee for some time, if ever.

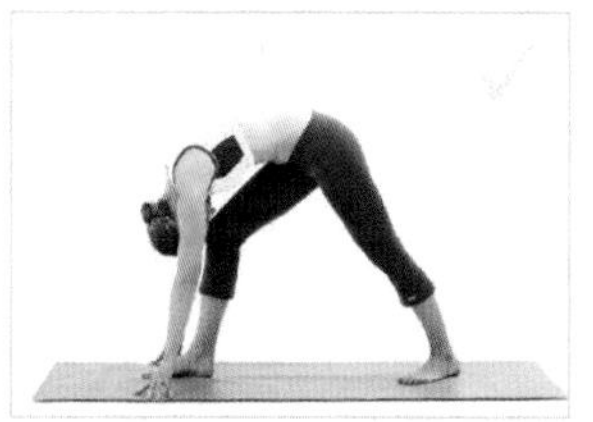

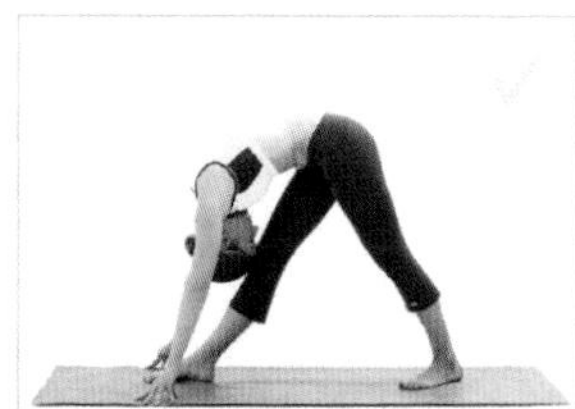

Back leg bent: Balance or very tight hamstrings may be the problem. Check your leg separation. Straighten the back leg and drive the heel into the ground. Feel that lovely stretch from the floor up through the leg, hips and down the spine!

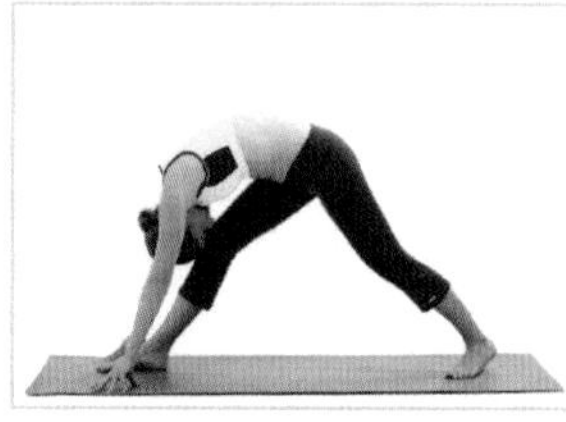

Forehead away from the knee: You will get better leverage and strength to round your spine if - while pushing with your hands on the floor - your head is on the knee. Actively push the knee back with the forehead. The very inflexible or injured may only get the nose or the chin there. Just try to tuck the chin, bend the leg and create the best compression possible.

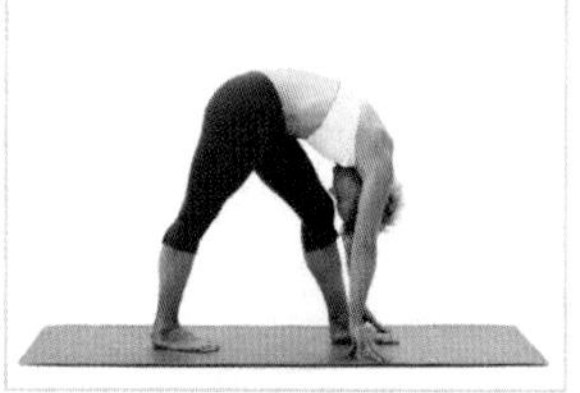

Uneven hips: Most commonly one hip stays up high, the other slumps down. The weight is mostly on the back foot. The main focus is lifting up out of the back leg to create a solid flat horizontal platform. Evenly plant the heels and big toes. Push the floor away from you with strong arms, and push with your feet while lifting out of your ankles. Ensure your back leg stays locked. Feel the neat swivel action where the back hip moves forward and the hip of your front leg lifts and moves back. The weight lifts up and forward becoming centered. Without square hips the hands should never approach each other to come into prayer position on the floor out in front of your foot. See the 'technique tip for perfect entry' on page 161. Keep the back hip forward on entry and exit.

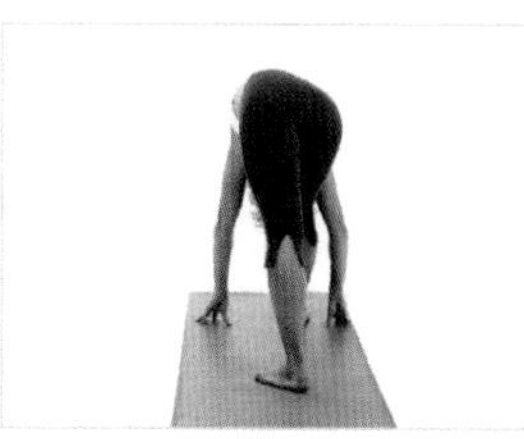

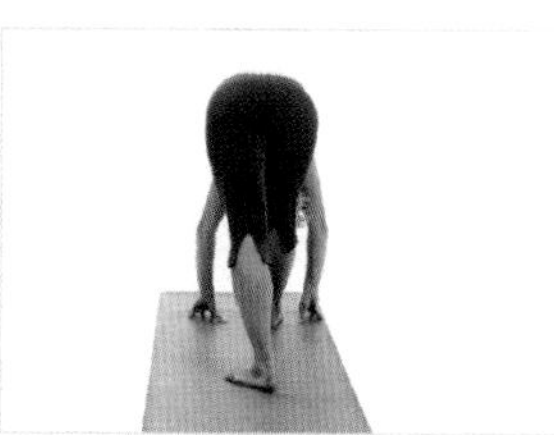

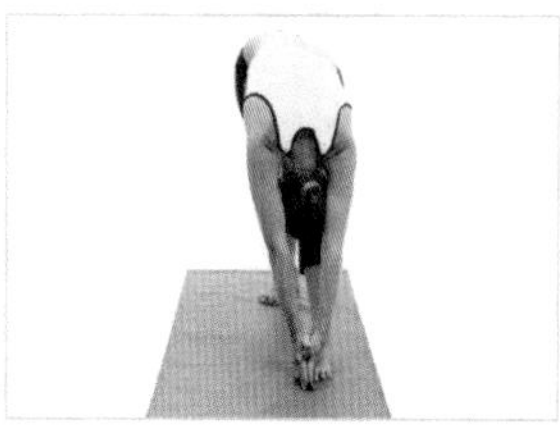

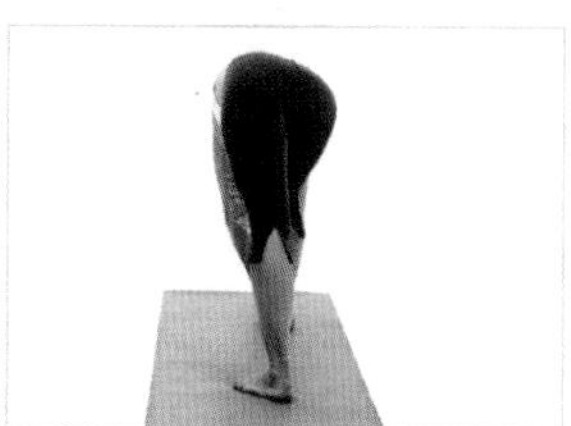

Hands in prayer position when hips are not even: See the above entry 'uneven hips'. Simply having locked legs is not enough to proceed to full pose. Hips must be square before hands move into prayer position. Push your hands firmly against the floor and swivel your hips into position. Normally too much weight is in the back leg, so even the weight distribution. If hips can stay set and solid then you may attempt bringing your hands into prayer position. I prefer that students have even hips AND locked legs before trying. Occasionally a strong well-aligned student may still have their front leg very slightly bent.

Leading with the chin: On your descent (and ascent) if the chin sticks out the rounding element almost disappears. You will engage your mid-upper thoracic back muscles instead of relaxing and stretching them. Some call this 'swan diving'. Keep the chin tucked to accentuate the rounding. Maintain a static relationship of your arms to your head and your chin to your chest, and then imagine curling up in a ball. On exit the chin comes up last.

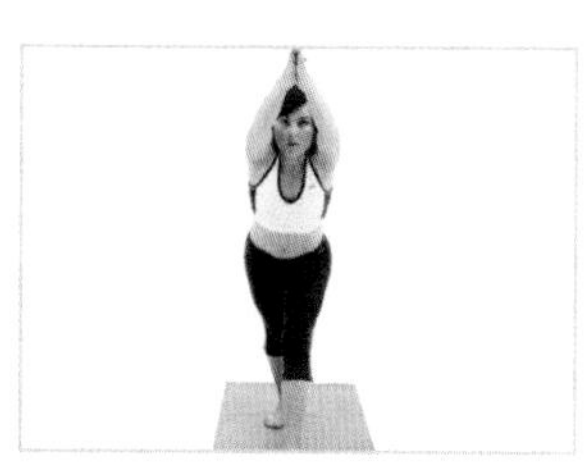

Forehead on shin: Forehead on shin or nose to shin is not head to knee! See 'Leading with the chin' above. Keep the chin tucked. Aim for the crown of the head on the quadriceps muscles and you will more likely get your goal.

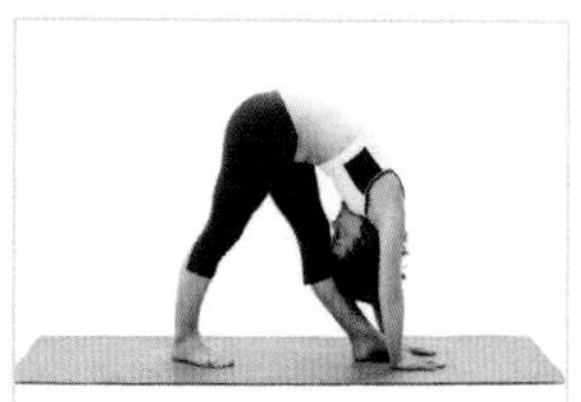

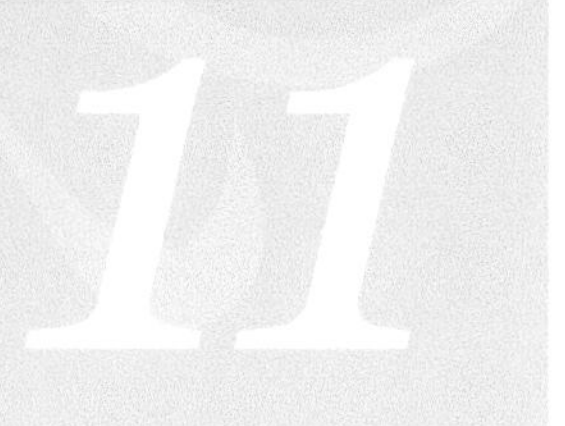

Dandayamana Bibhaktapada Janushirasana

Separate Leg Head to Knee

twisting hips and spine when releasing the pose to standing

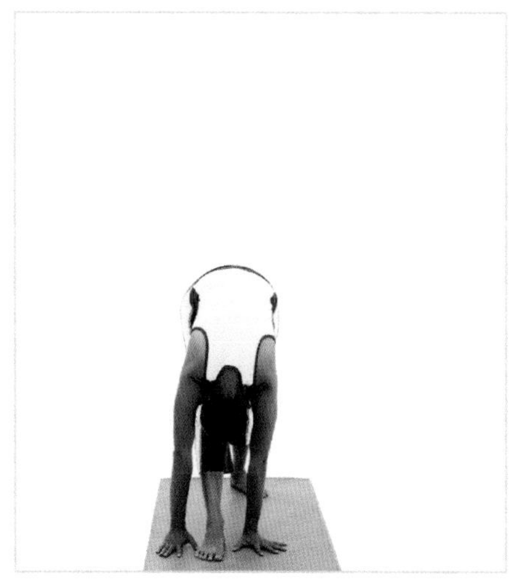

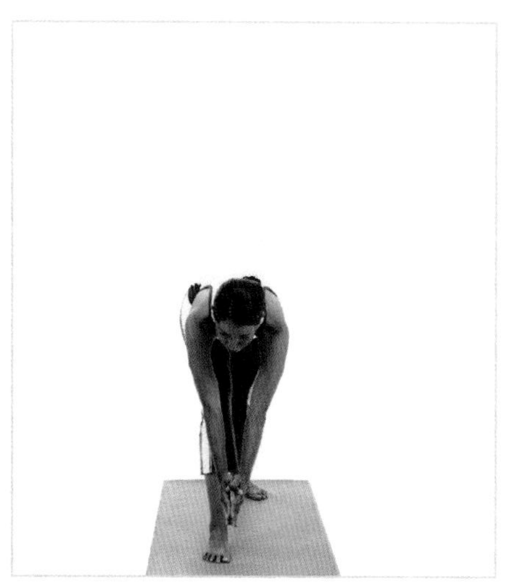

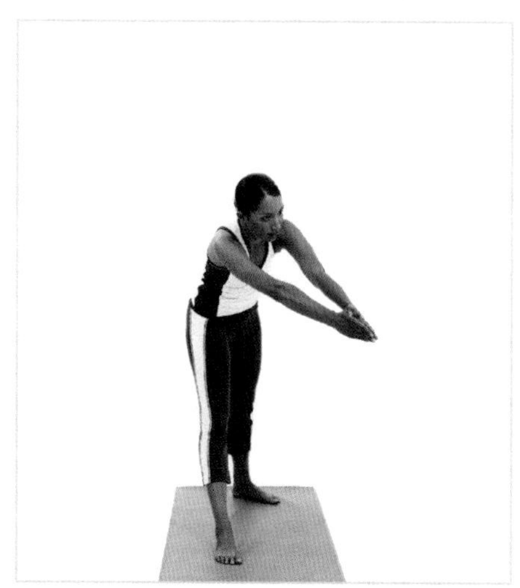

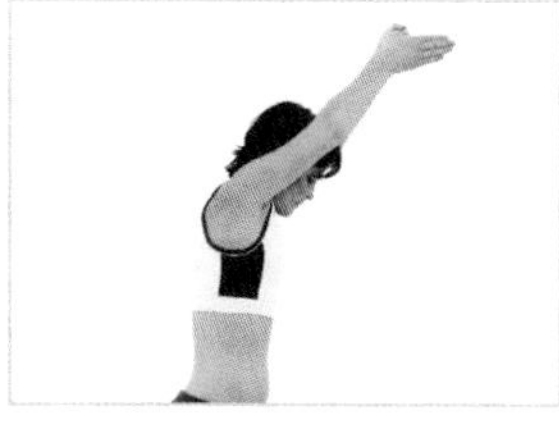

Bent wrists: Commonly wrists bend, causing fingers to point at a 20-40° angle to the arm. It can happen with the effort to squeeze the palms together, as a result of tightness in the shoulders or torso, or simply through lack of awareness. Facing the mirror it is difficult to see the angle at the wrists. There must be a straight line from shoulders, through arms to your fingers.

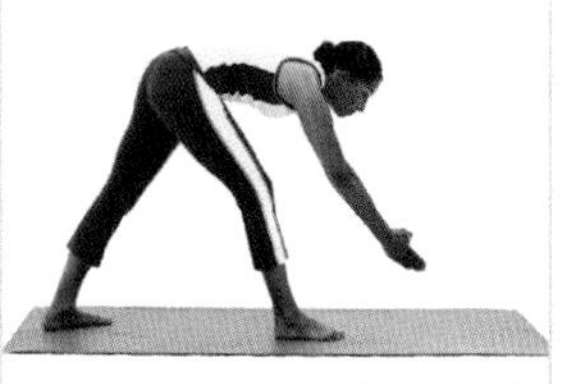

Arms away from head on entry or exit: It is always an error to separate the arms from the head going into or releasing from the pose. The mistakes present as follows; on entry the arms move down to reach the floor and the chin comes away from the chest. And for the exit the chin is not tucked, the head comes up first with the arms trailing. Often the arms do not even make it back up over the head where they started. These mistakes almost eliminate the spine rounding and the body moves by hinging at the hips. Ideally maintain your arms by your head and even behind your ears with chin tightly tucked. You must hold the shoulders down and back as always. A micro-bend in the arms is better than hunched shoulders.

Arms bend on entry: Sometimes this is unavoidable. If you have tight lats or neck or shoulder injury then round down with a preference for relaxed shoulders over straight arms. Still hold the arms by the head as best you can and definitely tuck the chin down firmly.

Pivoting on the toes: Pivoting on the toes to face the side walls seems harmless however it may make squaring the hips impossible if the heels 'cross'. Alignment and balance become more difficult. If pivoting on heels is difficult for you, then pivot one foot at a time to start. Heels should always be exactly aligned overlapping; neither crossed nor separated.

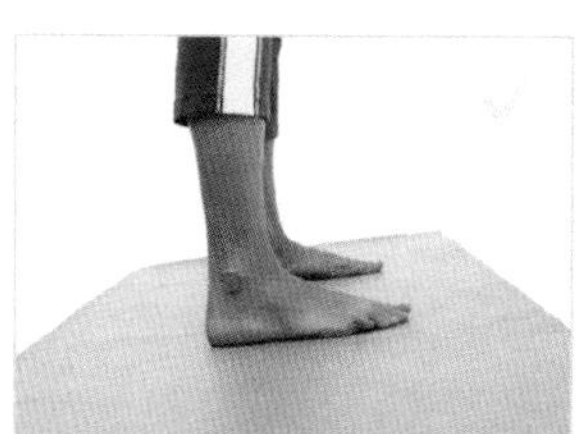

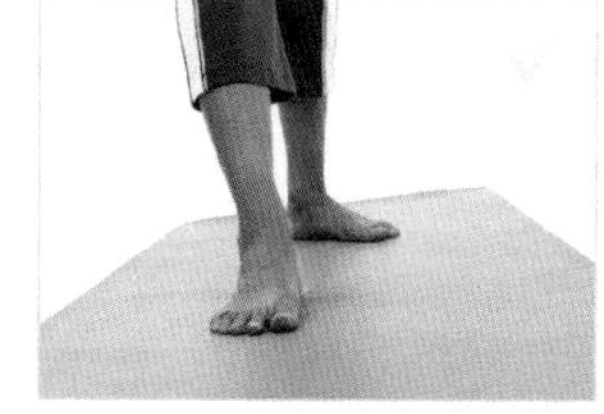

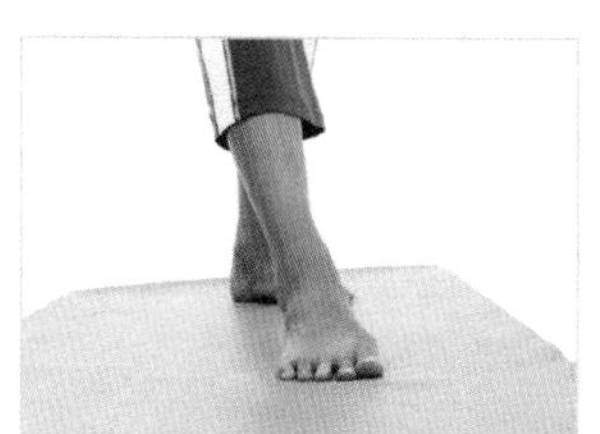

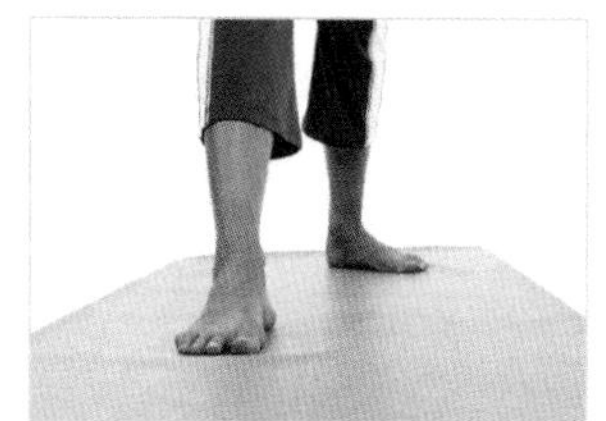

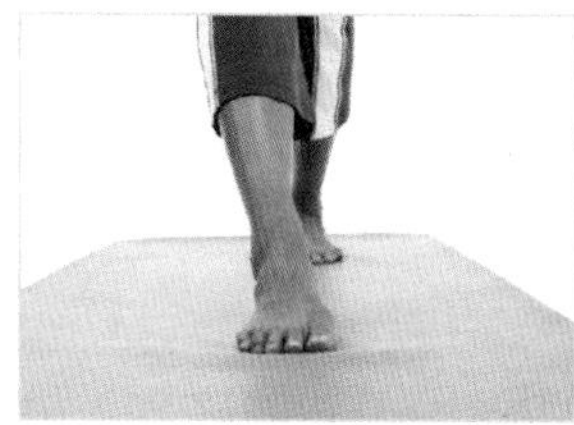

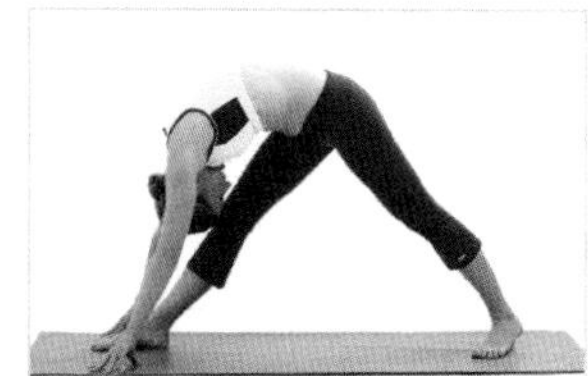

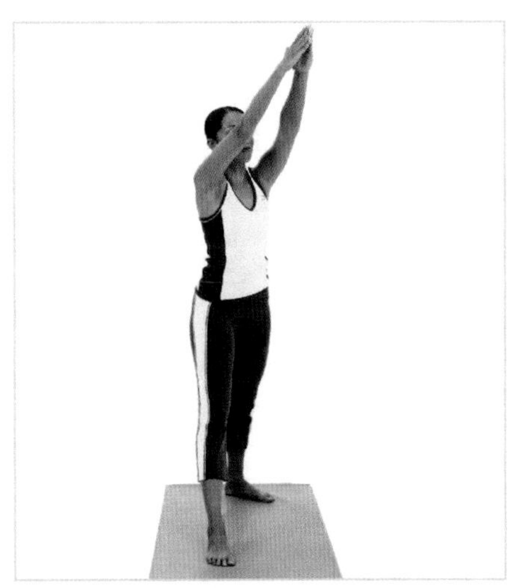

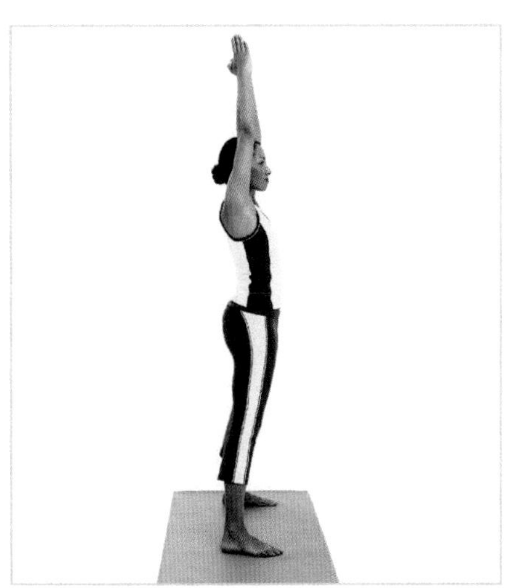

Feet parallel during pose: This is another problem of toe-pivoting. If your feet line up one behind each other in a line then balance will be extremely difficult. Hips won't square easily. Pivot on heels.

Can't square hips: Keep working on the basics. Pay attention to keeping the back leg long, strong and straight with the heel on the ground. Perhaps you need to adjust the leg distance apart.

Legs separated: Another pivoting problem. This time, it may be that your feet have been placed with the correct angles but the feet are laterally too far apart, as if they were on parallel tracks. The balance and correct hip positions are much easier to create with this particular misalignment.

This error is not as problematic as crossing your feet. In fact, I recommend introducing a small space as a legitimate modification for a tiny percentage of students who have extreme balance and tightness difficulties. The space is dependent on the student and can vary between 1-4 inches (up to 10cm). It is expected for you NOT to have great balance hanging upside down, legs apart with your head on your knee. Use your arms. They are on the floor to support you. Keep your heels aligned behind each other.

Crossed feet: Do not allow either of your legs to cross the midline and interfere with your foot alignment. See 'Pivoting on your toes'. Proper set-up will fix this.

Legs too far apart: Stepping out too far may prevent you locking out the back leg, driving your heel onto the floor, or getting perfect hip alignment. Your feet should never be 4 foot apart (1.2m). For regular height yogis the heel-to-heel distance is about 2½ (75cm). You can walk them in mid-pose.

Legs too close: If feet are positioned too closely then it will be too hard for inflexible bodies to get to the floor and achieve or even attempt head to knee contact. Conversely, it may make it too easy for the flexible, providing no challenge for the legs and hips to open. Straddle the mat or step out the correct distance.

Twisting hips and spine when releasing the pose to standing: It is extremely common for newer yogis to lift the body while swinging it around and forward, to face the mirror. See image sequence at top of this page. You risk compromising core strength and damage to your spine if you release by flying up and twisting at the same time. Inhale as you curl back up with hips square. Exit rolling back up, with your chin coming up last. This completes the uncurling to remain facing the direction that your front foot faces. Only then do you pivot on your heels back to the center turning your hips, body and head with arms simultaneously.

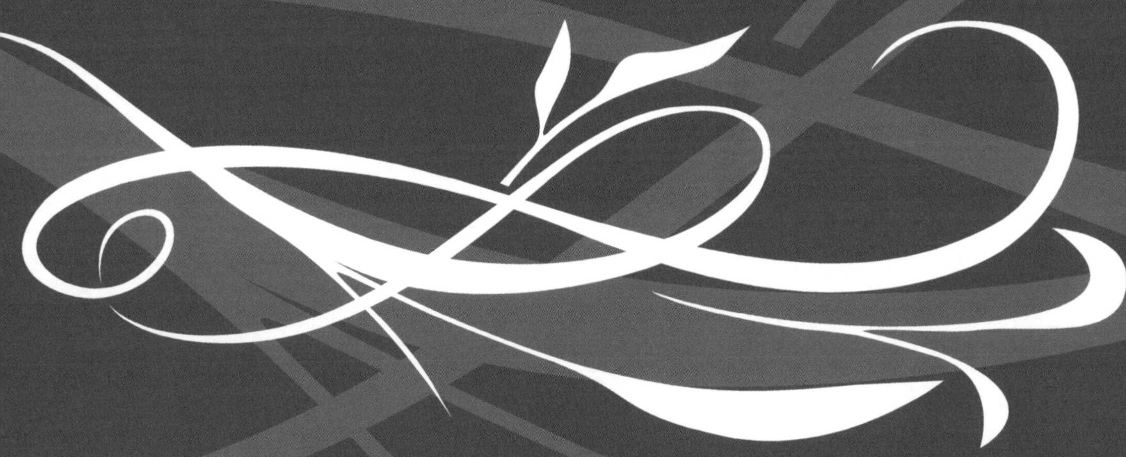

Tadasana

Life is just a mirror, and what you see out there, you must first see inside of you.
—Wally Amos

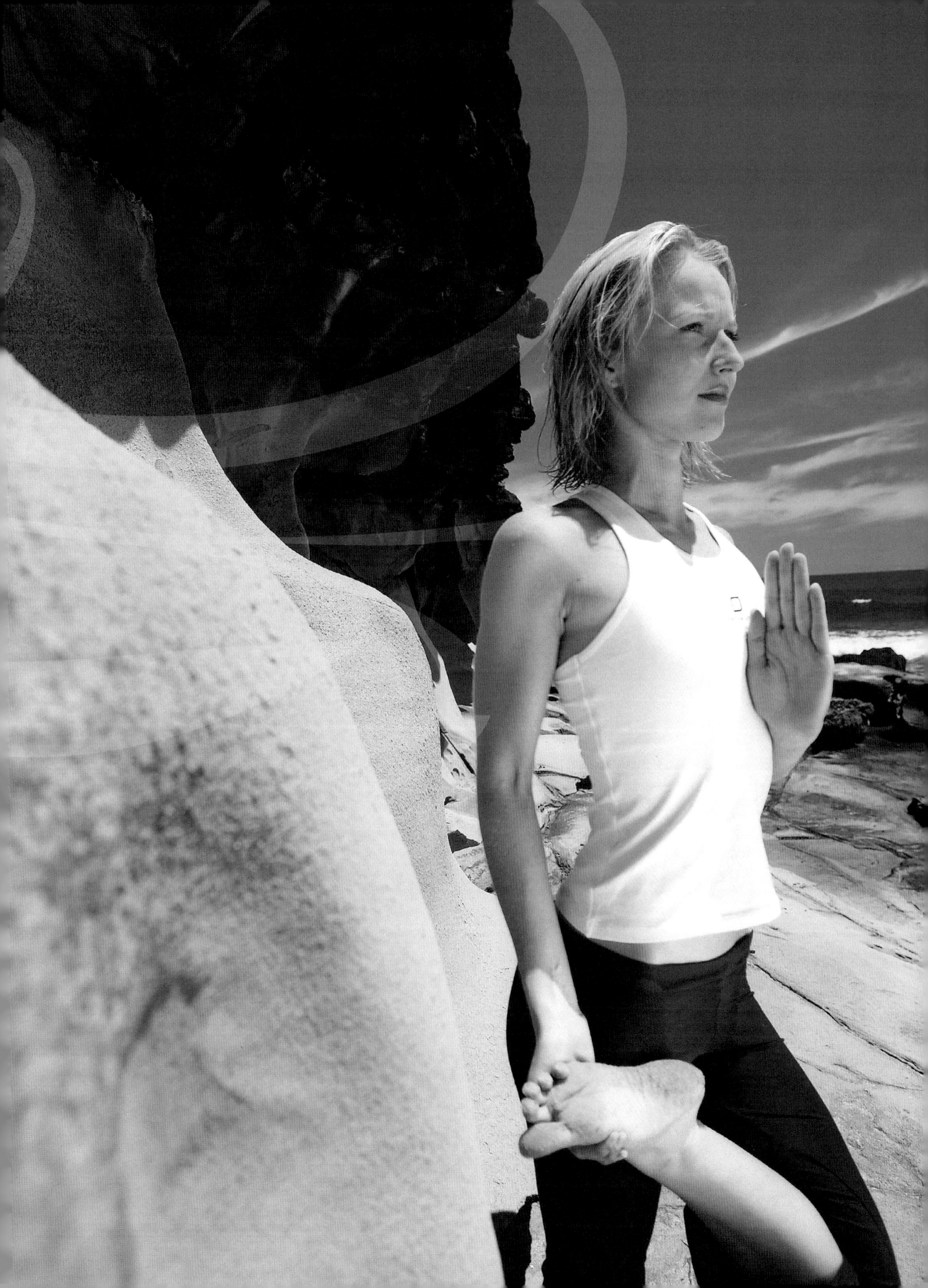

12 Tadasana

Tree Pose

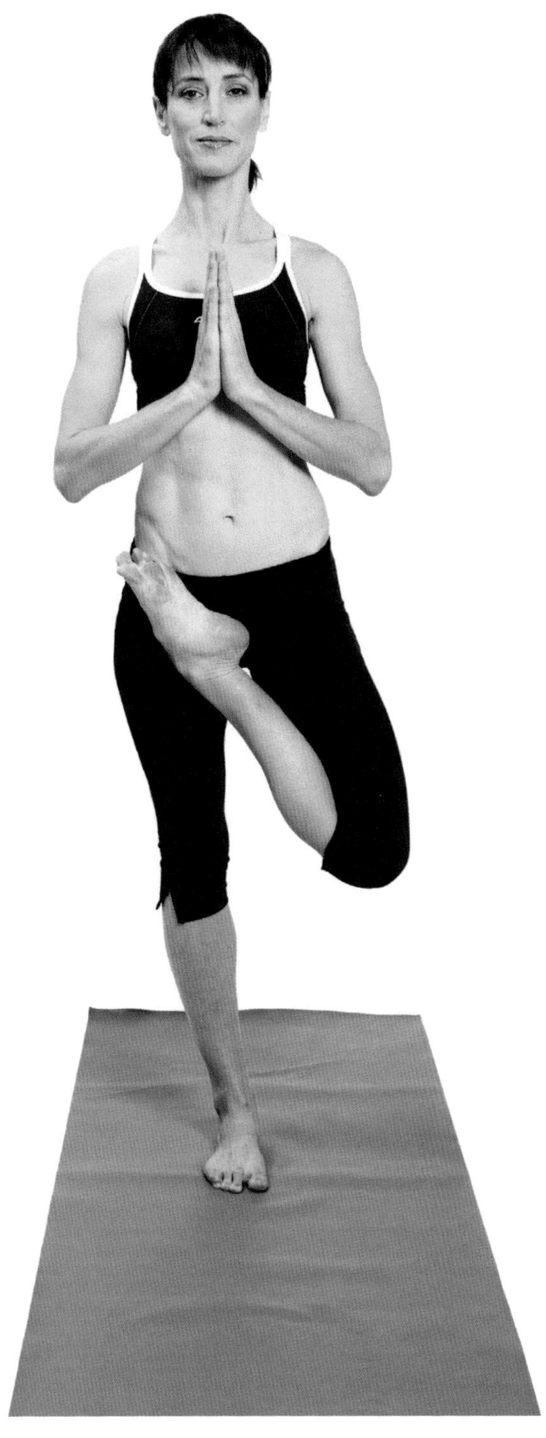

The essentials

You have almost made it to the end of the standing poses. The strong cardiovascular poses are finished with and the transition to the floor occurs with only Tree Pose and Toe Stand. These are less energetic and more calming on the circulatory system and bring a stabilizing focus to your practice.

These are good hip and knee openers. Very importantly, your steady direct communication in the mirror allows great feedback for your proprioception. You learn more about your posture, the way you carry yourself, perhaps even how you favor one leg over the other. As grounded as a strong tree pushes roots deep and wide into the earth, the crown of your head, and your body rise tall and proudly up heavenward. Balancing on one leg, you need to keep centering yourself.

What makes this pose so difficult to get right?

Physical limitations such as injured ankles, knees or tight hips will challenge your upper leg position, hovering above your one legged balance. Tight latissimus dorsi will tend to prevent you from standing as tall and straight as you would like. Above all, respect your knees, because this pose has the potential to cause a damaging twist. Have the humility to back out or readjust as and when necessary.

This is not a passive pose. You don't just pick up a foot and flop a hand in front of you – even though it can seem that way.

A word on knee safety

Make sure that discomfort never leads to excruciating pain. Although a simple hinge, the knee is a very complex nexus of muscles, ligaments and tendons. If your knee cannot bear the twist that occurs when you bring your foot to your hip then you may have to bring the sole of your foot to your inner thigh or lower leg. Never place this pressure directly against your standing leg knee.

Tadasana

Tree Pose

12

The technique

For these last two standing poses bring yourself to the middle of your mat. Roll your shoulders down and back, externally rotating your upper arms, with your palms slightly facing the mirror.

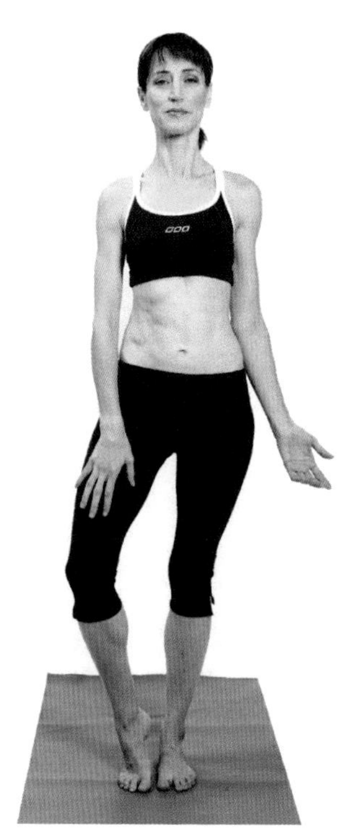

1. **Lock Your Standing Leg**: Solidly lock your left leg. Keep your hips even. Square them to the mirror and floor - no slumping, do not shift your weight to the standing leg.

2. **Lift Your Leg**: Inhale and bend your right leg up. I recommend that as you lift your leg you slide your right hand down the thigh, over the knee and then the lower leg so that you can gently bring your foot up (by grasping the ankle) to meet your left hip.

3. **Hold Your Foot From Behind**: Bring your right foot up to your left hip, your heel no further across your body than your left femur (thigh bone). Hold your foot from underneath with your left hand, with all fingers together. When you hold from behind your left elbow should point backward helping your shoulder draw down and back.

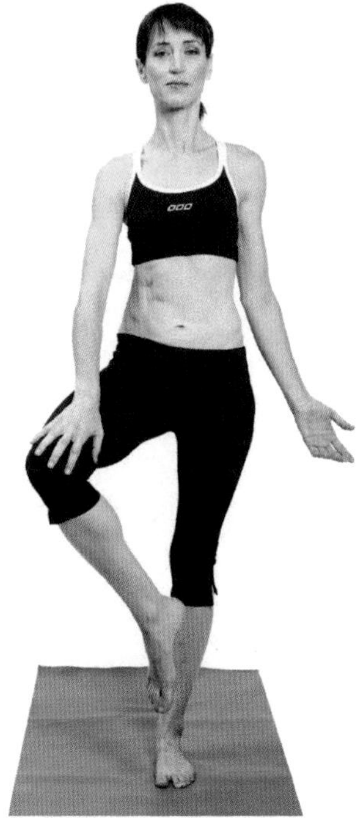

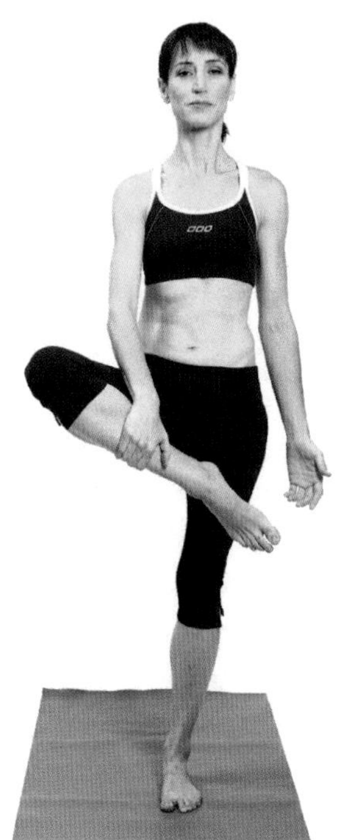

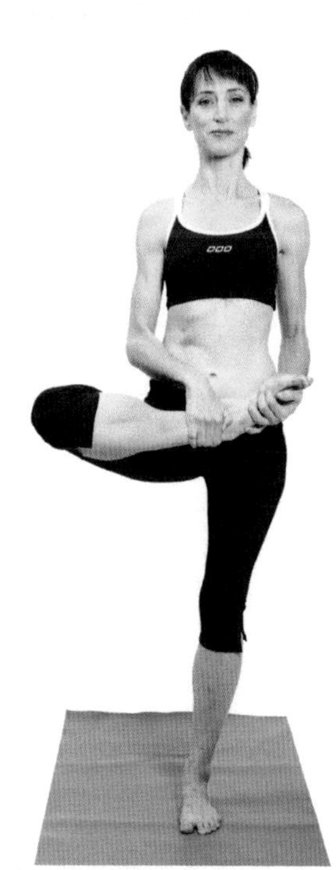

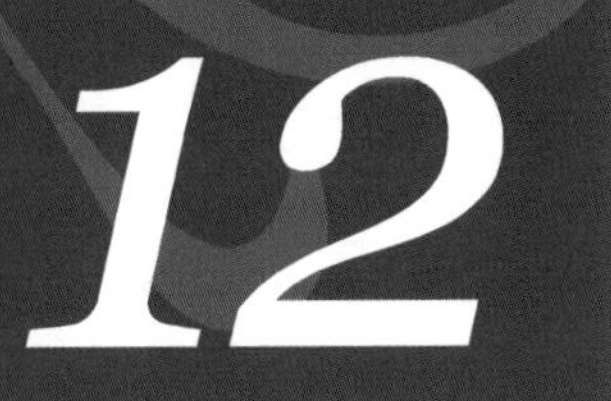

Tadasana

Tree Pose

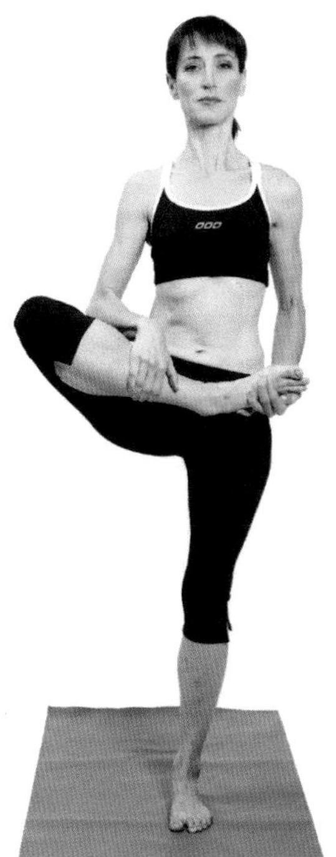

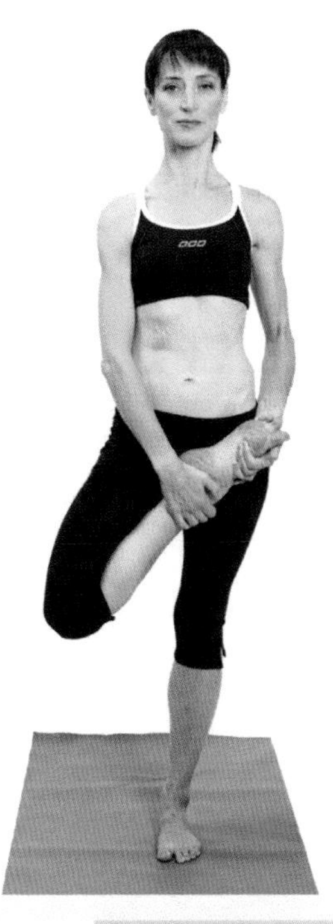

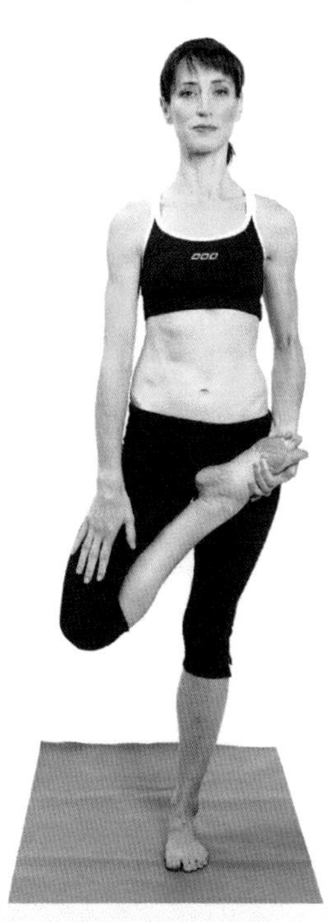

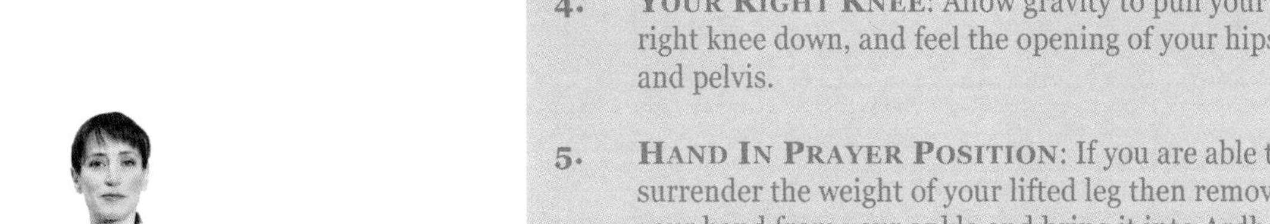

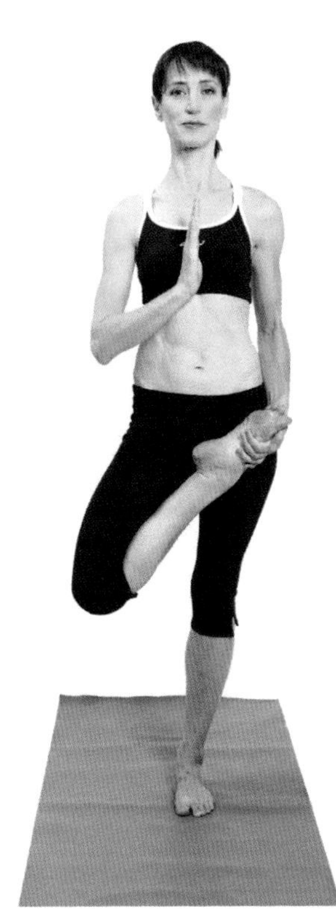

4. **Your Right Knee**: Allow gravity to pull your right knee down, and feel the opening of your hips and pelvis.

5. **Hand In Prayer Position**: If you are able to surrender the weight of your lifted leg then remove your hand from your ankle and bring it into Ardha Namaskar – or half prayer position.

6. **Create Traction In Your Spine**: Visualize growing tall against a strong grounded foundation. Every breath you take grow longer, with the crown of the head moving up. Every exhale, literally push the floor away from you. You will see space being created with your whole body and neck lengthening and your shoulders moving down your back.

7. **Your Body Opens**: Conscious intention is important to lengthen your muscles and open hips and knees. You will progressively move your knee down adjacent to your standing leg; with your tailbone neatly tucked under extending a beautifully straight back.

8. **Second Hand In Prayer Only If...**: If, when you release your foot hold, the leg surrenders easily to gravity, you can stand tall and your lifted heel is situated DIRECTLY underneath your belly button, bring your other hand up into prayer position.

 Release

Simply let go of your foot letting it come gently back down to standing position. Your hands come down to your sides. Stand in Savasana. Second side is the mirror image of the first side with no special instructions.

 The second set

The second set of Tadasana is either dedicated to a second set of Tree Pose or to attempting Padangustasana, Toe Stand.

 Common mistakes and how to fix them

Footprint at an angle: This may not seem critical – but a foot angled out to the side, even only by several degrees, decreases the amount of body awareness and correction required to balance effectively. Your pose instantly becomes substantially easier; unchallenging. Your standing foot must stay square on to the mirror. Just like walking in soft sand, your ankles and core muscles among others, have to work to strengthen and keep you stable.

Not able to grab the foot: Some literally cannot reach. You must try to hold your foot from behind. It helps resolve shoulder tension. Try grabbing what you can – maybe a couple of toes. Flexibility issues or an acute shoulder condition may prevent this. Transfer the grip to the front if this is your only option.

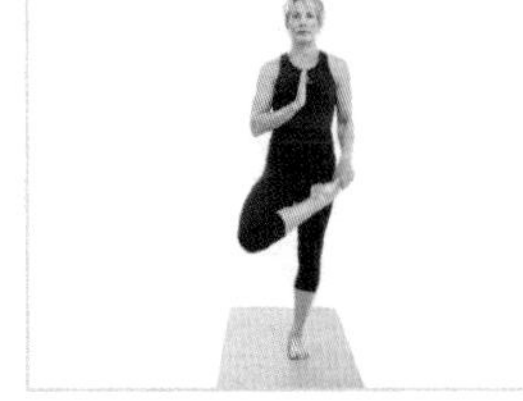

Heel crosses the midline of your standing leg: You can artificially get your knee down further by bringing your heel right across your hip, further from the midline. Ensure that your heel goes no further than the center of your femur. Your hand pulls your foot up, as gravity pulls your knee down creating safe traction to open your hip and knee. It doesn't matter if the knee is flying high near the level of your hip. What you need is to feel the leg surrendering and the hips opening.

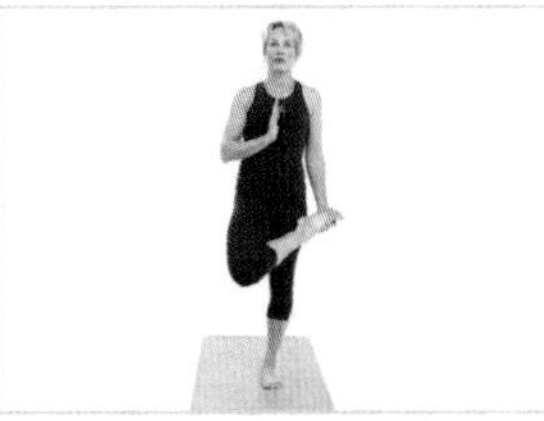

Hips slump: Hips slump when the body leans into one leg during the pose or set-up; or in attempts to get both knees parallel to the mirror. The hip and knee drop, the lumbar spine can arch and the bottom sticks out when you push past your current flexibility. Lift the hip back up again, tuck the tailbone under, to open up the hip and pelvis. Your knee will rise up but sacrifice the depth for the alignment.

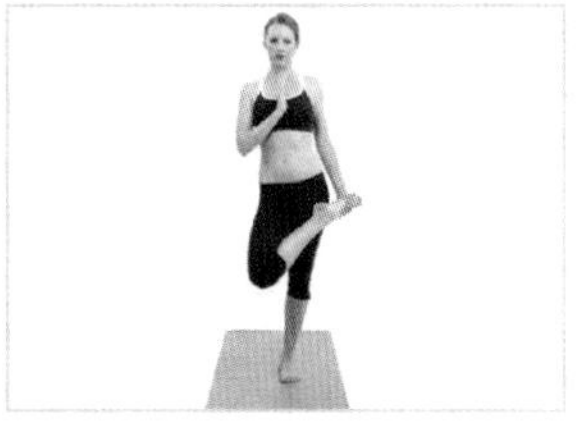

Elbow splays outward: If your elbow is out too far to the side the shoulder slumps forward, the chest rounds, the body leans to that side and it is difficult to balance and stand tall. Tuck your elbows in and center yourself.

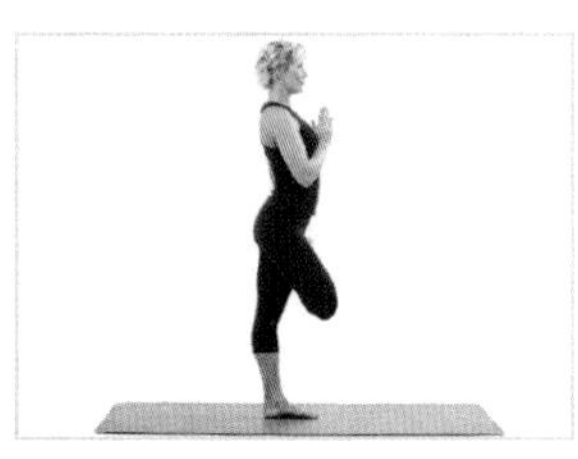

Sway back: If you push the bent leg down and back too far your spine will overly arch and the bottom may stick out. Tuck the tailbone under to lengthen the lower spine. Stretch up on the inhale, push the floor away as you exhale.

Half-prayer difficult: This is commonly caused by injury, hip or knee tightness, balance problems or rigid adductors. For an interim position; instead of bringing your hand to your sternum, lay it gently on your right inner thigh. This provides gentle physical guidance, aids gravity, while providing more symmetrically balanced forces.

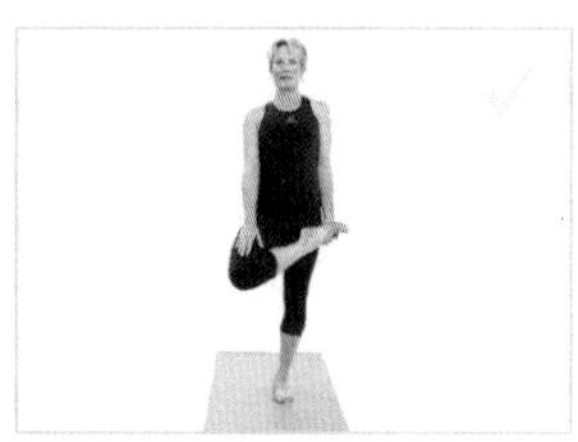

Bringing both hands into prayer before ready: Respect this rule: If the heel is not at the exact centerline of the body you have no business taking your hand away from behind your foot. When correctly and centrally positioned it will stay put. If it slips you are not ready. If you progress to Toe Stand for your second set then this rule is a little pliable; please see the next chapter. If you are doing two sets of Tree Pose never allow your foot to slip. Rather keep holding the foot.

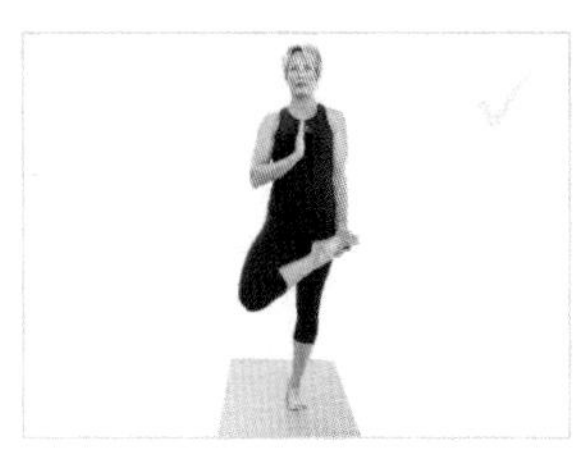

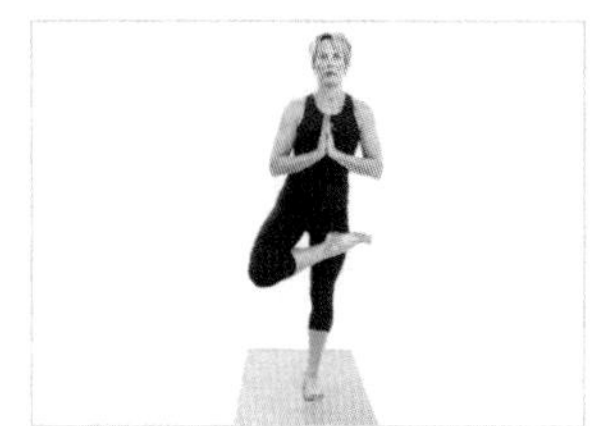

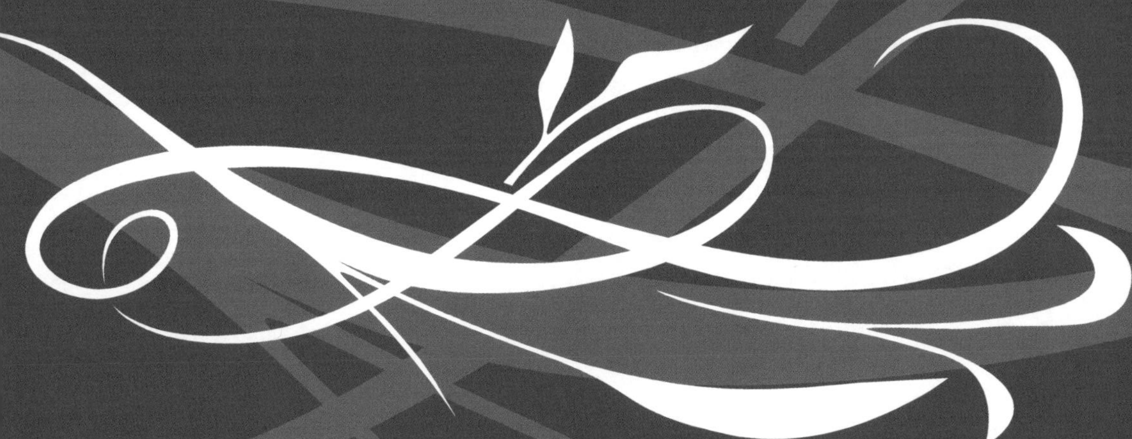

Padangustasana

When you dance, your purpose is not to get to a certain place on the floor. It's to enjoy each step along the way.
—Dr. Wayne Dyer

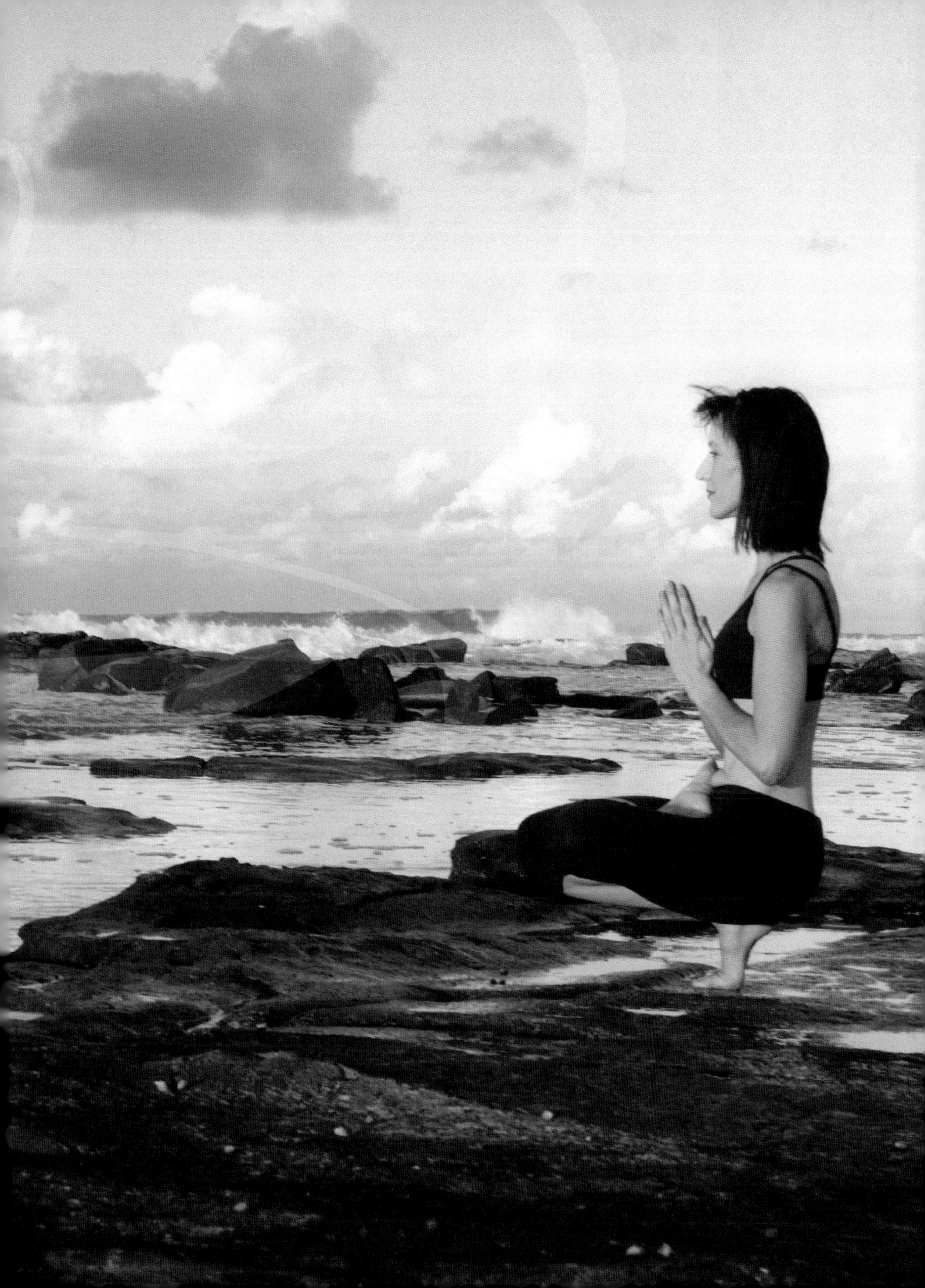

13 Padangustasana

Toe Stand

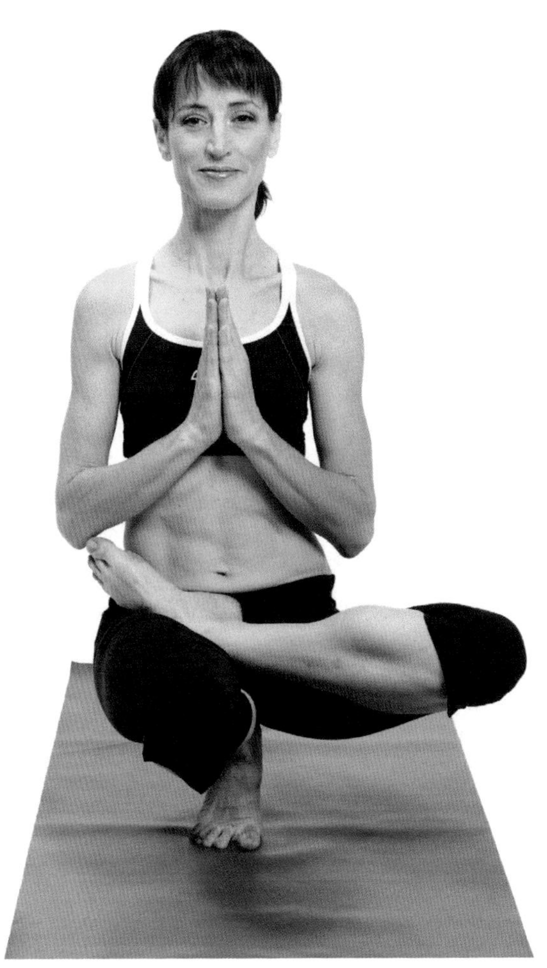

The essentials

This pose looks like an advanced pose – especially as it is introduced essentially as the second set of Tree Pose. It does look difficult. After all, there 'they' are balancing precariously on the toes of one foot attempting to bring their hands into prayer.

If we demystify it, you will see that it is just a natural progression from Tree, and accessible to many. Remember that if you are not attempting Toe Stand then a second set of Tree Pose is actioned.

What makes this pose so difficult to get right?

Toe Stand presents some physical challenges, but for the most part it is the mental challenge that confronts students. They often have to be coaxed into their first attempt. The pose doesn't have to be an 'all or none' proposition. It won't seem nearly as scary when we break it down into smaller components!

Body tightness or injury will hamper your ability to balance or get your knee down closer to the floor. You are aiming for both knees to be in a line parallel to the floor.

Padangustasana

Toe Stand

13

The technique

As a second set to Tree Pose you begin in exactly the same way with either one or two hands together in prayer position.

There are two ways to get into Toe Stand. The standard way which can be broken into stages depending on your flexibility, is used by most students and all new ones. It involves bending forward to the floor and using the hands for balance. The advanced method (used by less than 5% of students) is for those who have built sufficient strength to descend into final position without touching the hands to the floor.

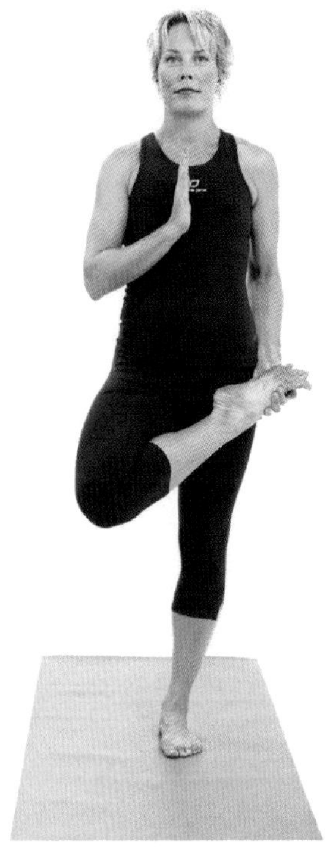

Standard entry:

1.1 **Hinge Your Body**: Exhale, draw in your abdomen and with your standing leg locked solidly, hinge your straight body at your hips to bring it toward the floor. One or both hands are in prayer position.

1.2 **Hands To Floor**: When close to the floor, let your hands rest there in front of you. Eyes look to floor, (not to legs) this helps iron out your spine.

1.3 **Open Your Sacroiliac Joints**: Hanging down in this way, with hands on the floor, is an excellent way to open your sacroiliac joints. Fully lock your leg. If you can't proceed any further, are having any lower back pain or need space here, you may choose to spend the whole time stretching, right here. Your lifted foot helps open the hip. But keep both hips square. Don't let the hip of the lifted leg slump.

1.4 **Bend Your Leg**: Your hands take the weight as your standing leg bends. Your heel rises up off the floor as your bottom approaches your heel. You are balancing thanks to the tripod made by your two hands and your toes. Make whatever adjustments with your arms to allow your knees to come down.

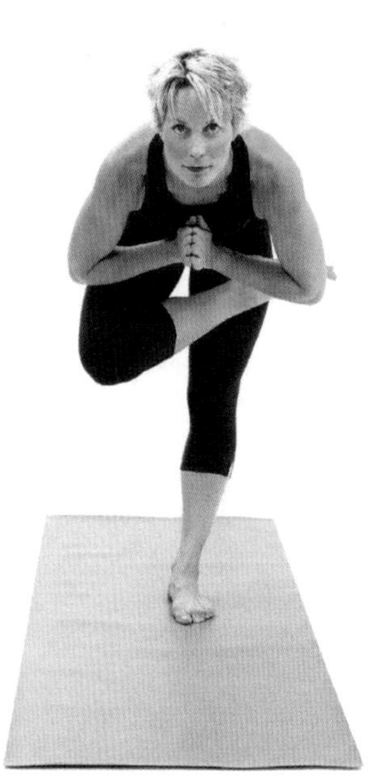

13

Padangustasana

Toe Stand

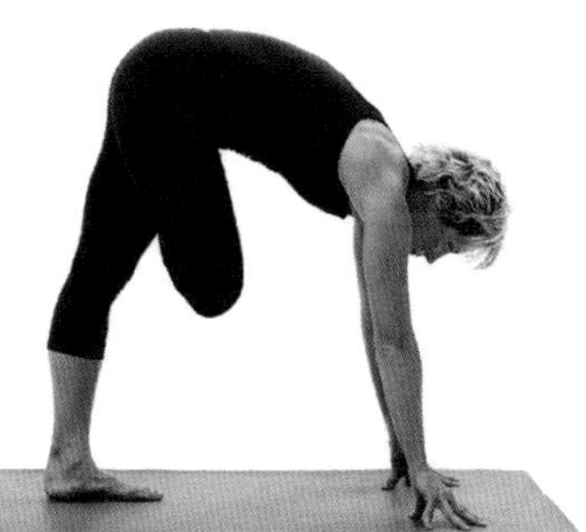

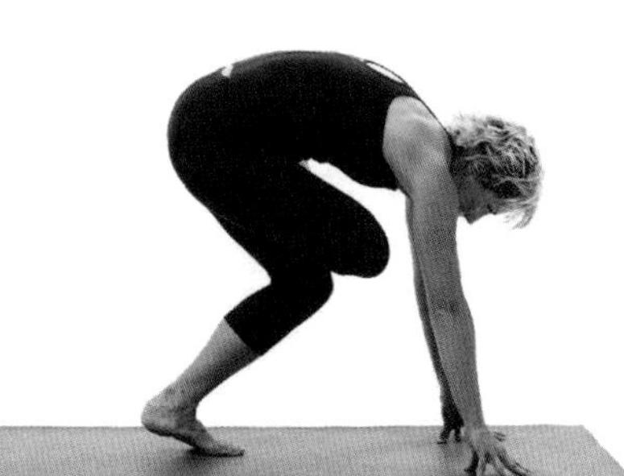

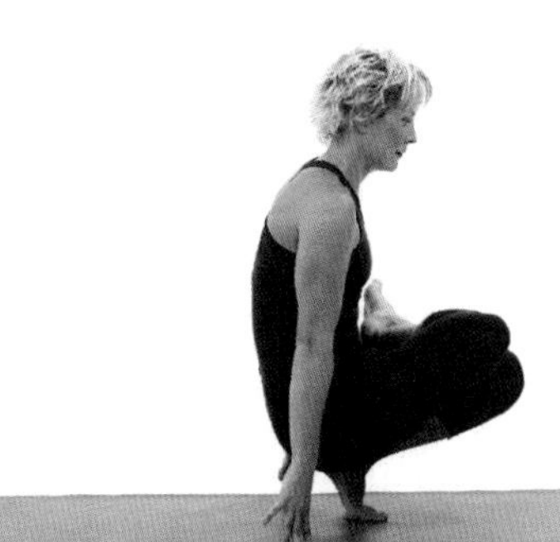

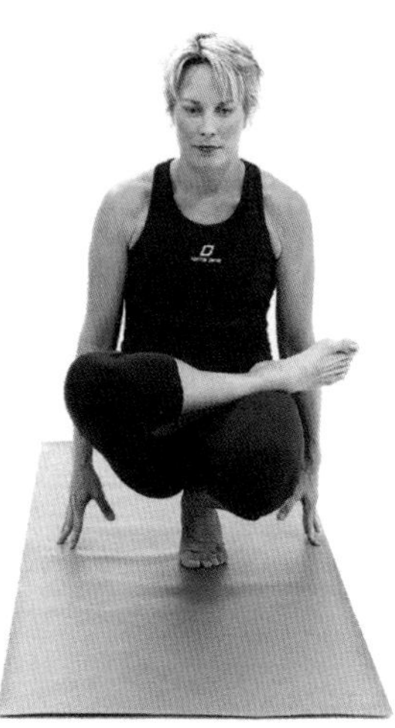

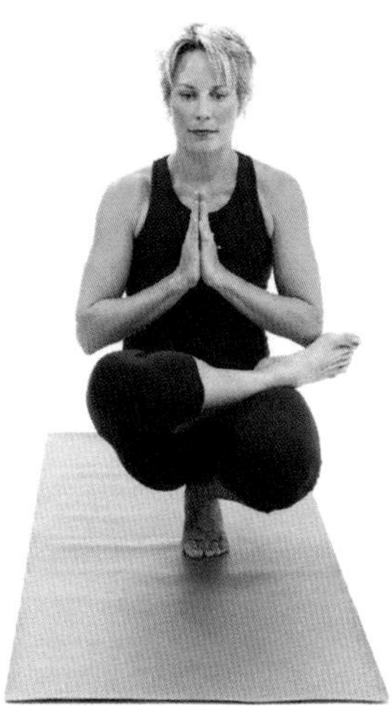

1.5 **Sit On Or Hover Over Your Heel**: In the beginning, you will rest placing your heel at a buttock or between them at the perineum. In time you will have the ability to hold space between the heel and body. The stronger your knees, ankles and core the more you can suspend your bottom above your heel.

1.6 **Remove A Balance Linkage**: Surprisingly, balancing with space between heel and bottom is easier than sitting on the heel. Just like links in a chain, there is instability at every link: Where toes meet the floor, the ankle and where the heel meets your body. When you have the strength to hover, you remove one of those weaknesses.

1.7 **The Process Of Balancing Without Hands**: Once the lower body is stable you will balance without hands and rely solely on your connection to the ground through the toes. The way you do this will depend on your body proportions.

1.8 **Those With Long Arms**: It's a 2 step process to final pose if you have long arms. One at a time place each arm behind you to support your now vertical body on straight arms. A steady forward focus assists your balance. Now bring one arm at a time into prayer position in front of your sternum.

1.9 **Shorter Armed Yogis**: The method described above is impossible for short-armed folk when the body cannot be vertical with arms behind. With 1 hand behind the weight shifts sideways, and it's hard to get back up. So leave the hands on the floor in front.

Padangustasana

Toe Stand

Keep a forward soft steady gaze. Lift your chest, gaze and hands at the same rate. The back raises and straightens as you calmly lift your hands up off the floor. Let your hands gradually approach each other to meet in the middle when your back is straight. This takes a little coordination practice, but it definitely works.

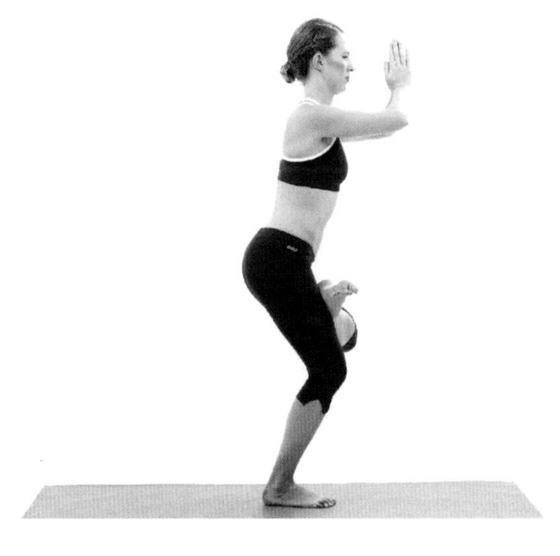

1.10 **Hands In Prayer**: The hands come together effortlessly and rest against each other without any perceptible pushing. When your hands are relaxed your shoulders and elbows can relax too. There should be no aggression in prayer.

Advanced entry:

The advanced entry is for those who can fairly easily stand in Tree Pose with both hands in prayer position and the heel at or close to the centerline.

A sense of humor, a strong body and mind are all needed. You may not have enough resources to succeed every time, so be prepared to incorporate elements of the standard entry (above) as needed. A word of warning: Don't even attempt this entry if you have knee problems.

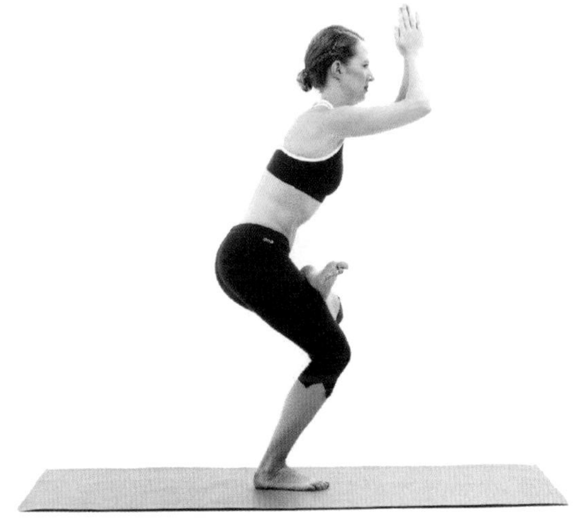

2.1 **The Descent**: Exhale, gather the strength in your core, and start to descend whilst holding your hands in prayer.

2.2 **Hands Push Together Strongly**: Actively push your hands together in prayer to help recruit strength and control in your descent. An upward movement of your hands feels as though your hands are cemented in space as you descend. It opposes the downward movement of the body.

2.3 **Heel Naturally Comes Up**: At some point - determined by toe and ankle strength and flexibility - your heel will come up off the floor.

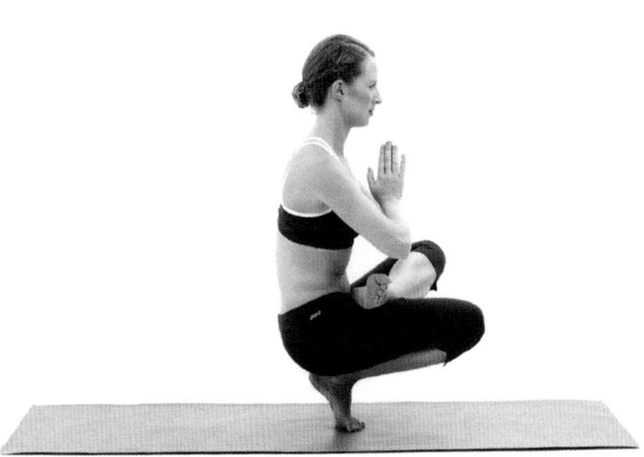

2.4 **Balance On Your Toes**: About half way down, when your heel is up and toes are taking the weight, the hands will descend into their final position. Gradually release the strong inward forces to finish in a real passively-placed prayer position.

2.5 **Work On Hovering**: If you have the strength to descend hands-free then you tend to have the ability to hover. Balance is easier in these circumstances. It is very rare to descend hands-free and rest on the heel.

Padangustasana

Toe Stand

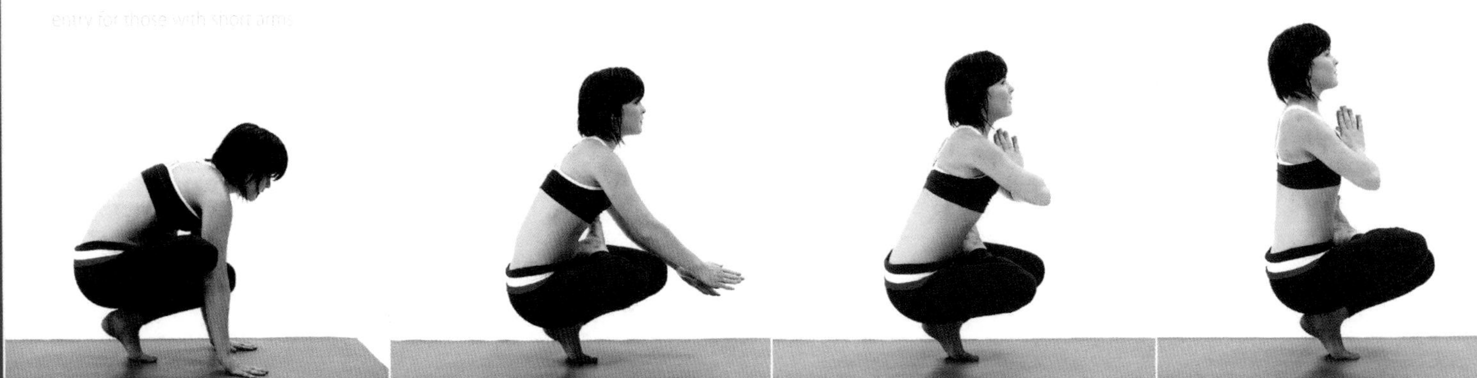

Where do your eyes look?

- Look forward in the mirror when standing.
- Your chin is away from the chest when you are in your big forward bend and opening your sacroiliac joints. This gives extension to your spine rather than rounding.
- For 'long-arm-entry' into prayer position: Beginners keep focus on a fixed target. Look forward a couple of yards/meters on the floor.
- For 'short-arm-entry': Your mid-range soft focus will float up at the same rate as you unhinge your body into vertical position. Fix your focus when you are stable.
- The more competent you become at Toe Stand the more you will raise the object of your focus. Over time fixing your target or gaze will graduate to focus on your body, throat chakra, or directly into your own eyes.

Release

It's obviously harder coming out of this one than going in. Reversing the pose might not be feasible especially if you entered using the advanced technique. You are tired, and moving against the forces of gravity. Whichever way you decide to come out, there are usually balance issues as you haul your body back up off the ground, trying to keep your hands in prayer. You need a strong core and you need to know when to simply let your hands do more of the work. Make considered conscious movements and come up safely.

3.1 Release your hands onto the floor. They will either land to the side or you will fall forward onto your hands.

3.2 Either way you will need to push off from the floor, with your fingertips in front of you about shoulder width apart for maximum leverage.

3.3 Straighten then lock your lower leg and bring your heel to the floor as you push up and straighten your arms. Keep your lifted leg heel in position on your upper thigh.

3.4 Come up to standing with one or both hands in prayer position.

3.5 Release your leg to the floor and then your arms down and stand in Savasana.

Release from the hands-free entry method is more difficult and is rarely seen in class. Students usually require help to propel themselves off the floor, in the form of an upward push of the elbows or support of the hips. If you are at this level (less than 1% of students) then request occasional assistance so that one day you can do it on your own. More commonly however, you can enjoy the standard release and use your arms.

Common mistakes and how to fix them

Going down before you are ready to progress from Tree Pose: You are not ready to proceed if:

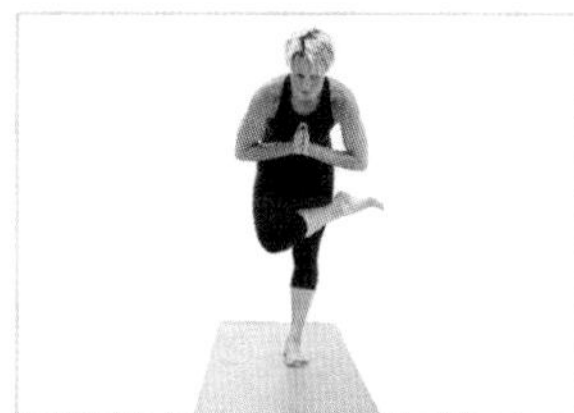

- Your lifted heel travels across your body past the center of your standing leg, or femur. Stay in Tree Pose for both sets because your hips are insufficiently flexible. Not only will you will stand with less symmetry and strength but your foot is likely to slip off your leg. Work on your hip flexibility first to place your heel slightly inside of your femur before attempting Toe Stand.
- You can't take your hand away from your foot without it falling (to your knee or beyond). It is usually OK if your foot settles down your leg only an inch or two.
- Your knee 'floats' up in the air when your foot is in position.
- You can't balance on one leg.
- When you try to bend forward, your foot slips to the floor.
- When you bend forward your hands cannot reach the floor.
- Your knee bends to reach your hands to the floor. See below for exception.

Knee bends to get to floor: Usually the best scenario for Toe Stand attempts is when you can reach your hands to the floor with a completely straight and locked out standing leg. This is not a hard and fast rule as there are those who have sufficient body and core strength to descend on a bent leg yet still lack sufficient flexibility.

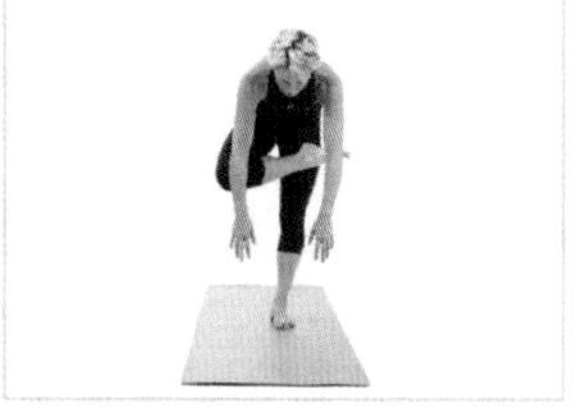

For the most part I want my students to have developed enough power in their quadriceps muscles and have no trouble locking out their legs for long periods of time. If you have a weak core, or a weak lower back then a forward bend to the floor while on one leg could spell trouble. Have the sense of humor and humility to develop your core and leg strength from the other poses and leave Toe Stand for another time.

Leaning: The body may lean sideways or forward when you are sitting on your heel or attempting upright balance. Build strength. Work on activating your legs to support you and check if you have tension in your upper body.

Settling onto the heel: This is not a huge mistake. It is rather a stepping stone to success. Your ideal outcome is to hover so don't be content to go into position and sit on your heel. When you sit down it can be difficult to balance because you introduce an extra link to the balance chain. But more importantly when you sit, your muscles surrender and then you must re-activate them to ascend and exit from this pose. Ascent is far easier if your leg muscles are in a state of engagement even with little or no space between heel and hips. Build your strength and space over time.

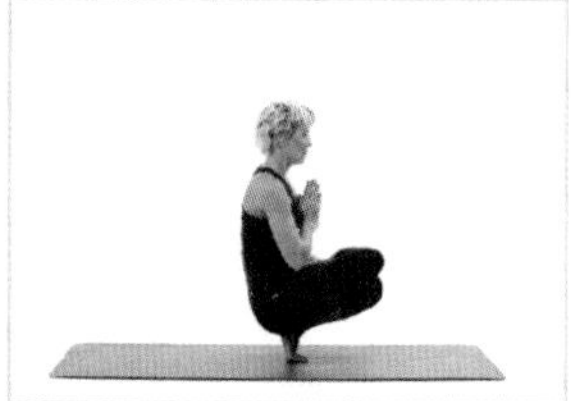

Forced prayer: Pushing your hands together at the chest creates numerous possible outcomes; tension across the chest, elbows lift up and out, shoulders tighten, neck tenses, teeth clench, balance is more difficult, the pose becomes fraught with struggle. You will lose the battle to gain control over your stiff unyielding body. Take the fight out of the pose, allow the hands to settle together and the elbows to drop in final position passively, relaxedly, calmly. Feel tension melt away.

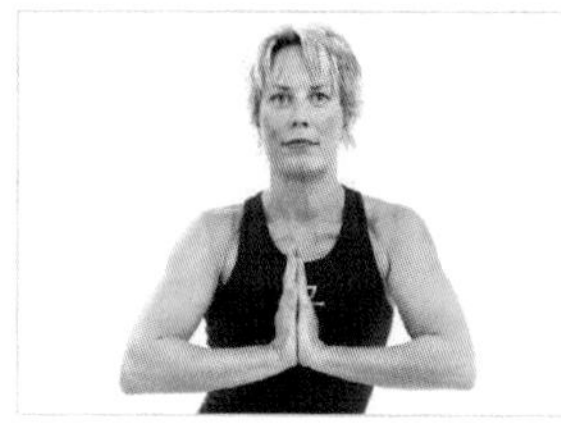

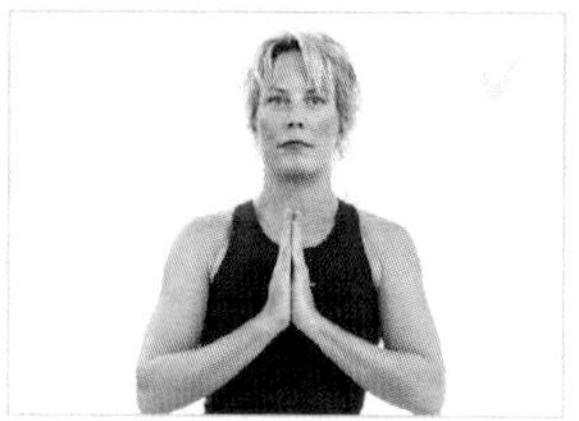

Tight shoulders and splaying elbows: These are signs of a forced prayer position.

Chin down: Dropping the chin drops the gaze and you are more likely to fall. Where your eyes go your body follows. So draw your gaze forward and out in front of you. If you are experiencing balance difficulties then look at something completely static like the floor a couple of yards/meters ahead. Gradually move your focus up to rest on your own eyes in the mirror.

Thinking too much: Trying to balance is a different proposition to creating balance. Work and take your attention to your breath. Relax your body.

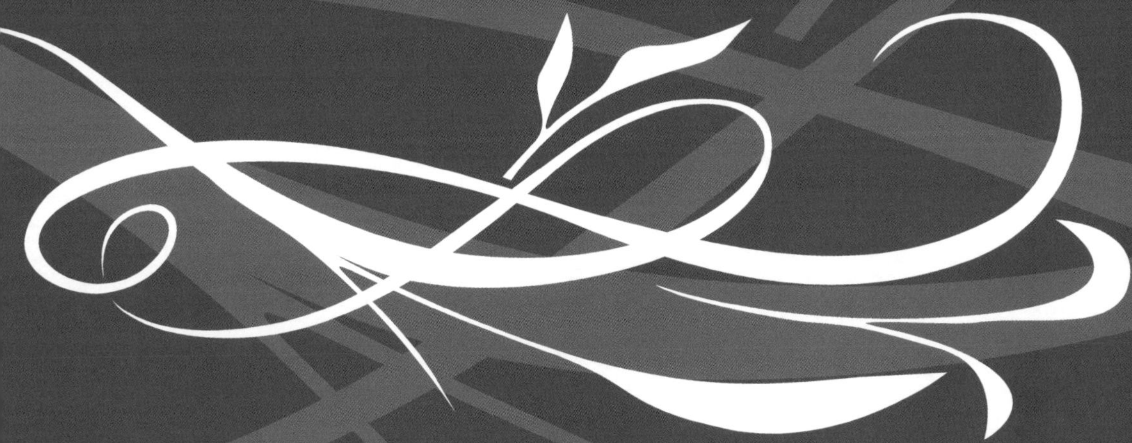

Savasana

There is more to life than increasing its speed.
—Mohandas Gandhi

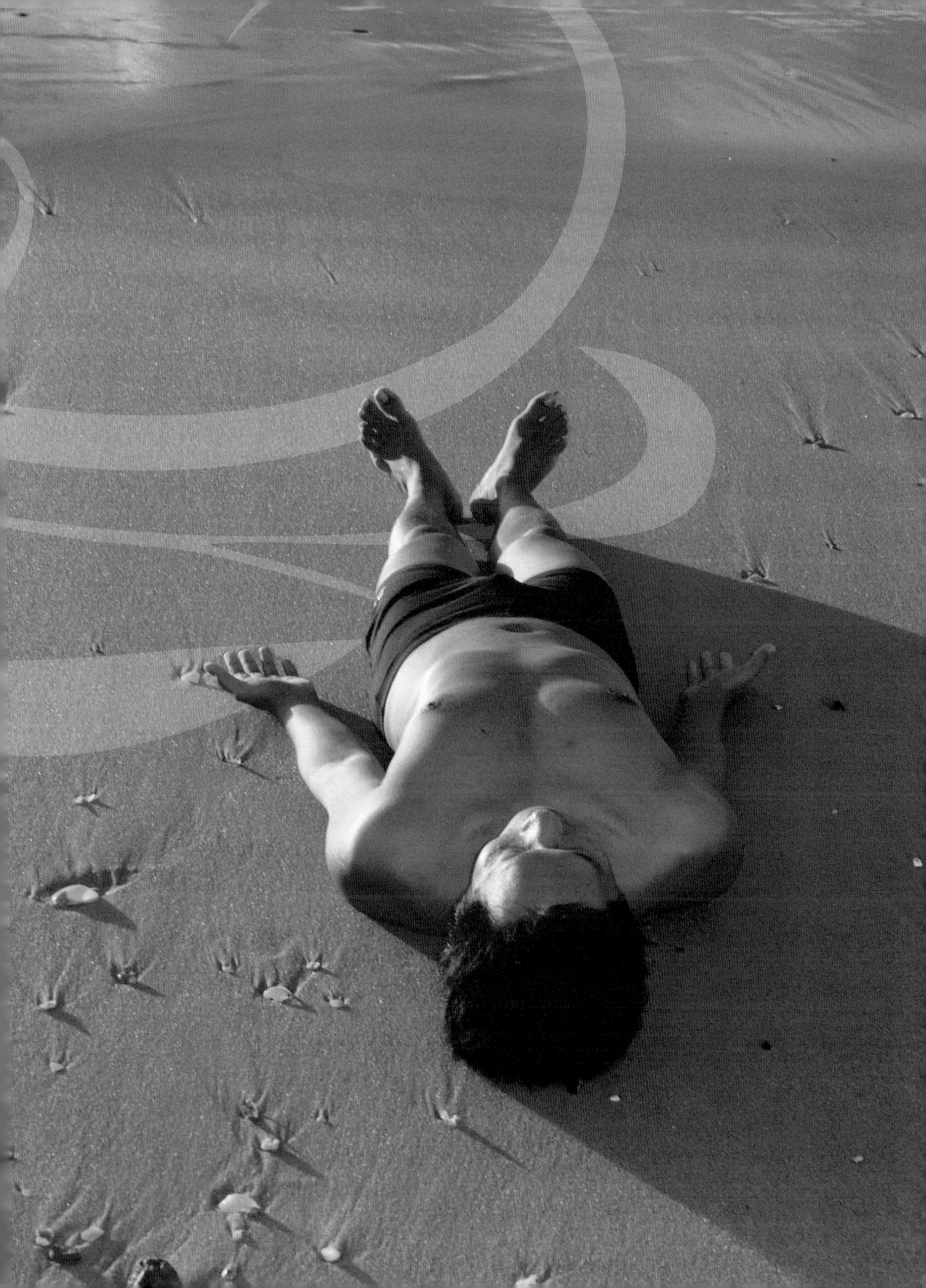

14 Savasana

Corpse Pose

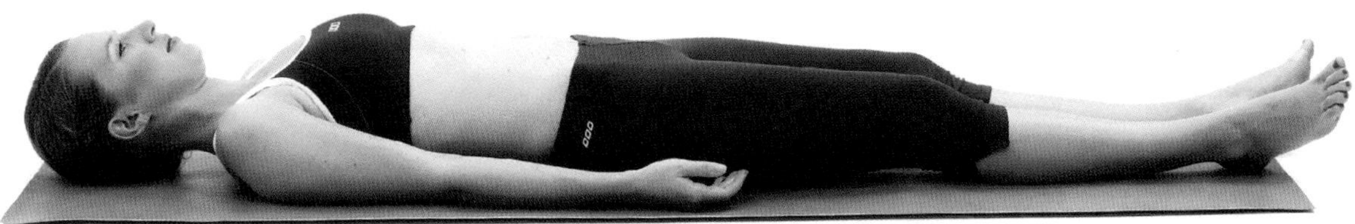

The essentials

It feels so good to arrive at this point. The stronger more cardiovascular 'half' of the class is over. You deserve this two minute break to settle your heart rate back down and regroup your energy. Move efficiently. Use as little time as you can to get into position and then lie there and breathe deeply. Focus your attention on the breath to bring you into the present moment. Even the novice meditator would recognize this as a primary technique in gaining stillness.

We'll take a look at the other rest positions in this chapter; the Savasana of the belly-down poses, and another that may be useful for you if you have injury or illness, or if you are pregnant.

What makes this pose so difficult to get right?

When we first start yoga we all think that this is an easy pose. After all, you just lie there. Right? Uh uhhh. It seems crazy that lying still would be so difficult. However, you have just spent the better part of an hour using your body's movements to help quieten your mind. In effect your conscious mind has been distracted by the poses, into a kind of lull or stillness, leaving little time for thought.

You will realize how profound the effect is particularly on days when you cannot find the stillness. The mind chatter can literally be unbalancing and you fall over and out of poses much more often. Let those thoughts go and hey presto, you find your center again and the class flows for you.

Up until now, the momentum of the class has kept these breaks short, sandwiched between periods of physical exertion. Now without the activity, it is up to you to keep your body AND mind still. Perhaps surprisingly, this may be your biggest challenge yet.

Savasana

Corpse Pose

The technique

Remember first and foremost that relaxation is a learned skill. You can facilitate it, nurture it and practice it. A constant return to Savasana will act as a trigger for progressively deeper relaxation. The more efficiently you get there, the quicker and more deeply you can reach your chilled-out state.

In a live hot yoga class the teacher will usually talk for the two minutes with the aim of guiding your meditation and awareness in a thoughtful manner. This technique serves to bypass your conscious mind and steer you away from unnecessary or extraneous thoughts (like your next meal, the work you are supposed to have got done, etc) and helps you zero in on your breath. Sometimes you will hear concepts on which to focus, other times you will be left in silence. Stretches of silence are usually where you need to muster more self-control to attain body and mind stillness.

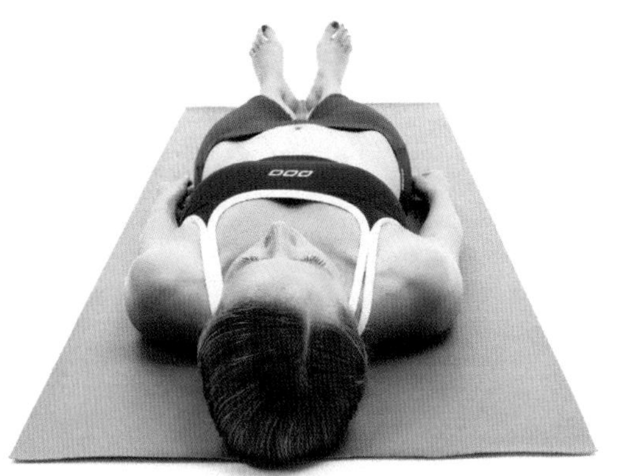

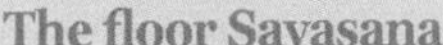

The floor Savasana

1.1 **Acknowledge Your Effort, Stand In Savasana**: Finish your last standing pose. Take a few moments to meet yourself in the mirror and really acknowledge your fine efforts up to now. I invite you to be more conscious. Let your shoulders hang down and back and palms face forward slightly. Chin up, eyes forward, feet together. Then, adjust your towel if necessary, drink if appropriate, and lie down in your first supine Savasana.

1.2 **Get To The Floor In Good Time**: Be quick and fuss-free but don't rush. Take the minimum time and you gain the maximum available seconds to benefit. After the standing poses however, you can buy a moment or two to get some leverage on your most important pose in yoga.

1.3 **Lie Down**: Lie down on your back, completely square to the room, with your head closest to the mirror and feet to the back wall.

1.4 **Arms By Your Side**: Your arms are relaxed close to but not touching your sides, palms facing the ceiling.

1.5 **Legs Together**: Bring your feet together, let your toes fall out to the side, your heels may or may not end up touching. The relaxation extends from your hips right down to your toes. Feel the adductor muscles (your inner thighs) soften.

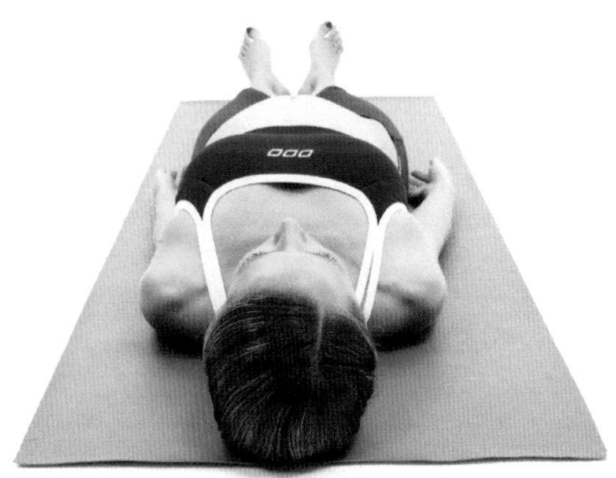

shoulders shimmied under

Savasana

CORPSE POSE

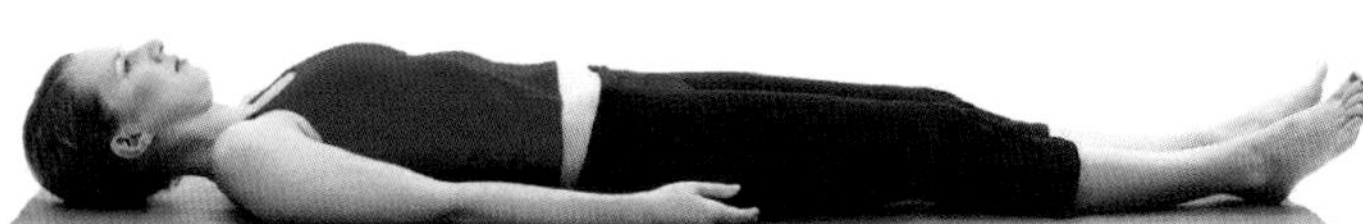

abdomino-diaphragmatic breath
inhale, belly rises

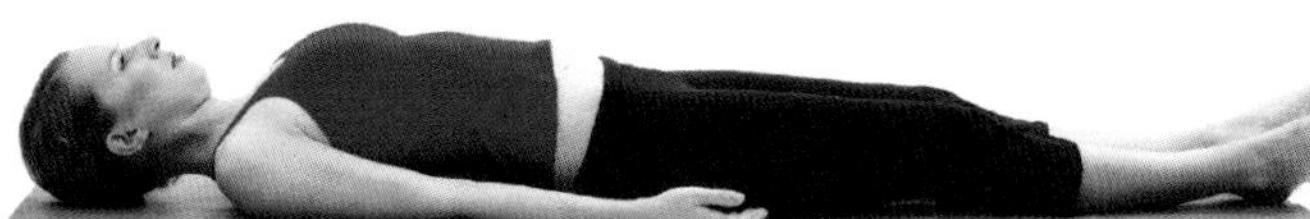

exhale, belly falls

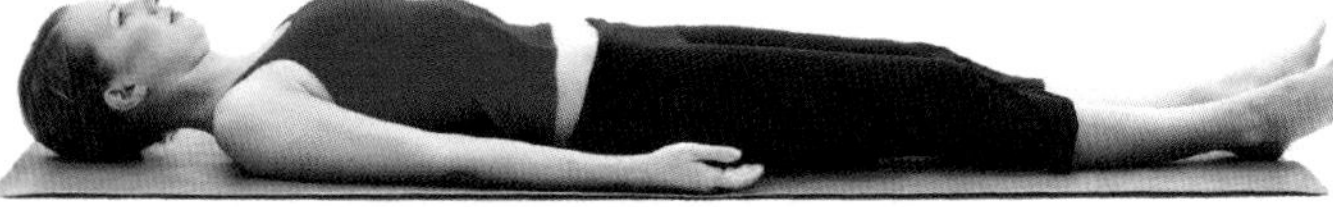

1.6 **SHOULDERS UNDER**: Shimmy your shoulder blades toward each other underneath you to relax your shoulders down away from your ears. More importantly it physically balloons your ribcage from a 'collapsed' state to an 'inflated' one. The belly relaxes and it makes drawing air in and out of the 'space' very easy. Your belly rises and falls rhythmically and your lungs fill more fully with your abdomino-diaphragmatic breath.

1.7 **LENGTHEN YOUR CERVICAL SPINE**: Tuck your chin to instantly lengthen your neck and cervical spine on the floor. Your gaze is slightly angled down. Avoid looking directly above you, and instead gaze at a point on the ceiling more or less above your feet or beyond.It helps you connect with your physical and emotional being allowing you to really take inventory of every moment. You can feel yourself settle in quite comfortably.

1.8 **RELAX, YIELD, SURRENDER**: You need to relax into the floor. Yield to the forces of gravity and submit to the floor simply holding you up. You are heavy and your muscles are molten. Lie still without even moving a muscle. This means no twitching of fingers, moving of feet, no adjusting your hair or your yoga wear, no drinking, talking or thinking! There is nothing else to do but breathe.

1.9 **OBSERVE YOUR BREATH AND YOUR SENSATIONS**: The idea is to focus on your breath moving in and out of your nose. Explore the sensations at play; how the air moves in and out; is it warm or cool; does it move with more ease through one nostril; feel it swirling through your nose, down your trachea into your lungs; feel the movement of your abdomen up with every inhale and down with every exhale. Meanwhile, remain aware of the other sensations in your body. Perhaps you can sense a spreading relaxation in your body; where is it spreading from and going to? Are there any areas of tightness or discomfort, maybe even pain? What happens when you breathe into them and then exhale right through to dissipate them?

1.10 **BE IN THE MOMENT**: There will be times when you can embody these principles and truly be 'present'. Be the observer, explore each and every moment as it comes, neither burdening yourself with memories of the past or expectations of the future. Welcome to the greatest gift you can give yourself – and without which there is nothing – your breath.

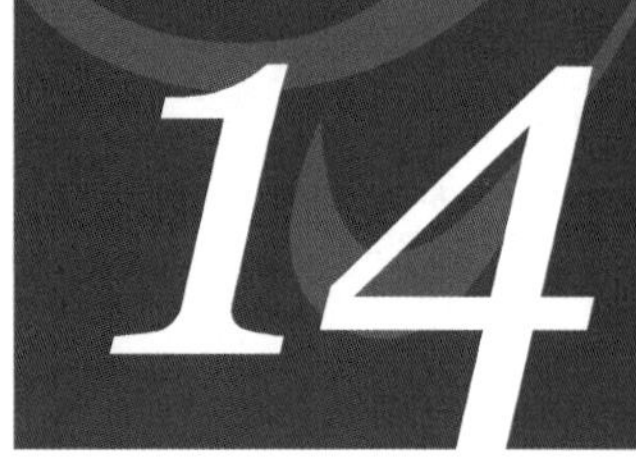

Savasana

Corpse Pose

Why 'shimmy' the shoulders under?

There are teachers who would say just to lie in the manner that you find yourself without adjusting the shoulders. I do not agree. A tent without a pole in the center has a reduced volume. Prop up the middle and you have instant space with the same amount of canvas. Do this with your chest by bring your shoulder blades further under. Your chest 'props' open your lungs and more air will effortlessly passage in and out, getting to out-of-reach areas.

The belly-down Savasana

This rest position is used from Cobra through to Floor Bow during the floor-facing Spine Strengthening poses.

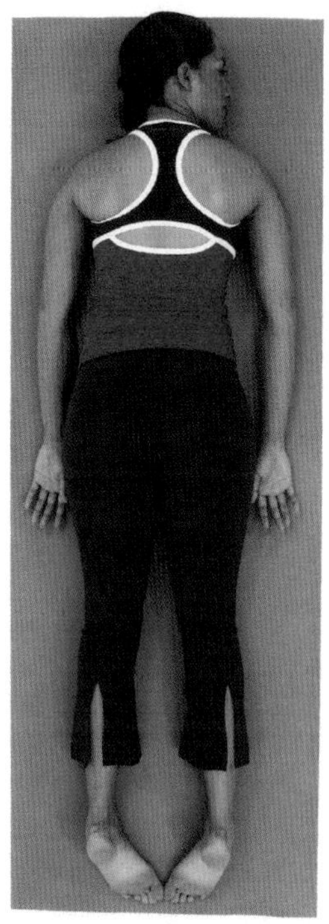

2.1 **Release Your Pose**: When you exit, your chin will contact the floor again, along your central axis keeping your spine in a neutral position.

2.2 **Turn Your Head**: Support yourself with your hands while you lift and turn your head to contact your ear on the floor. Keep your chin up to keep your spine straight.

2.3 **Arms By The Side**: Bring your arms to your sides, relaxed. Your palms face upward, allowing a natural slight curve to the fingers.

2.4 **Legs Soft**: Bring your toes together touching. Allow gravity to draw your heels out and down to the sides. This particularly releases the lower spine and your bottom and inner thighs soften.

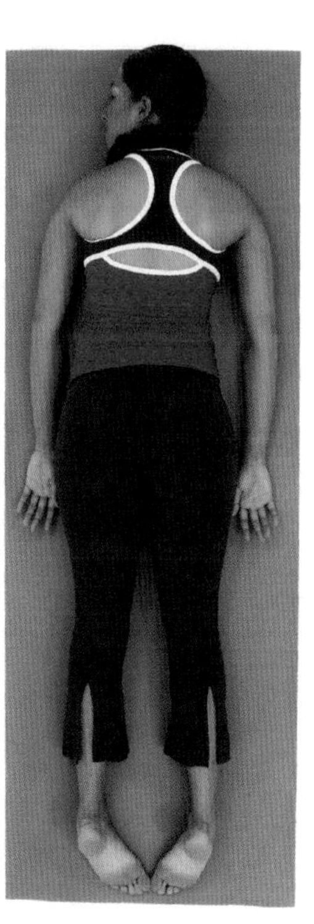

2.5 **Soft Gaze**: Look only as far as the edge of your mat or towel, no further. You can more easily keep inward attention, focusing on your breath and sensations without distraction.

2.6 **Breathe And Massage**: Feel your belly rise and fall with your every breath. Your spine muscles are massaged by the hydraulic pressure of your organs as your fluid-filled abdomen pushes against the immoveable floor.

Savasana

Corpse Pose

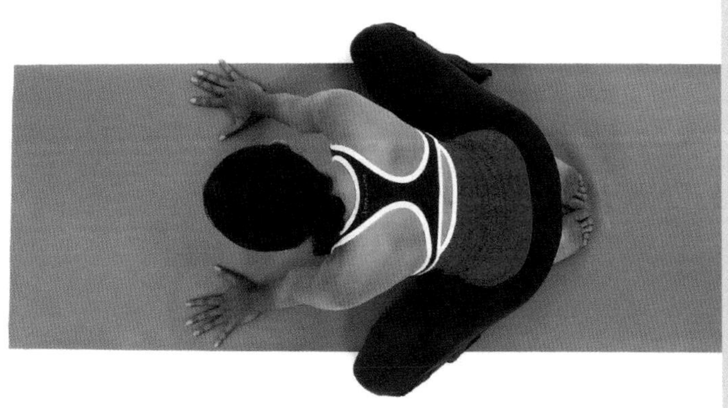

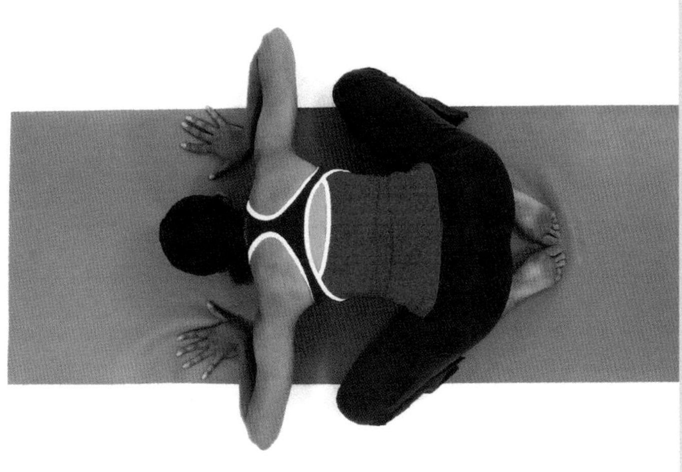

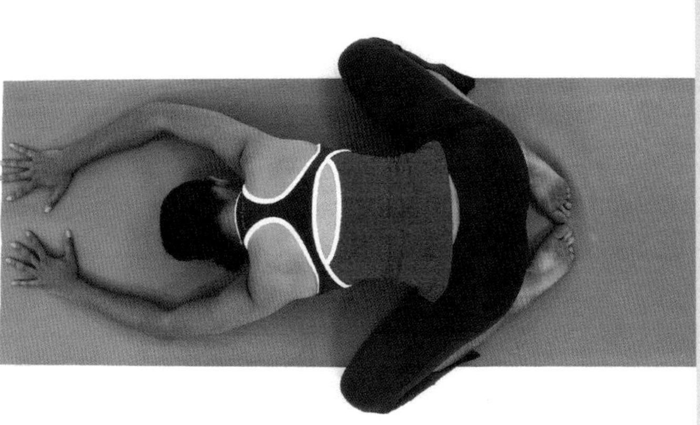

Alternative Savasana positions

Some people can't lie comfortably on the floor. They either can't get there easily at all or they suffer acute pain. I teach some alternatives to those who take too long to get onto and off the floor. But keep these as a tool for after Supta Vajrasana. I always advocate attempting to lie down on your back for the 2 minute Savasana.

Lying in lateral position

Lying on one's side is an alternative Corpse Pose that is seldom used. It is for people who really can't lie on their backs, are injured, or for pregnant women who exercise their choice to take Savasana like this. Legs bend and the palm of the upper arm, which is placed near the chest, supports the body from rolling. Although useful, if you have severe difficulty in getting in and out of Corpse Pose then I invite you to consider the next two options. There are definite problems created by getting off the floor in an incorrect fashion. Please see the chapter on the Sit-Up.

The floor facing Savasana

This pose is superbly restful and restorative. I introduce it to students with acutely painful conditions of the back, shoulders, or neck, or if they are experiencing extreme difficulties with sit-ups or fatigue. They constantly travel to and from the floor in pain, risking further damage and without benefit of a Savasana.

Instead, this alternative allows them to rest and recover, providing relief and an opportunity to fully participate. It opens up the sacroiliac joints particularly lengthening and giving space to the lumbar and sacral areas. It feels fantastic.

Pregnant students also benefit greatly. It is especially good for lower back relief. Additionally and by virtue of the softened tendons in the expectant mother, this position assists in a good pelvic opening helping to prepare the body for childbirth.

Always lie down on your back for the first 2 minute Savasana so that you are ready for Wind Removing pose. Do not use this pose until after Supta Vajrasana when you are sitting upright.

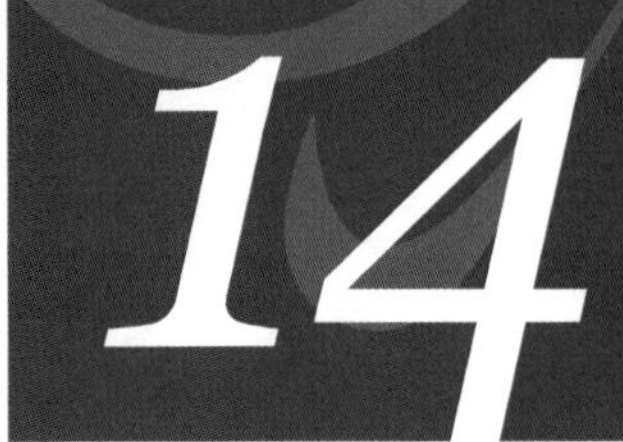

Savasana

Corpse Pose

Here are the steps:

3.1 Bring your big toes together under your bottom.

3.2 Widen your knees as far apart as you can. Feel your adductors stretch.

3.3 Your legs fan out, knees pointing toward the room corners.

3.4 With straight arms place your palms on the floor ahead of your shoulders, to take your weight.

3.5 Your elbows move out sideways as you bend your arms to lower your body.

3.6 Keep your spine straight and your head still.

3.7 When your head touches the floor you have 2 options depending on your comfort level.

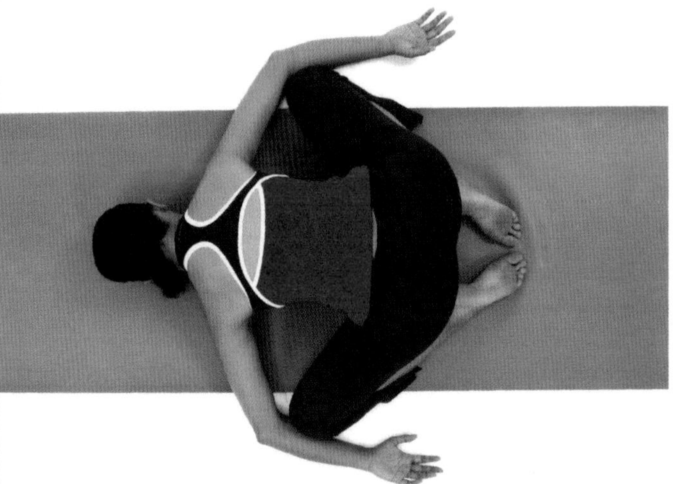

Forehead to floor:

It may be all you can do to simply rest your forehead on the floor. Stabilize your position, lift your hands and allow them to trail around your legs, hands resting behind you with your palms up. Your elbows will slightly bend. If you cannot get your forehead to the floor you may extend your arms forward to support you while you lengthen. Now relax, and continue to breathe deeply and through your lower spine. Use your breath to lower your hips to your heels. Allow yourself to be fully supported by the floor.

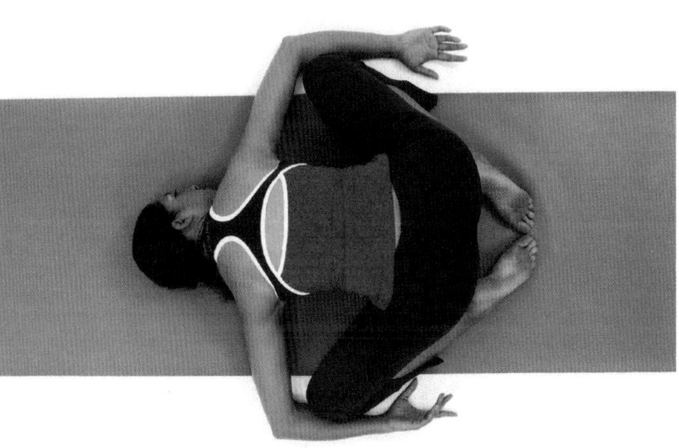

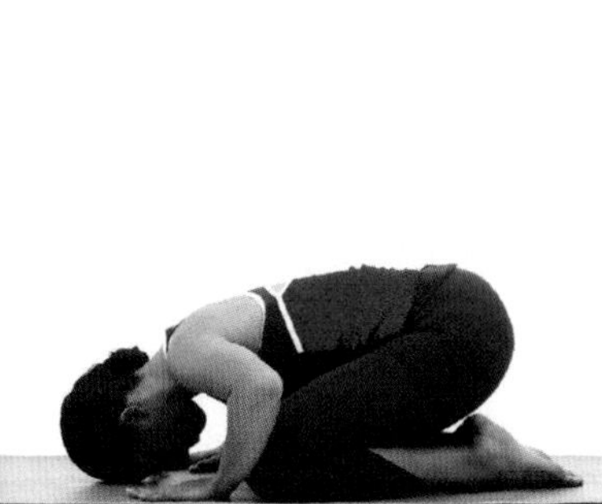

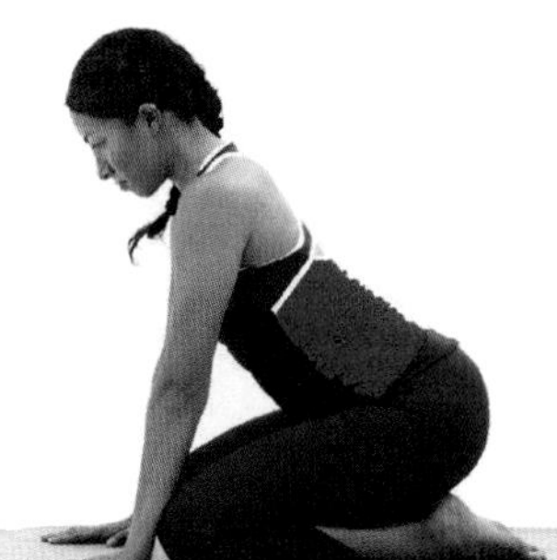

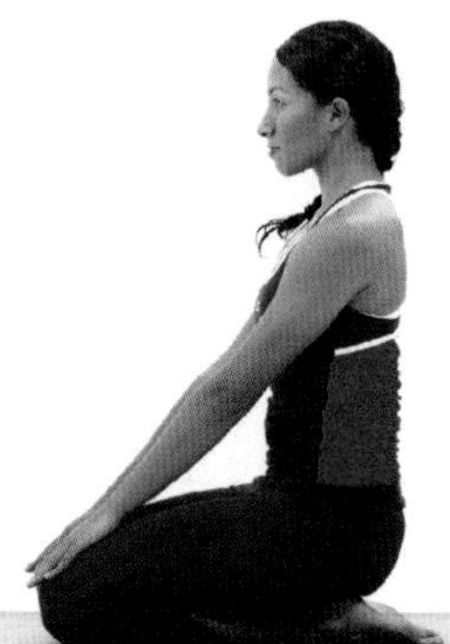

Ear to floor:

You may be flexible or comfortable enough to take this one step further. Get your forehead to the floor. Keep the weight on your palms and lift your head sufficiently to turn to face the right, for the first set. Second set you are to face the left. Aim to get your ear on the floor and look no further than the edge of your mat. Bring your hands off the floor and then trail your arms out and around your knees, palms up, fingers to the back wall.

Release from Corpse Pose

There are several ways to get up from the floor after Savasana. After Floor Bow you will push up off the floor before Suptavajrasana. The Sit-Up and alternative movements are examined in the Sit-Up chapter.

Release from the alternative Savasana

Entering into and coming out of this Savasana wastes no time at all. There are no potentially damaging movements and your spine is always in a neutral position. Simply place your palms down in front of your knees. If you are looking to the side then support yourself as you lift and turn your head to the spine-neutral position; forehead on the floor. Take the strain in your arms as you straighten them to support your body up to vertical. Then set up for your next pose.

Common mistakes and how to fix them

Too fast: Never be in a rush to get to the floor. You may be losing your last chance while standing to gain a meaningful connection in the mirror. Practice mindfulness of movement. Despite any emotional intensity or the overwhelming desire to lie down, simply meet yourself in your reflection. Learn to be comfortable with what you see.

Ritualizing your passage to the floor: Do you routinely do the same thing every time you finish Toe Stand? Always take a drink? Adjust your towel? Or fix your clothing? Whatever it is, perhaps you have your own little routine to get to the floor. These are distraction techniques and ways to avoid self-confrontation in the mirror. Finish your pose, meet yourself, do what you need to do and get to the floor with efficiency and conscious awareness. Avoid engaging the same set of conditioned responses every single class. Maybe you will find you really aren't thirsty!

You move, you lose: You guessed it. If you move you lose the benefits. Settle yourself in and then resist every temptation to move even a muscle. No twitches of your littlest fingers, and no modesty checks of your yoga wear. Don't fuss with your hair, wipe sweat or jiggle around.

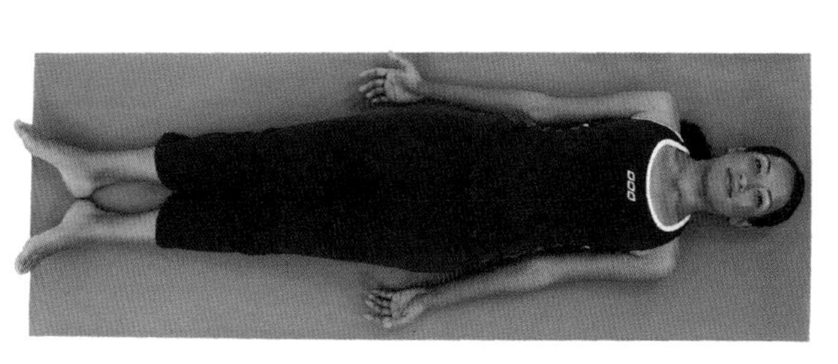

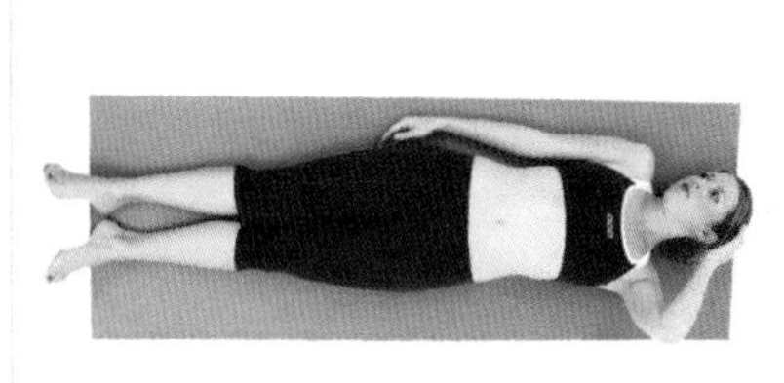

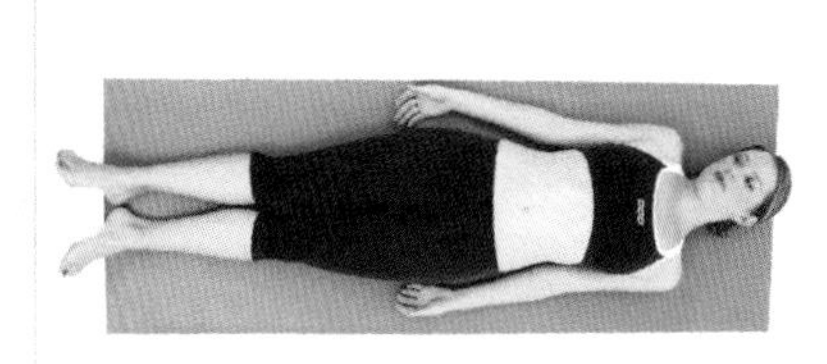

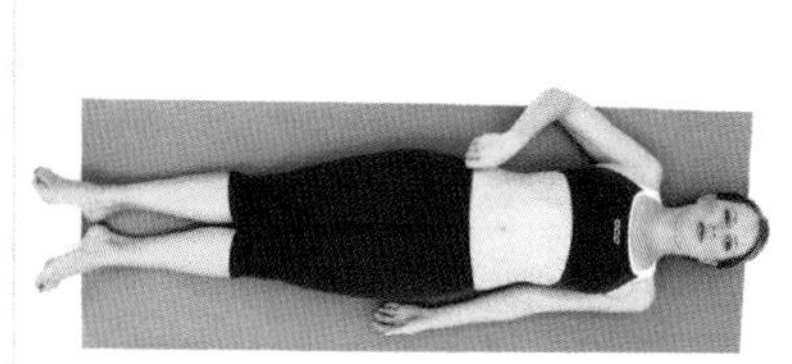

Savasana

Corpse Pose

14

Review the tourniquet effect, pages 29-30. The asana is the work, the release is the cleanse. The more effectively you work, the greater the cleansing effect on the body. For your circulation to access the body's peripheral and stagnant areas you need to stay completely still in your Savasana. Every unnecessary movement introduces blockages to the refreshed circulation and cleansing action.

Eyes move: Creating stillness in the body and mind is hard. If movement or your environment draws your eye, then find a spot and keep looking at it. Tuck your chin and gaze as described above. Let your gaze soften, focus on your breath and observe your body. For belly-down Savasana only look as far as the edge of your mat. Keep your gaze and therefore your thoughts internal. Minimize distractions and breathe.

Worried about flashing: If you have problems with flashing your bits at anytime during class then you are wearing the wrong gear. You have to question your motivation for wearing it in the first place if there are body parts peaking out at inopportune times. Your yoga practice is not about exploring your egocentricities and narcissism. Get real, get practical and wear something appropriate.

Lifting head up to listen to or look at the teacher: Savasana is about introspection so you should never look at your instructor, even though under normal social conditions it is courteous to look at a speaker. Familiarity with your practice, ability to focus as well as tune out distractions will change your habit.

You may find it difficult to hear. Or you may need or want to read lips for better comprehension. Having to look at a person talking is usually indicative of hearing loss. Work out what you need. Approach your teacher for them to talk more clearly, or loudly if necessary. Let them know you are hearing impaired so they can better direct their voice no matter where you are, or come and make specific requests of or for you when necessary. Sort out your hearing needs as it is unhealthy to strain to hear a speaker.

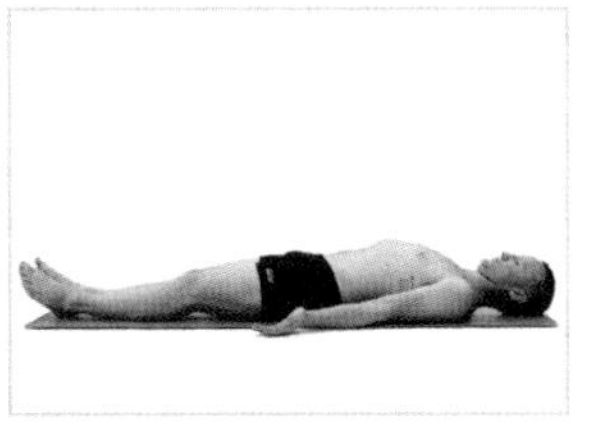

Stiff legs: Many students find it difficult to dissipate leg tension whether lying face-up or face-down. One thing is for sure, relaxation is a skill and must be learned and practiced. Face-up, heels are together, so gently move your knees. Face-down, toes are together. Gently shake or wobble your thighs on the ground to facilitate dissolving stiffness. Then lie still.

Body shape and flexibility can determine if your heels or toes touch together when 'setting up' your Savasana. The most important aspect is release and surrender. Heels or toes do not have to touch in this pose. Approximate your feet and then let go. Never force it.

Cheek on the floor: When face-down you turn your head in alternate directions. You are improving and giving back natural range of motion to the spine. Improving neck flexibility will eventually bring your ear to the floor.

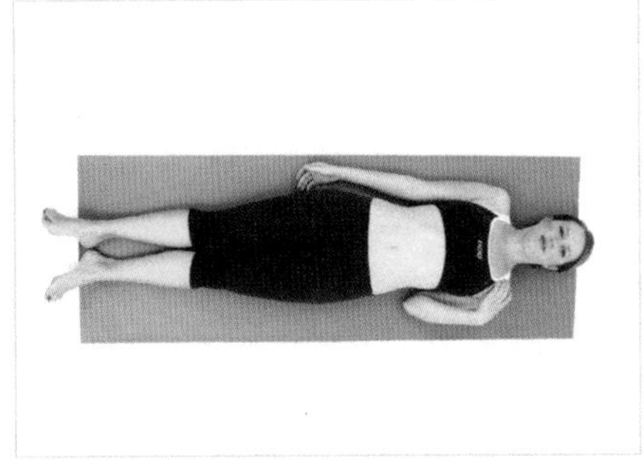

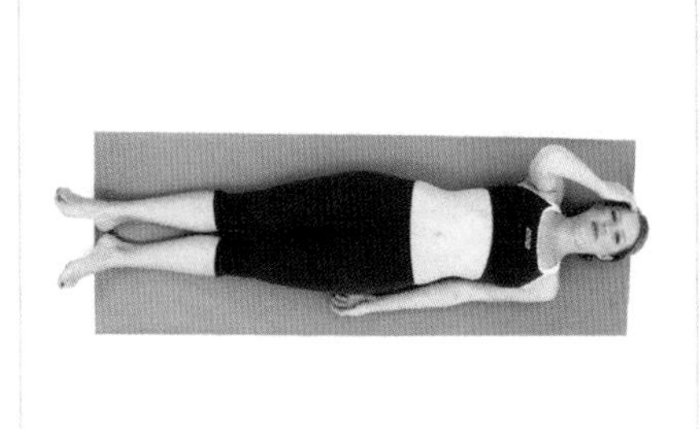

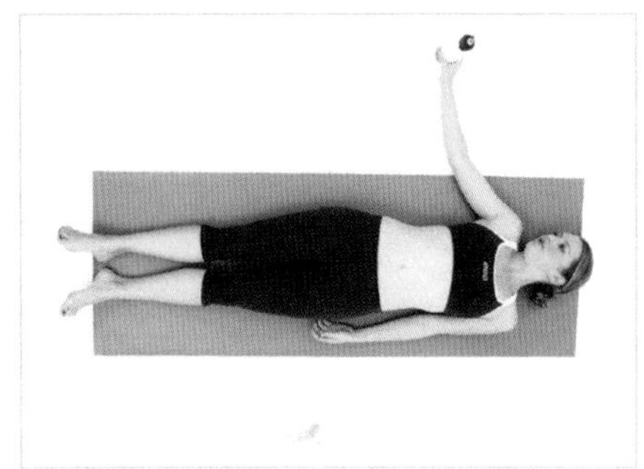

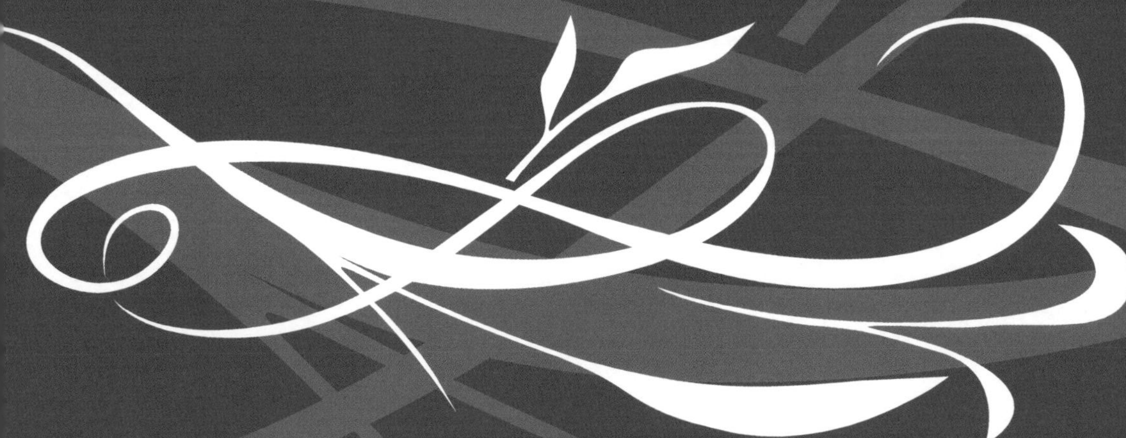

Pavana Muktasana

You have to give 100 percent in the first half of the game. If that isn't enough, in the second half, you have to give what's left.
—Yogi Berra

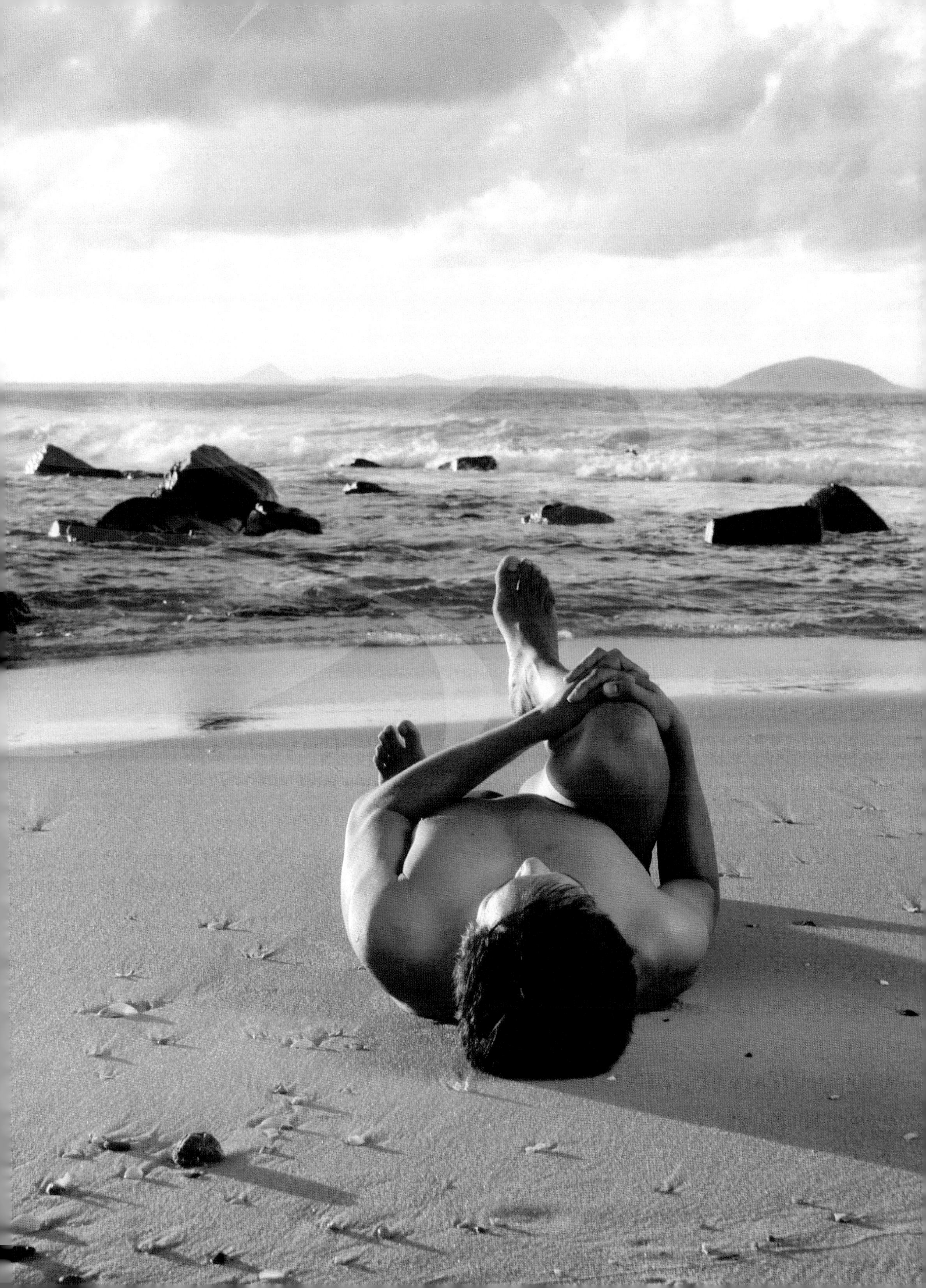

15 Pavana Muktasana

Wind Removing Pose

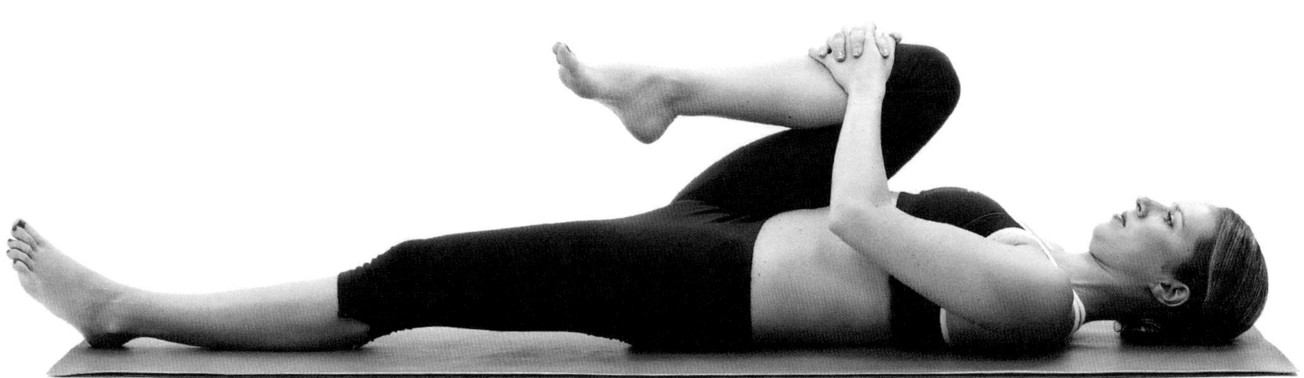

The essentials

Simple in concept, the primary focus of the first active floor pose is abdominal compression and hip opening. It helps iron out spines and is particularly useful for those with scoliosis.

Compression in the abdomen has a cleansing and flushing effect on your gastro-intestinal system. The massage of the intestines also provides a physical softening of the bowel contents making your wastes easier to process. This pose is named 'Wind Removing' for a reason.

Your metabolism gets a kick start with deep regulatory work on the thyroid and parathyroid glands. Engaging the abdominal muscles also provides a massage for internal organs and spinal muscles. Draw in your abdomen as you breathe very deeply through each of the single and double leg lifts. It further enhances every one of the effects and benefits.

What makes this pose so difficult to get right?

This pose is in itself not difficult beyond physical limitations due to tightness or injury. There are nevertheless definite misunderstandings about how to release from both the single leg and double leg parts. Correctly done the release is an extension of the pose, incorrectly it not only hinders the pose but reverses your ability to benefit fully.

Pavana Muktasana

… Removing Pose

15

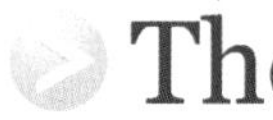

The technique

After your two minute Savasana, inhale and bend up your right leg.

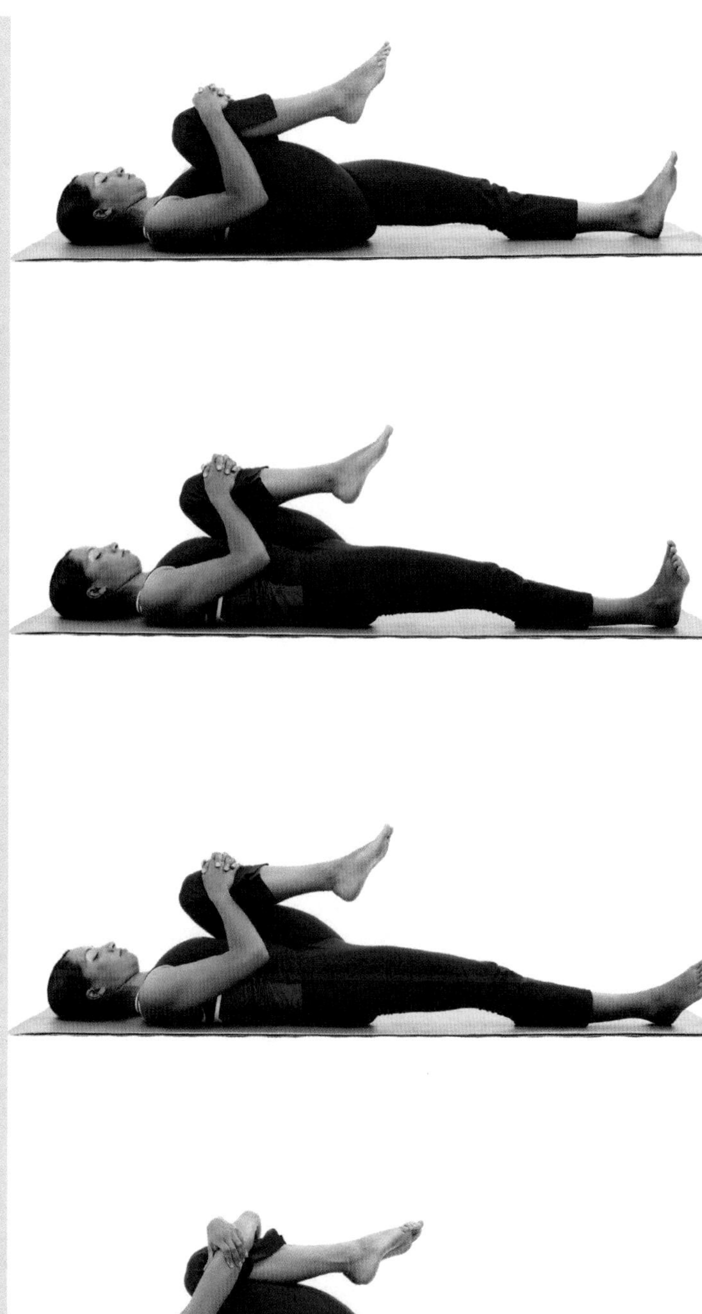

Single knee to shoulder

1.1 **Draw Knee Toward Chest:** Bend your leg and bring your knee toward your chest. In one movement you bring your interlocked hands to draw your knee down toward your shoulder, gripping firmly just below the right knee.

1.2 **Knee To Shoulder, Colon Compression:** Draw your knee toward your shoulder, moving it out to the side sufficiently, to avoid ribcage compression. Your upper thigh compresses against your intestines. Massage the ascending colon with the right leg, the descending colon with the left, and the transverse colon when both legs are held to the chest. Improve the massage and compression by drawing in the abdomen and breathing deeply.

1.3 **Shoulders Down, Elbows In, Pull With Biceps:** Hold both shoulders down evenly on the ground and isolate the effort to your arms and hands. Hold your elbows in and point them down toward your hips.

1.4 **Fingers Work:** Your hands pull down against your knee, compression occurring in your knuckles and fingertips. You are flushing, cleansing and strengthening your fingertips as a result of this grip.

1.5 **Relax The Lifted Leg:** Completely leg go of your leg against your strong hands. Your relaxed foot simply hangs and is not flexed at all. Consciously release the muscles in your bottom, your hips and pelvis. Feel incremental opening as your knee approaches your shoulder.

1.6 **Flex The Extended Foot:** Only activate the straight leg and flex the foot momentarily if the calf muscle is not on the floor, then release it. Keep pulling on the knee.

15 Pavana Muktasana

Wind Removing Pose

1.7 **Strong Chin Tuck, Eyes Down:** Press your chin as strongly as you can to your chest. Look down your centerline. Not only do you lengthen your cervical spine flattening it to the floor, you are compressing and toning your thyroid and parathyroid glands vital to normal metabolic function. Your gaze helps eye muscle tone and deepens mind-body connection.

1.8 **Pull Without A Break, Feel The Stretch:** Pull without letting go: No grip adjustments, no hip or leg shifting; not even for a micro-second. To maximize the tourniquet effect you must pull on the knee continually. The deep hip stretch is enhanced by consciously releasing the muscles around the pelvic girdle. Feel extension down your lifted leg hamstrings and into your buttocks. The extended leg allows a beautiful stretch from the thigh across the pelvis up to the target shoulder. Focus on shoulder symmetry. This pose has great potential to balance and realign your spine.

Knees to chest

2.1 **Palms Down, Bend Up Legs:** Place your palms down on the floor and bend up both legs at exactly the same time.

2.2 **Bear Hug:** Hug your knees against your chest by enveloping them with your arms. Wrap the right arm first then the left arm. You will swap this order wrapping left then right for the second set. Take hold of each elbow. The tightest body hug is required here so try first to grab your elbows. Failing that, try to grasp as close to your elbows as possible. You may need to grab your lower arms, wrists or your hands.

2.3 **Squeeze And Pull:** Pull your knees in toward your chest continually. Also squeeze your knees together for the duration. Continuous force is key.

2.4 **Hips Down:** Release your hips as you roll your lumbar spine and your sacrum down toward the floor. Eventually your hips come closer and closer in contact with your mat as you iron out your spinal column onto the floor. This movement together with the pull on the knees delivers incredible traction.

2.5 **Chin To Chest:** Tuck your chin again elongating the spine and getting thyroid compression. Eye gaze is down through your centerline.

2.6 **Deep Breath:** Keep drawing in your abdominal muscles while breathing deeply into your belly to facilitate a deeper massage and compression.

2.7 **Active Stretch:** Create traction with the pull of the knees against the push down of both hips to the floor.

The advanced pose

What happens when there is more hip flexibility available and nowhere for your knee to go? There is a further position to enhance the pull, the hip stretch, the finger strength and the cross-body stretch.

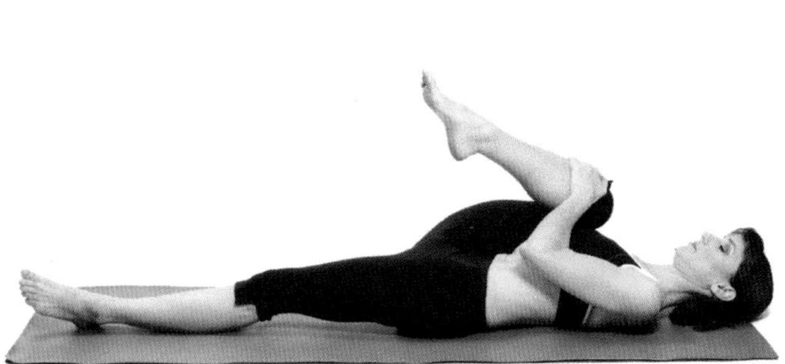

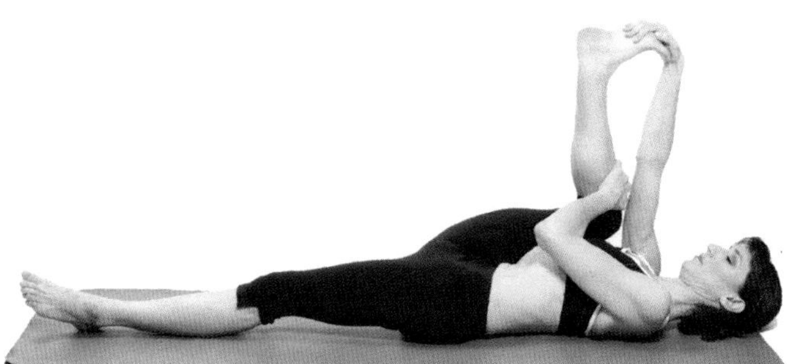

Pavana Muktasana 15

Wind Removing Pose

Needless to say that it is only those with very open hips who will be able to attempt this position. If this is you, then you are probably feeling that you can't get the best leverage out of 2 sets of this pose. All you need is some simple guidance with the grip one or two times.

This modification is never to be practiced in the first set, only ever in the second set. There is only an alternative for the single leg lifts. The double leg lift remains identical. The example below is for the right leg.

3.1 **Knee Up To Chest**: Inhale and bring your bent leg up. Once again avoid the ribcage. Your right knee comes to your shoulder. Move your upper leg to lie as close to the side of your chest as possible. You can help hold it there with your right hand for the moment.

3.2 **Left Hand Grip**: Bring your left hand across your chest and with all fingers together grab just below the right knee. This is a very important action to accomplish first. It stabilizes the hip joint, draws the leg in and holds it in position.

3.3 **Adjust Your Left Arm**: Settle your left shoulder down by moving your left elbow down toward your left hip. Women may need to negotiate their elbow crook around the breast.

3.4 **Lower Right Leg**: Flex the right foot, the leg is at right angles.

3.5 **Right Hand Grip Along Foot**: Your right hand comes over the top of and along the length of your right foot. The extent to which you have the grip is determined by your flexibility, strength, and arm length. Feel a firm and positive contact as you pull down through the ball of your flexed foot. You may only be able to hook the fingers over at first. Over time you may be able to push through the palm on the ball of your foot, and then with the seat of your palm on your toes.

3.6 **Right Arm Position**: Draw your right shoulder blade to the floor and your elbow down (rather than out to the side wall or backward at an angle). The force through your hand pulls your flexed foot and bent leg down, stacking your ankle and knee vertically. Make room for the approaching knee.

3.7 **Stabilize And Pull**: The left arm stabilizes the leg's position. It pulls the knee across as the left shoulder stays anchored to the floor. The right arm does more of the work to open and stretch the hip and leg. The right shoulder draws down to help resolve neck and shoulder muscular tension.

3.8 **Left Leg And Pelvis**: The left leg is passive and likely to be in full contact with the floor. Just make sure that all destabilizing forces are kept at bay: Keep the leg down and remove any twisting component of the body.

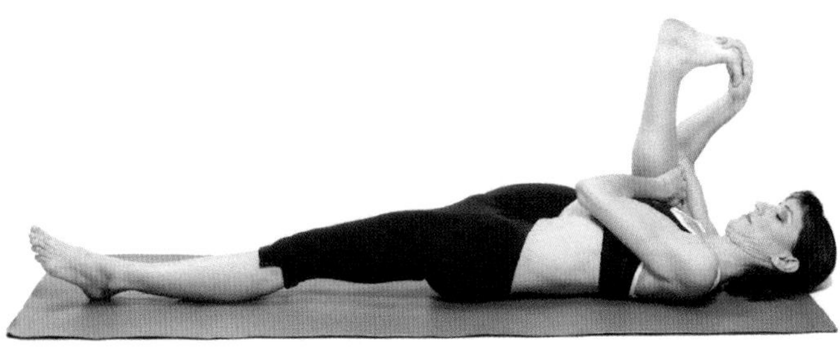

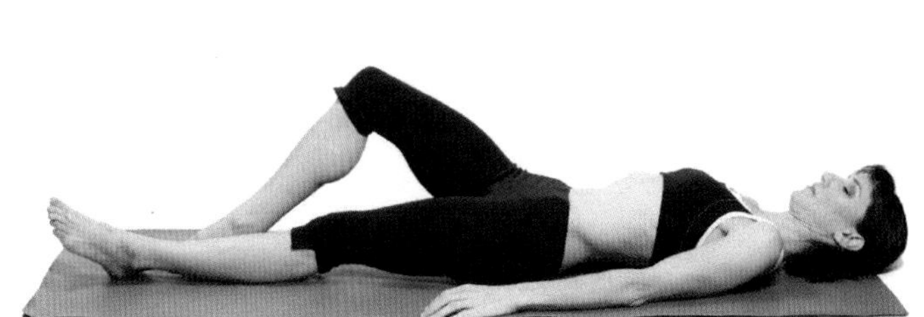

15

Pavana Muktasana

WIND REMOVING POSE

 Release the single leg

Reverse the flow. Let go of the grip on your knee and allow your leg to unfold onto the floor. The best way to accomplish this is to simply release the bent leg and allow your foot to effortlessly touch the floor near your buttock as it hinges around the hip. Then slide your foot to the back wall until your leg is resting on the floor.

Release the double leg position

Simply release your arms. Your feet will naturally just fall to the floor near your bottom. Your legs are relaxed. Just let them slide out toward the back wall. Let your arms and legs resume position for your Savasana. Slightly release your chin so that your cervical spine is still extended flatly. There is no forced compression of the throat. Lie completely motionless and breathe.

 Common mistakes and how to fix them

Uneven shoulders on single lift: When the right leg is bent to the right shoulder the left shoulder has a tendency to lift up and round forward in an attempt to deepen the stretch. This also twists the spine. Holding your opposite shoulder down here may give you the impression that your knee moves away from the shoulder slightly but the spinal alignment remains solid and strong with both shoulders in a symmetrical position. The irregularities in the spine are likely to resolve more easily.

Elbows out: Pulling with elbows out will involve your shoulders moving them toward the ceiling. Bring them right in close to the body so you can pull with your biceps.

Sweat causes hands to slip: When I first embarked on my hot yoga journey my hands used to slip a lot. This is part of just about every student's path. The first thought is that the body sweat generated is the root cause of the sliding. This is absolutely not true. You will look back in a relatively short time to see that no matter how sweaty you are you can hold your leg there as your fingers become strong. Don't blame it on the sweat. You don't need a hand towel at all. Be patient and cultivate your hand and finger strength.

Hands overlap instead of intertwined: One intention of the grip is to strengthen fingers. Overlaying hands is not nearly as effective. It makes it harder to employ your biceps muscles.

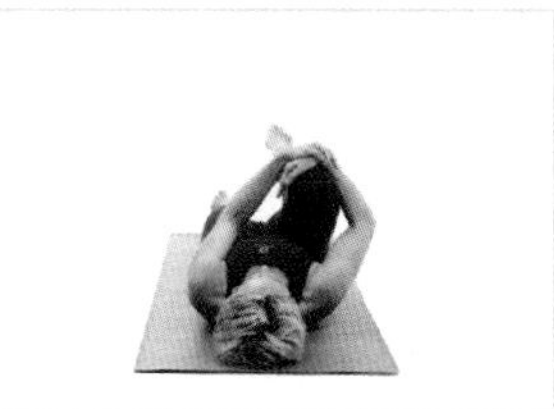

Chin away from chest: You lose a good deal of the benefits if you are only focusing on the abdominal compression. Hormonal regulation is assisted with the chin firmly pressed to the chest. It also lengthens the spine onto the floor and provides a good bolstering effect.

Rolling into a ball: The double leg lift brings the knees into the chest, but keep the head back down on the floor to lengthen the spine.

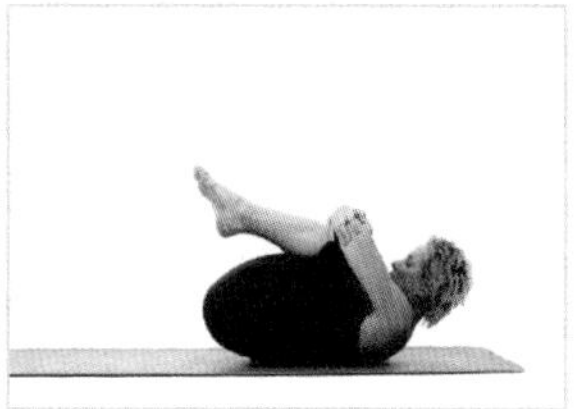

Knee to chest: The instructions are to pull the knee as close to the shoulder as you can without compression of the ribcage.

Letting go of the grip mid-pose: If you continually grip and re-grip the knee then the pose becomes a stretch and you will remove any tourniquet benefits out of the equation, so STAY STILL and PULL. Furthermore, after about 10 seconds or so the body starts to recognize the safety in the stretch and releases even more. This is why you can feel your body yielding to the pull and your hip and leg opening up. The longer and smoother the pull the better the results. Just as in Savasana, 'you move, you lose!'

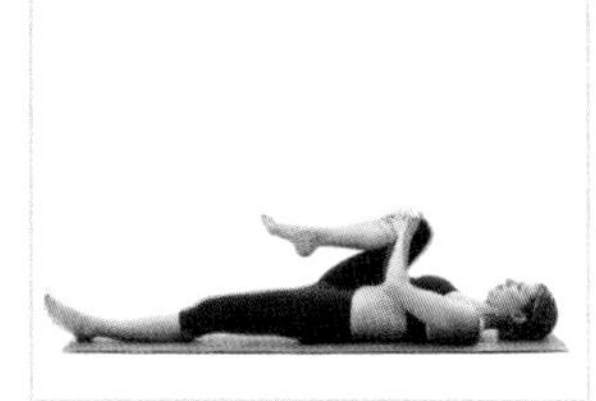

Pavana Muktasana

Wind Removing Pose

Releasing from pose by lowering active straight leg(s): I remember when I started hot yoga that like many others, I extended my leg(s) straight up in the air and lowered it. I was thinking I was doing myself a favor by strengthening abdominal and core muscles. I was just a sheep, unthinkingly copying the experienced yogis, just like every other beginner always and understandably does.

After applying yogic logic I came to the conclusion that the 'straight leg release' is wrong. The benefits are largely eliminated when releasing in this contrived way (which is also why you don't let go of the pull mid-pose). Actively lowering your legs uses muscles that should be relaxed and being flushed, and it blocks the 'tourniquet effect'. Review from page 28 about the principles of Savasana.

Pull hard and unwaveringly for the compressive effects of the thigh against the body. Maximize the tourniquet and then simply and passively release the leg(s) to capitalize on your hard work. Let the heel(s) contact the floor near your bottom and slide your foot/feet away from you. Exit correctly to receive the flushing, cleansing and healing effect in the stillness of your Savasana. Let go of ego, and just let your leg(s) get to the floor.

Scissoring legs up: Bring both legs up simultaneously. Do not bring them up in a scissor action. Place your palms face down and your arms will automatically exert just the right amount of pressure on the floor to protect your lower spine. No conscious arm pressure is required if palms are down. Just bend up your legs.

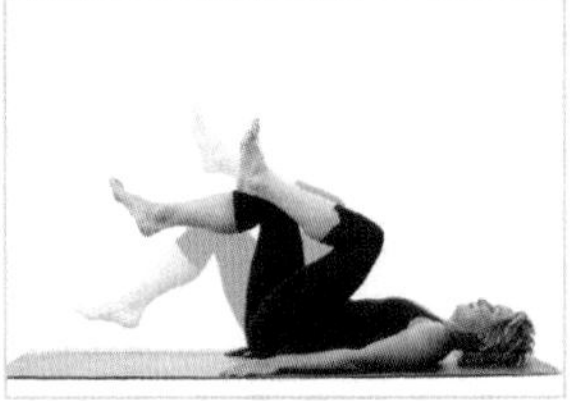

***Can't grab elbows**: Grab as close to your elbows as possible. You may need to grip your lower arms, wrists or your hands. In the rarest of cases each hand holds the knee of the same side.

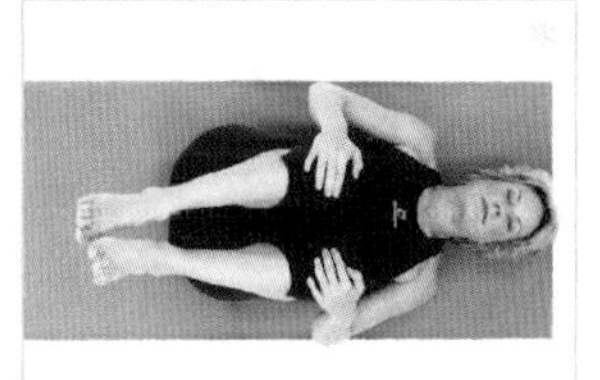

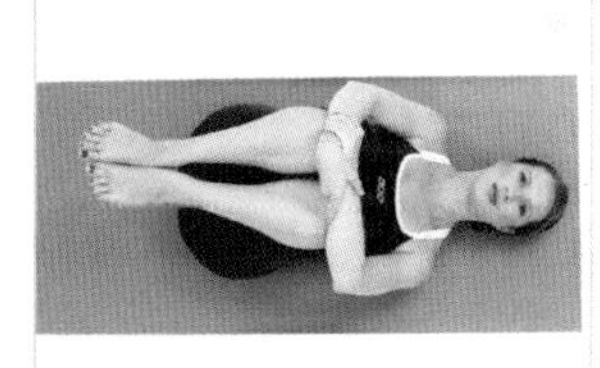

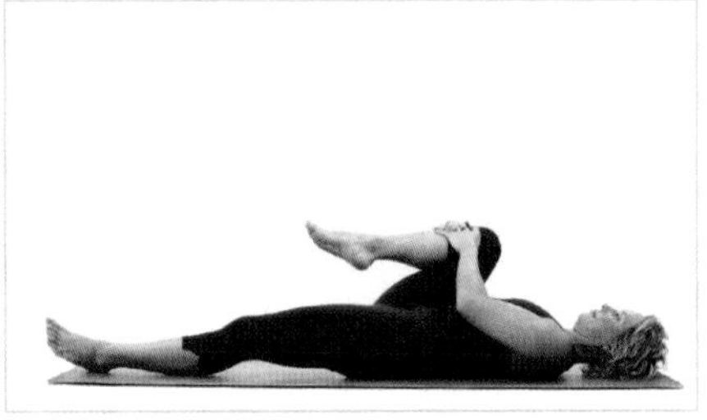

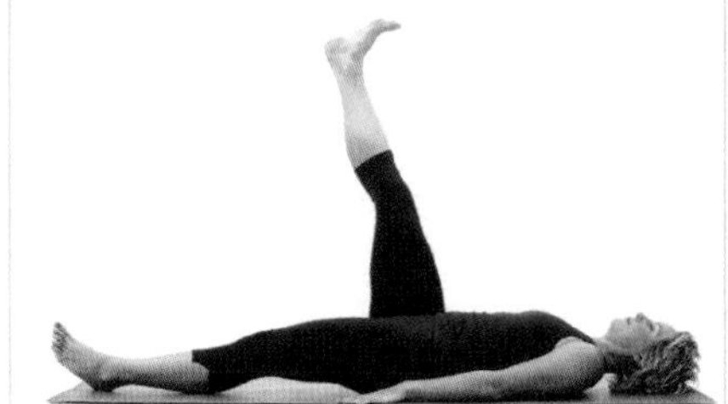

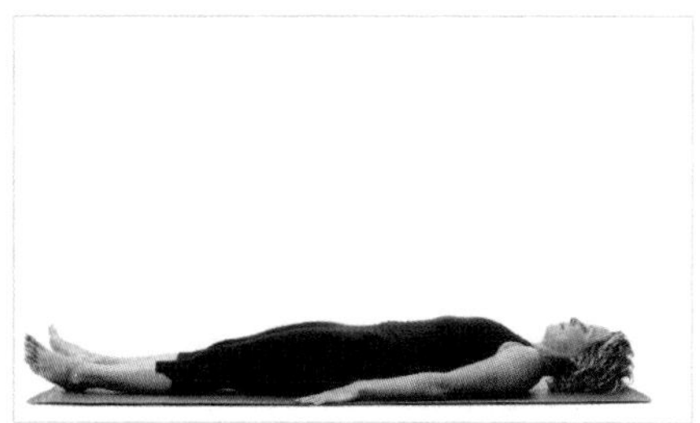

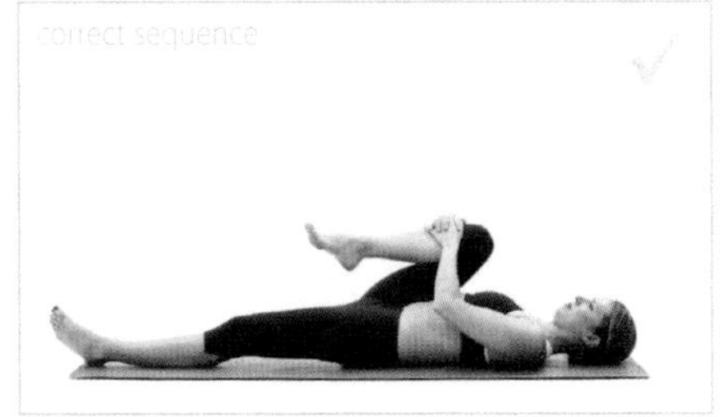

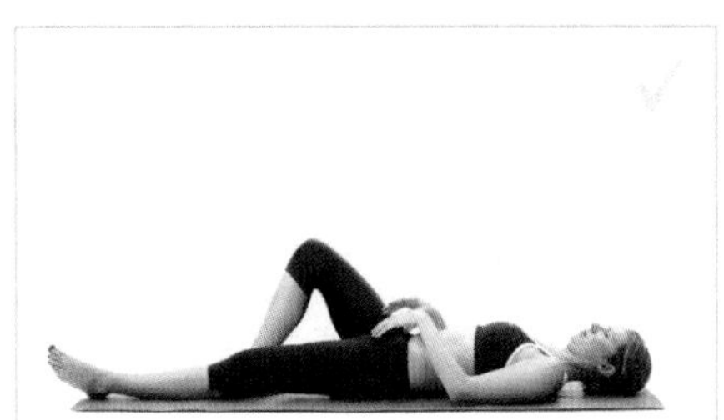

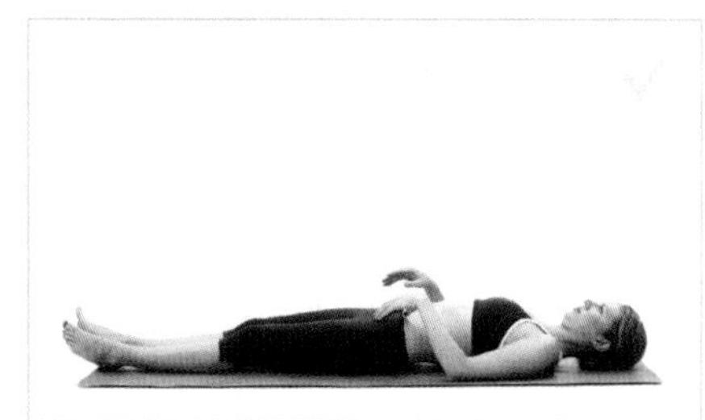

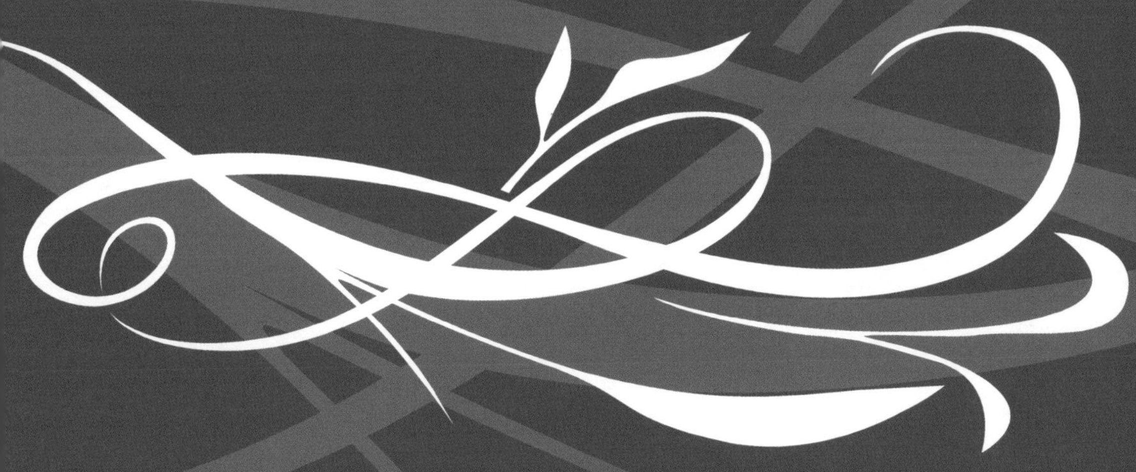

Sit-up

Age is something that doesn't matter, unless you are a cheese.
—Billie Burke

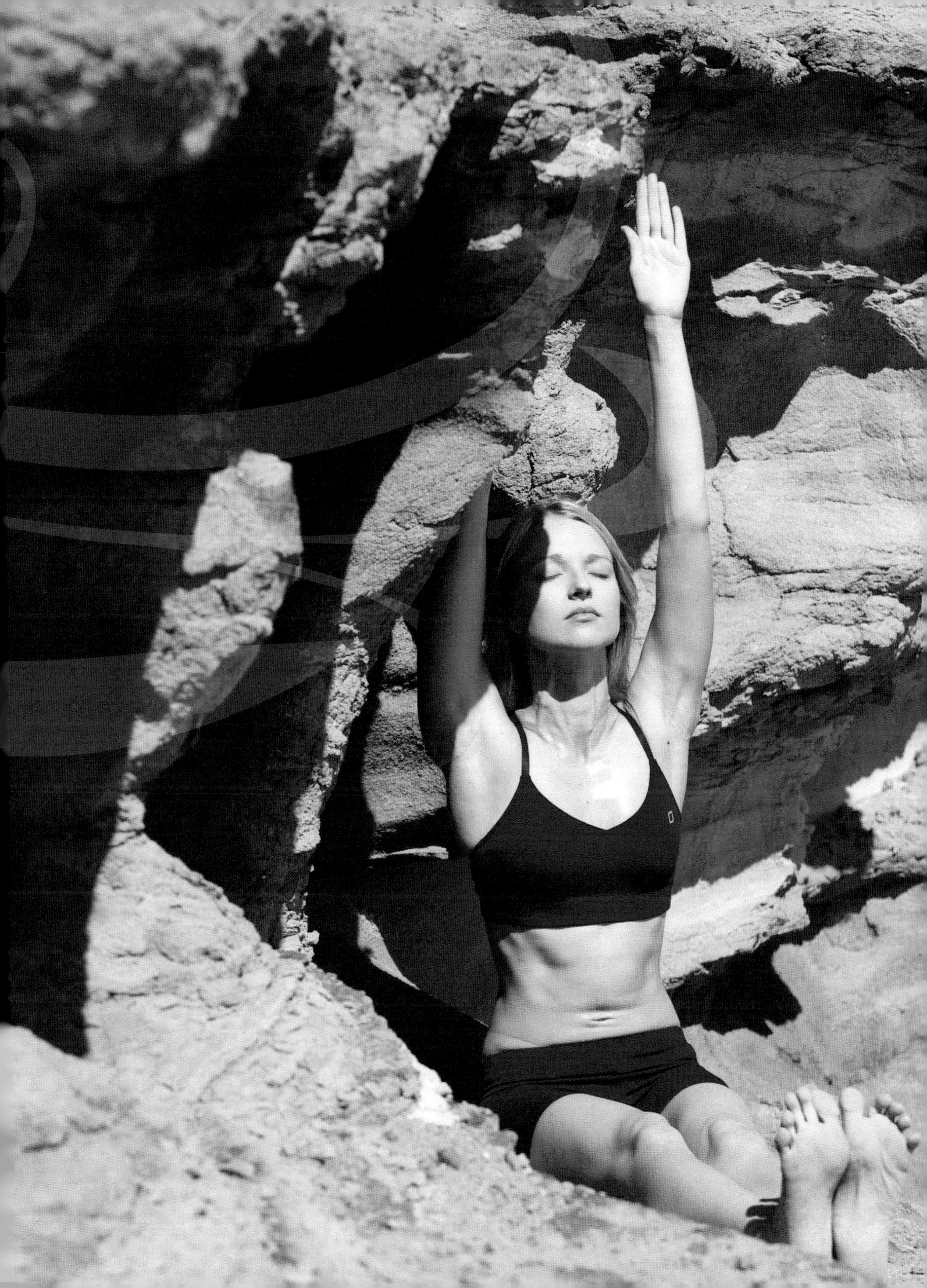

16 Sit-up

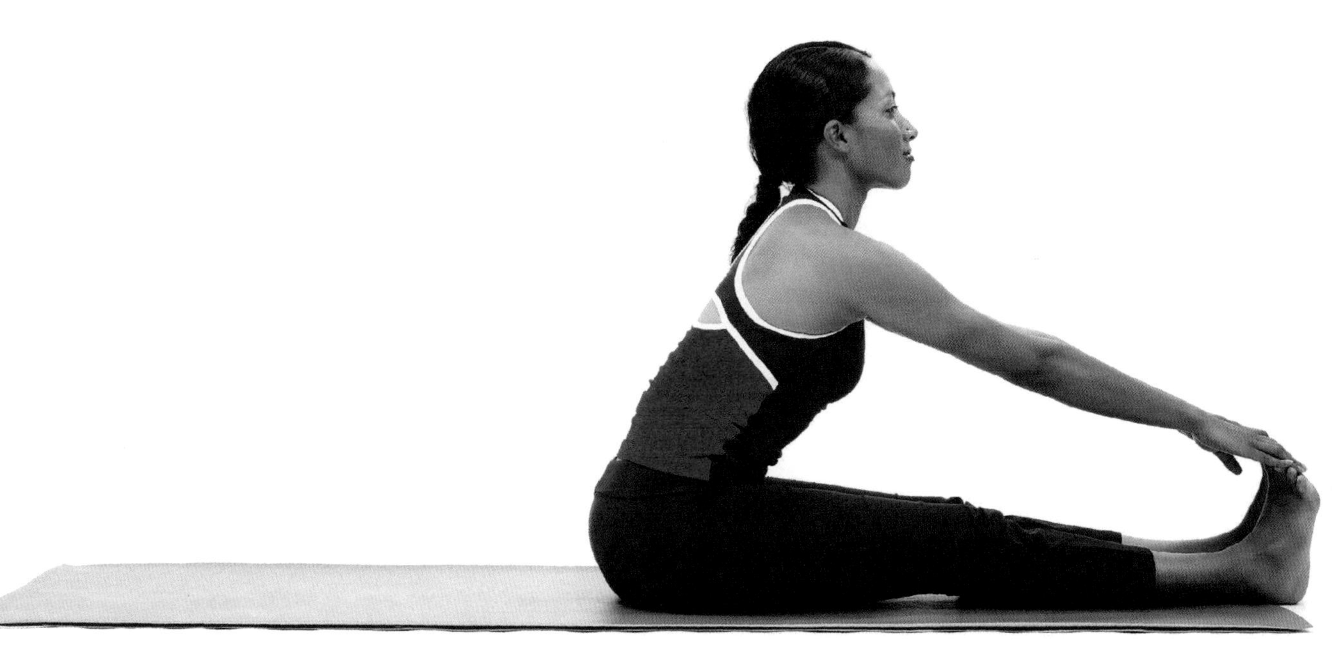

The essentials

There is no Sanskrit for 'sit-up'. It is a great energizer between many of the floor poses and gets you up off the floor into next pose readiness. You get to improve your strength and flexibility. For safety's sake you need to ensure you have sufficient back/core fitness to perform your sit-ups. There are some alternative ways to segue into your poses. But first let's look at the classic sit-up, and in fact the two commonly used methods. I will also outline why I teach one and not the other.

What makes this pose so difficult to get right?

A poorly performed sit-up is a risky proposition. It strains the cervical spine, and the hip flexors – which are attached to your lumbar spine – 'yanks' on your lower back to lift your torso up without the supportive efforts of your abdominal muscles. Lower back pain is a sign of abdominal weakness. So improving abdominal and core muscle tone will assist you greatly. Having the right sit-up technique is critical to prevent risk to your spine.

For many years the sit-up was done in a certain way. Recently there has been a practice wave changing the norm. I will show you both, but recommend only one. The reasons are compelling: You will literally feel safer and stronger. The benefits of the work and support in one method far exceed those of the other.

The sit-up is meant to consist of two parts. You are supposed to come up to an L-sit on the first partial exhale and bring the body forward over the legs on the second partial exhale. However one method lends itself to combining the two parts which further dilutes its effectiveness and increases the chance of injury. First up I would like to briefly discuss the differences.

Here is where the 2 methods differ:

Method 1:

Method 1 is a risky proposition. I will briefly describe it for diagnostic purposes. I do not ever recommended it because; it does not have clear landmarks, does not work with the body, the cues are indistinct and are open to wide (mis-) interpretation, it causes damage, prevents development of, and worse, weakens core strength.

This poorly constructed sit-up asks you to cross the thumbs or connect your hands in some way; then inhale as you fling yourself off the floor, then exhale twice in quick succession as you bounce your rounded back over your straight legs, looking down. Arms then pull against the toes. The arm/hand positions encourage neck, shoulder and back strain and the legs often lift from the floor as part of the propulsion mechanism.

Method 1 students use the forward movement of the arms and head (largely using neck muscles) to initiate movement, propelling themselves off the floor, risking damage (to neck muscles and spine). Mostly just the superficial muscles of the trunk engage from neck to pubic area which overrides engagement of the core.

But that's not all. The momentum of this poor movement causes a sharp tug on the lumbar spine by the hip flexors. If you have lower back pain (usually from abdominal muscle weakness) then you will cause damage. Many students also end up with their toes forward and heels closer to their bottoms which shortens leg muscles.

According to physiotherapists, chiropractors, osteopaths, martial artists and fitness experts there is risk of damage and very little to gain from throwing oneself forward from a fully laid-flat position shortening muscles in the abdomen and legs and diminishing your control.

Experts agree that Method 2 is a better way to do a sit-up. You'll feel a firmer connection with the floor to support you. You'll find step by step details over the page and discover a method that links the inhale and exhales to physiologically sound actions and makes it safe and allows the body to open and get stronger.

Method 2:

In complete contrast to the first method, the Method 2 sit-up has overall benefits that help you in the rest of your practice. The 2 parts of the sit-up are completely distinct and each movement occurs with each exhale. The whole back side of the body lengthens from the heels right through the back and cervical spine and the muscles in your core are strengthened too. You continue your lengthening and strengthening work, plus it is an invigorating way to come up off the floor.

I teach this method to every student in my studio. If there are any new students or beginners in the class then I do a physical demonstration of the different options available to them. I don't want anyone damaging their spine or muscular support mechanisms under my watch.

A sit-up is like brushing your teeth. Everyone thinks they know how to do it. They don't remember how they know, they just know because they have seen it being done or have done it for years and years. In fact, egos sometimes get a little bruised when it is suggested that they could learn how to do it differently or properly.

I know because as a qualified dentist I have taught thousands of patients how to brush their teeth. Many of them have been in their 40s or 50s and have thanked me for being the first one to have taught them how to do it properly.

So you get my point. It pays to have some humility to take on these new skills. Every student deserves a proper debunking of the sit-up myth; to be shown a better way. What you must do is recruit the correct muscles to bring you up off the floor at the same time as strengthening your back and anchoring your legs. Done incorrectly you can throw your back out. The main difference is that at all costs you will maintain a straight back coming forward from L-sit, bending your legs in preference to rounding your back.

If you don't know what I mean try this little experiment. Sit on the floor with your legs together, your knees bent, feet flat on the floor and your hands resting on your knees. Sit with a rounded slumping spine. What do you have to do to straighten up your spine without putting your hands down on the ground?

You must tilt your pelvis forward. You will also feel your hands pull backward on your knees. You have used some traction in your body to sit forward and up with a straight spine by creating length and tilting your pelvis. The same forces are at play in your sit-ups and all of your Paschimottanasana poses.

This experiment gives you the key to Method 2 and what to do if you cannot reach your feet.

16 Sit-up

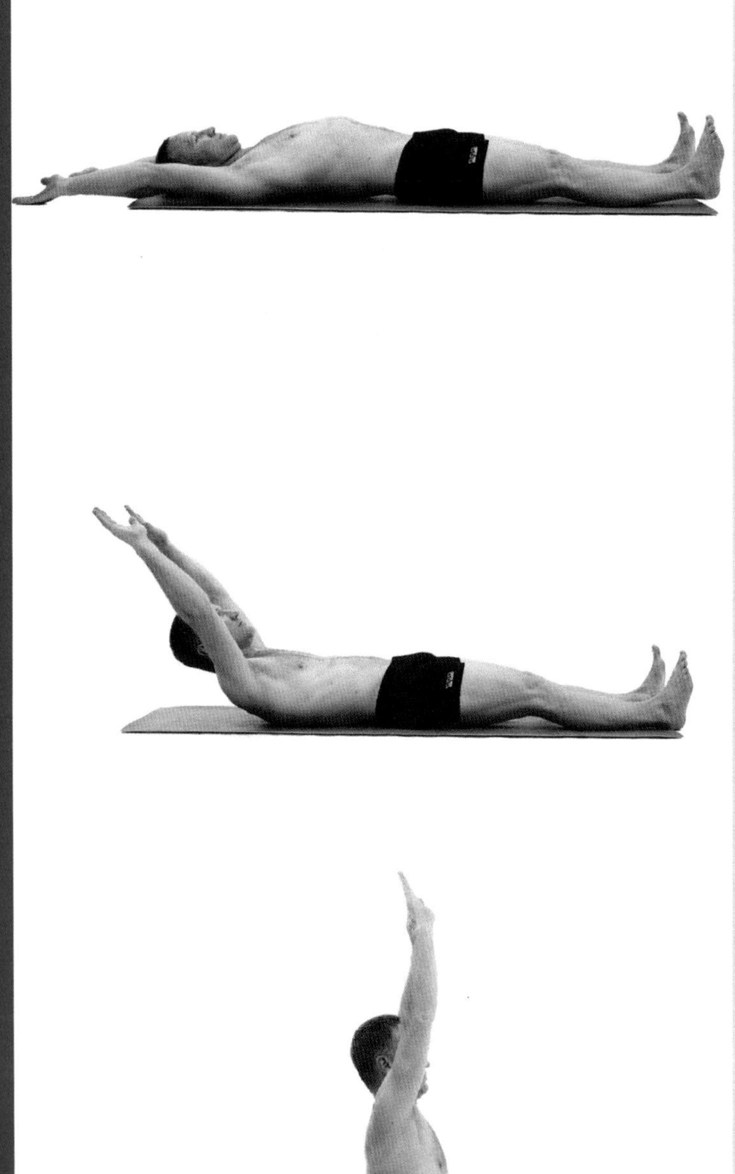

The technique

You are lying in Savasana on your back on the floor, completely yielding to gravity and totally still.

1. **Flex Feet And Strongly Lock Legs:** Bring your feet together and flex them strongly: Extend your heels away from you and point your toes back toward your face. Lock your knees and engage your thigh muscles. Your totally active legs and feet will assist you off the floor in a stronger and yet lighter fashion.

2. **Arms Up:** Inhale your arms up over your head. Extend them directly up from your shoulders, so that they are parallel and shoulder width apart with hands apart and palms up.

3. **Bed Your Shoulder Blades Down:** Keep your shoulder blades down in firm contact with the floor. This provides vital support for when you come up off your mat. If your hands are together then your shoulder blades are only in partial contact and so support is lessened.

4. **Come Up In 2 Stages; The Exhale Is Important:** The sit-up proper happens in two parts, each part attached to a short sharp exhale. Draw in your abdomen. An open mouth and slight throat constriction helps force the air out, cleanses the lungs, and also recruits extra strength and support for your spine by the activation of your abdominal muscles.

5. **The First Exhale:** You move off the floor with your first open-mouth exhale. Do what you can to preserve the straight line from your hips to your fingertips as you move into an L-sit with arms vertical. Keep your arms active, long and separated and your shoulders down. Look up to the ceiling rather than toward the back wall. This simple crucial change in visual focus makes it much easier to sit up correctly. There is the slightest almost imperceptible roll of the vertebrae as the spine and muscles bed themselves down into the ground in turn from neck to hips. This is why the shoulder blades need to broaden to create a solid platform. The next partial exhale, you extend your arms toward your feet.

6. **Second Exhale**: Exhale again from L-sit. On your second exhale bring your arms down to grab onto your feet, palms down and fingers pulling back against the balls of your flexed feet. Look forward over your feet to the back wall to help keep buoyancy in your body – your chest up. Keep the chin up. Above all your priority is to maintain a straight back.

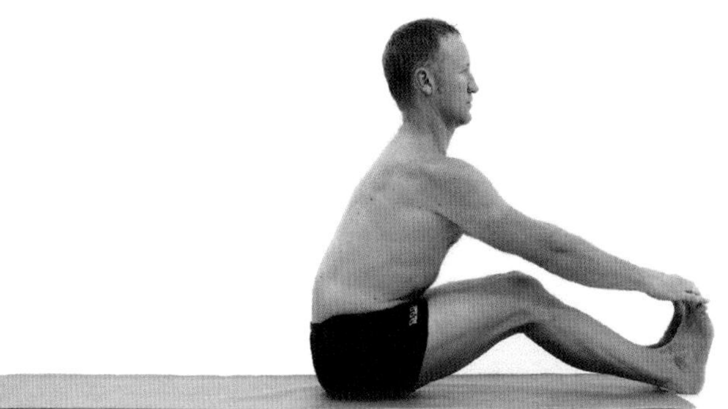

7. **Straight Or Bent Legs? Divide And Conquer**: Making a strong separation between the two movements means that if you know you can't grab onto your feet with straight legs you can coordinate your forward movement of your upper body with a bend of the legs. Keep your arms straight and feet flexed. Then bend your knees and grab your toes with long arms and chest lifted. The traction that you create in your straight spine improves the higher you lift your chest and the stronger you pull with your straight arms. The technique is the same for everyone. The back and arms are straight and the legs are either bent or straight.

8. **Stretch, Stretch, Stretch**: Pull on your feet with your arms straight. Feel the satisfying tractions as your body works itself open. Pull back on your toes as you pull your shoulders down and lift your breastbone forward and up against your straight arms. When you 'get' this you will definitely feel a pleasing slight compression as you arch your lumbar spine. It is almost as if you are pulling your chest forward through your shoulders.

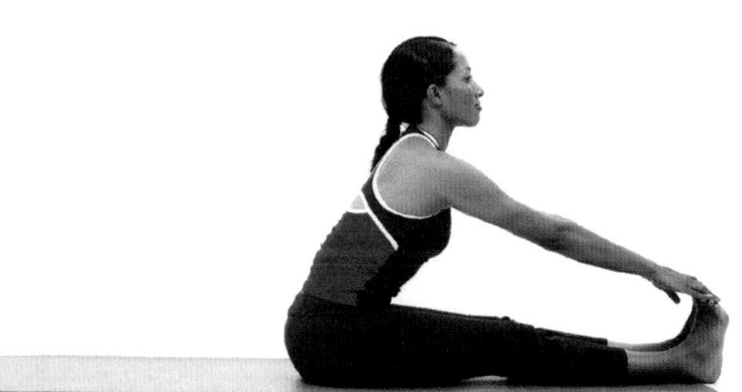

9. **Rule Of Thumb**: When your arms and your back are straight you will find yourself either with bent legs or straight locked out legs for the 3rd side of your 'triangle'. Keep pulling against your feet with straight arms. Only bend your elbows if your back is completely straight with no sign of rounding; your legs are extended and fully locked out. Think stretch not rounding. With your fingers against the balls of your feet, palms facing down your elbows will point down and your shoulders will stay down too.

16 Sit-up

 Release

Hold the stretch for a couple of breaths by pulling back on your toes. Release your arms, lift your body up and come to a sitting position. Roll to one side onto the thigh. Turn around in an energy-efficient manner to face the mirror for your next pose.

 Balance your efforts

As you become familiar with your poses you will recognize the need to balance your physical body and to free yourself of unconsciously habitual or repeated body movements. Each of us prefers to interlock fingers, cross arms or exit poses in a certain way.

For example if I am coming out of Savasana into the first set of a pose I move onto the right side and then spin around. When I finish my first set I lean to the right again and then spin back to my Savasana. I go to the left before and after the second set. I am mindful about it but neither side is preferred anymore. You too can achieve this kind of balance in your practice. It is a small but significant consideration.

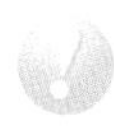 When not to do a sit-up

You must know when you should not attempt a sit-up. Weak or tender lower backs are more sensitive and need to build strength before the sit-up is attempted. Most students will know when they are lacking the resources to even try. Avoid them for as long as you have to: Have the humility and know that it is OK to do some and not all of the sit-ups in a class.

Being a big burly guy with a strong and muscly upper body doesn't mean you will find sit-ups easy. I see a very typical scenario with men in their 30s, 40s or 50s who seem physically strong yet have terribly weak lower backs. One day their upper body strength can no longer compensate for their poor core strength. They bend forward to get in the car (for example) and whammo, they are laid flat and out of action. They wonder how this could happen when they are in such good condition. If this describes your predicament, then skip the sit-ups for a while. Start to introduce them as your whole body strengthens.

 Coming off the floor without a sit-up

Side exit:

1. Bend up your knees.
2. Roll to the side in one motion. No twisting: you roll at the hip so don't lead with your legs.
3. Place your palms down on the floor adjacent to the shoulders, at about shoulder width apart.
4. Look at your hands.
5. Push yourself away from the floor. You straighten your arms while looking at your hands.

Why look at your hands? Because this is a safety mechanism that will protect your back. Looking down will make you push your body up away from the floor using your arm strength. The reliance on your back will be minimal. Years of teaching and observation have prompted me to introduce this important detail.

Students who don't look at their hands tend to use one hand behind them to help them up off the floor; they recruit and strain their neck, back and abdominal muscles. They lead with their chin and often rock themselves up with their legs with a constant bend at the hips. They may as well have done a sit-up incorrectly!

Exiting floor-facing Savasana?

Later on in the class you may be resting in floor-facing Savasana so you won't be doing a sit-up. This has already been explained along with photos in the Savasana chapter.

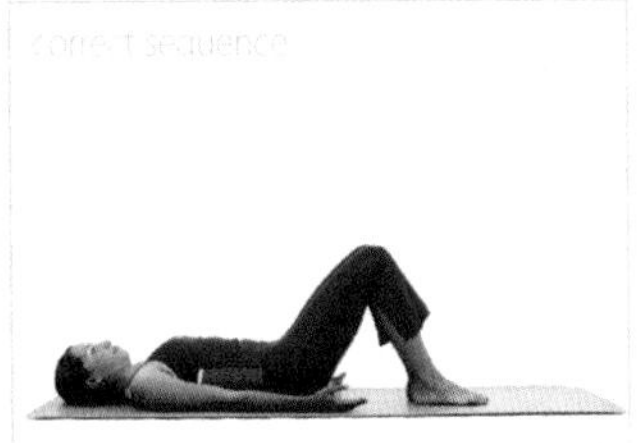

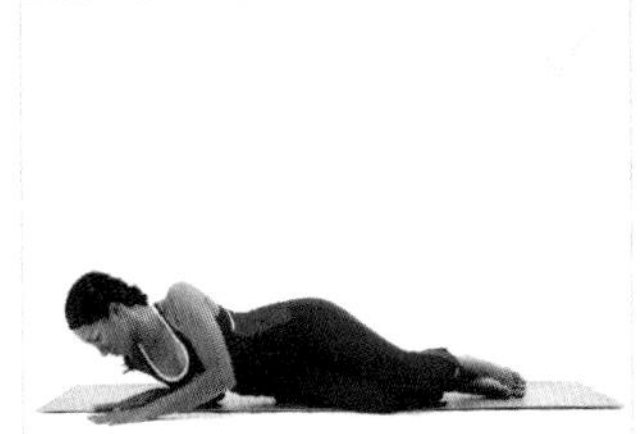

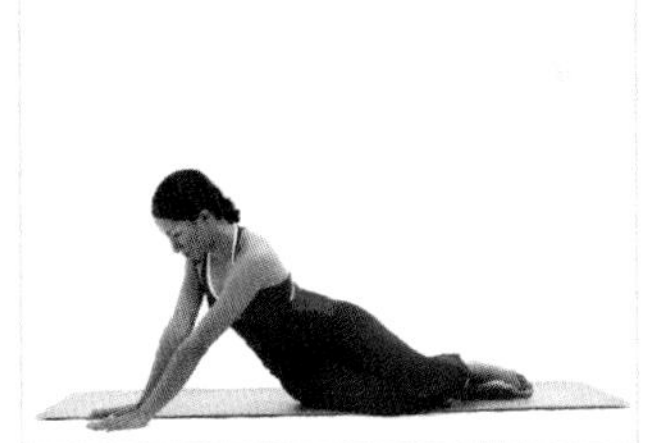

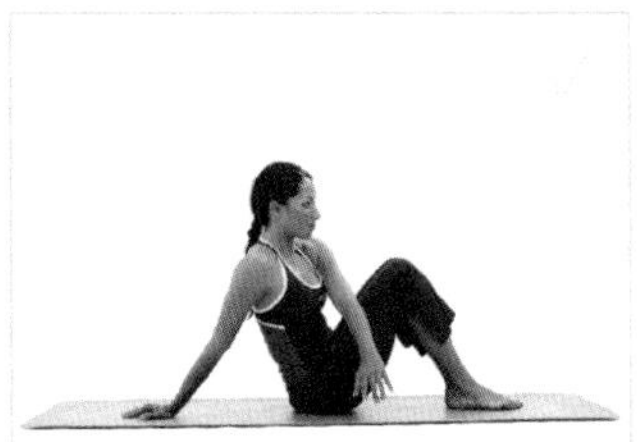

Common mistakes and how to fix them

Thumbs link: Bringing your hands together or linking your thumbs makes your sit-up more difficult and less effective. Students fling themselves up off the floor without good shoulder support, straining abdominal and neck muscles. They lead with the arms, often throwing the head forward.

It does seem as if you are being asked to get off the floor from lying flat to L-sit without changing the relative positions of your arms and head and body. But, a sit-up is not strictly a hinge movement from the hips. The body's muscular and connective tissue systems will assist you off the floor so even though you are trying to maintain a plank-like upper body and arms, there will be some muscular engagements that will support you by creating a 'wave' kind of movement.

Your arms, shoulders, back, abdominal and core muscles are deeply involved. There will be some slight rounding of the spine for a moment at the shoulders and mid-back as you project yourself upward. Your shoulders need to 'bed down' into the floor to get the support. This is why your arms right up to your fingers have to be at shoulder width. If they are together you cannot exert this pressure into the ground and your shoulders may even shrug.

In fact, try this right now. Bring your arms up over your head and extend them directly up from the shoulders. Activate your muscles: Find arm extension at the same time as drawing your shoulders down away from your ears. Notice how your shoulder blades feel more sturdy, broad and strong in this position.

Now link your thumbs. Notice how your shoulders now lift a little, your neck compresses and it is harder to keep that strong warrior-type sensation across and projecting through to your fingers. There is a noticeable loss of strength and support. Unhook your thumbs and broaden your shoulders and strengthen your arms again. With your arms apart, contact of the shoulder blades on the floor is preserved for longer, making your sit-up better and safer.

Grip around the feet: The best grip is with the palms facing down and the fingers reaching over and pulling hard against the balls of your feet, toes pointing back. Work your foot flexion as you push your heels away to deepen the stretch against the pull.

Pulling with bent arms when the back is rounded: Bent arms will accentuate a round spine. Only bend your arms if your back and legs are both completely straight.

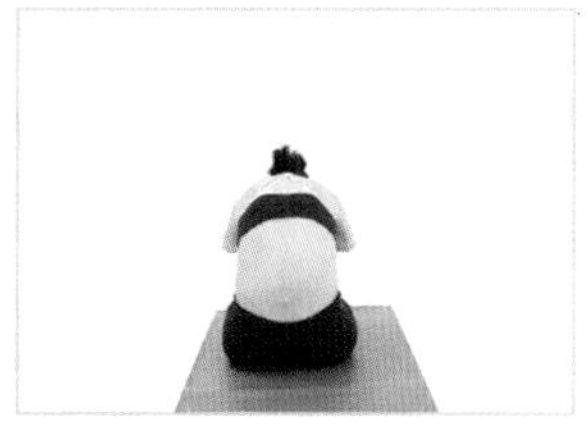

Wherever you are you will pull your toes back, extend your heels, lift your chest and straighten your spine. You must feel the traction.

Toes pointed: Pointing toes shortens the backs of the legs, just where you need a lengthening stretch. The arms get pulled forward with the forward moving toes instead of straightening against flexed feet as the chest lifts. You must lift your breastbone and arch your spine while pulling back on your toes.

Can't reach your feet: Most students cannot reach their toes and still maintain a straight back. You have to decide whether to round the back or bend the legs.

Using your yoga logic (and the results of the experiment above) you will bend your legs. Why? Because you want to take EVERY opportunity to avoid a rounded back, to stretch open your vertebrae and elongate your torso. Bend your legs in preference, don't slump your back, keep it straight.

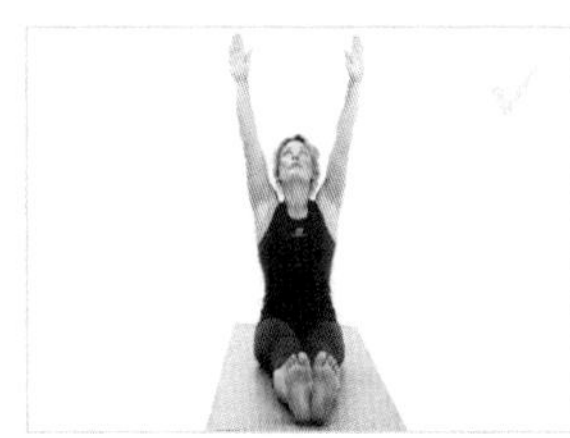

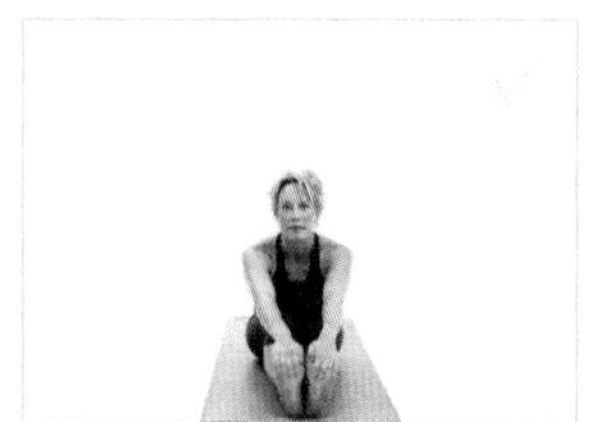

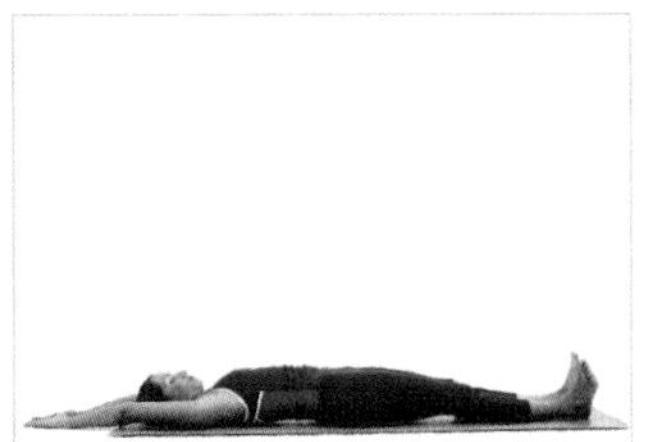

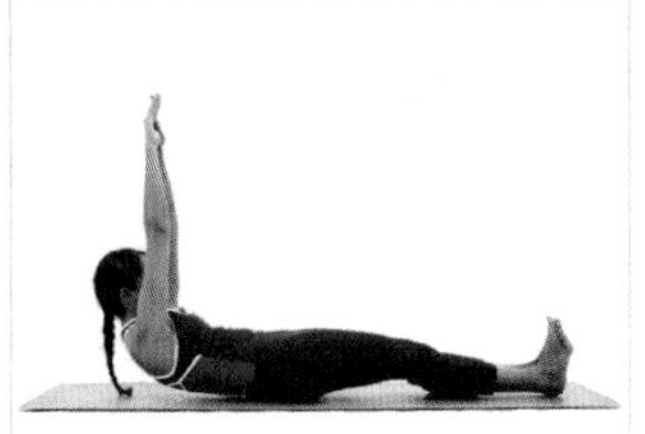

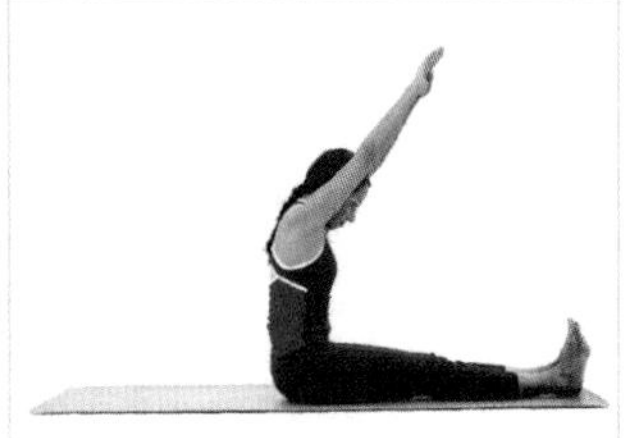

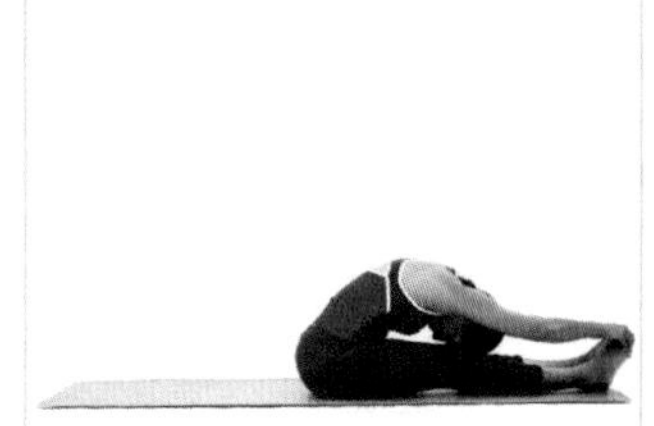

Bhujangasana

You are never given a dream without also being given the power to make it true. You may have to work for it, however.
—Richard Bach

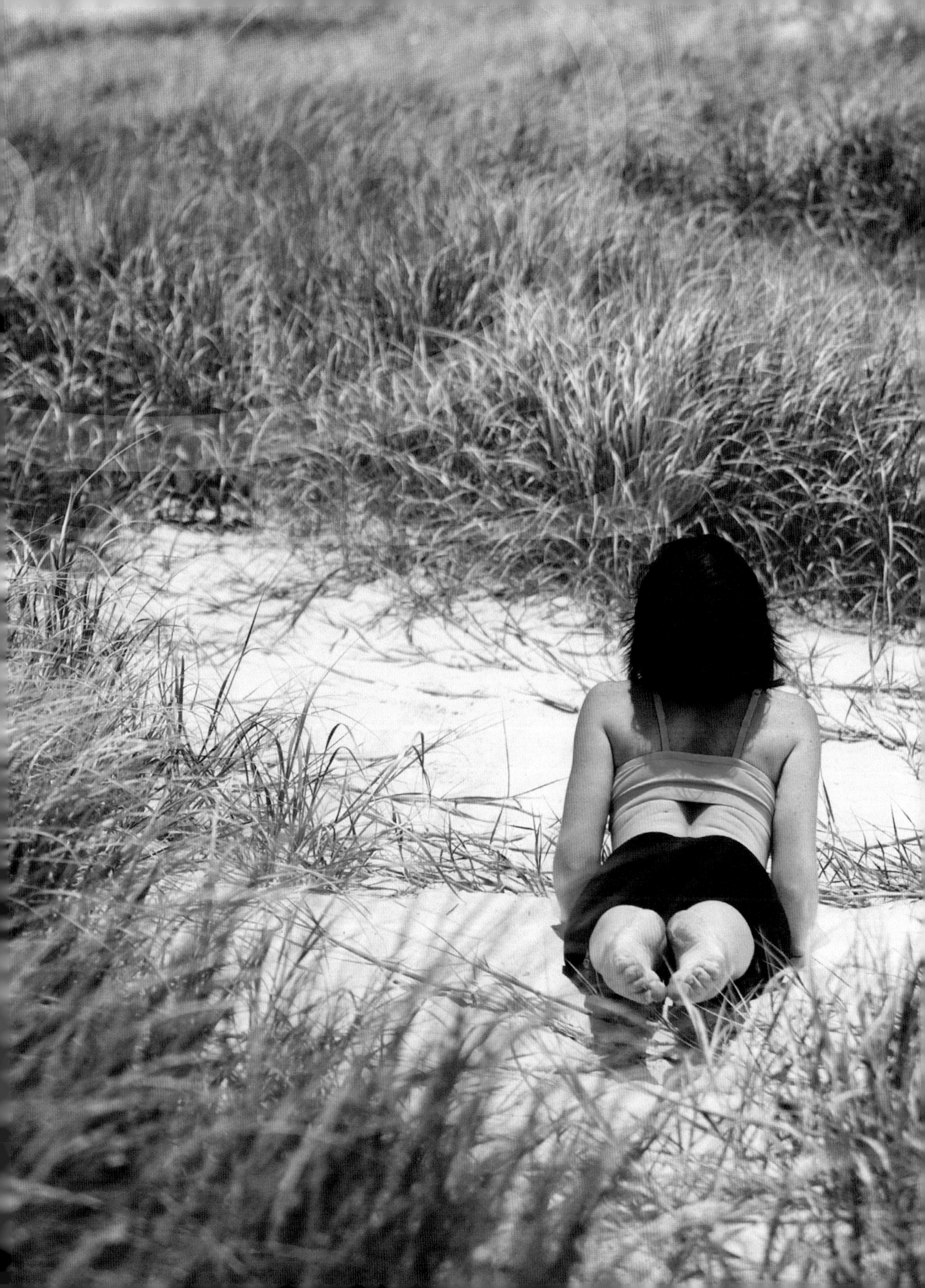

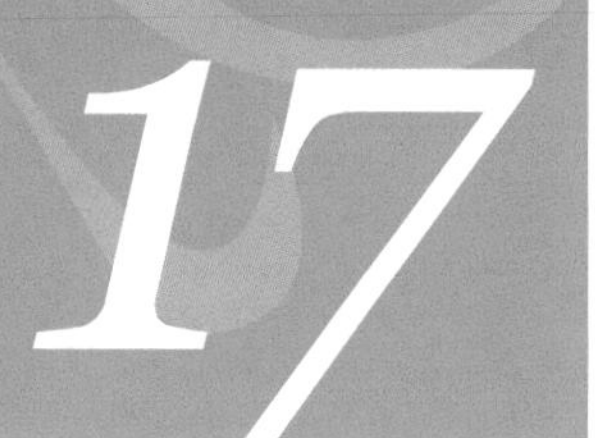

Bhujangasana

Cobra Pose

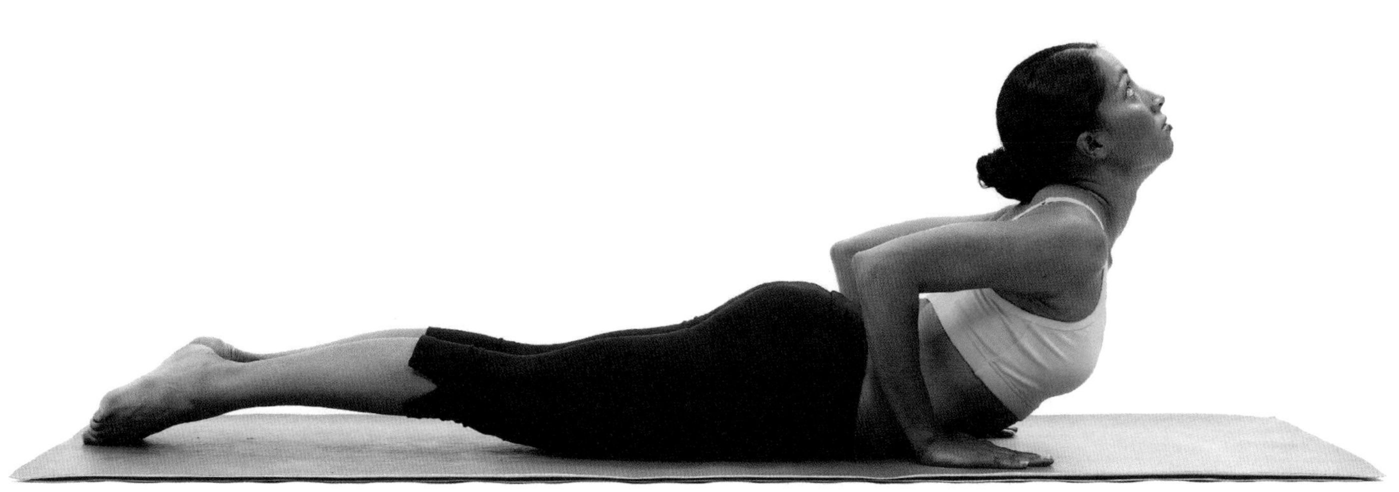

The essentials

The great thing about Bhujangasana is that every *body* can do it and benefit. Only the degree of lift and the arch in the spine will differ. It can be performed without having warmed up at all. As lower back pain is often a sign of lower back weakness, I recommend this one for any student with lower back pain. It can be practiced in isolation, at any time of the day, as often as desired or possible.

Cobra is the very first of four spine strengthening poses where you face the floor belly-down. The main focus is lifting the upper body off the floor using only the muscles of the spine, simply supported by your strong lower body. Although you cannot isolate the different muscles in your back to work separately, Cobra does preferentially strengthen the lumbar spine.

What makes this pose so difficult to get right?

Just about every first time Hot Yoga student will either confuse this pose with a push-up or a similar Cobra pose from other yoga styles, and use their arms to push their body off the floor. Who could blame them? Their arms are there, bent and primed with palms down looking and feeling every bit like they are going to be asked to use them. If you do use the arms for anything other than support you will find a huge dilution or reversal of the effects and benefits.

Bhujangasana

Cobra Pose

The technique

Having been on the floor on your back, you will most likely do a sit-up and then turn around to face the mirror. Place your palms down near the top of your mat at shoulder width apart and then lower yourself to the floor.

1. **Body Square To The Room**: Align your body at 90° to the mirror, lie completely straight with your chin forward on the floor. You are trying to look in the mirror and in doing so are creating length in your neck, straightening your spine and creating other benefits of compressing local glands.

2. **Palms Down, Fingertips At Or Behind Shoulders**: Your palms are under your shoulders with your fingers pointing directly onto the mirror. Depending on your body, your fingertips are at or behind the mirror-most extent of your shoulders. For better lift, place your hands as far back as you can while maintaining the heels of your palms firmly connected to the ground.

3. **Elbows And Shoulders**: Your elbows are bent up and your arms are held closely to the sides. Keep your shoulders relaxed down away from your ears creating space.

4. **Legs In Correct Alignment**: Ensure spinal integrity by verifying in the mirror that your legs are extended in a straight line. If necessary or on rare occasion, momentarily bend up your legs to see if your heels rise symmetrically over your head. Now relax the tops of your feet on the floor, toes extended backwards.

5. **Lock Legs**: Bring your legs and feet together. Exhale as you squeeze your bottom, lock your legs and point your toes.

6. **Look Up And Lift**: On the inhale, look up and peel your upper body off the floor, only recruiting the muscles in the back. Your body will follow where your eyes are looking. You aim to raise your chest through to your abdomen, up off the floor.

7. **No Hands**: No weight is taken on the hands. They are resting gently against the floor and balance you by completing a stable tripod of support for your body. Focus on looking back and lifting.

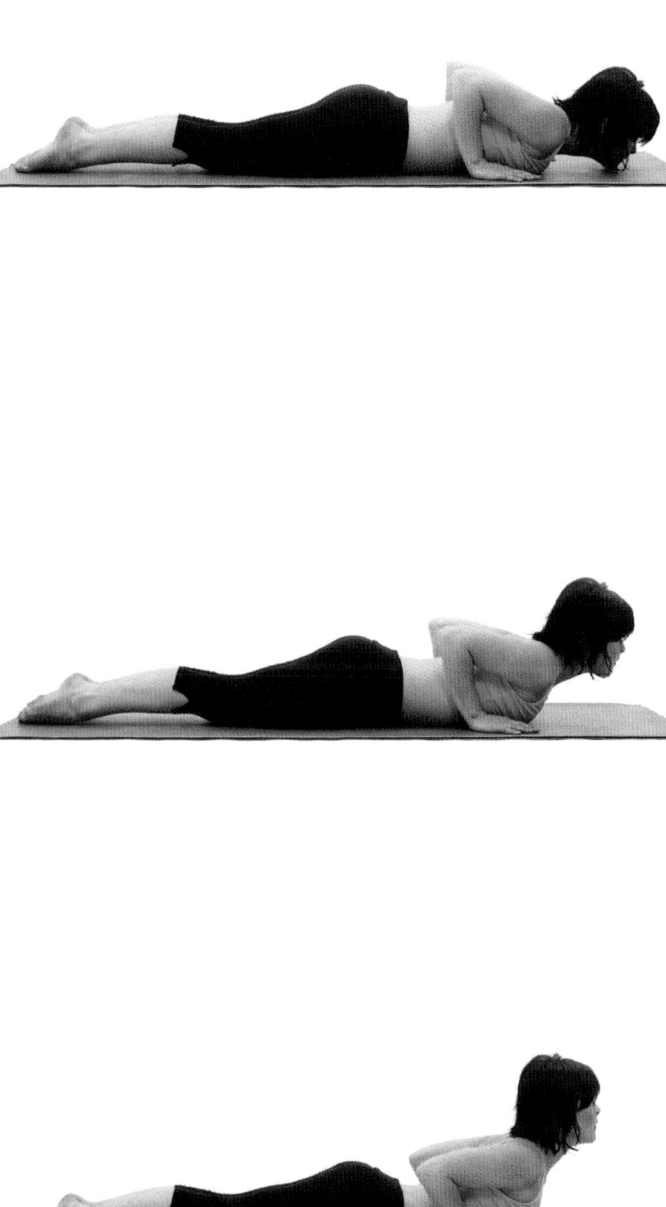

17 Bhujangasana

Cobra Pose

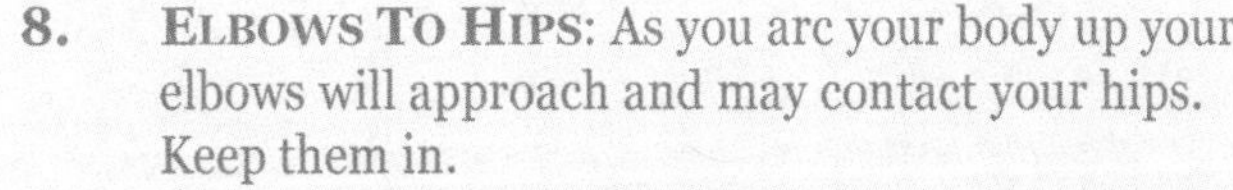

8. **Elbows To Hips**: As you arc your body up your elbows will approach and may contact your hips. Keep them in.

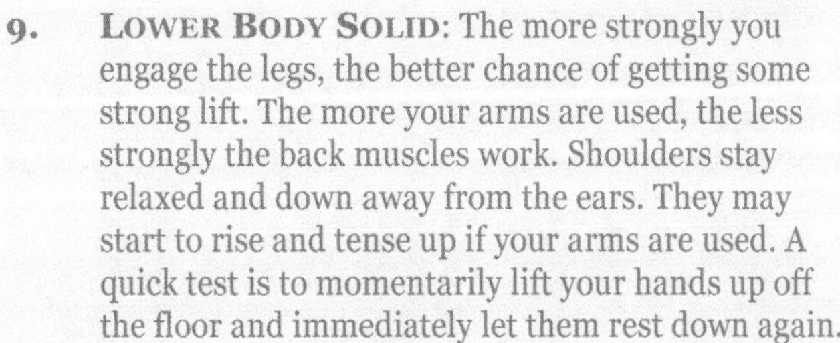

9. **Lower Body Solid**: The more strongly you engage the legs, the better chance of getting some strong lift. The more your arms are used, the less strongly the back muscles work. Shoulders stay relaxed and down away from the ears. They may start to rise and tense up if your arms are used. A quick test is to momentarily lift your hands up off the floor and immediately let them rest down again.

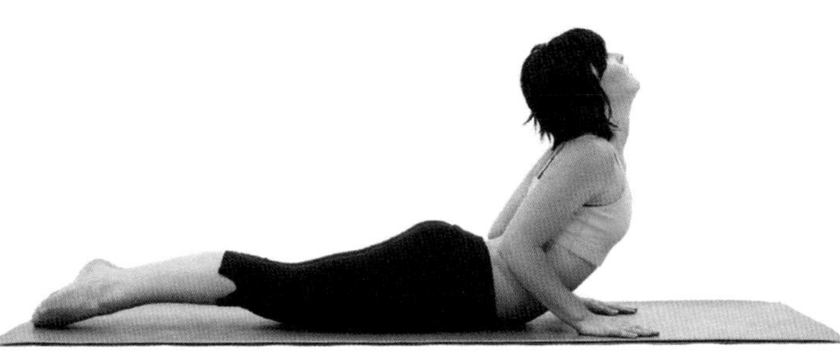

Great tip 1, for better lift: As part of your set-up lengthen your abdomen on the floor before placing your palms down. Positioning your fingertips a little posteriorly will help this elongation.

Great tip 2, visualization: Of course it will be easier to get up higher for those with stronger and more flexible spines. I remember a movie with Leslie Caron in which she was ballet dancing. On the floor she lifted her entire torso up to 90° from a flat position without using her arms which were extended out to the side and back as if wings. I have never seen such an amazing back lift without assistance. This visualization definitely helps me aspire to greater heights!

Release

Exhale as you lower your body and bring your chin down to the floor with your neck extended. Your hands stay in position. After chin contact use your hands to push against the floor to lift your head and turn it to face the right side and bring your left ear to the mat. Second set you will face the left. Now take your arms to your sides, palms up. Bring toes together and let your heels fall out to the sides. This action will help you release and relax your legs, hips, thighs and lower spine. Keep your chin away from your chest to maintain a straight spine. Assist your meditation by lying motionless in your Savasana extending your visual focus only as far as the edge of your mat.

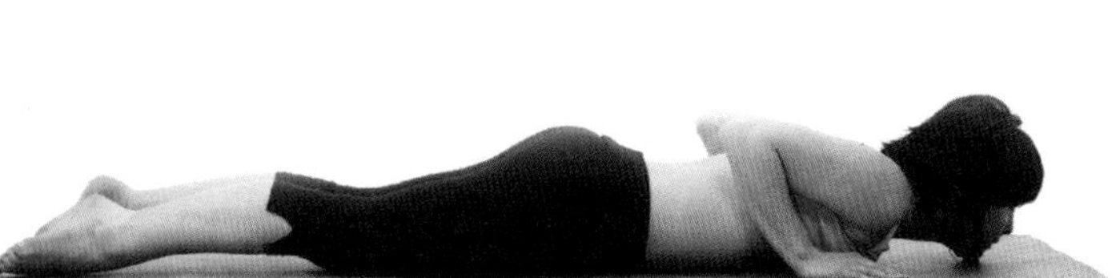

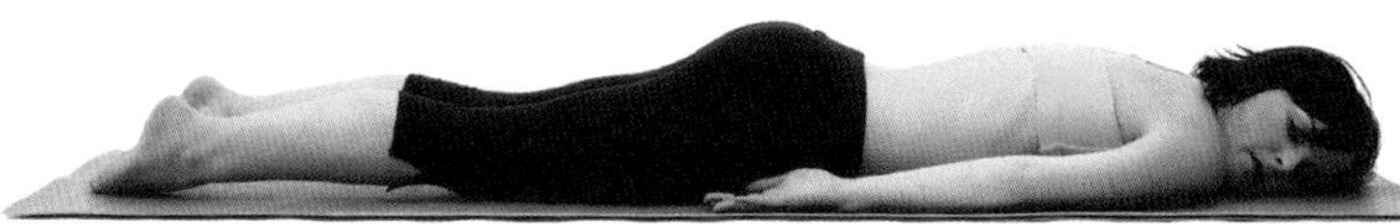

Common mistakes and how to fix them

Using the arms for the lift: Everyone has done this at some stage and to varying degrees. Most commonly it can be a little downward pressure through the hands and can even be unconscious or unintentional. Maybe your energy resources are down even for a moment or two during the 10 second lift. The mistake may be much more obvious and involve the complete straightening of the arms with accompanying shoulder hunching.

In every case, this dilutes and minimizes the work that your back has to do to lift your body off the floor. The gross error is easy to spot and easier to correct. The subtler hand pushing needs attentiveness. From time to time you can test your arm muscle use by lifting your hands up off the floor for a microsecond – no more. See below.

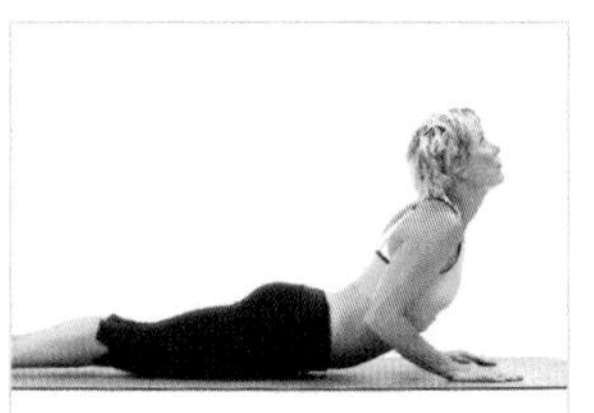

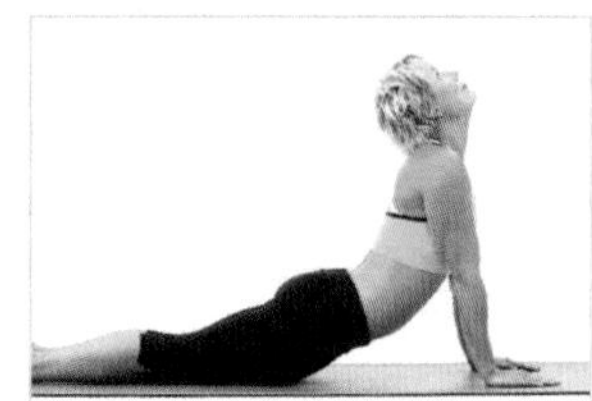

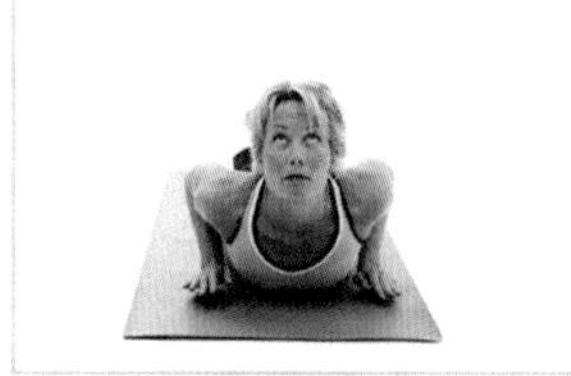

Incorrectly applying the hand-lift test: The problem with suggesting students lift their hands off the floor is that too many students take the wrong lesson from it. What some do is lift hands and then let them hover above the floor for seconds, or worse, for the entire pose. This is not supportive and strains the neck and shoulder muscles.

The test lasts only a fraction of a second. Additionally it is not recommended on a regular basis. The purpose is to gauge any arm involvement, let the body settle and then replace the hands. Learn to lift recruiting your back muscles only. Whether the body settles or not, you are to replace your passive hands back on the floor, immediately.

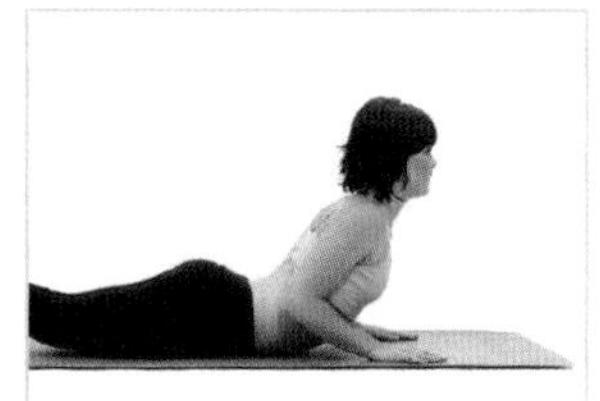

Eyes looking in wrong direction: Either the student will look at themselves in the mirror or they will look up insufficiently. Look up and back as much as you can without undue strain and you will be rewarded with greater lift.

Eyes closed: Lift is compromised with closed eyes.

Flexed feet: Do not bring your toes digging into the floor under you. This causes flexing at the ankle and difficulties in strengthening the legs. Make sure the feet are extended, touching and toes pointed.

Incorrect hand placement: Setting up with fingertips at the shoulder edge is the most commonly taught instruction. It doesn't take into account different hand plus finger lengths. What you want is a position that will optimize your lift, by bringing your elbows close to the hips, and making your arms feel light.

Everyone has an optimum palm position. Smaller hands lining up with shoulders, or fingers placed forward of the shoulders, make the arms and shoulders take more weight for the lift. And you know you have placed your hands too far back if your palms are not flat on the floor.

Playing around with placement I discovered the further back you can place your palms completely flat on the ground, the better. It all depends on your wrist and shoulder comfort and flexibility. Further back, your hands will feel a little charged during set-up, but not for the lift. Your shoulders will stay down and relax more easily and your elbows will skim your hips as required. You will lift your upper body higher.

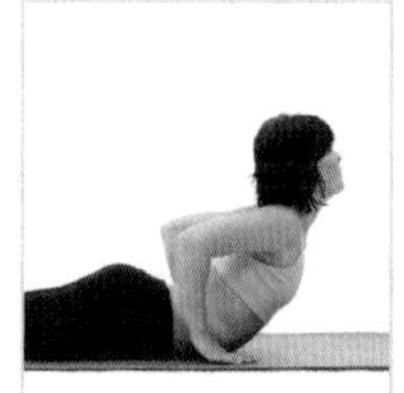

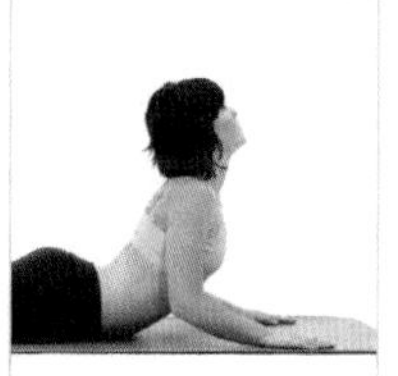

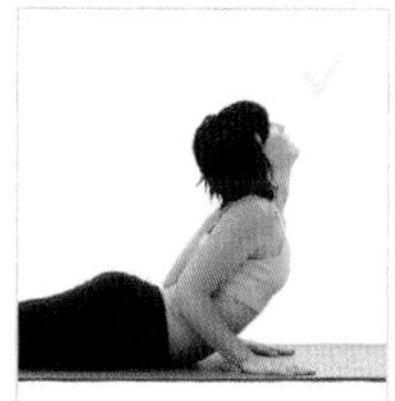

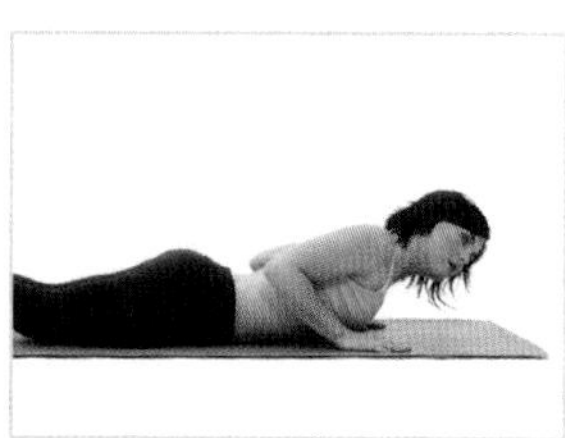

Twist on release: Muscular and spinal integrity is lost by turning your head as you release. Anticipating your Savasana means you lose the physical and mental benefits of correct pose reversal and the opportunity to be in the moment. See 'Release' for detailed guidance into your belly-down Savasana.

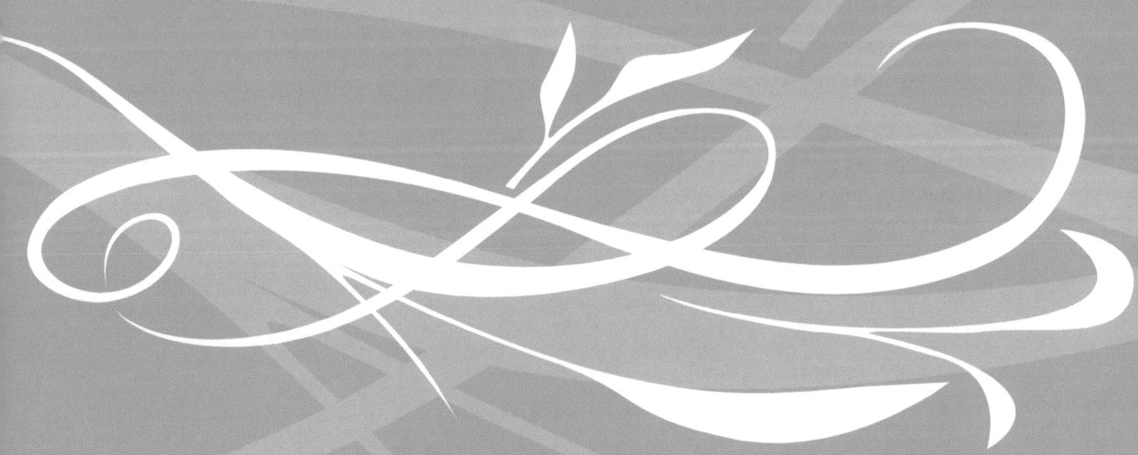

Salabhasana

Start by doing what's necessary,
then what's possible, and suddenly
you are doing the impossible.
—Francis of Assisi

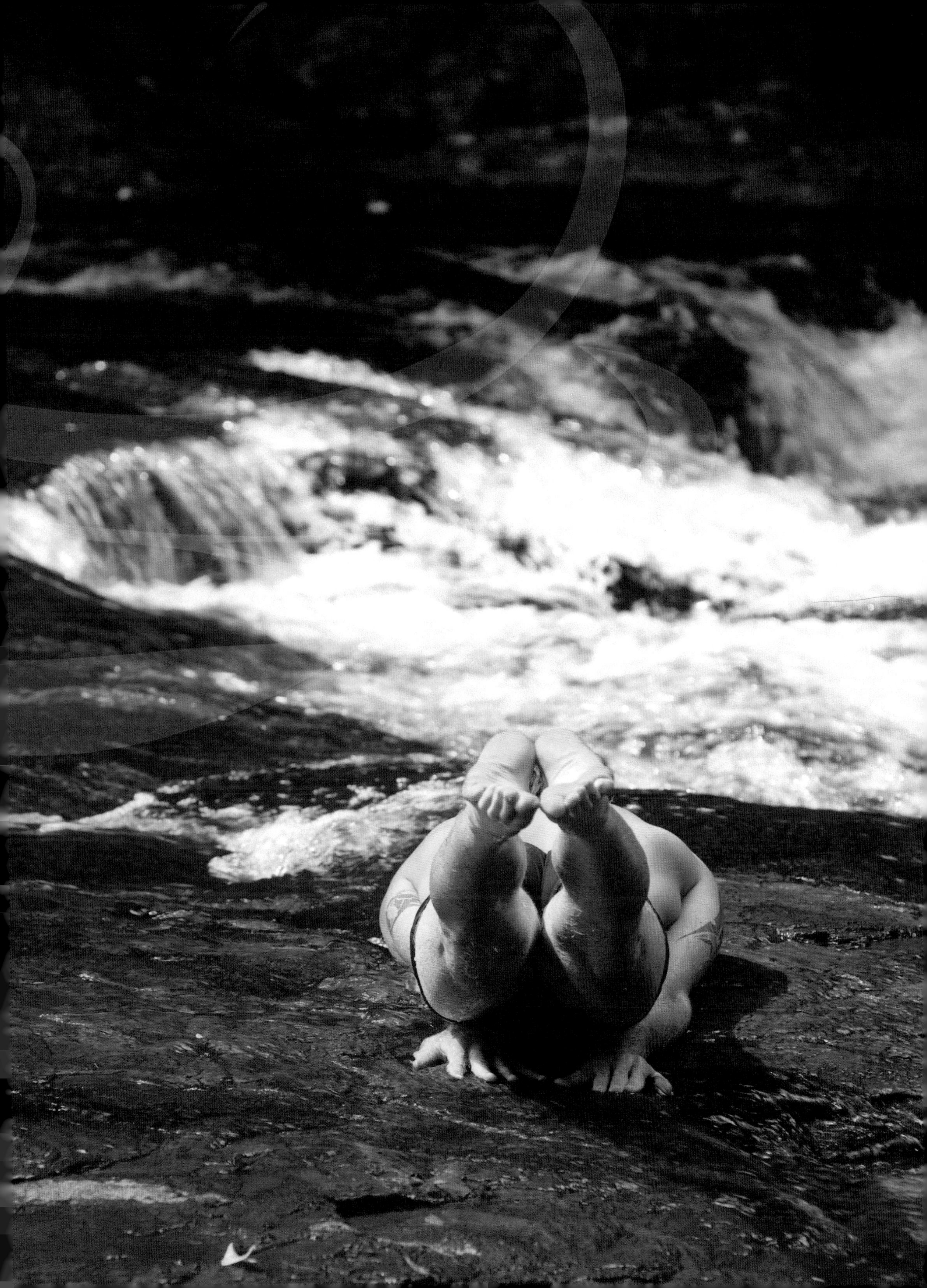

18

Salabhasana

Locust Pose

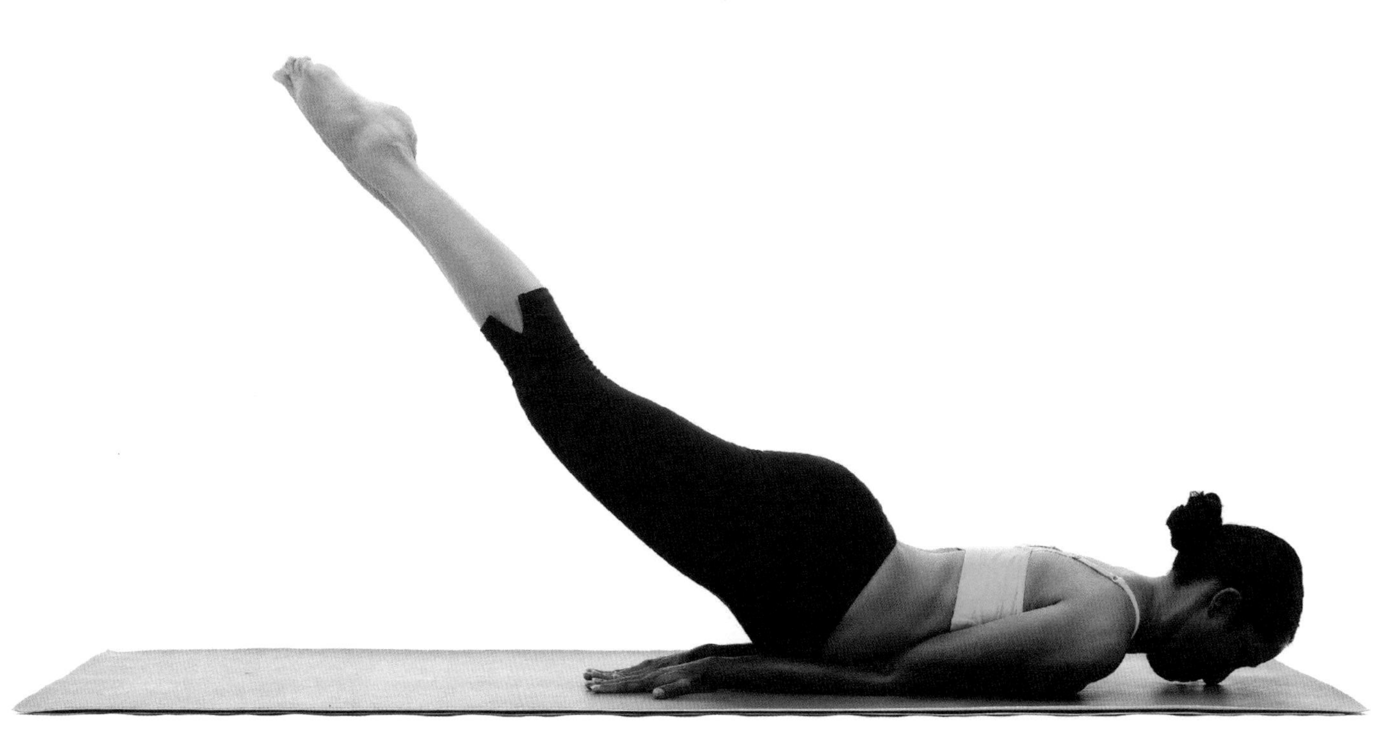

The essentials

Locust has both single and double leg lifts. Your work will strengthen the upper spine in the vicinity of the shoulders. That in itself is difficult for many to fathom because of the apparent focus on leg work. As with all the belly-down poses Salabhasana helps to realign the spine.

Many of the actions and benefits center around the positioning of the arms underneath the body. The double leg lift could well be one of the strongest hot yoga poses both requiring great reserves of energy and building excellent strength.

What makes this pose so difficult to get right?

Even though the two parts of the pose are performed chronologically and in quick succession most students don't 'get' the strong interrelationship. The biggest error is not using the arms sufficiently in the single leg lifts. When it feels easy to lift the leg, it is usually because we are unconsciously bracing the lower leg to gain stability and forgetting to use the arms until the double leg lift. Learning how to use the arms will help you strengthen the upper spine.

Salabhasana

Locust Pose

18

The technique

The single leg lift

Having just finished second set of Cobra your head is facing the left and you are lying exactly square to the mirror. Come out of Savasana and place your chin forward on the floor and bring your arms underneath your body.

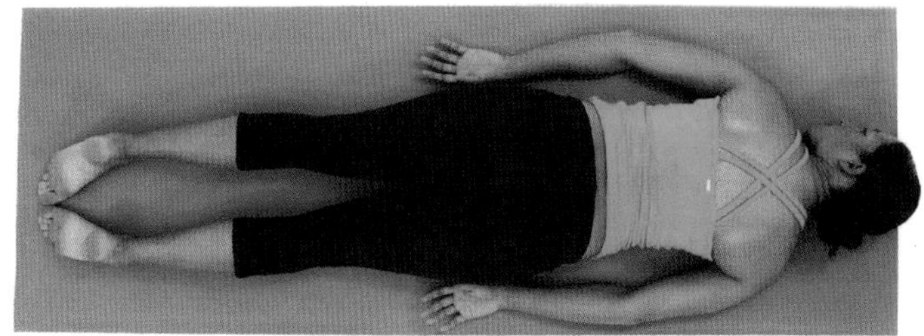

1.1 **Lift Your Hips**: The best way to bring your arms under your body is to lift your hips up centrally. You push your flexed feet into the floor behind you to support your lifted body. Then bring one arm under and then the other.

1.2 **Place Your Arms Symmetrically Under The Body, Palms Down**: Each arm is placed as centrally and as closely as possible to the other with the palms down on the floor elbow points toward your stomach. Stretch your arms out straight. Perhaps the hands will line up touching but it's not essential. Broaden the area between your shoulders by externally rotating the arms which further allows the elbows to approach each other.

1.3 **Chin Forward**: Elongate the neck and place the chin forward on your mat. In this way you can observe your alignment.

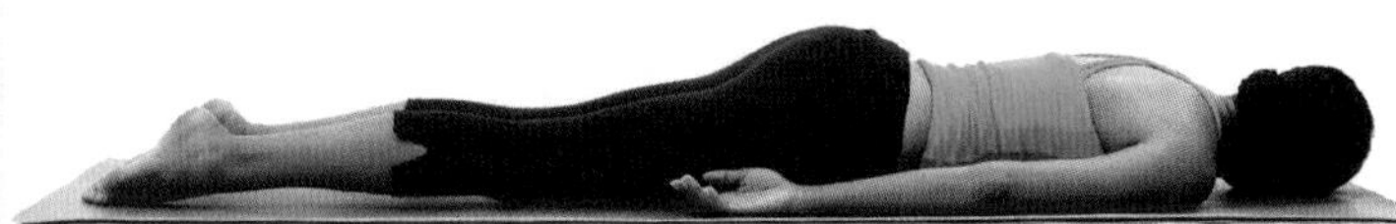

1.4 **Wrists And Elbows And Shoulders**: This is one pose where any teacher will tell you that it is OK and very normal to put up with some elbow and wrist pain. It is through this pose that you will break up scar tissue and deposits in the joints, reinvigorate the circulation and create better movement. Pretty soon you should notice that there is no pain and less to no resistance.

1.5 **First Side, Relax Your Left Leg**: Let your left leg go completely.

1.6 **Lock And Extend Your Right Leg**: Exhale as you completely lock out your right leg, extending your leg back from hip to pointed toes actively stretching your leg toward the back wall. This action may result in your leg slightly lifting. On your inhale, press the arms down and lift your active right leg up. Pivot it at the hip in order to solidly seat the right hip on your forearm.

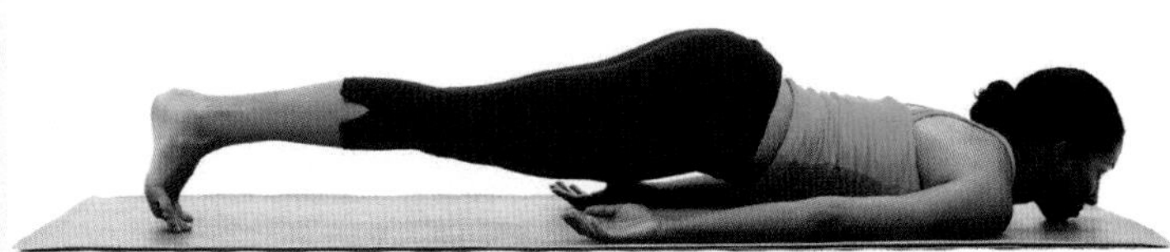

18 Salabhasana

Locust Pose

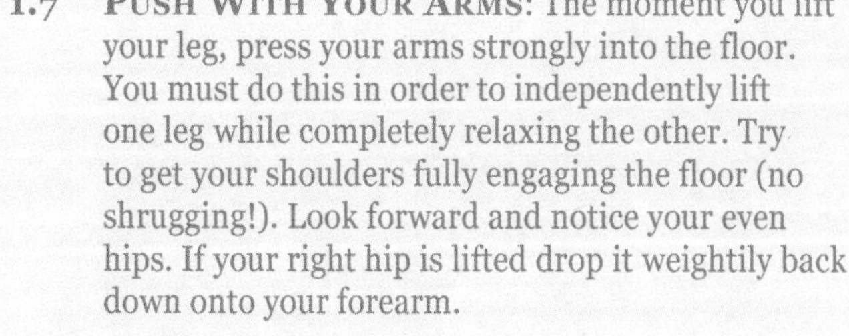

1.7 Push With Your Arms: The moment you lift your leg, press your arms strongly into the floor. You must do this in order to independently lift one leg while completely relaxing the other. Try to get your shoulders fully engaging the floor (no shrugging!). Look forward and notice your even hips. If your right hip is lifted drop it weightily back down onto your forearm.

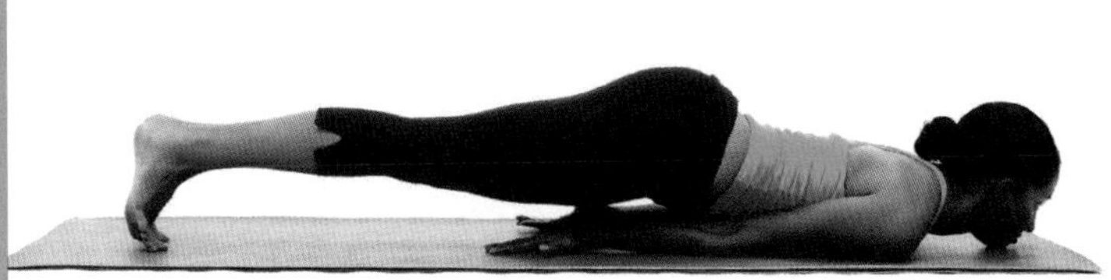

1.8 Lift To 45 Degrees: The aim is to lift your extended active leg to 45° while keeping the hip firmly planted and the other leg absolutely relaxed. Keep the breath flowing and continue pushing with the arms.

1.9. Release: Maintain sufficient pressure through the arms as you release so that your lower leg stays relaxed and the upper leg stays active as it descends. Resist letting go and flopping your leg down. Keep your chin forward and arms beneath. Once on the floor, relax your right leg completely allowing your heel to fall to the side to release your hip and thigh. Repeat for the left leg.

The double leg lift

Your arms are still in position. But you will make some changes to help increase support for the lift.

2.1 Your Head: Tuck your chin in order to bring your lips to the mat. These will act as suspension, cushioning the forces into the floor and balancing your body through the lift. Keep your head like this until your feet lower to the floor again.

2.2 Rotate Your Arms Closer Together: Believe it or not, there is a right and wrong way to do this. It is not simply a question of bringing your arms more closely by drawing your shoulders together under you toward the midline. You want to reproduce the movement that you create when you stand in Savasana relaxing your shoulders down and back (with palms slightly forward). When facing the floor you bring about similar conditions by externally rotating the arms. This brings your elbows closer together and at the same time draws the shoulders apart, flattening and broadening the area on the floor between your shoulders. Your shoulder blades will move closer together and open your chest. You now have a firmer broader platform against which to lift your legs and support your body.

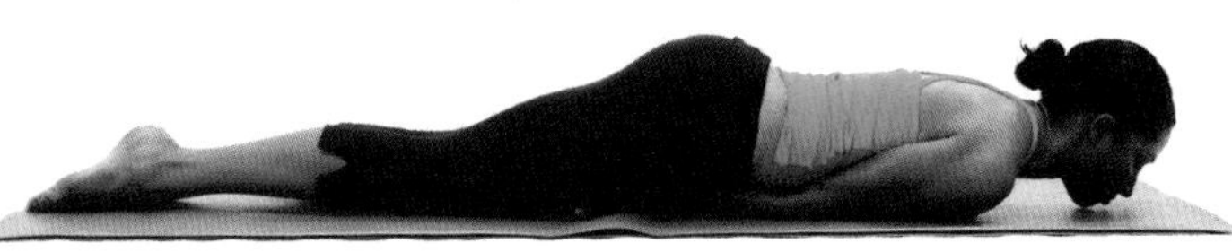

2.3 **Activate Your Legs**: Extend your legs together along the midline right down to the toes and activate them strongly, locking the knees. Always do this before you enter into the pose. Activated legs usually come off the floor slightly before the lift.

2.4 **Lift As You Exhale**: Exhale and lift your straight locked legs up as high as you can by pushing your arms strongly into the floor. Strong exertion works better on an exhale. Keep your breath calm, deep and slow to allow full gaseous exchange and focus on smooth steady effort. You are not rocking your legs up in a movement akin to that of a caterpillar. The stronger your core the higher up the body the hinge or fulcrum will be. You can visualize hinging at the shoulders as your legs and body lift off the floor like a long straight plank.

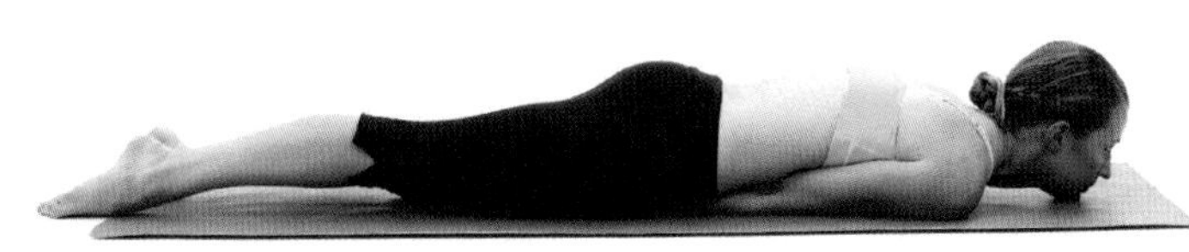

2.5 **Legs Unbending**: While you aim for a 45° angle of your single lifted leg, you simply try to lift both legs as high as you can. It is the effort and not the height that is important, so don't worry if your legs don't even clear the floor. Just keep them strong, straight, legs locked and active and push through all this intensity no matter what height you achieve.

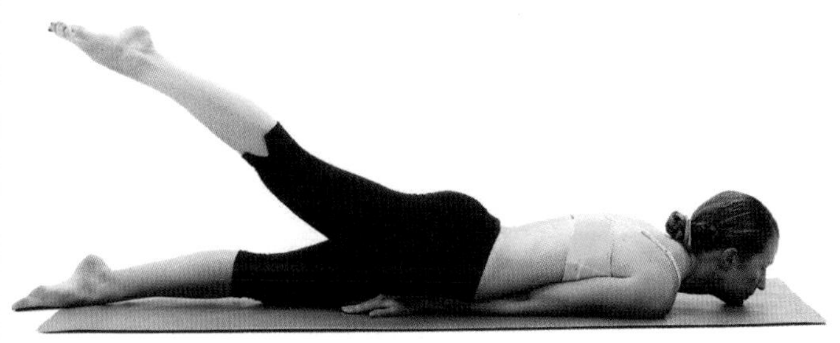

Advanced double leg lift

There is an advanced pose for Salabhasana. Not many manage the strength to lift their body and legs to reach an almost vertical position. Not surprisingly these yogis have great upper body strength and can often be surfers. I recommend doing the normal pose for the first set; the advanced pose in the second. The chin stays placed forward on the ground. Lift your body and legs with both arms under you pushing into the floor. The stage after is to bend the knees and allow the feet to hover over or even contact the head. Definitely ask for guidance from your teacher.

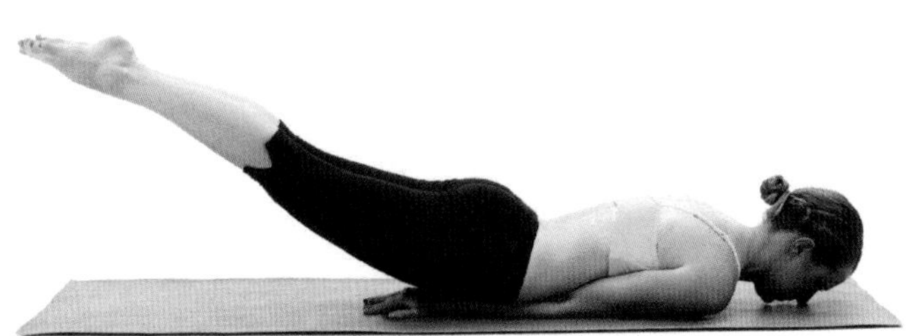

18

Salabhasana

LOCUST POSE

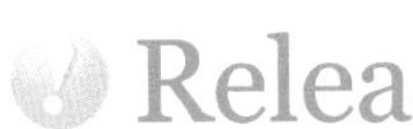

Release

This is a controlled lowering of both legs metered by the strength in your arms and legs. Don't let them collapse down. After all that effort it is hard to find extra strength to slow the descent against gravity. You will be glad you did – you will feel strong and certainly safer.

When your legs touch the floor, allow them to relax enough to lift your hips and remove your arms out from underneath. Enter your Savasana with mindfulness and avoid twisting the spine (no flailing legs).

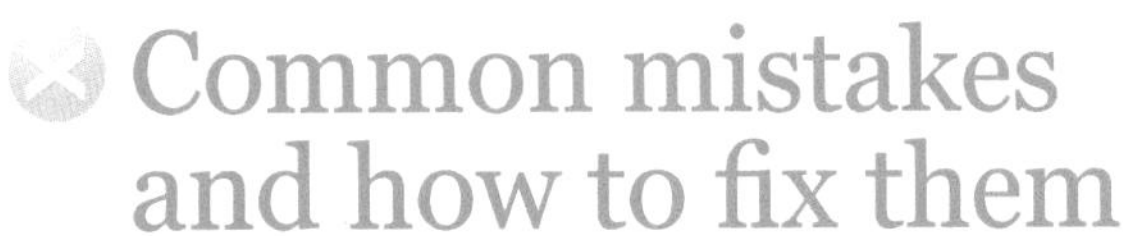

Common mistakes and how to fix them

Getting your arms under you: Many students don't lift their hips the right way to get their arms under. They bring their feet up off the floor and rock their bent legs over, twisting one side up off the floor to place one arm down. They then reverse the movement rocking their feet over to the other side, twisting the body up for the second arm placement. This movement is neither mindful nor efficient and risks potential damage as the central axis (spine) is twisted from the knees up diagonally through the torso. You see bodies flopping and legs flailing – not pretty!

The best way is to flex your feet, push them into the ground, engage your legs straight behind you and lift your body up once, and be done with it. You can now position both arms either separately or simultaneously. If this is too difficult, then the following method is acceptable. Keeping both feet contacting the floor, keep your spine straight and untwisted, use some arm pressure to lift up the shoulder, hip and knee on one side. Try bending your knee a little for support and added hip height and bring one arm underneath you. Repeat for the other side. *

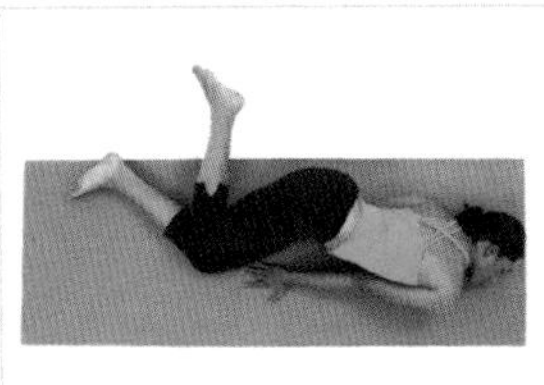

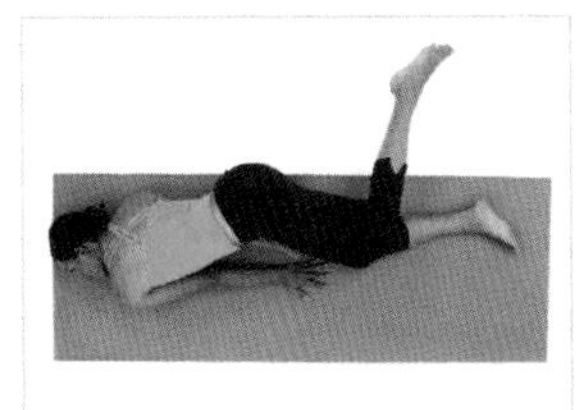

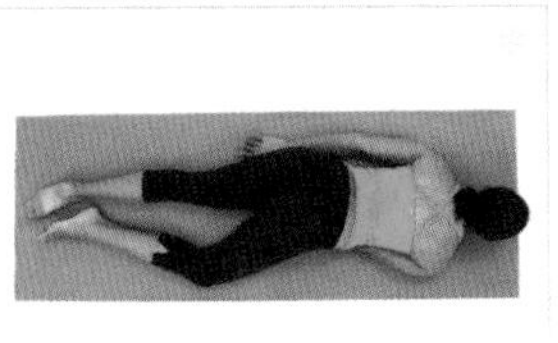

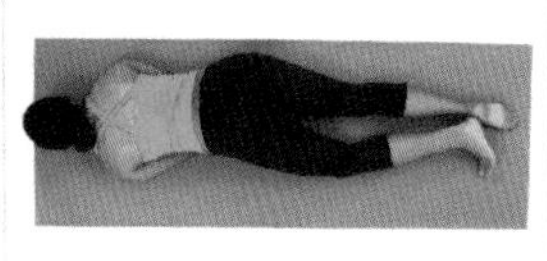

Palms up: If not corrected by the teacher this palms-up position will make it impossible to exert the downward force needed to relax your leg while the other lifts. Your shoulders roll in and cannot broaden to create that supportive platform to protect and build strength in your spine. Externally rotate your arms to bring palms onto the floor.

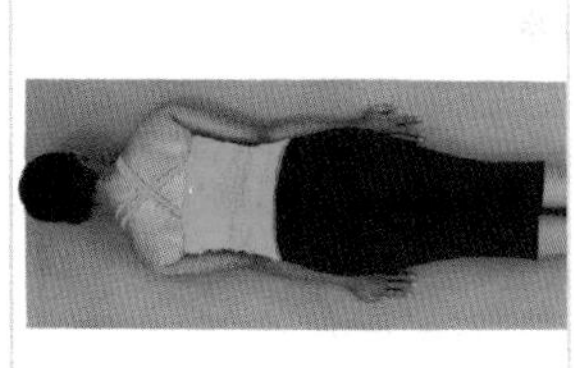

***Can't get your arms underneath**: Occasionally some cannot get their arms under the body at all. No doubt someone will tell you that getting your arms underneath your body is essential and that it is OK to be in pain here. Yes and no. Do you force a student with recent shoulder reconstructions to bring about a painful, impossible or damage-causing position? Is it really no pain, no gain?

Hopefully you are familiar with the pain/discomfort balance. It is wrong to go beyond your own threshold and be in excruciating pain. Be sensitive. Pushing your edge without damage is a process with no particular timetable. This pose really gets in there like a broom to break up scar tissue helping recreate movement in the wrist, elbows and shoulders.

If you have injury or tightness, your arms may start out alongside the body. Maybe the smallest fingers will be tucked in at the thighs. Symmetry in placement is crucial to create proper support and balance regardless of injury. Push your edge and bring your arms closer together over time.

Forgetting to use your arms: In the single leg lift many students are so focused on lifting their leg that they bring little or no attention to the pushing force of the arms into the floor. Although Locust appears to be a leg exercise, it is designed to strengthen your upper back. If you want proof, try lifting both legs together, without using your arms by bringing them passively out by your side!

Use the single-leg lifts as a rehearsal for the double-leg lift. If you don't use maximum downward force with your arms, then you will not be able to relax the other leg on the floor during the lift. Who cares how high your legs go? What matters is your 100% dedication to lock out your leg or legs. The more you harness the energy in your arms, the better.

Locking the extended leg(s) at the moment of the lift: Locking your single leg as you lift it means you have no choice but to recruit the muscles of your supposedly relaxed leg. If you don't engage both your active legs before the double-leg lift you are more likely to bend your legs to get them up. The height your bent legs reach is an artificial reading and only reflects the height of your toes, not your straight legs. Your core muscles and your upper spine are not utilized as much when the legs are bent.

When you lock your leg(s) before the lift, your leg(s) is active and may already be slightly off the ground. You get the whole 10 seconds to engage and work the leg. The same goes for the release. Don't flop out. Keep the leg(s) locked out until you have reversed all the way to the starting position again.

Legs bend: Keep the appropriate leg locked for the duration.

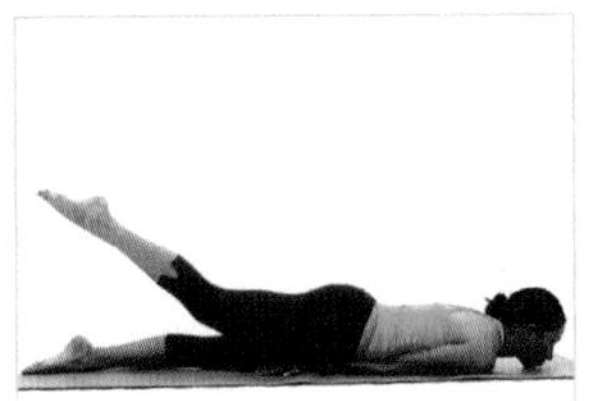

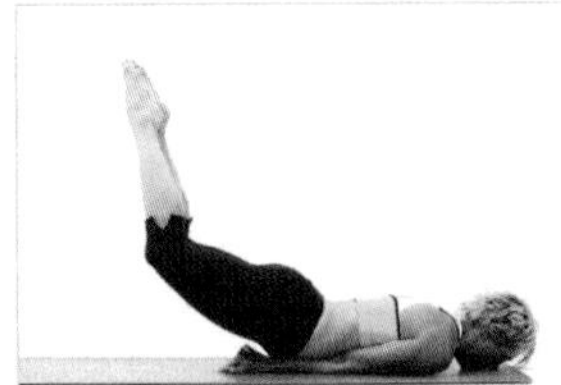

Hip lifts: The aim is not to get the single leg as high as possible. This classic new student mistake causes a central axis twist as the hip lifts off the forearm. Press the hip of your lifted leg down as you simultaneously extend and lift the leg to 45° only.

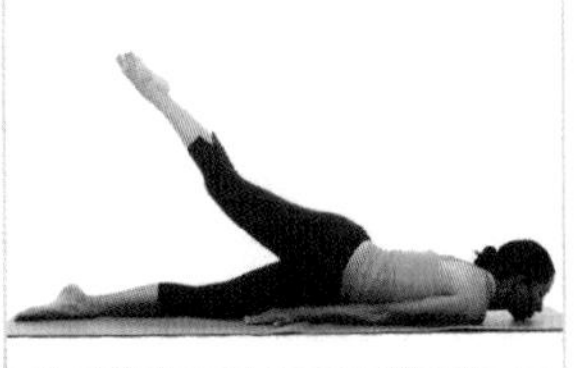

Can't get your shoulders on the ground: Some people will never get good (or any) shoulder contact for the double-leg lift. For example this pose will be more difficult for you if you are an amply endowed woman. Sometimes too, you are asked to move your palms closer to your knees to help you with the double-leg lift. This is poor instruction as it only works for those who have shoulders on the ground.

Externally rotate the arms to bring them closer together and create space between the shoulders and a solid platform through the chest against the floor. Think of pressing the heart into the floor. Push with the arms and keep your legs solid and unbending. You will progressively grow your core and spinal strength.

The outward rotation of the arms will draw your elbows closer and bed your shoulders more broadly as well as more firmly down. Your hands will therefore settle somewhere along the midline in no particular common position.

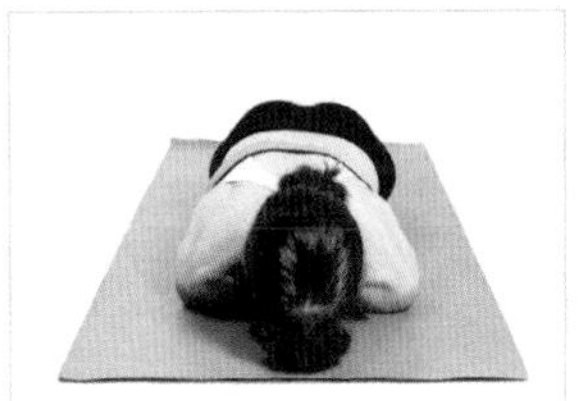

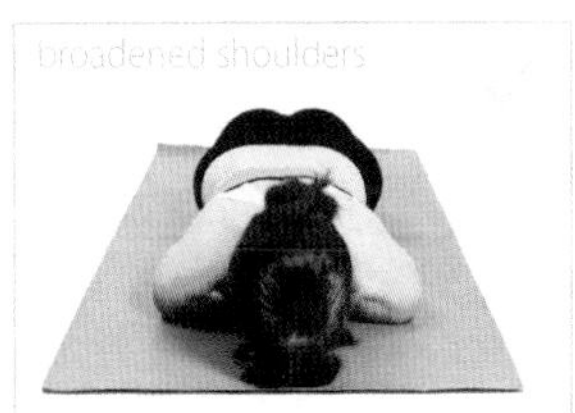

Holding the breath during exertion: Commonly newer students hold their breath during this energy-hungry pose. Once you have a few classes under your belt you may have the bandwidth to start to slow your breath and make it more rhythmic and deeper than the common shallow (and anxiety-inducing) breath.

Legs separate: Often with the exertion of the double leg lift the legs erroneously drift apart. Squeeze your legs together as you activate and lift them.

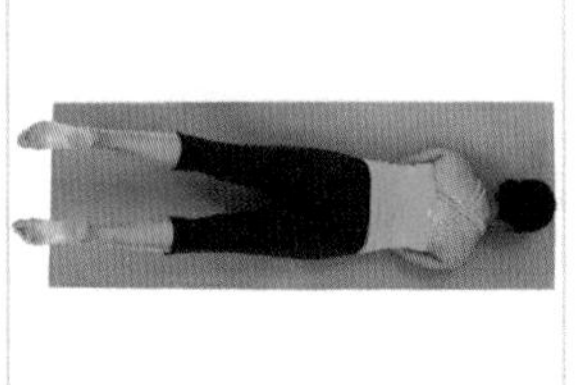

Looking to see your height: Many sneak a peek to check out the height of their double leg lift. Remember it is essential to keep your head down to gather strength in the neck and shoulders and protect your spine. Never look up. If you need to know, let the teacher be your eyes, or have a photo taken.

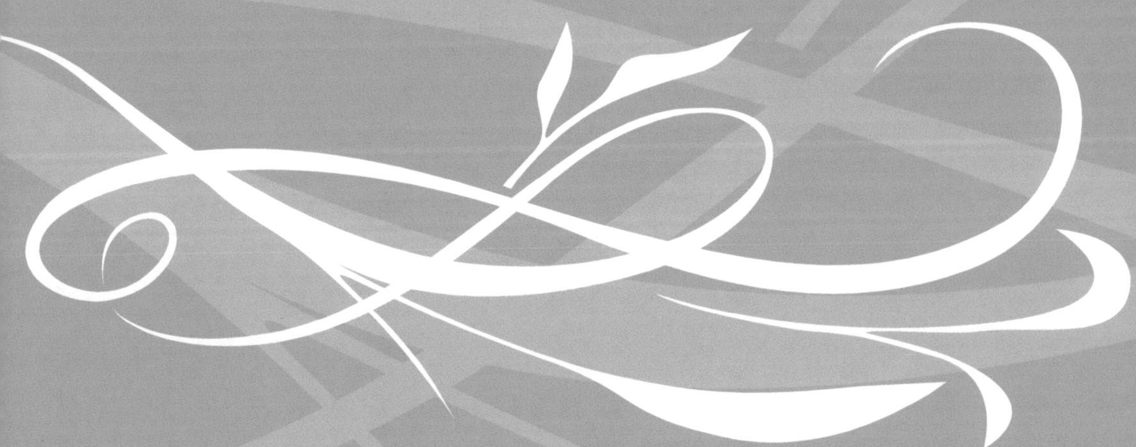

Poorna Salabhasana

When one door of happiness closes, another opens, but often we look so long at the closed door that we do not see the one that has been opened for us.
—Helen Keller

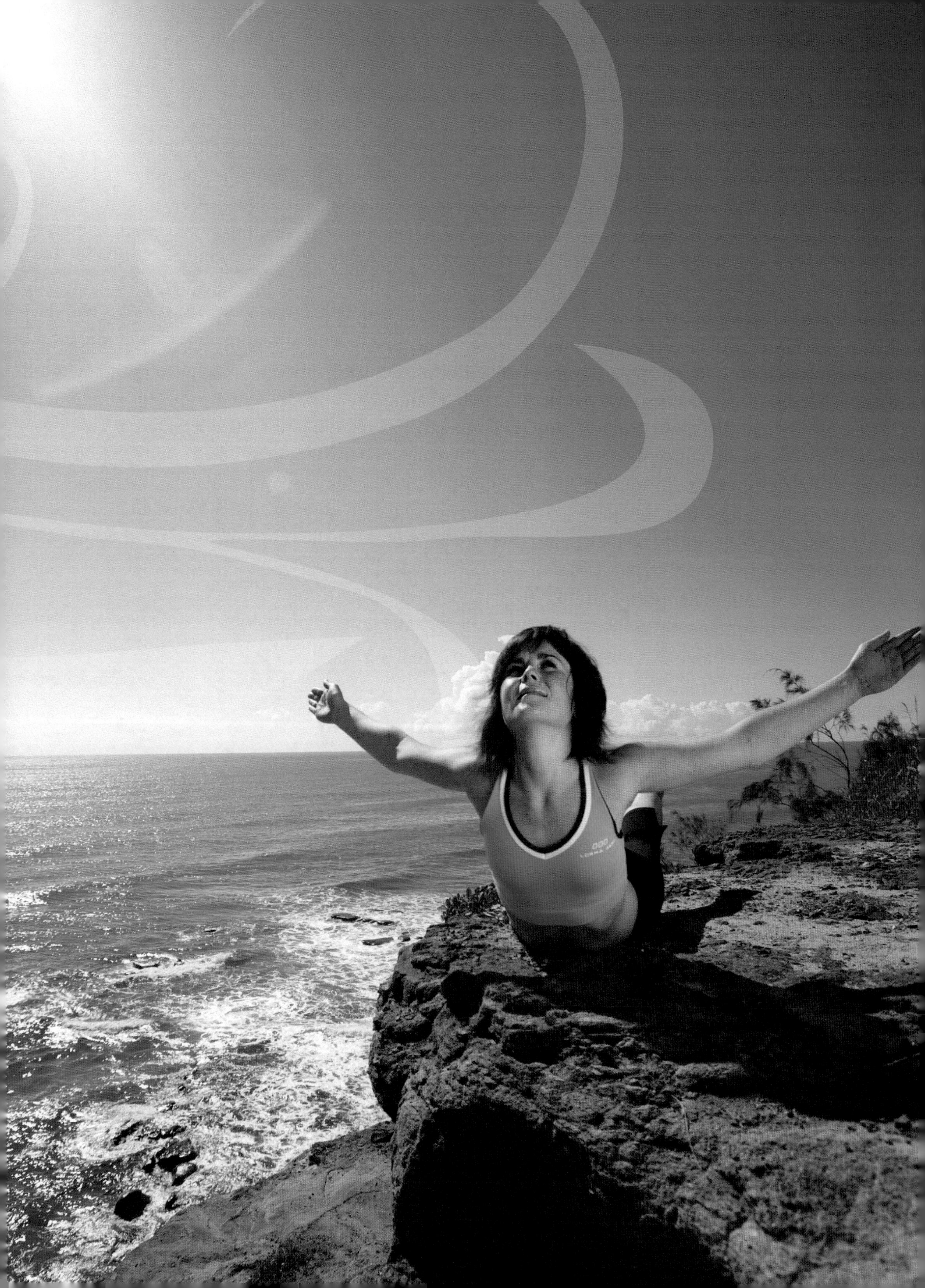

19 Poorna Salabhasana

FULL LOCUST POSE

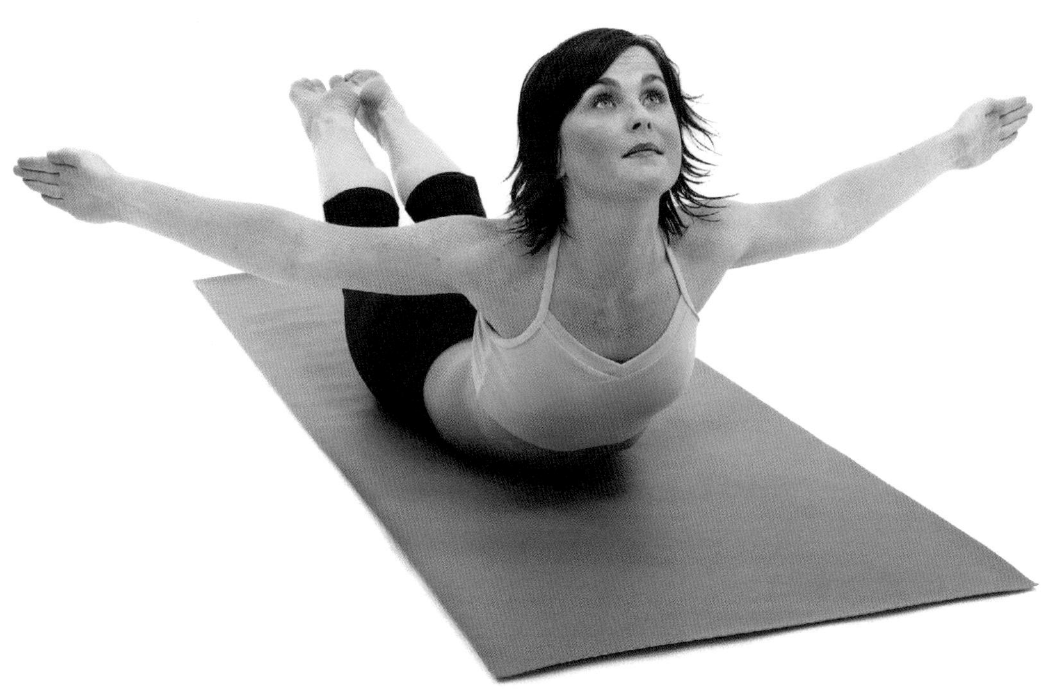

The essentials

For such a simple pose it can be surprising that this can be such a challenge. Remember when you were a kid. Well this pose and the next (Bow pose) were things we did for fun. Remember that, if you find yourself getting caught up in struggle. Basically you activate your body both lengthwise and crosswise and then you lift everything up off the floor as high as you can. I told you it sounded simple.

What makes this pose so difficult to get right?

So long as you look where you want to go (up!) and you keep a constant orientation of your arms plus palms with your shoulders and not with the floor, then you will find extra lift.

Poorna Salabhasana

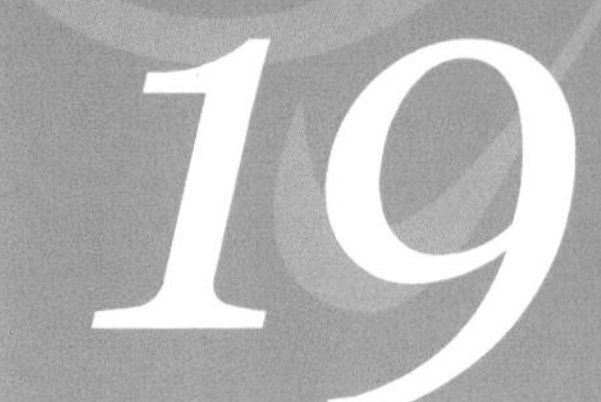

Full Locust Pose

The technique

Center your head with your chin as far forward as you can, so that you can look forward in the mirror, throat flat on the floor.

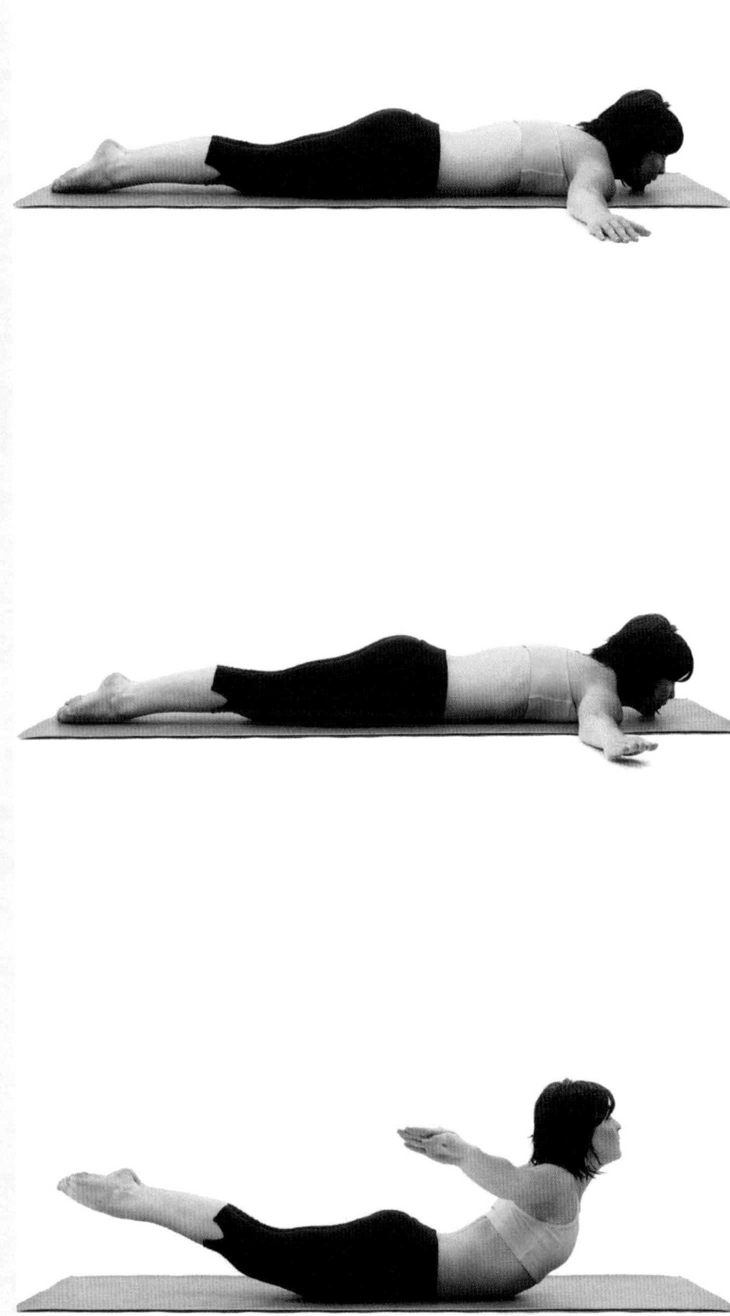

1. **Your Arms**: Extend your arms as far laterally as you can into a T-position, walking your fingers towards each wall to create arm length and space in the shoulders. Your palms are down on the floor and your fingers are together.

2. **Lock Legs**: Legs come together and are locked out completely to raise your knees off the floor. Feet are together and toes are pointed.

3. **Exhale, Activate Your Muscles**: You have locked your legs already, but most students neglect the next little detail. As you exhale, lock your arms out, activating your muscles all the way to your fingertips. Arms will slightly lift off the floor. Your lift will become easier and more effective now that both arms and legs are energized.

4. **The Lift**: On your inhale look up to the ceiling and behind you. Simultaneously lift everything up off the floor to create an upward facing arch in the spine. Your aim is to bring your head, hands and feet to the same height. You will be anchored, making floor contact between abdomen and thighs, ideally balancing only on your hips. Your spinal strength, your stamina, your flexibility and the degree to which you can create the lift while locking out your legs and arms will all determine the height you reach.

5. **Keep Finding Lift**: As you get further into the pose gravity can tire your extended limbs and they tend to settle. Breathe constantly, calmly, deeply. Keep lifting up and looking up. Open your chest and squeeze your shoulder blades together. The palms should start and stay in the same relative position facing the same direction as the front-facing area between the shoulders. Continue to lift your long, strong, activated legs and arms. Legs must stay locked and together.

19

Poorna Salabhasana

FULL LOCUST POSE

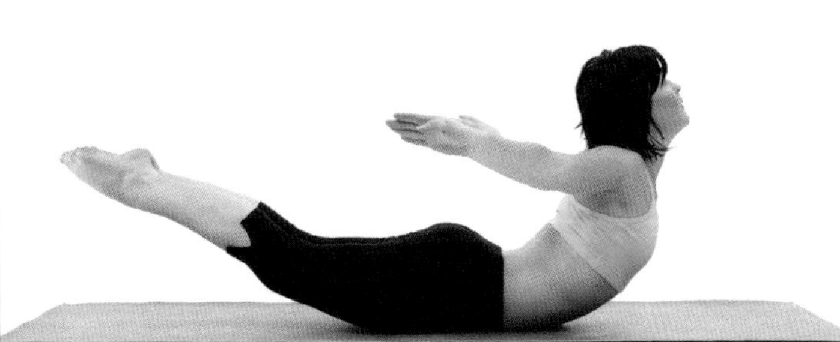

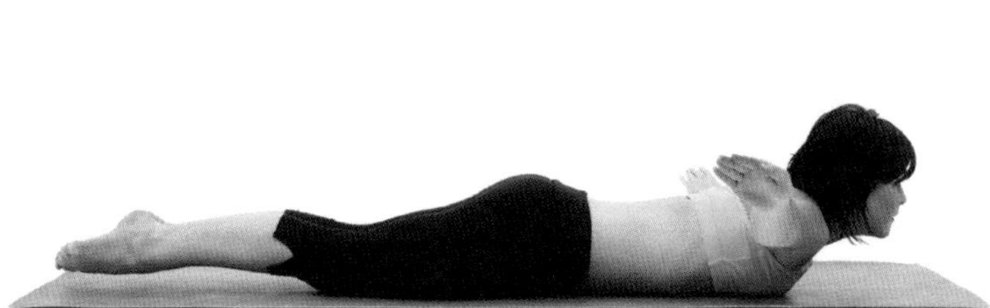

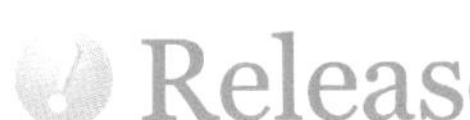

Release

In a nutshell, you lift everything up for 10 seconds and then you reverse it. Work on your lift through to the end of your last inhale. Exhale as you release and engage your muscles to avoid slumping to the floor. Come down with control. Contact the floor with your arms and legs at the starting T-position bringing your chin to the floor on your centerline.

Then (and only then) lift your head and turn to the right with your left ear on the floor (change direction for second set). Then bring your arms to the side of the body, palms up, toes together, heels apart. Relax. Savasana.

Common mistakes and how to fix them

Your arms start in a 'V' to the back wall: Some students actually start with their arms down on the floor already in a 'V'. The starting position is a 'T', which means one straight line through fingertips and shoulders.

Your arms move to a 'V' to the back wall and palms stay facing down: Probably the most common mistake is when students consciously move their arms back into a 'V' shape when they start the ascent. During a poorly executed Full Locust pose students will lift the chest and arms but keep the palms facing the floor. Their arms form a strong 'V' shape, backwards from shoulders through to fingers.

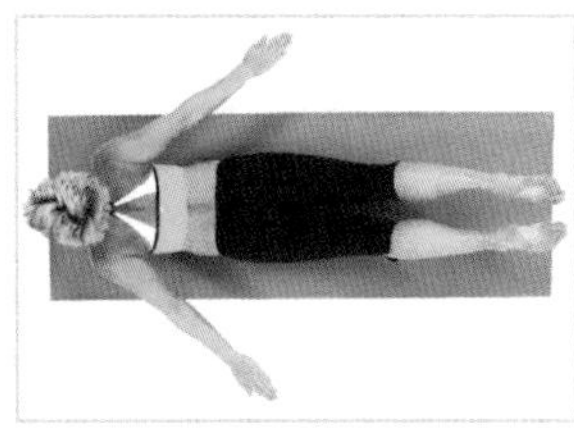

To do this you must wrongly cause an internal rotation of the shoulder and arm, which rolls the shoulders down and forward. This has a physically constricting effect on your ability to breathe deeply. The potentially damaging movement creates tension and strain in the shoulders, shoulder blades and neck.

The 'V' shape does appear in the properly executed pose, but it is almost an illusion. If you were to lie down on the floor and only lift the arms up from the 'T' position (leaving the legs and body down), then you would raise them in a purely vertical movement, anatomically described as posterior.*

The corresponding photograph illustrates the constant relationship of the arms to the shoulders and body. When you raise the upper body up off the floor you must preserve this relationship at all times whether you lift up a little or a lot. This means that there is no rotation through the shoulders.

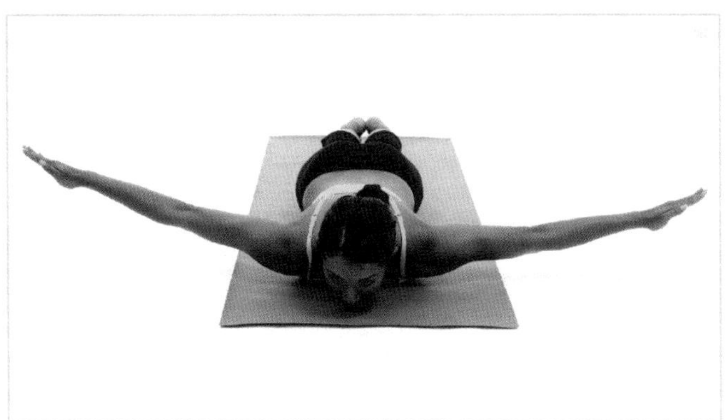

Poorna Salabhasana

Full Locust Pose

19

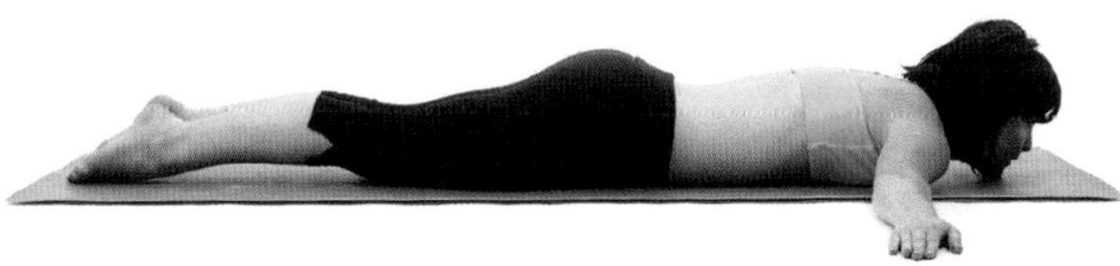

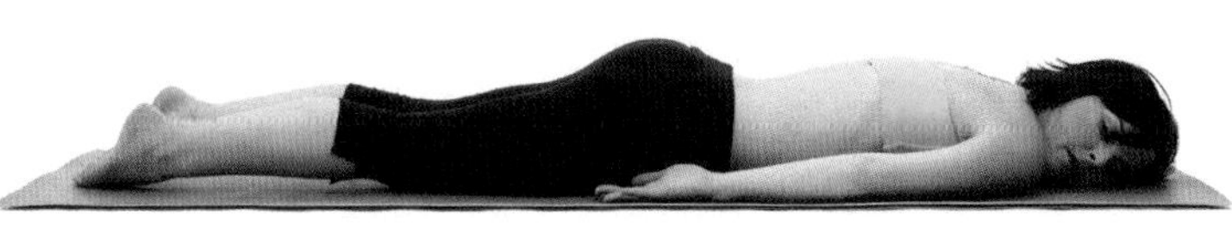

In other words, the higher your shoulders lift up due to your backbend, the more your palms will face the mirror. The more you can lift your arms posteriorly as in the photo example, the more exaggerated the 'V' shape will appear. Together they create the illusion that your arms are wilfully moving towards the back wall.

You can understand why the new student would wrongly perceive this as backward movement of the arms with downward facing palms. Read the chapter on arms for more hints and tips to proper movement.

Extend and lift your active arms without rotation as your shoulder blades come together in a squeeze.

Even though the following suggestion is not entirely correct, it would be better for you to imagine the backs of your hands (rather than your fingertips) approaching the back wall to fix this problem.

Your eyes: Look where you are going! Look up. Still, this is one very common place for students to watch themselves. And in some very wise words often uttered in class: "If you are looking at yourself now, then you are watching yourself doing the wrong posture".

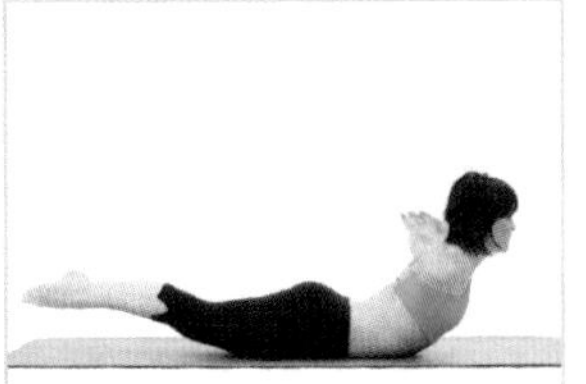

If you find it very difficult to look at the ceiling, you may need to free up introduced neck tension. Correct any arm rotation. Check that your palms are still in line with the fronts of your shoulders.

Your legs bend and separate: Often with the attempt to move legs higher, the feet move apart. Try to keep them together. The other error is to bend the legs rather than recruiting and building leg strength. Legs apart is the lesser of two evils. Primarily ensure that the legs are locked out and activated, then lift them.

Bypassing the release to get to Savasana: Students often release and go straight from their lifted position to their Savasana. Avoid bypassing the proper release: Check that you are neither turning your head to the side, nor angling your arms backward to your sides, as you descend. Simply reverse your pose.

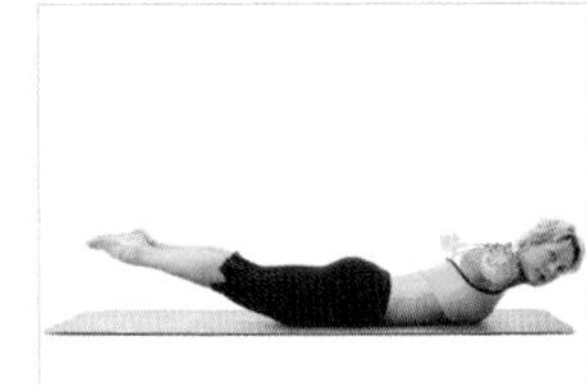

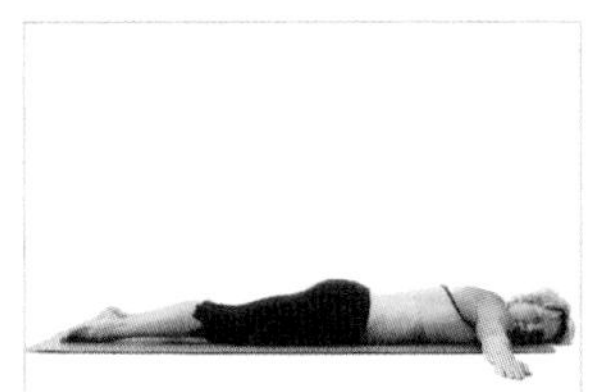

Dhanurasana

Some people think it's holding on that makes one strong; sometimes it's letting go.
—Sylvia Robinson

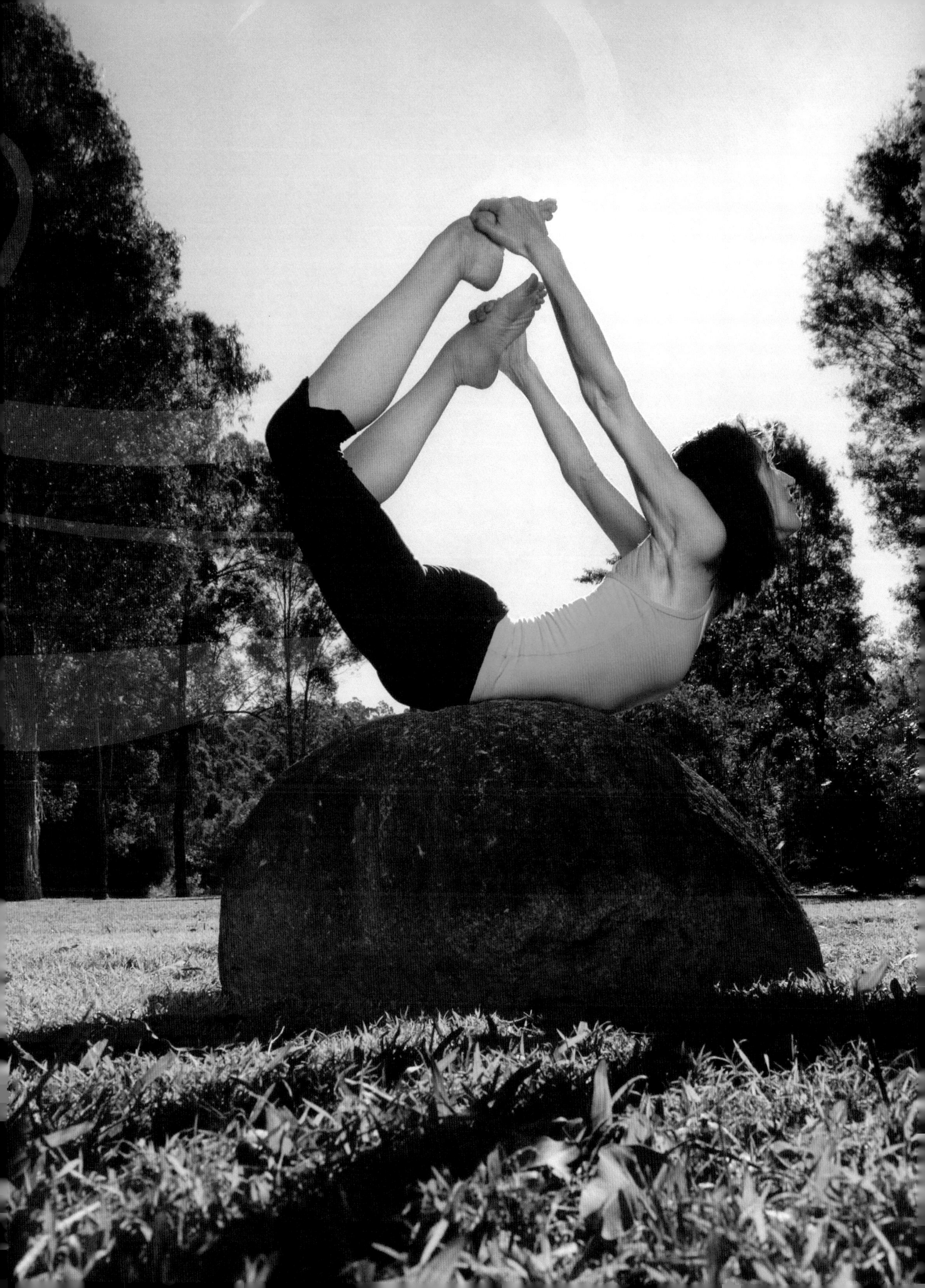

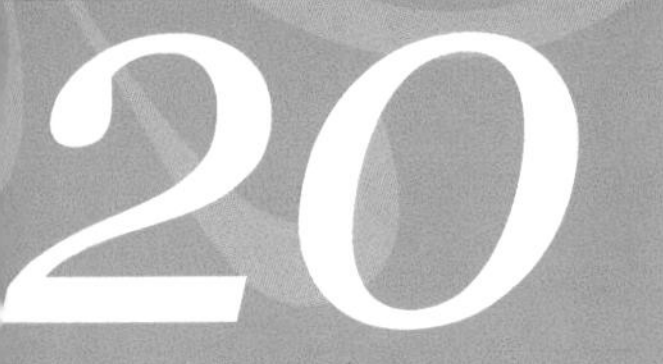

20 Dhanurasana

Floor Bow Pose

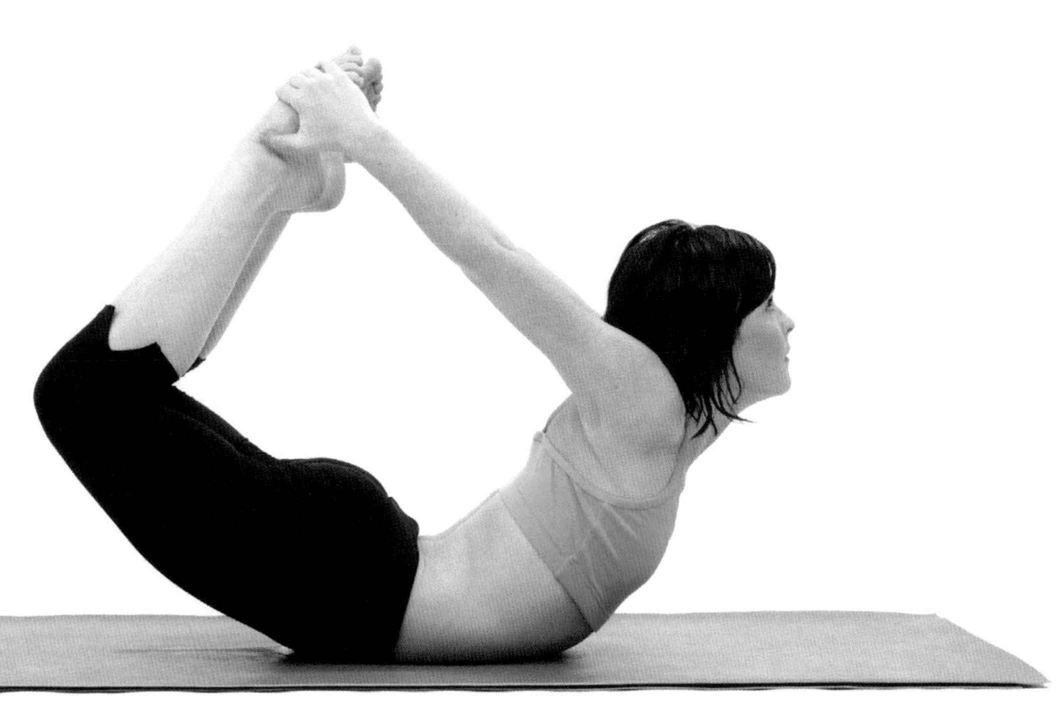

The essentials

This is the very last of the belly-down postures. By this stage in your class your muscles are usually very tired. Thankfully, this opens you up to yoga's transformative effects by diminishing your body's and mind's resistance and providing you with the potential for incredible breakthroughs. You carry these with you beyond class and it does translate to real and yet possibly unconscious skills in your life.

The last few seconds are crucial and need your committed staying power. It is through your great effort and mental determination that you find the way to be one with your body: The movement of breath; the stinging sensation in your kicking thighs; and the intensity in your hard-working muscles.

Don't think; breathe, do and breakthrough.

Representing beauty in balance, Floor Bow is as much about strength and kick, as it is about yield and release. Surrender to the breath and settle into a slower deeper rhythm and be surprised how quickly 20 seconds will pass. Find a sense of calm – not struggle – as you work hard through a calm slow deep breath.

What makes this pose so difficult to get right?

Somehow the impending effort combined with current flagging energy can have students dreading this strong pose. Procrastination may be more apparent around performing this pose than any other. Students may muck around and take longer to get the grip, they start late or finish early, and in doing so, reduce their practice to a set of physical exercises.

For some the hardest part is to actually grip the feet. A number will require the teacher's assistance. Most find challenge in overcoming feelings of tiredness, finding the wherewithal to push through their mental and physical limitations and really work hard. Many will find it hard to consciously allow their arms to lengthen and shoulders to release allowing a beautiful heart opening.

Dhanurasana

Floor Bow Pose

The technique

Bring your chin forward on your mat and bend up your legs.

1. **Your Legs**: Bend up your legs so that your heels are over your buttocks and your knees are close together.

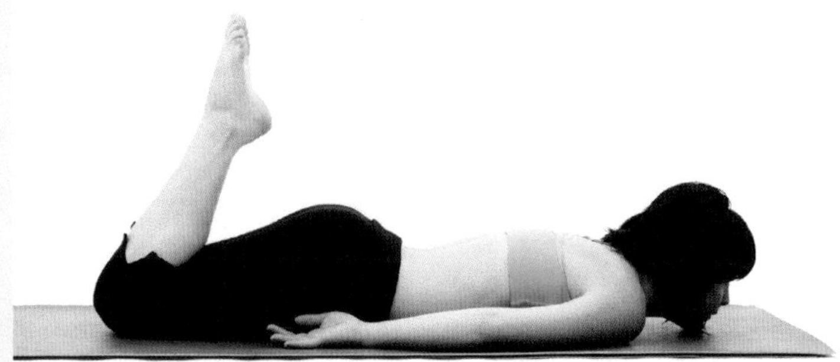

2. **Your Arms**: Reach back and grab each foot from the outside with all fingers together. Hook your hands around adjacent to the ball of the foot. Do what you can to relax your arms and shoulders to feel traction in your relaxed and lengthened wrists.

3. **The Kick Drives The Pose**: Inhale buoyancy in your chest and look up. On the exhale, strongly kick your feet back and your knees up, at the same time. Allow your body to come up off the floor. It is as if you are trying to kick your legs straight behind you but the grip on your feet is stopping you. The arms are quite passive – there is traction all the way from the shoulders to the hooked hands.

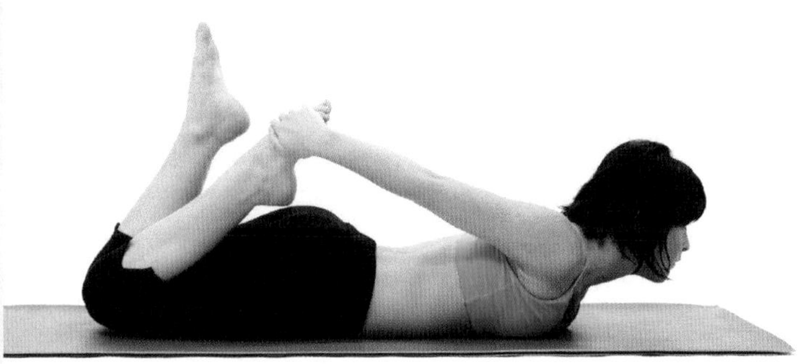

4. **Creating The Bow**: You can now feel why this is called bow. Your arms are part of the bow and the legs are the string. The increasing tension in the bow is replicated in the forceful kick of the legs. Feel them kick up off the ground to drive your feet further and further up over your head. Grow your ability to drive your thighs upwards. Naturally your spine arches in response to the effort.

5. **Your Bottom**: While you will squeeze your bottom to help you drive this pose allow the activation of the legs to take your focus. This way your lower spine will be free to create increasing freedom and flexibility. You will feel a pleasing compression in your lower spine too as your thighs burn a bit from the kick.

6. **Yield And Roll Forward**: Surrender to and continue working the kick. Consciously let the force of the kicking legs pull the shoulders behind you and roll forward onto the area between hips and ribcage. The more you kick, the more the arms and shoulders will open. Keep concentrating on looking up and further driving the legs up, right 'til the very last moment.

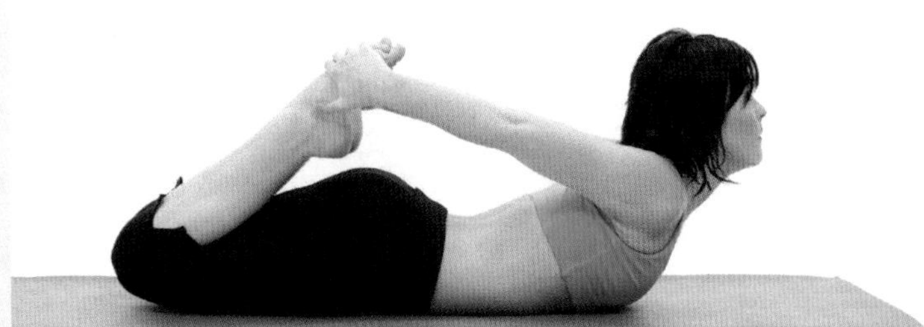

7. **The Wheel**: You may hear that legs and arms together form two parallel sides of a wheel. This analogy shows why the legs should not flare outward but stay in close at about hip distance apart.

20 Dhanurasana

Floor Bow Pose

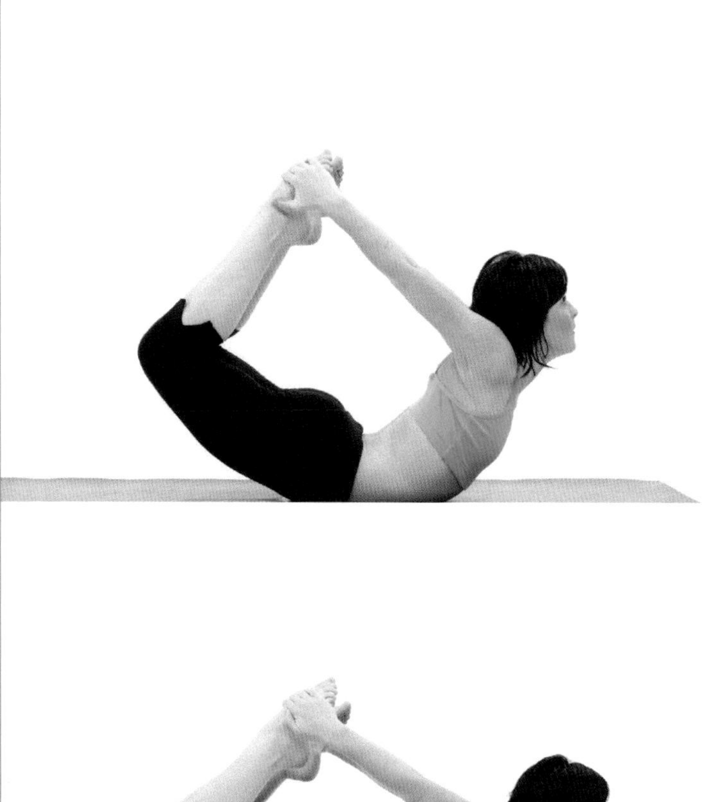

An advanced pose

If you managed to directly see your feet over the top of your head (and NOT just the reflection in the mirror) then you have an advanced pose to attempt but only in the second set. Bend up your legs. Extend your arms backward with an external rotation, your elbows in and palms facing out. Use your thumbs and forefingers to grip around your big toes.

On your inhale look up, and on your exhale press into your hands and simultaneously pull on your feet. Bend your elbows and bring them forward toward the mirror. Your arms will come toward each other, eventually parallel and possibly touching together at the elbows.

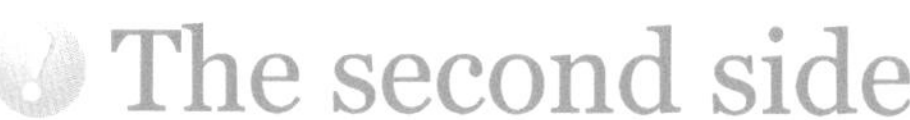

The second side

There are no special physical instructions. If you fell out early, try to push past where you were and take it right to the very last second. Check that you are using your eyes looking up and back and slowing your breath down. And of course kick, kick, kick.

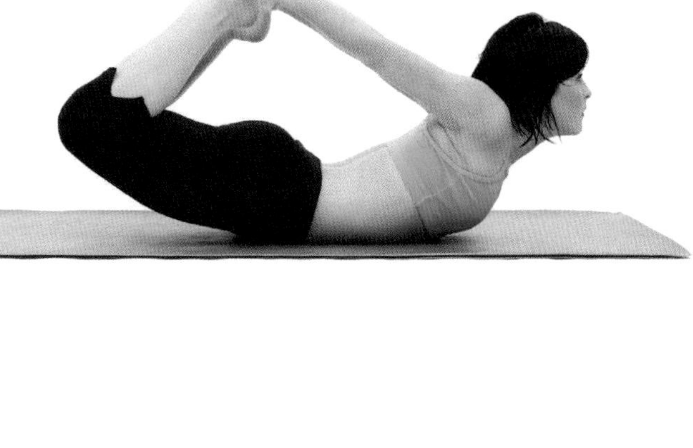

Release

Maintain a slow, deep and steady breath. Keep kicking with your strength while surrendering to the opening in your shoulders. Maintain the strength of your kick and work your legs even higher right to the last instant.

Then on release, keep your hands in position and allow your legs to come down with control, assisted by gravity. Don't flop out, don't let go of the grip, or drop your legs to the floor. Bring your head down to the floor so that the chin contacts centrally. Release your hands from your feet and allow your feet to come back down to the floor, toes together and heels apart. Feel that tremendous release in your lower spine and bottom. Let your arms relax and turn your head, your ear on the mat for Savasana.

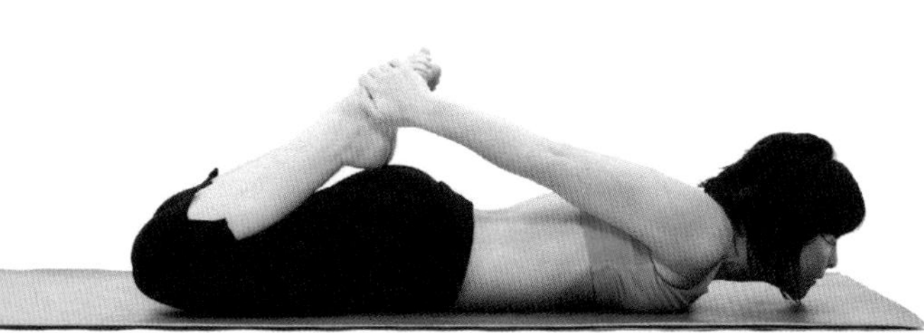

Common mistakes and how to fix them

Bending the arms: Pulling your arms against the kick to try and muscle your way into Floor Bow, is absolutely the wrong thing to do. It creates tension in the shoulders and neck. Kick against the hands so that the shoulders and arms are lengthened backwards in traction.

A range of incorrect grips: Do not grab at the toes, the arch or the ankle and do not allow the thumb to reach around onto the sole of the foot. Flexibility or injury may not allow the best grip, just do your best. Fingers and thumbs are together in a hook allowing the fingers to strengthen and the arms to lengthen in traction.

When you hold opposite the ball of the foot you create powerful traction from knees to toes. The difference in the ability to kick upwards powerfully is measurable. You feel an amazing stretch through the ankles, as your whole leg opens from hips through to toes.

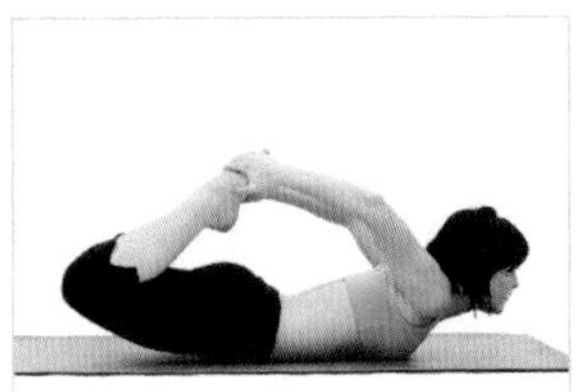

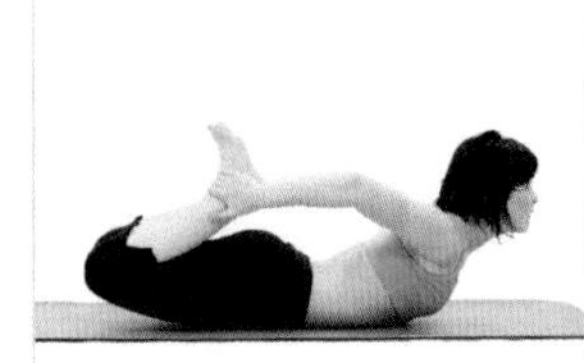

Flexing the feet: This is counterproductive. Try it once to see why you must try to point the toes. Flexing the feet causes you to hold at the ankles. And conversely, holding at the ankles causes you to flex the feet.

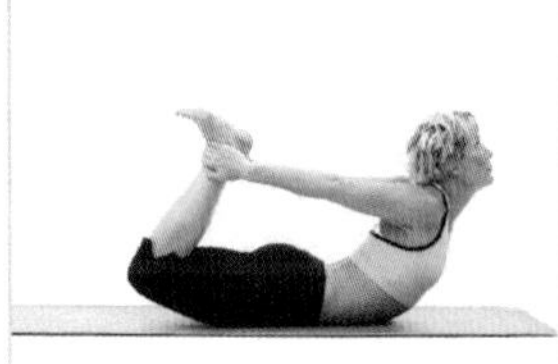

The kick involved in both the Standing and the Floor Bows, can be broken down into a backward kick involving the lower leg, and an upward one, driven by the thigh and the hip.

Because the ankle flexes, a downward force is introduced, working against the upward power of the thigh. This can make it difficult to move the knee away from the floor as far as you would like, and harder to move the leg upwards.

Can't reach your feet: You may need to get the assistance of a teacher to gently press each foot toward the buttock as you reach back with each hand. If you really can't reach then you may need to lay a rolled towel under your ankles and lift and draw your legs into position as you readjust the grip on the towel.

A small problem with this approach is that if you don't get help with the final towel grip, there will always be extra slack in the towel. Your feet will flex when gripped in this way. See above. The towel grip forces biceps involvement and the arms to bend outward in a way that goes against the pure technique described above. Just do your best to minimize unnecessary movements.

As a beginner, reaching back on your own can be risky as you have to twist your body to reach the towel. Be careful, and try to make your movements symmetrical.

Your knees: Flaring knees out to the side should be avoided. Aim to kick them high off the floor, keeping legs parallel.

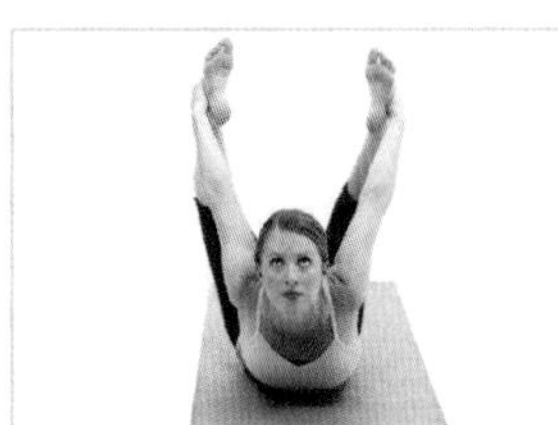

Procrastination and anticipation: The poses of most effort are the ones that people are most likely to delay getting into or come out of early. Cut out the thinking and do the yoga. It is not at all in the spirit of meditation to ponder any thoughts. Focus on your breath. I find it easiest to slow down the breath and keep it moving. The slower the breath the less number of breaths to get to the end of your 20 seconds, the faster the time seems to pass.

Looking at yourself: Don't look forward into your own eyes or check out the height of your legs. Otherwise you are watching yourself doing the wrong pose. Look up and behind you toward the ceiling or back wall if possible.

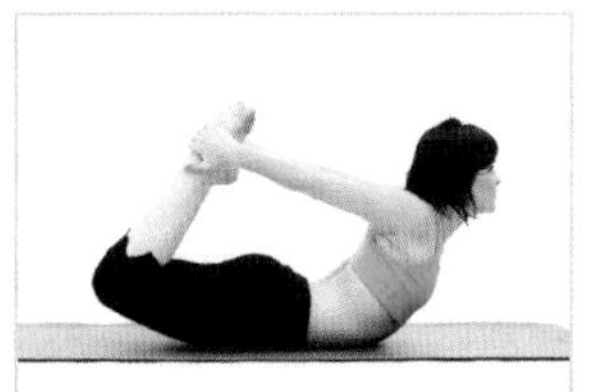

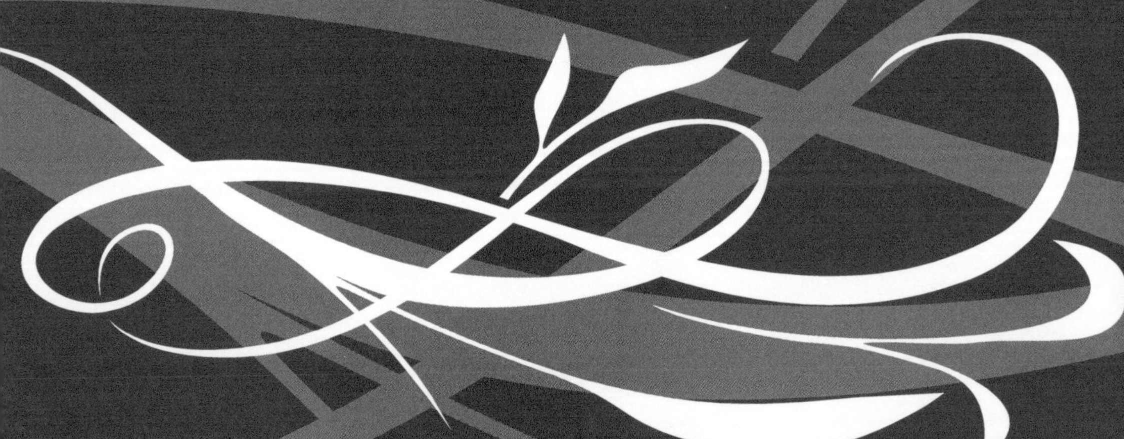

Suptavajrasana

Difficulty is the excuse history never accepts.
—Edward R. Murrow

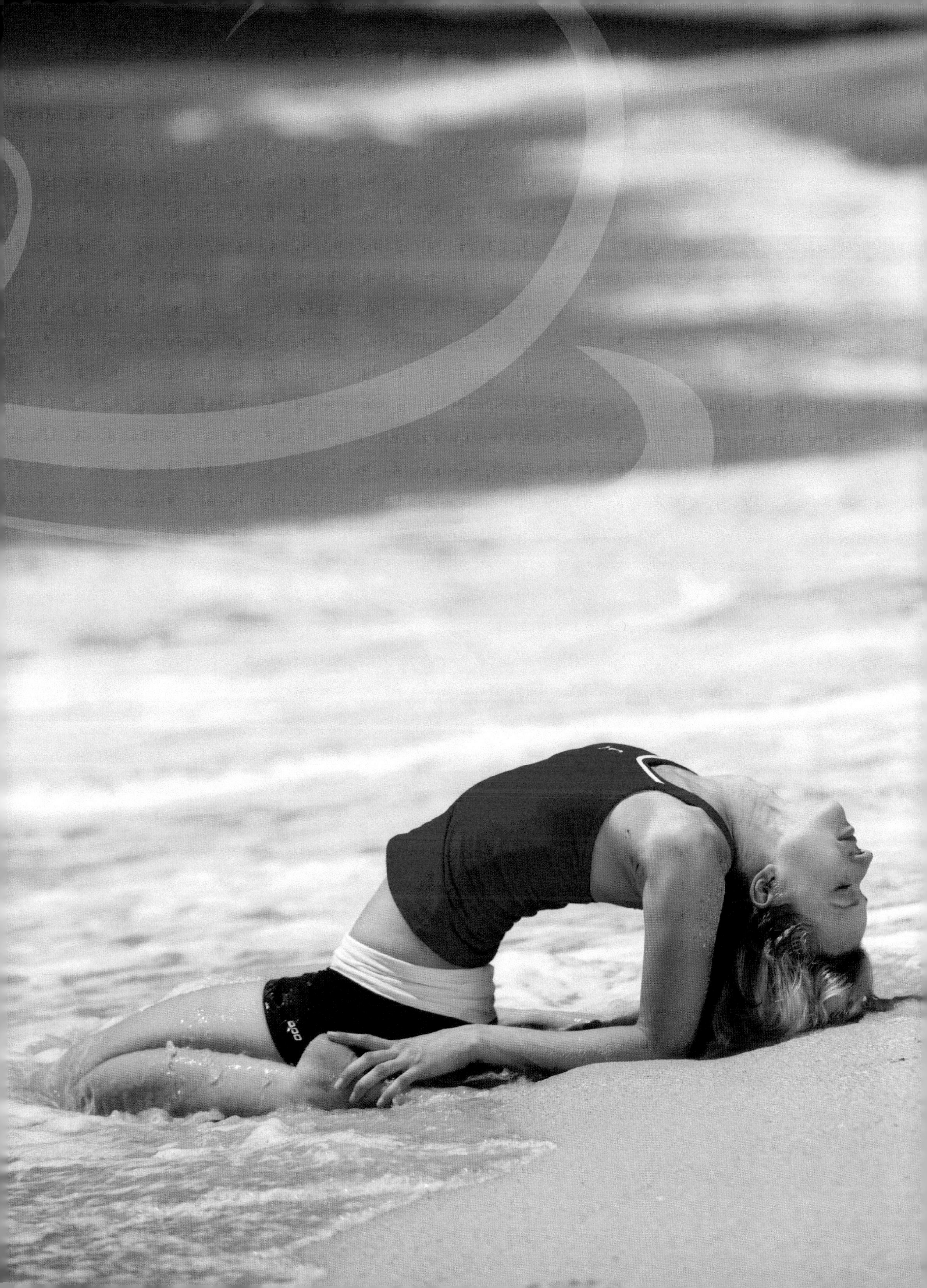

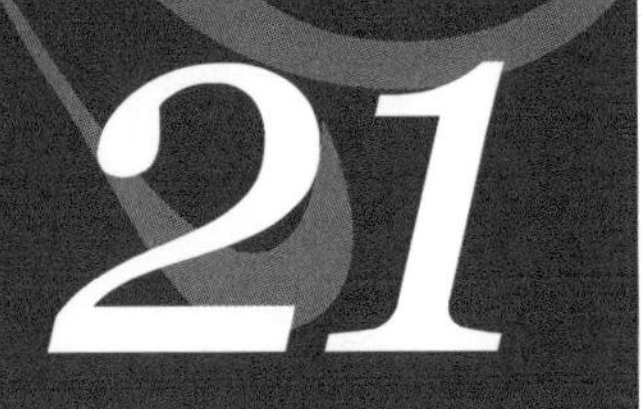

Suptavajrasana

FIXED FIRM POSE

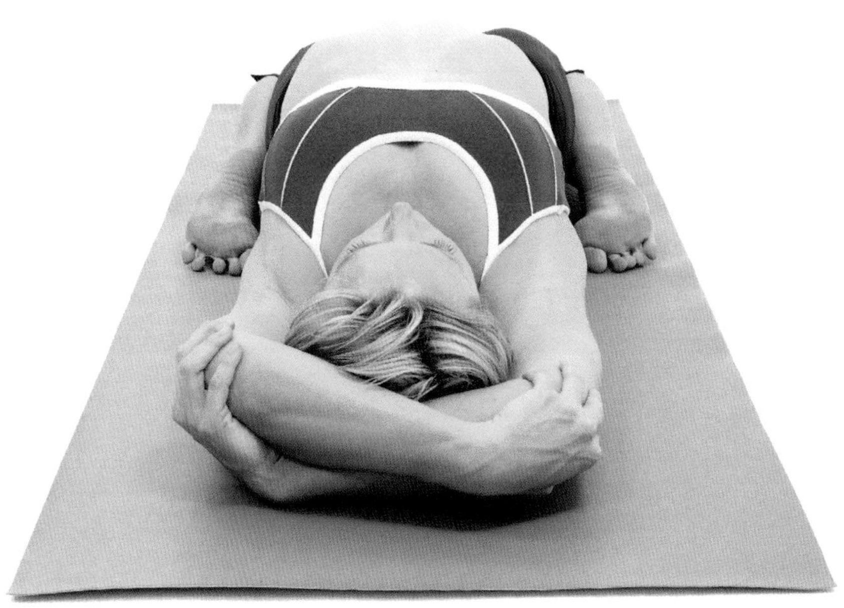

The essentials

There are four distinct stages to this pose. Each part has certain critical elements which must be achieved before proceeding further. The aims are; to open shoulders, hips, ankles and knees; to create a backbend and a powerful stretch down the front side of the body; and work strongly into and regulating many hormonal systems squeezing and compressing various organs including kidneys, pancreas and thyroid glands.

Apart from yoga and dancing there is really no other way you are going to get that fantastic ankle stretch spanning your toes and shin. I have had countless students who have proclaimed through tears of joy after surprisingly few classes (sometimes only three) that it is the first time in 20 years that they can once again sit on the floor with feet facing backwards.

What makes this pose so difficult to get right?

The most challenging element is to get the leg positions correct. These may be difficult due to injury or illness, or the relationship of feet and hips could be wrong due to lifelong habit. A major focus will be to protect your knees from over-twisting.

Remember that the final destination is not as important as respecting where your body is supposed to be. So at any stage you must stop if you have too much resistance to proceed. Your ego can be your biggest enemy. Don't let where you want to be get confused with where you ought to be.

Interestingly, what can complicate matters is the fact that the exit of this pose is not the exact reversal of the entry.

Suptavajrasana

FIXED FIRM POSE

21

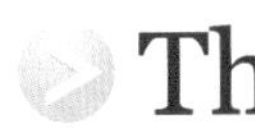

The technique

Moving out of Savasana

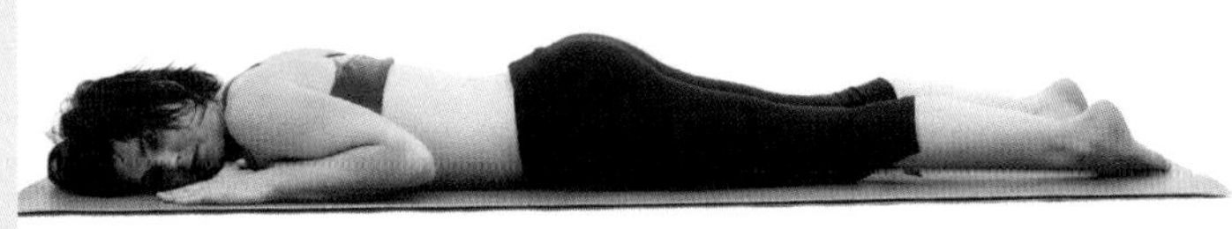

Fixed Firm completes a set of five strong backbends. So how do you get to your knees without introducing an unwarranted forward bend and counteracting the solid backbend work of the belly-down poses?

Some contention exists over the way many students place the bottom back onto the heels (as if on a prayer mat). It does feel good to do it but it is unnecessary and is borne out of habit alone. There may be occasion where this extra movement has merit but on the whole simply move from lying to sitting as described below.

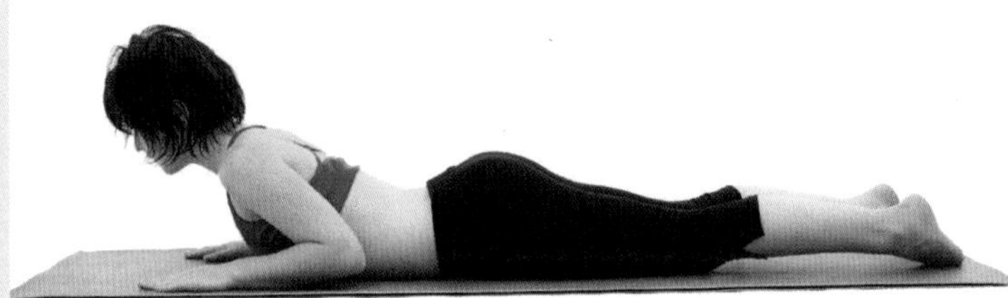

You can get up off the floor in one of two ways.

1. Push up from the floor with your arms, with palms down under shoulders. Look up, squeeze the bottom and legs and get a great frontal stretch. Now raise the bottom off the floor so that you are momentarily standing on all fours. Almost simultaneously, walk on your knees to the top of the mat.
2. Or you can do the same as above without the big backward stretch. Simply push off the floor and get into position.

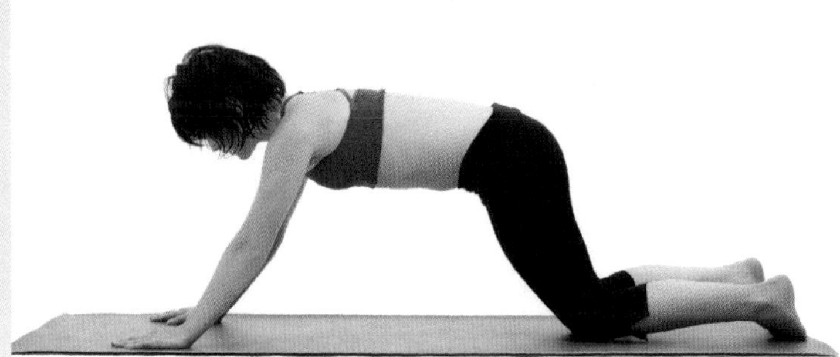

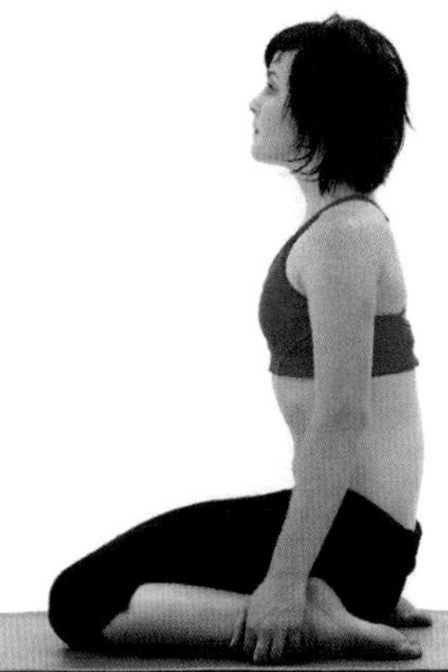

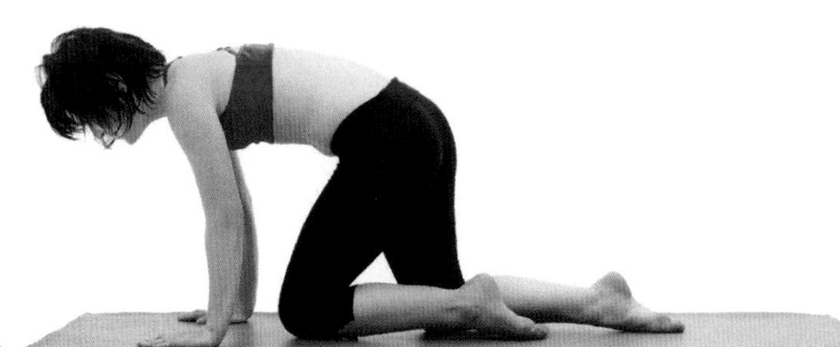

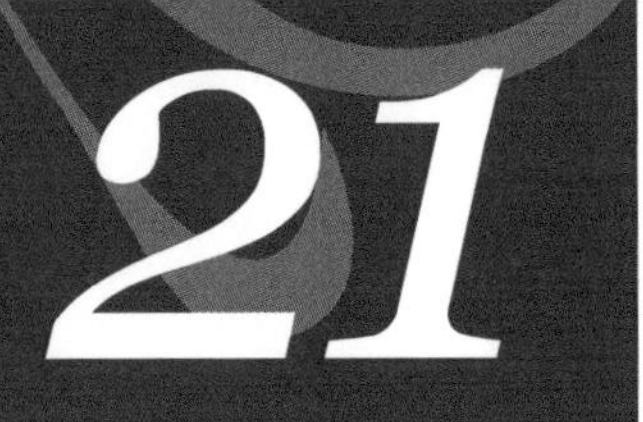

Suptavajrasana

Fixed Firm Pose

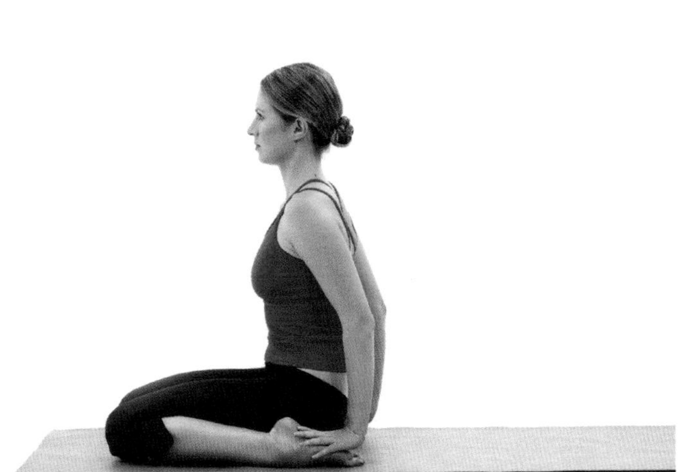

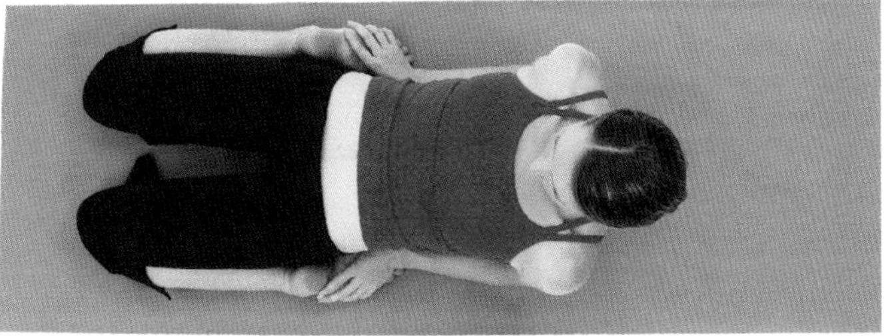

Stage 1: Sitting in fixed firm pose.

Now that you are up at the top of your mat you are to sit on your knees.

1.1 **Sit, Your Heels Touch Hips**: Sitting in fixed firm pose means that you sit down, bottom on the floor, with your knees ahead of you. Your heels MUST be touching your hips no matter what. Space between hips and heels brings an unnecessary and potentially damaging knee-twisting element.

1.2 **Your Feet Point Back**: Ideally your feet are parallel and face backwards. More correctly however because not everyone can sit with knees together, the feet extend a straight line from the knee through the ankle to the toes.

1.3 **Your Ankles Flat**: The fronts of your ankles are stretched open and lie flat against the floor (neither rolling in nor out).

1.4 **Your Knees In Or Out**: Knees can be as far apart as they need to be, but hips must always be touching heels.

1.5 **Your Bottom Down**: Your aim for the first part of the pose is to work your bottom onto the floor between your heels. This is a PREREQUISITE for proceeding any further in the pose.

Checklist for proceeding to Stage 2

In order to proceed further you must fully comply with all four points below.

- No pain in knees (remember comfortable discomfort is normal and good)
- Your hips are touching your heels
- Your knees may be apart (you can work on moving them back together in time)
- And your bottom is on the floor.

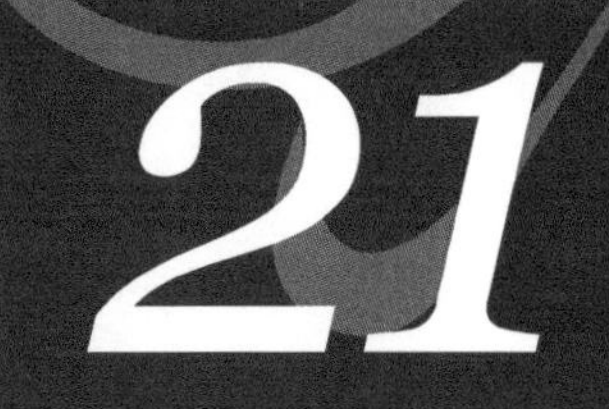

Suptavajrasana

Fixed Firm Pose

Stage 2

2.1 **Hands On Feet**: Place your hands on your feet. Your fingers face forwards toward the mirror and thumbs on the inside.

2.2 **Support Yourself On Your Elbows**: With hands in place, slowly bring your right elbow down to the floor directly behind you, lowering your body down on that side. Then bring your left elbow down.

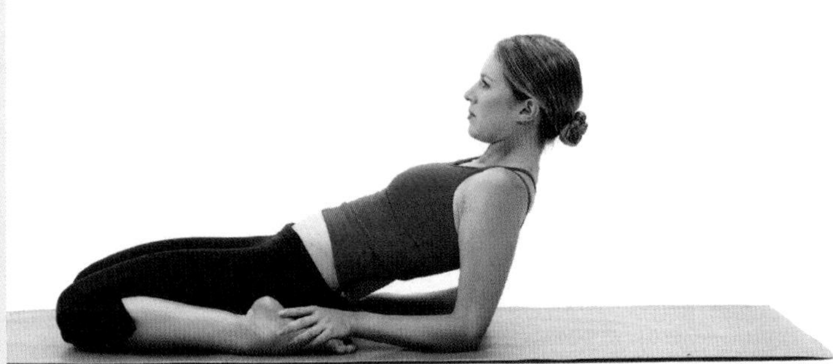

2.3 **Your Neck Relaxed**: If both elbows are down and there is no undue tension through the legs, hips or back, allow your neck to completely soften. Let your head go back and look back, trying to get your head to touch the floor.

2.4 **Your Head To The Floor**: This is the gateway to Stage 3. Stay here developing sufficient opening in your body to eventually rest your head on the floor. If you can do so with your knees anchored on the floor then you are safe to go further.

2.5 **Going Back, Bottom And Knees Down**: If your knees and/or bottom lift off the floor then stop and reassess. Either come out a little way or adjust your knees outward to provide optimal support. Often all it takes is to move your knees further apart to get your head down and feel more stable. Remember, as long as your hips are touching your heels - with tops of feet flat on the floor - your knees should be safe.

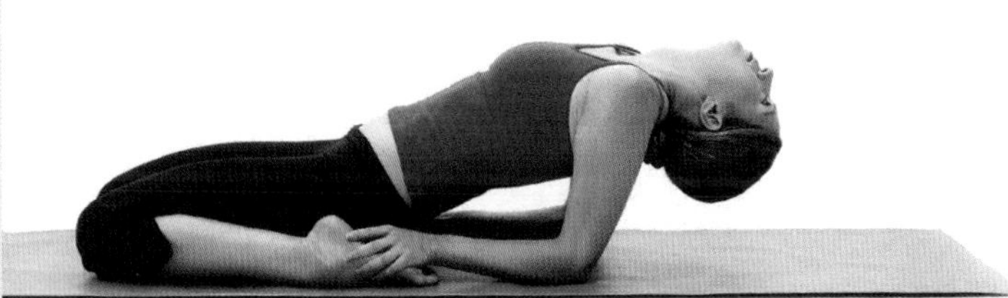

Stage 3

3.1 **Move Your Elbows**: When the top of your head touches the floor start to move your shoulders and the back of your head to the floor, by allowing your elbows to move away from the body.

3.2 **Arch Your Spine**: Arch your spine as high as you can between well-anchored shoulders and hips. Feel the enormous traction and stretch on the front side of your body.

3.3 **Your Knees Contact Floor**: The knees must be in contact with the floor. As long as the feet are in good position and the bottom is on the floor, the knees can be at any distance apart.

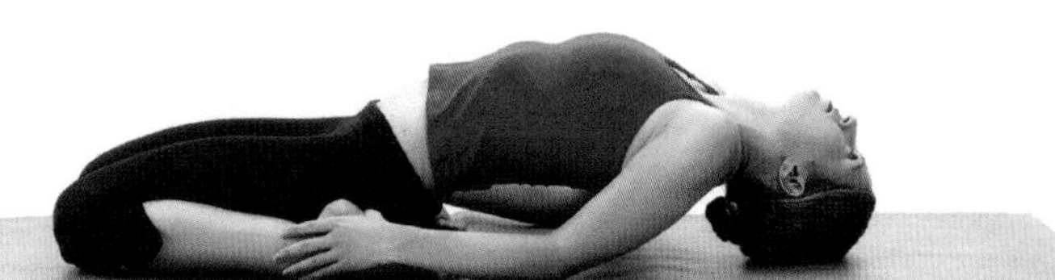

3.4 **Tuck Your Chin**: The aim is to tuck your chin to lengthen your cervical spine and further anchor your hips and shoulders. You get tremendous thyroid compression here.

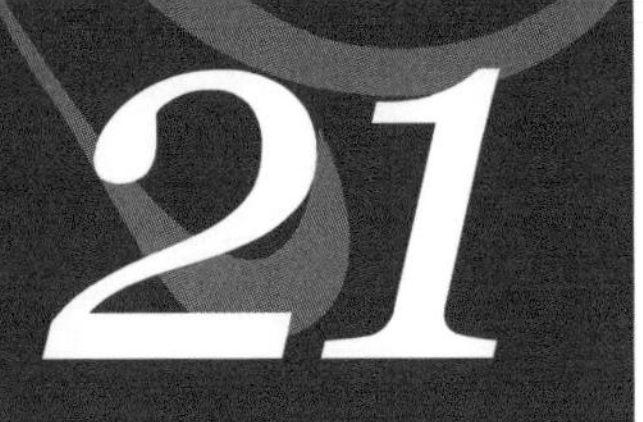

Suptavajrasana

Fixed Firm Pose

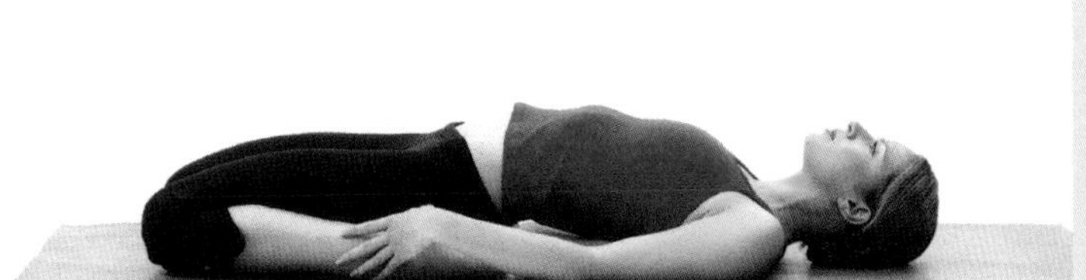

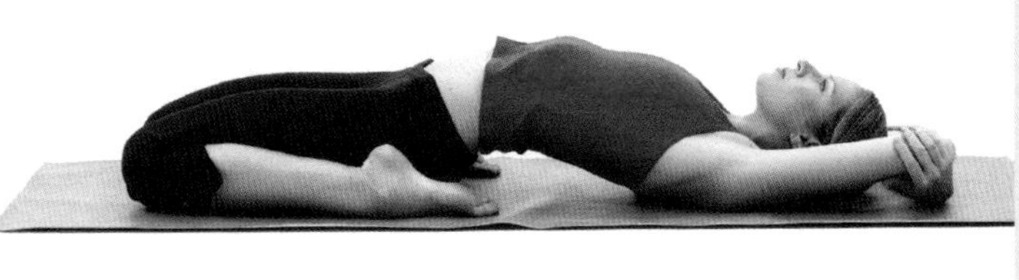

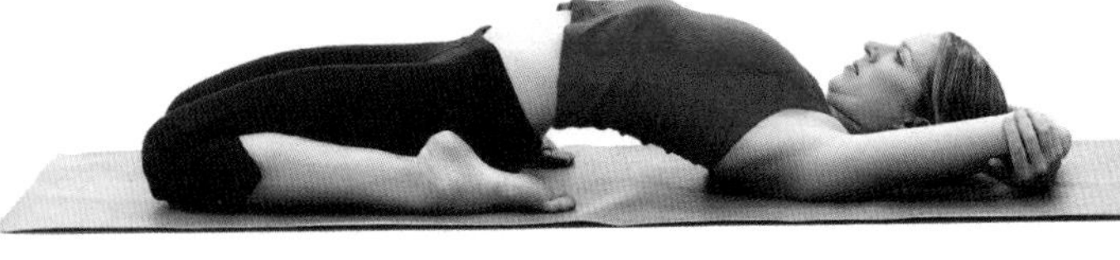

3.5 **Easy Slow Breath**: It should be quite easy to slow the breath down and breathe directly into your belly. Tucking the chin may hinder the breath somewhat but the more experienced you are, the easier it is to work through this slight impediment.

3.6 **The Comfort Factor**: You are lying back on the floor. For some this pose is difficult. They really feel the stretch and the discomfort, and for some, the pain as they progress through the stages. With persistence comes reward and comfort! If the discomfort is too great then briefly see if widening the knees helps. If not then either stay put or retreat to the last pain-free position. Once you make it to the floor it is a pleasing repose and often so comfortable that students don't want to come out! If 'comfortable' then proceed.

Stage 4

4.1 **Your Arms In A Square**: If you are not struggling now and are 'comfortable', bring your arms over your head and grasp your elbows. The elbows and shoulders form the corners of a square. Imagine 4 sides firmly pressing down into the floor.

4.2 **Draw Your Shoulders Closer To Your Hips**: Push your elbows into the floor. Work your shoulders away from your ears, closer to your hips and your shoulder blades more broadly and positively pressing into the floor. It surprises some that this posture is not about laying your spine flat on the floor. A maximally arched spine like a bridge in the torso is what you are aiming for. The proximal supports are the hips and the shoulder blades, strongly connecting with the floor.

4.3 **Tuck Your Chin**: Tuck the chin to elongate and decompress the neck. You will more easily and forcefully draw down the elbows and shoulders.

4.4 **Plant Your Lower Spine**: Keep planting your sacrum into the floor. Feel the opening traction between your shoulders and your hips.

4.5 **Your Knees Together And Down:** The eventual aim is to have maximum spinal arch and positive contact of the shoulders, hips and knees on the ground; with knees as close together as possible. The moment knees come off the ground, move them apart just enough to reaffirm contact. Do not let the knees come together if the lower spine comes up off the floor.

Release

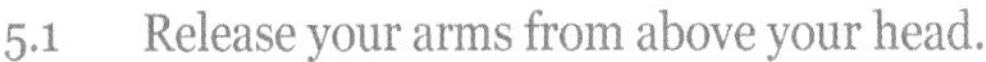

The exit from this pose is not an exact reversal of the entry so extra care must be taken in order to stay safe. It is crucial to leave your head back behind you as you bring yourself up from the floor with your body completely supported by your arms and balanced by your legs. Precise details follow.

To exit:

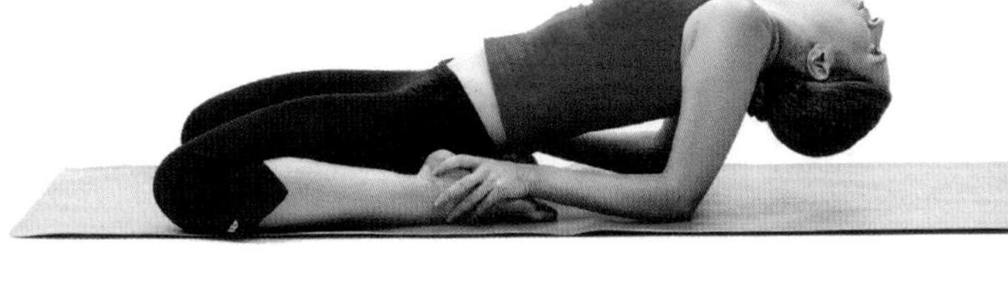

5.1 Release your arms from above your head.
5.2 Bring your hands onto your feet, fingers forward.
5.3 Bring yourself onto your elbows again, letting your head stay dropped back on soft neck muscles.
5.4 Widen your knees (further) at this point. Spreading the knees brings your center of gravity forward (shifts your hips), plants your knees so you can spread the load to bring yourself safely up off the floor.
5.5 When you are halfway you may need to reposition your hands behind your hips to support your torso as you ascend.
5.6 Bring your head up last and make contact. Slide onto your right leg and spin around as you extend your legs to the back wall. Then simply and efficiently lie down in Savasana.

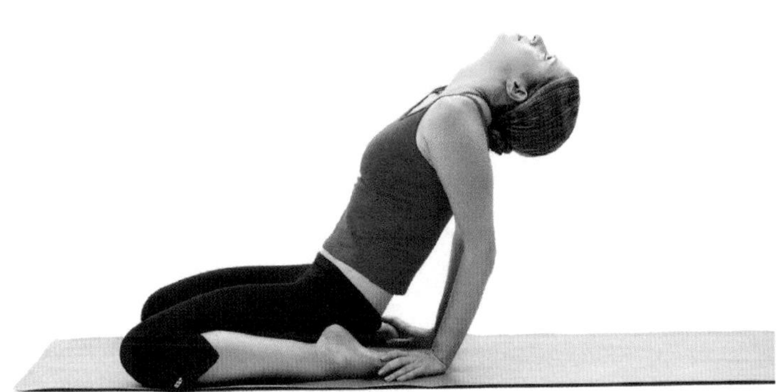

Your sit-up brings you into the second set. On releasing out of second set, slide onto your left side and move into Savasana. If you are genuinely unable to do your sit-ups please refer to the Savasana chapter which details the floor-facing rest pose.

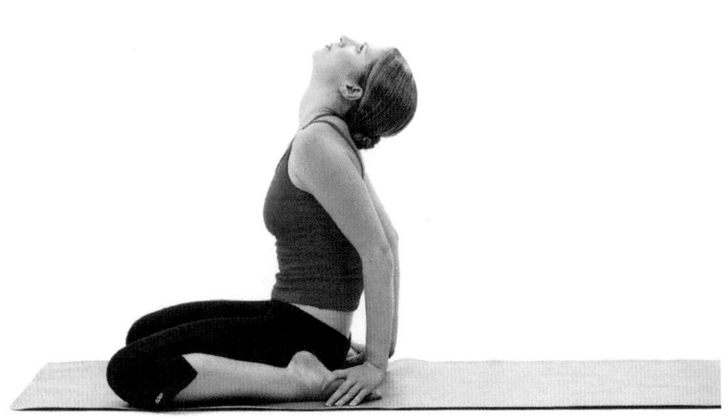

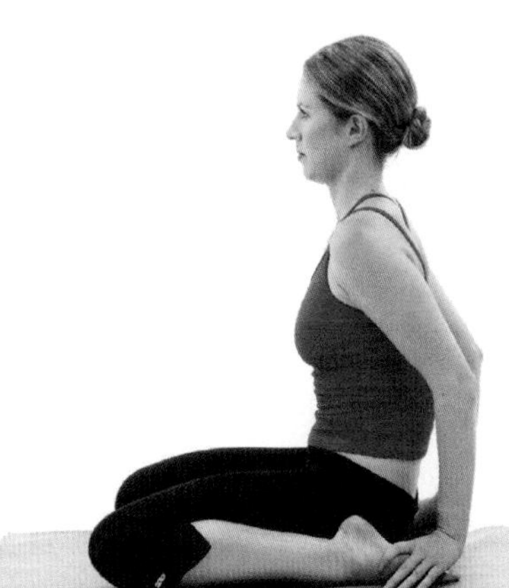

21 Suptavajrasana

FIXED FIRM POSE

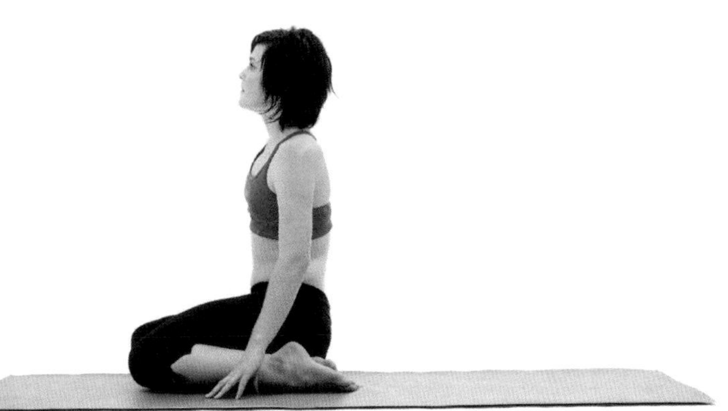

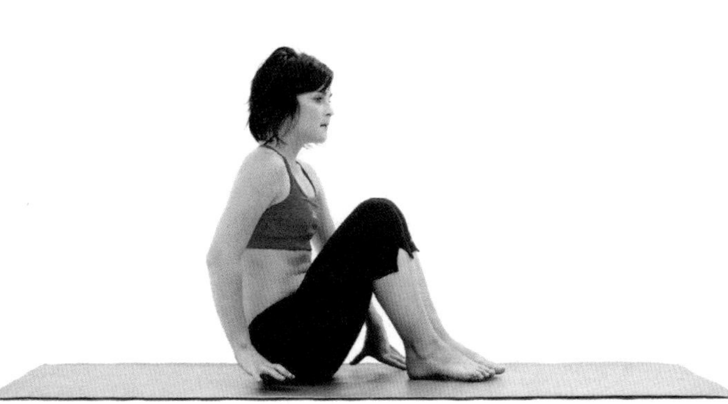

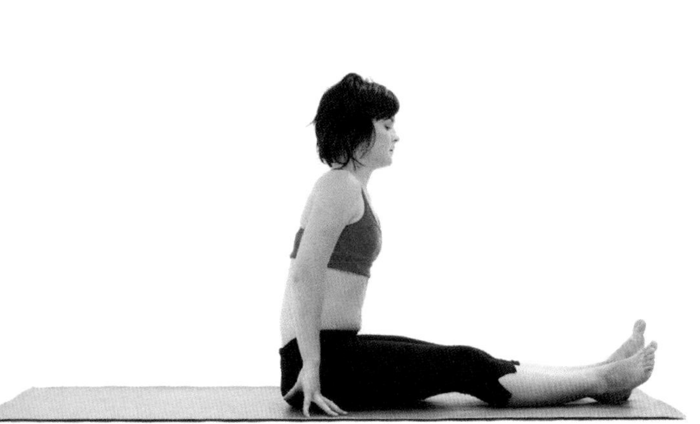

Common mistakes and how to fix them

Pain in your knees: If you are feeling pain in your ligaments, particularly on the inside edge of your knee (medially) then you can try two different things. Firstly try to move your knees apart keeping your heels touching your hips. You should feel more comfortable and more stable. The feet will no longer be parallel so keep a straight line from the knee through the ankle to the toes. For second solution please see directly below.

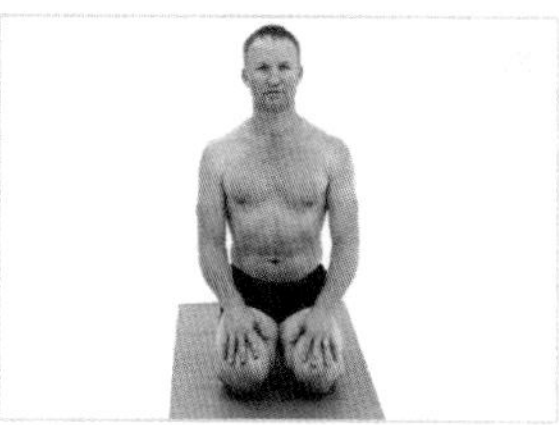

***A restorative pose for the knees**: If you can still feel that pain (not just discomfort) then sit in a true kneeling position by drawing your knees and feet together. This is a very strong and restorative pose for the knees. It will counter the severe and damaging knee-twisting forces that you felt. Keep this up until your knees stabilize.

One point to emphasize: If you are kneeling then your bottom is obviously not touching the floor. This means you must stay in Stage 1 of the pose. Breathe through the opening of your knees and ankles. Be patient.

Little by little, over time move your heels apart to create the space for your hips. Move your knees apart as required. Use your hands against the floor for support to buffer any pain. Stay strong and tall sitting on your ankles. Regardless of your ability to take your body back, you are to stay with your body vertical until the day your bottom touches the floor.

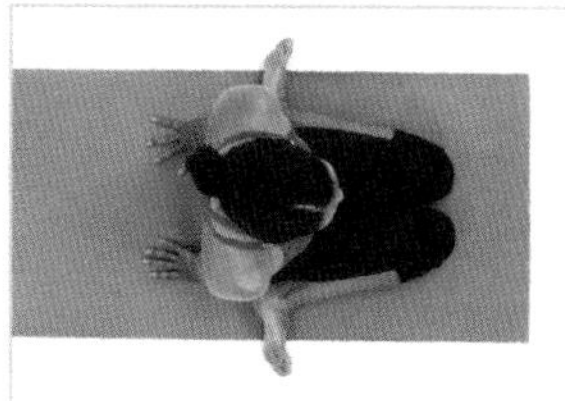

Inside of flexed feet against floor: Sitting with your legs and feet in a 'W' formation (with the insides of your feet contacting the floor) is a dangerous position. This is normally a habit carried through from infancy. It underlies problems of knees and hip support, and indicates leg weakness. The tops of your feet must be on the floor regardless of the ease in which you get into the wrong position. It may take quite a number of classes (even simply kneeling) to work the opening into your ankles and sit correctly. You will have to take a lot of the strain with your hands on the floor to stop you sitting too heavily at first.

Leaning back on your hands to get bottom to floor: Your bottom must get to the floor without performing this little trick. Get firm contact without the use of your hands and preferably with a tall straight spine (not slouching). Patience again, and not ego, is the key.

21 Suptavajrasana

Fixed Firm Pose

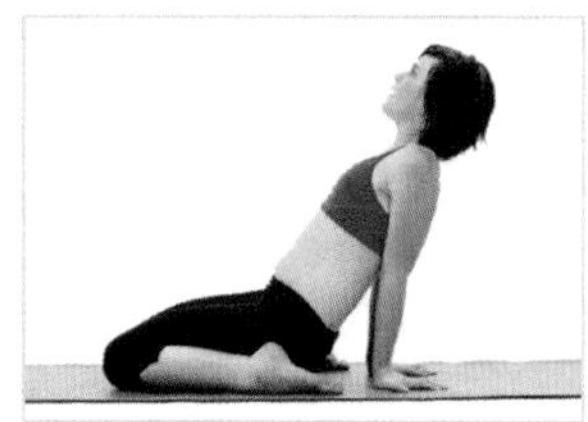

Fingers face backwards when leaning back: If your fingers face backwards then your arms can only be straight. This means that support is an all-or-nothing proposition. Your arms must have the capacity to bend when lowering your body in Stage 2. Fingers forward means your arms can amply support the body all the way down to the floor as the elbows bend, allowing you to back out safely if needed.

Bottom lifts off floor: If your bottom lifts at any time, then you have proceeded too far in one or more basic pose elements. Moving from Stage 1 – 2 you may have to reverse your body off the floor. You must act to re-establish bottom contact (and knees on floor). Try first to widen your knees. This shifts your center of gravity forward and grounds your hips (and will re-establish knee contact if they too are airborne). You will feel your sacrum and shoulders drive into the floor as the arch in your spine deepens creating better stretch and traction.

Knees together but feet away from hips: The reverse of this mistake is far better on the body. Try bringing the knees apart and slide the feet back into hip contact. Maintain the straight line between toes and knees through ankles.

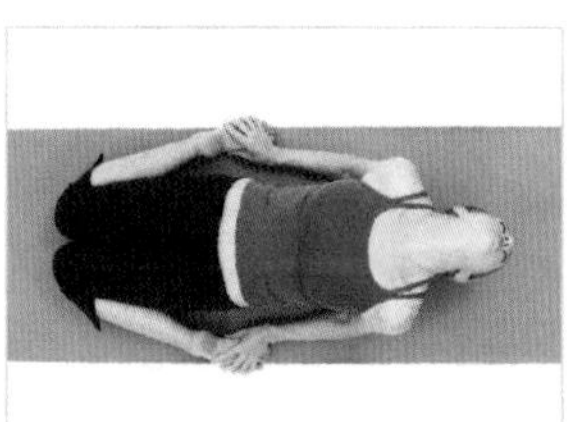

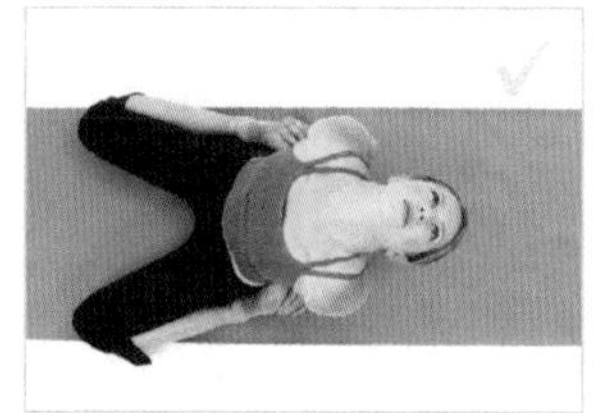

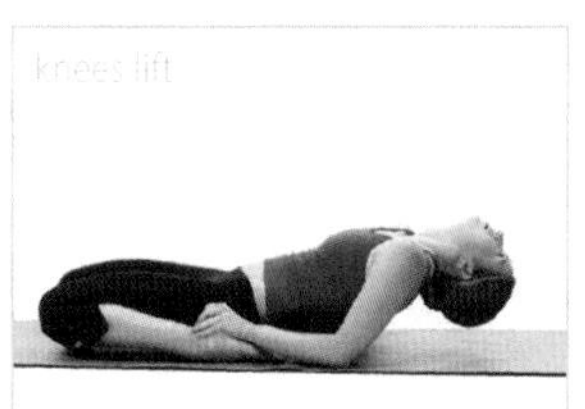

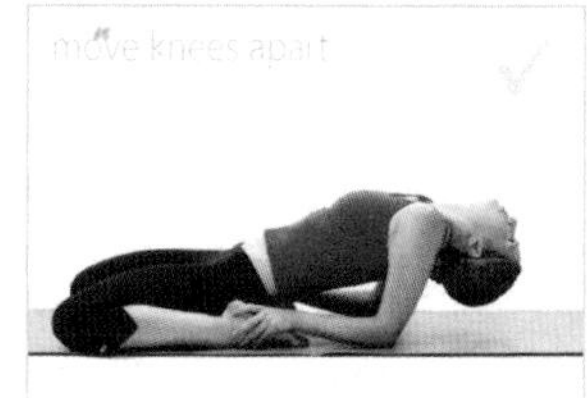

Knees lift: If your knees lift when trying to get your elbows or head to the floor then adjust the knee distance and bring your body back up a bit. If you are all the way back, arch your spine more and check if altering knee distance helps you. Draw your shoulders closer to the hips and feel your pelvis tilt forward.

Shoulders come off floor: Usually this will happen when you enter Stage 4, bringing your arms up over your head. Think of your task requirement as bringing your shoulder blades to the floor and tucking your chin. Not only is it more clearly defined but you work on moving your shoulders closer to your hips and resolve neck tension. No shrugging!

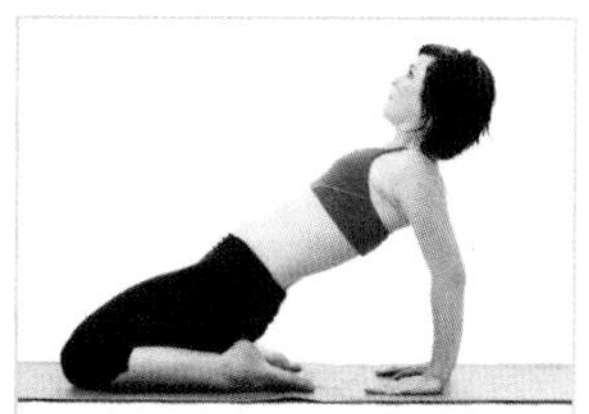

Letting ego get the better of you: Often, students who have been trying to proceed further for a long time (from any stage), typically allow their ego to drive the depth of the pose. The most common is going from Stage 1-2 without the bottom on the floor. Less commonly they move from 2-3 without their knees (or bottom) on the floor; and from 3-4 without their shoulders (or even knees or bottom) contacting.

As a teacher it is frustrating to see students go further without the basics. I am sure they are thinking "I should be there by now, so damn it, I'm going". Back off and do it right. Letting the ego take over obviously dilutes the benefits. Take the struggle out, proceed with care and patience.

Hanging out comfortably: Those comfortable here can still work hard in this pose. Hanging out is easy, so provide some extra challenge. You could simply breathe deeply and mindfully follow your breath. What better way to enhance your meditation and be in the moment? On a physical level you could work on contacting your 'bridge' abutments into the earth, shifting your arms and shoulders towards your hips and driving your lower spine and knees downward, to create improved traction.

Neck stiffens on entry and exit: Holding your head up with tense neck muscles can strain a cocktail of muscles. Besides compromising your lower back (making it work when it doesn't have to), the muscles in your neck and down the entire front of your abdomen all tense in response as they try to help you up. This negates your good effort and the benefits of your following precious Savasana.

The purpose of this pose is to s t r e t c h the muscles down the front of your body. Leave your head back and use your arms to lower or raise you. You will keep your neck muscles passive, as the posture requires.

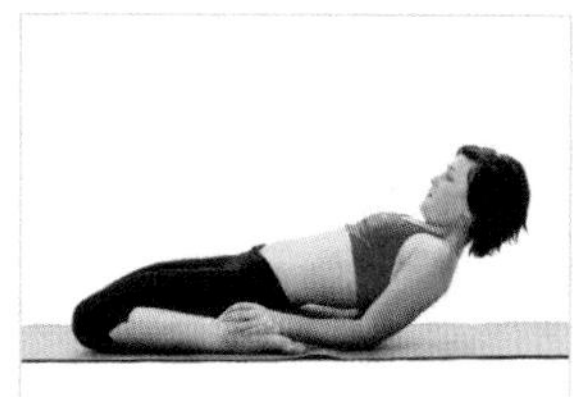

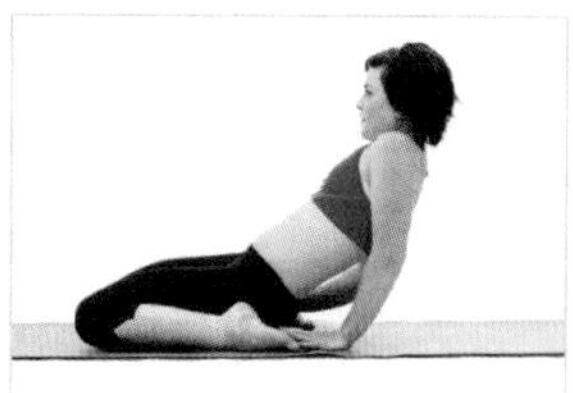

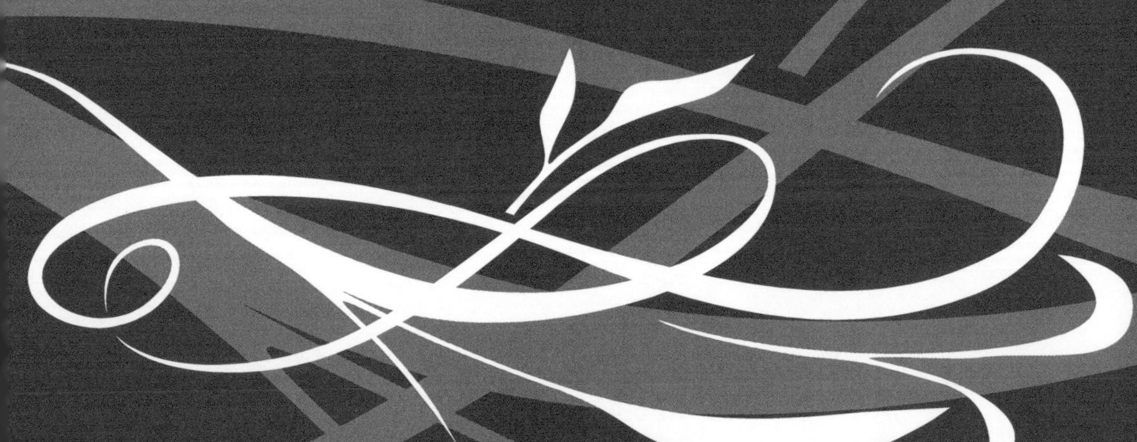

Ardha Khurmasana

Do not dwell in the past,
do not dream of the future,
concentrate the mind on the
present moment.
—Buddha

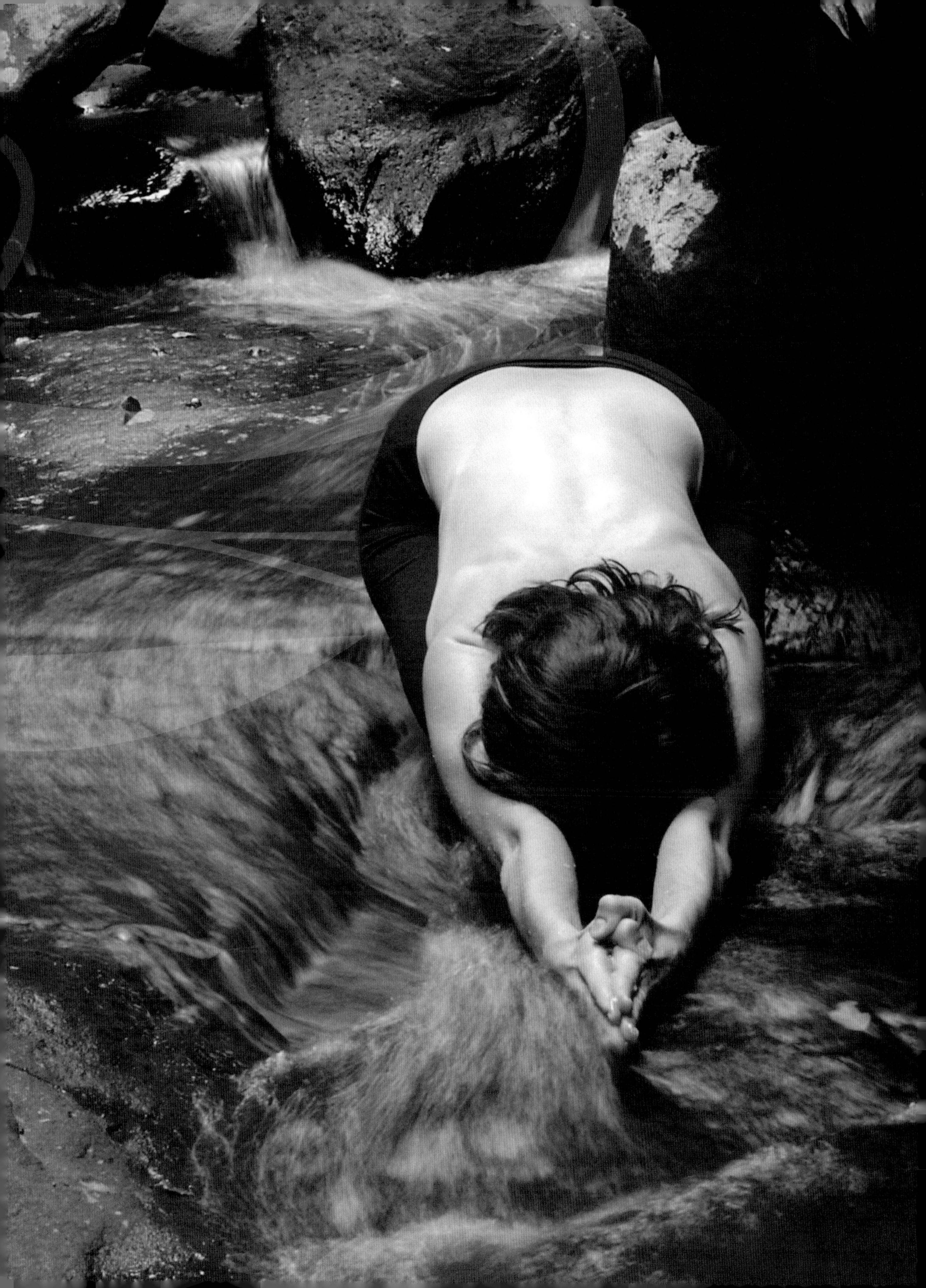

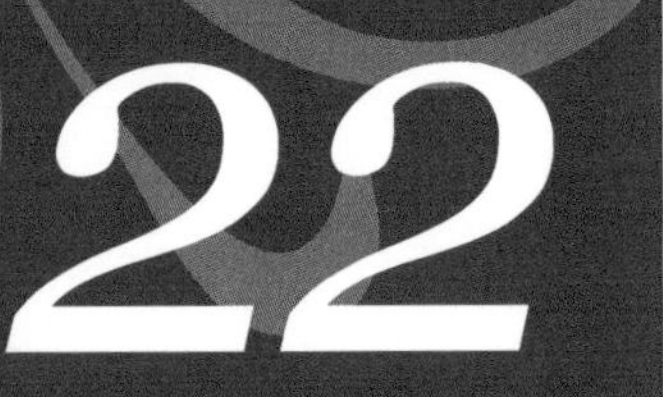

Ardha Khurmasana

Half Tortoise Pose

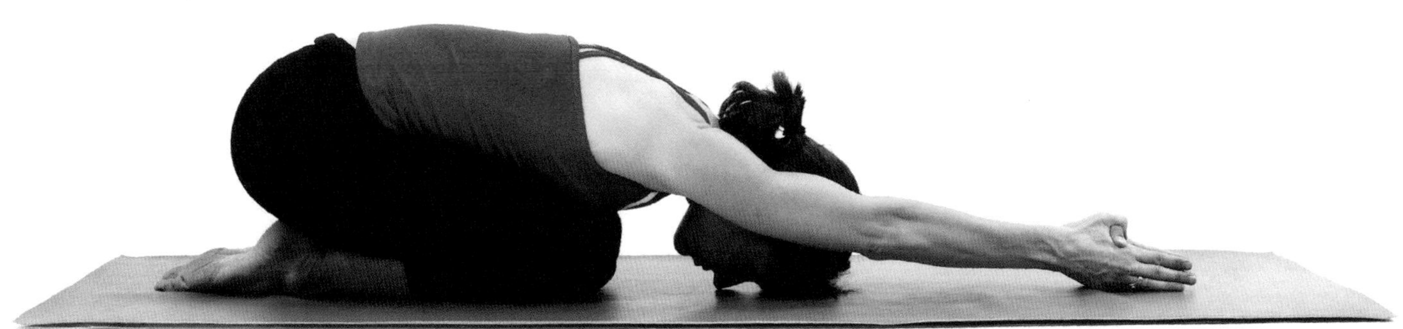

The essentials

Half Tortoise Pose is one of those positions where gravity helps reduce our real effort and improve the results. Even though it can be difficult for a number of us, for the most part it provides a welcome physical and mental rest.

There are certainly those that 'hang out' in this pose, but the opportunity to really work the traction is great. Many benefit with yet another chance to iron the kinks out of latissimus dorsi and serratus anterior, providing relief and length, countering shoulder tightness.

What makes this pose so difficult to get right?

Beware! This pose looks deceptively simple. It seems to be easier for the flexible and those with open shoulders, ankles and hips. If you have tight shoulders, tight latissimus dorsi and other torso muscles, lower back issues or are even carrying quite a bit of extra weight then the entry to this posture can prove to be one of the most challenging of your practice. Once you are at the floor however, most can feel themselves ironing out and lengthening.

Ardha Khurmasana

Half Tortoise Pose

22

The technique

After your sit-up position yourself at the base of your mat.

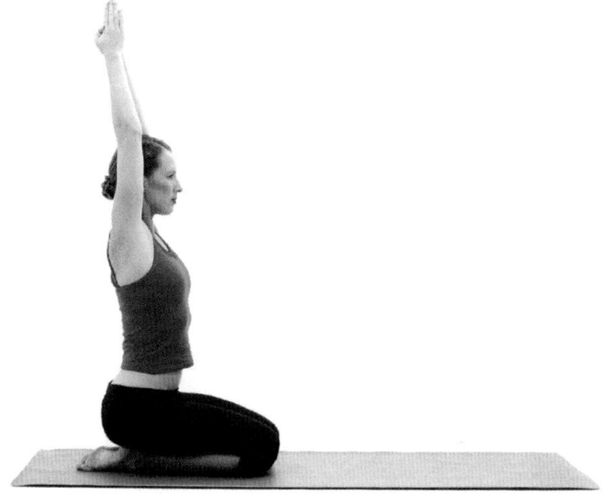

1. **Kneel**: Kneel with knees, heels and toes together, sitting on your heels. Some classes progress more quickly than others allowing you varying times to get out of your Savasana. Be sufficiently patient that you settle and sit, and make eye contact even momentarily, before commencing.

2. **Arms Up, Palms Together**: As you inhale lift your arms up over your head. Bring your palms together so that your hands contact from the wrists all the way up through to your fingertips. Cross your thumbs for a more positive effect.

3. **Arms Back**: Bring your locked out arms back as much as you can to facilitate open shoulders.

   If you find your shoulders hunch, slightly draw your arms away from your ears by decompressing your neck. In anatomical terms; you need to relax your levator scapulae. In this way you will find length in your neck muscles and prevent your chin dropping below parallel to the floor.

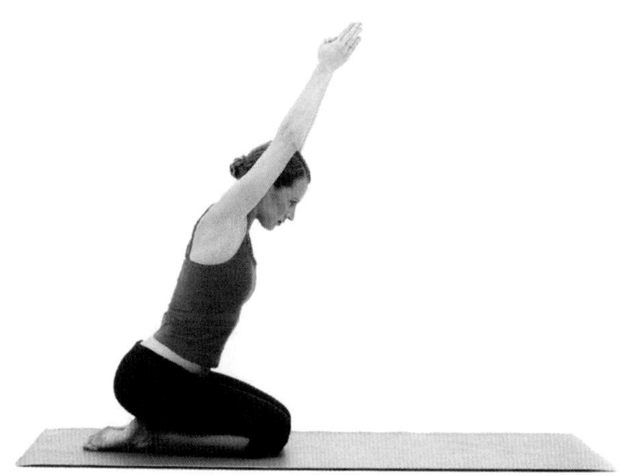

4. **Your Body Is A Plank As You Enter**: Feel a strength in your body as you firm up everything from the hips to your fingertips. It is as if your body takes on the form of a solid plank. Everything gets set in cement right down to the angle your chin makes with your neck.

   As you exhale aim to keep your hips seated on your heels, draw in your abdomen, and in one plane of movement hinge your body/head/arms from your hips. Create length in your body as you bring your head toward the floor; forward, out and then down.

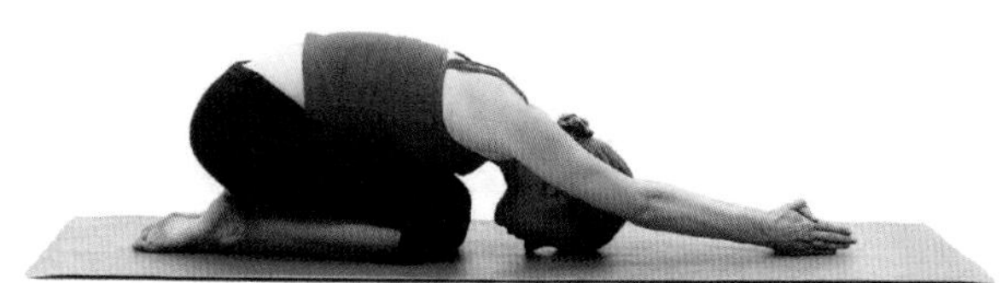

5. **Your Forehead To Contact Before Hands**: Your job is to land your forehead as far in front of the knees as possible. Along with keeping your arms and head in constant relationship, this will keep your chin in the best possible position and continue to lengthen the spine on the way down. Although most cannot manage, try to touch your forehead to the floor before the hands do.

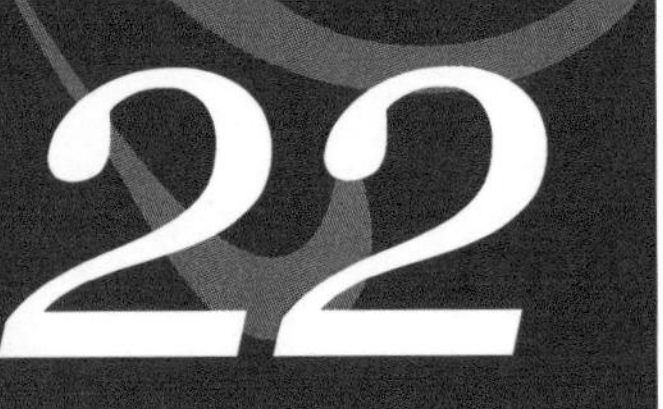

Ardha Khurmasana

Half Tortoise Pose

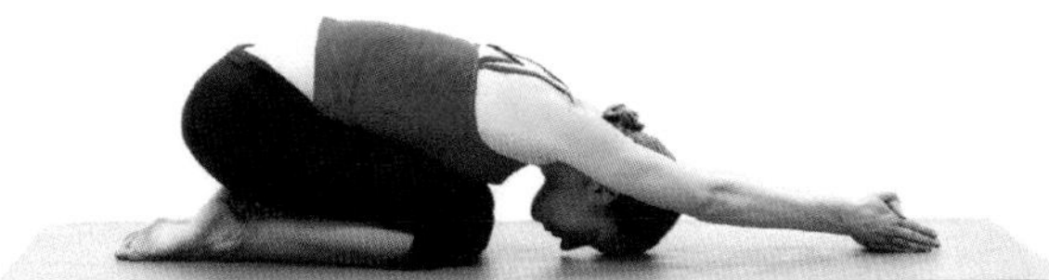

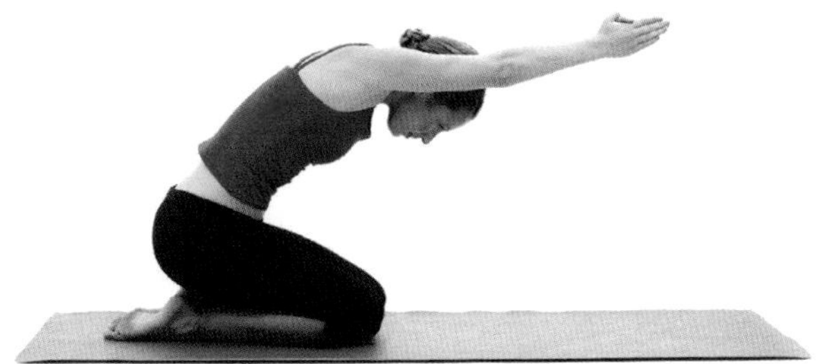

6. **Edge Of Hands To Floor, Lift Wrists And Elbows**: The edge of your glued hands along your smallest fingers and possibly also the fingertips of your 3rd, 4th and 5th fingers will contact the floor. Continue squeezing your head with your activated arms while lifting the wrists and elbows off the floor. Make sure your palms stay strongly together for the entire pose.

7. **Progressively Create Length With Breath And Traction**: You are creating spinal length through traction between the two anchor points of your hips and fingertips. On every inhale edge your hands forward. On every exhale settle your hips down further to your heels as you surrender to the stretch. Keep lengthening your body with your strong deep rhythmic breath.

8. **Create Traction In The Arms**: As you move your hands forward you broaden your shoulder blades. Rotate them internally, away from the ears to create further traction from the shoulders to the fingers and create space in your decompressing neck.

9. **Forehead Flat**: Preserve the forehead flat on the floor during the length creation process. You may feel your head slide back and forward. Perhaps your nose will squash against the floor. The chin must stay away from the chest. You should always find yourself looking at the floor and not your knees.

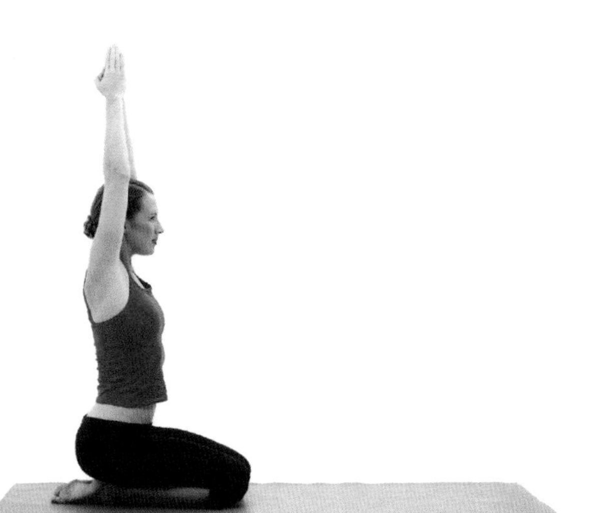

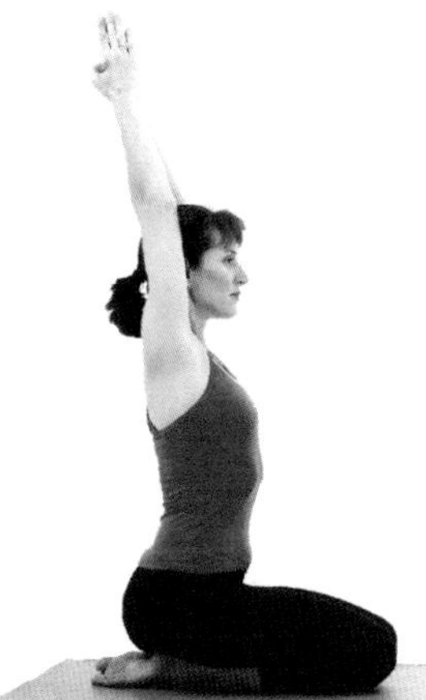

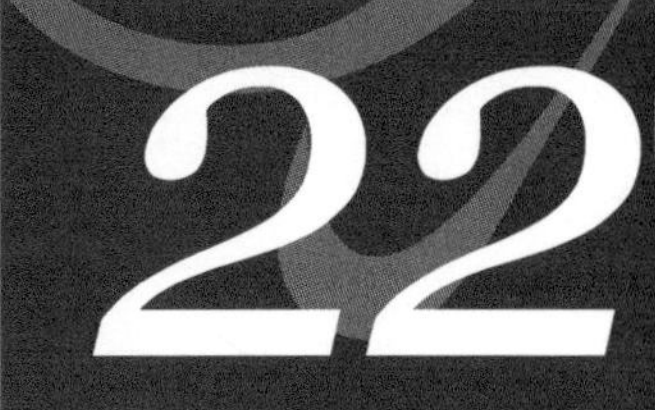

Ardha Khurmasana

HALF TORTOISE POSE

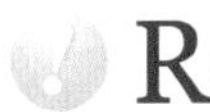

Release

Draw in your abdomen and strengthen your core muscles. Now strong, start inhaling and then lift up your firm 'plank form' (with arms, body position and chin constant) as you continue to inhale. Aim to keep your hips seated on your heels as you raise your entire body up to the starting position. Make contact in the mirror. Exhale as you calmly bring your arms down by your sides again, then turn around and lie down in Savasana.

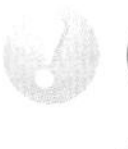

Getting your forehead to the floor first

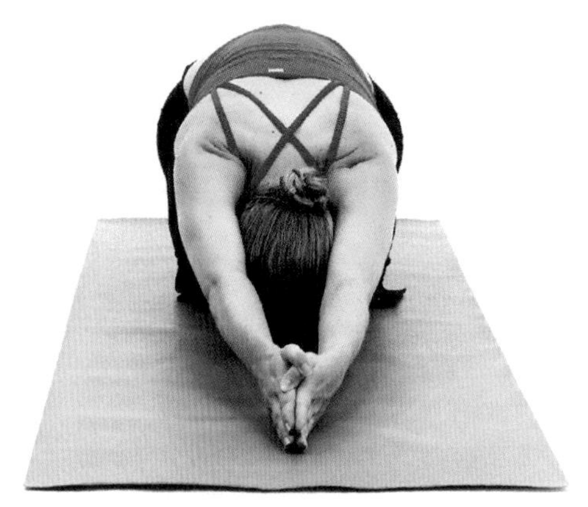

The four photos sequenced below illustrate what is probably this pose's most elusive goal. First and foremost you will need a good balance of strength and flexibility, an open torso and shoulders as well as a strong core. Your target is to descend from the seated position to touch your forehead to the floor before your hands make contact. Equally challenging is to keep your hips seated firmly on your heels. Practice a calm fluid breath.

You must maintain a straight line from shoulders to fingertips without changing the orientation of your fingers along the way. You may have an inadvertent habit of pointing them up away from the floor as your head approaches, so please be careful to keep the wrists locked out. If your shoulders allow it (and can stay down) squeeze your head with your strong arms and lock your head into position. Aim to land your forehead as far away from your knees as possible. This has the effect of preserving the correct angle of your chin and will continue to lengthen your spine as you descend.

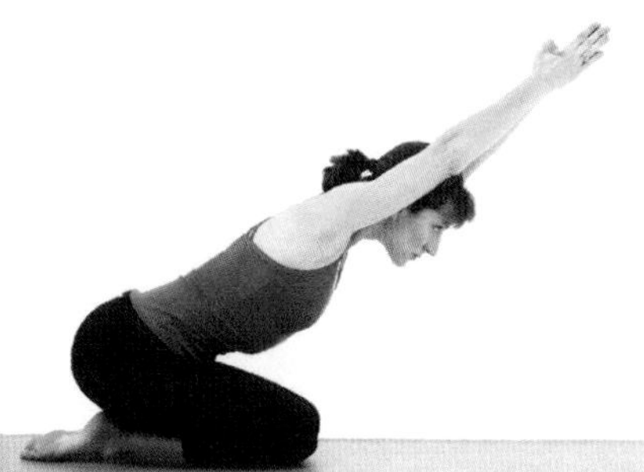

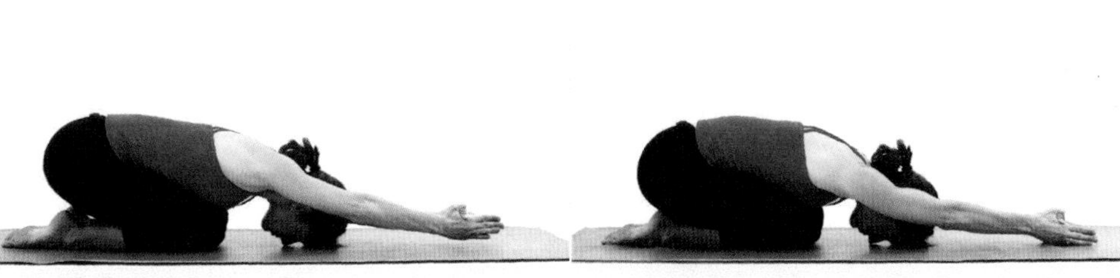

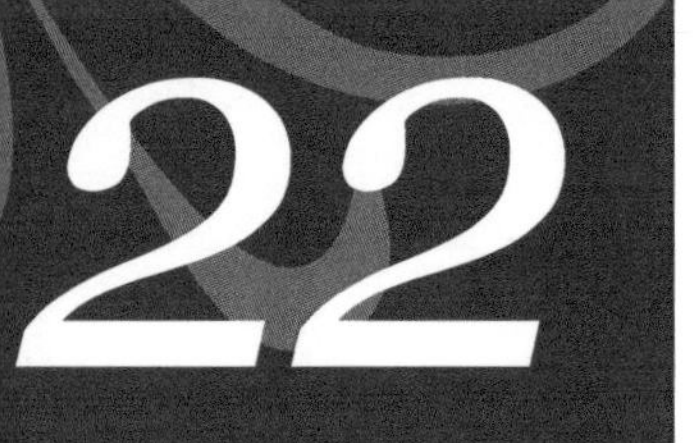

22 Ardha Khurmasana

HALF TORTOISE POSE

Common mistakes and how to fix them

Arms come down before head on entry: Abandoning the 'plank' position to get to the floor could be a sign of tightness, laziness, fatigue or unfamiliarity with the pose. The arms and chin drop and the student rolls to the floor rather than extending out and down. Attention to detail may be the fix!

If your problem is not simply technique related it could be that your physical state (size, injury, flexibility) may be standing in your way of performing this asana. Please see the next error.

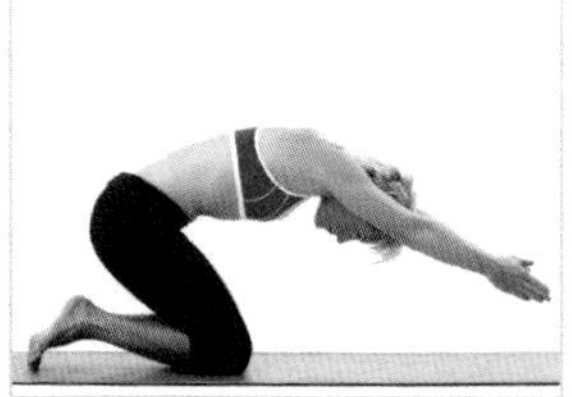

Difficulty on entry and exit: A significant percentage of students never find any ease in getting into or out of Half Tortoise. Some are physically unable to preserve the solid starting position of torso, chin and arms.

If you are particularly inflexible or have damaged shoulders, ankles or vertebrae, tight torso muscles, ankles or hips; then this pose will be far more challenging.

There are many ways that your current body form could be preventing you from entering or releasing from this pose with relative ease. You could be experiencing the following difficulties:

a) When the body descends, the spine rounds and the bottom flies up high off the heels. It feels as though you are falling to the floor with almost no control.
b) When the bottom moves back to seat on the heels again the head comes off the ground.
c) When you try to get the head on the floor the arms bend and separate.
d) If you have to enter with palms on the floor ahead of you the head stays up off the ground and/or the bottom hovers in the air as the finished pose.
e) In order to get your arms to the floor your chin tucks in instead of being flat on the floor.

Sometimes it just seems like a no-win situation. The good news is that once you are down the forces of gravity help stretch you out.

Remember persistence with all and not just isolated poses in your practice is the key to your progress. Don't ever get caught up with any one pose. Do the work. Make your observations and then just move on. Just like a tennis player needs to work on the basics if she wants to improve her game, so too will you have to work on the foundational necessities of your practice. The fancy stuff will come later!

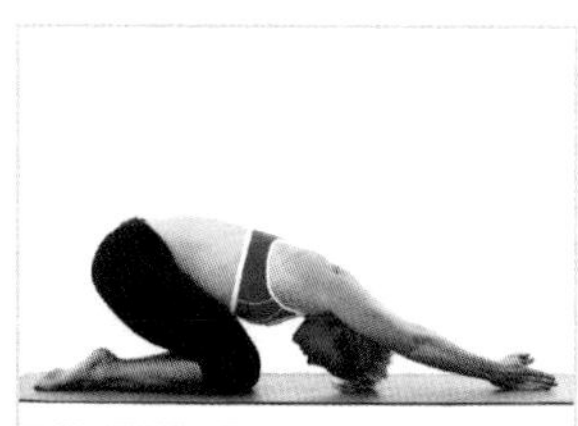

Can either get bottom to heels OR head to floor, never both: If you feel like a seesaw, then use the first set to get your hands and head to the floor. Use the second set to seat the hips onto the heels.

Round spine: On the way to or at the floor, you may find that your back rounds and you are looking at your knees. This is either due to physical limitations or to technique issues. Regardless of cause you can try transforming your body by:

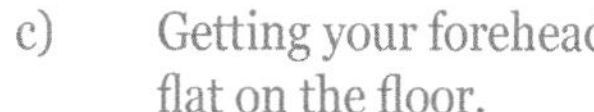

a) Lifting your chin away from your neck on entry.
b) Squeezing your head with your arms, on descent.
c) Getting your forehead flat on the floor.
d) Looking at the floor and not at your knees.

Shoulders hunch to try to squeeze arms to head: This is particularly common given the difficulties inherent in this face-down pose. Instructions can be confounding because you are asked to:

a) Lift your wrists and elbows.
b) 'Walk' hands forward and squeeze the arms to head.
c) Create length in the spine and neck.

None of this is possible if you are hunching. Don't move your shoulder blades towards your ears without rotating the scapulae. It is a sure-fire method of creating tension, chin tucking and neck damage.

To lengthen your body broaden your shoulders down and away from your ears. Your shoulder blades rotate toward the midline and the upper outer corners move toward the mirror. Paradoxically, you create far more space in the neck, through the whole spine and more length in the arms.

Ardha Khurmasana

Half Tortoise Pose

You may find that the arms don't at first squeeze to the sides of the head quite as strongly but you will find it easier to lift the wrists and elbows. Locking the wrists may be easier and occur before you can lock the elbows. You will however, create greater traction from hips to fingertips.

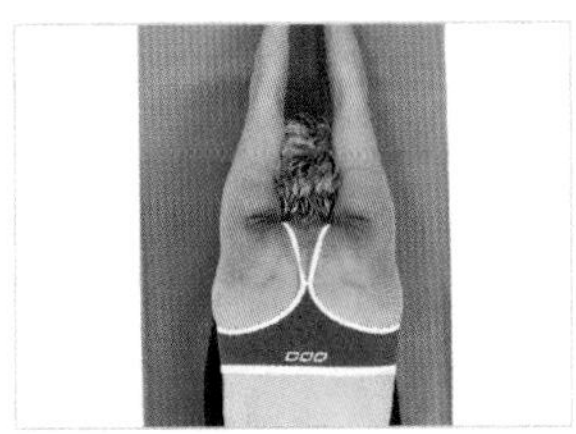

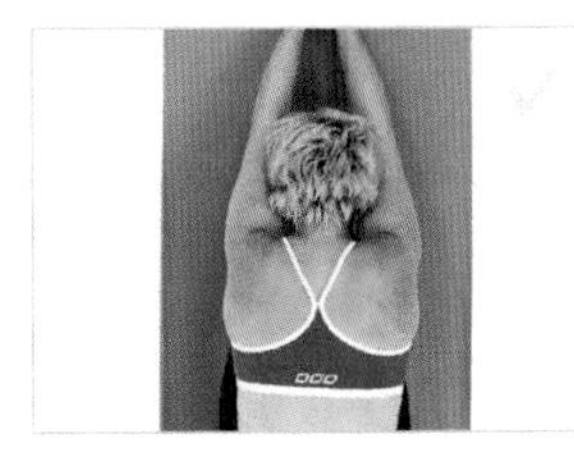

Palms and outstretched fingers on floor: You may hear instructions to 'walk your fingers forward'. I used to say that but I always saw too many students separate the hands and place their palms on the floor. This can be a useful or even essential alternative for students who are nursing acute shoulder pain, recent shoulder reconstructions and for whom bringing the palms together is just too much, and causes shrugging.

As a teacher what I really want to see is the maintenance of that same plank position, with the same chin/throat relationship. As a student you want to feel length creation and shoulder ease and space. Over time your arms and torso will start to lengthen and you will feel strength build in your arms and shoulders to make this a much more active and powerful pose.

Looking at knees: You are rounding your spine if you are looking at your knees because your chin is tucked. Creating length in the spine includes your upper vertebrae, that is, your neck. Get your forehead flat to the floor.

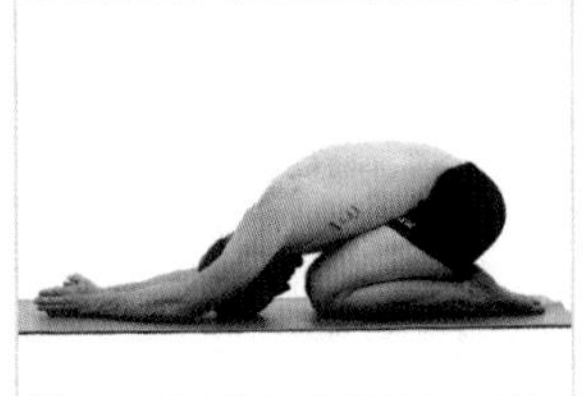

Arms not straight: If the torso is tight and entry is difficult the wrists often bend and the fingers point down toward the floor. Mostly it springs from the effort to keep the arms squeezed in tightly to the head and to minimize the struggle during a somewhat uncontrolled descent.

Conversely, if you are more adept at the entry to Half Tortoise you may find that you bend the wrists up away from the floor. This could be an unconscious attempt to get the forehead to the floor before the hands.

Hands and fingers should always aim to extend directly through the long axis of the arms.

Chin moves to chest: Mistakenly, the head often pivots at the forehead and the chin moves to the chest as the student aims to stretch out in this pose. This also causes the spine to round.

The process of lengthening the body and arms coordinates with the breath cycle. Move the hands forward on the inhale and hips back on the exhale to tease length into your body. As you lengthen the spine you must slightly lighten the head's contact on the floor so that the forehead can move and you can avoid the rounding of the spine that comes with chin tucking. Continue with the aim of getting your forehead as far away from your knees as you can, keeping a straight spine and getting the extension.

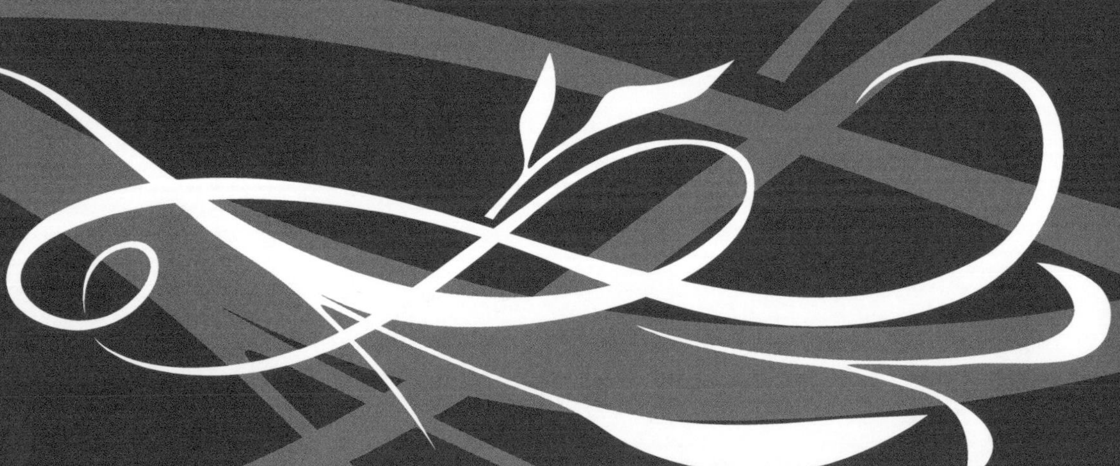

Ustrasana

Nothing in life is to be feared.
It is only to be understood.
—Marie Curie

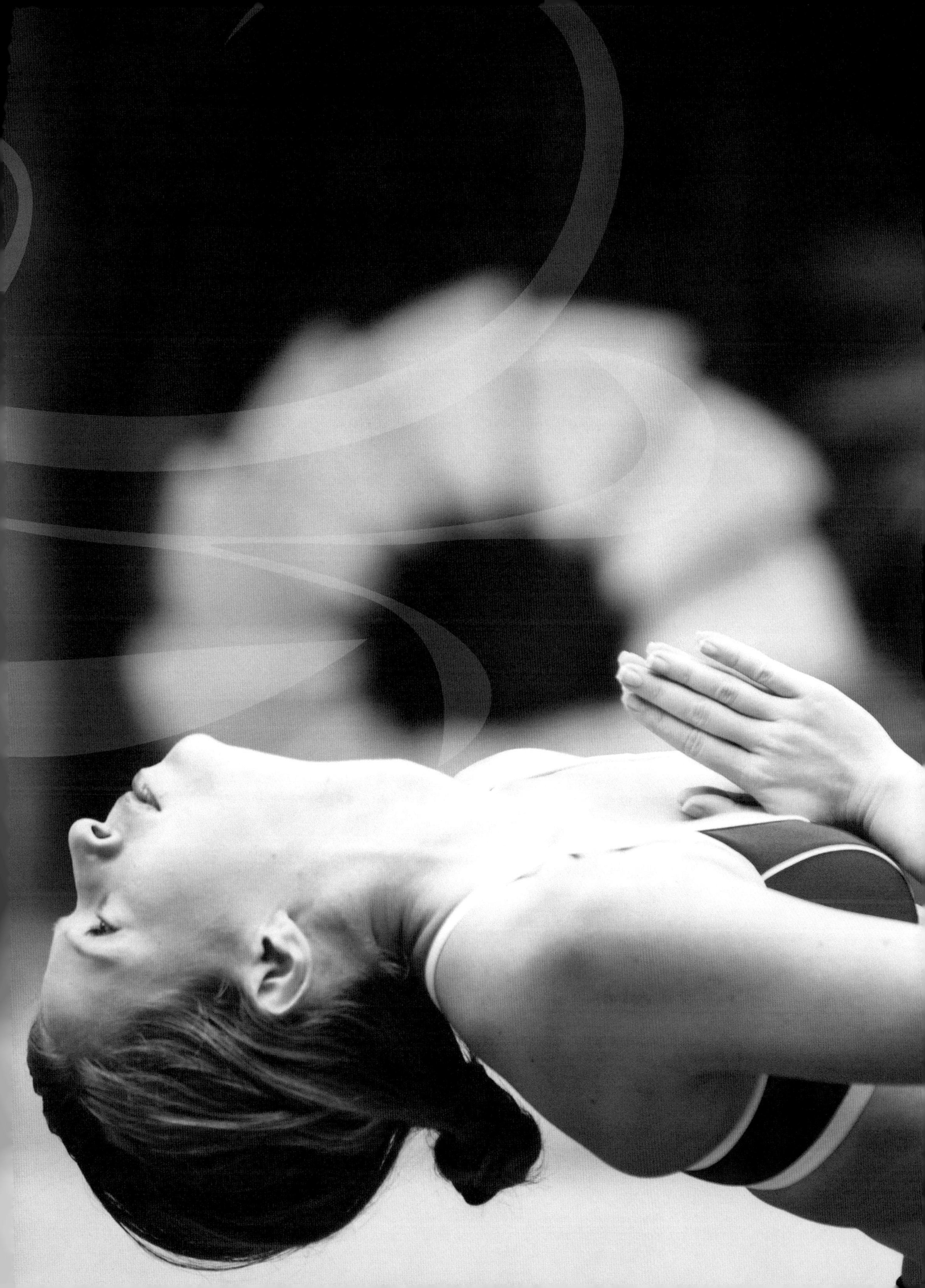

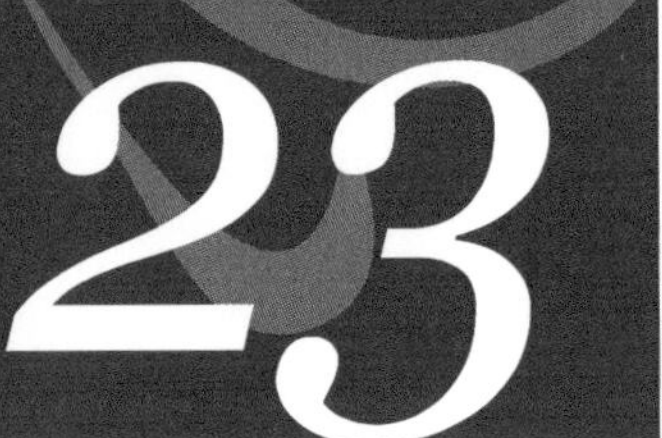

Ustrasana

Camel Pose

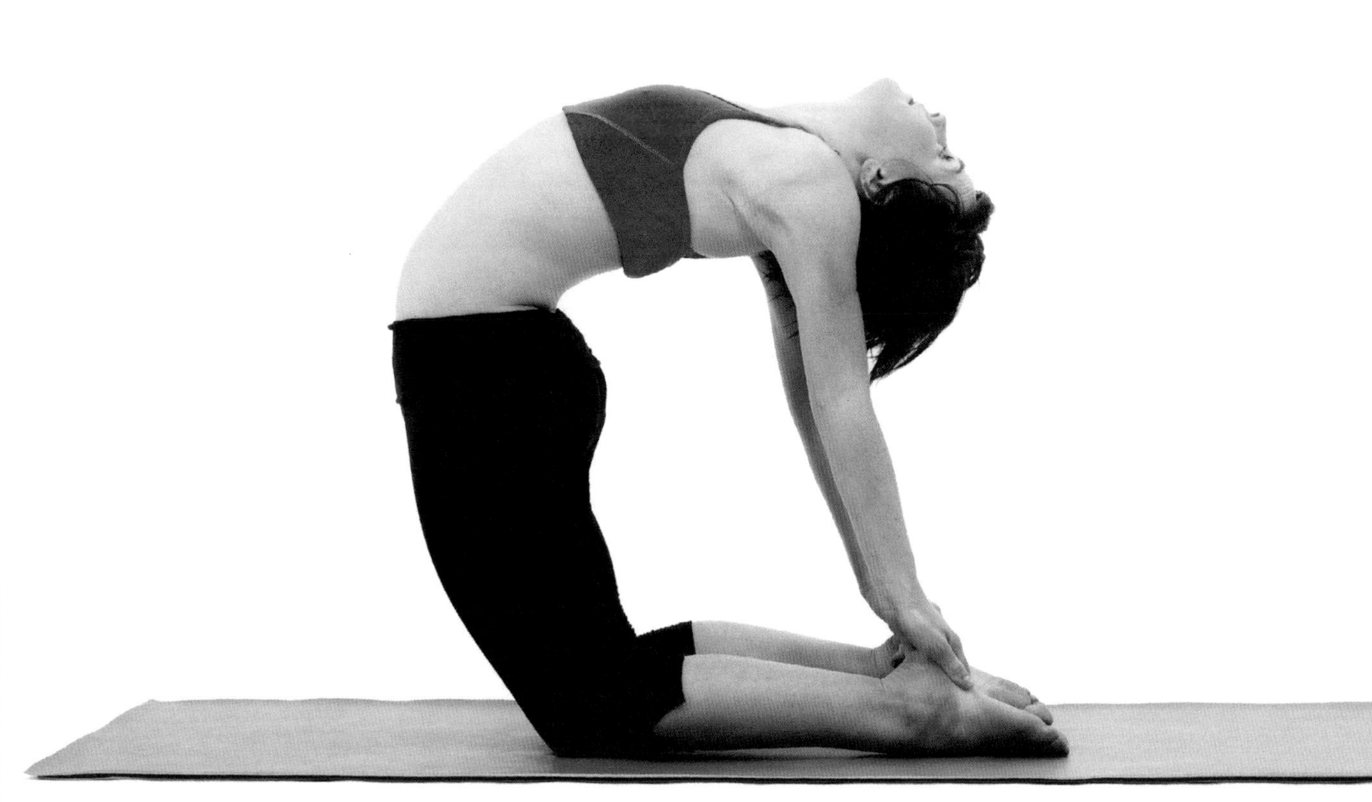

The essentials

It is often said that these next 2 poses - Camel and then Rabbit - are what all your work has led you to. A note on personal safety: It is best that the body is warmed right through before you attempt this posture. Placed at this point in your class you can be assured that this is the case. Hard work and muscle tiredness means that resistance of your muscles is very low allowing you to go deeper and achieve greater opening than if this were placed at the beginning of class.

Camel is great for calming the central nervous system. It allows for space and free-flowing movement of neural messages through the spinal cord and brain. So the longer you are in it the better.

What makes this pose so difficult to get right?

This is a very strong backbend. In any backbend, most humans will feel unprotected and vulnerable, baring vital organs and 'exposing' them to real or perceived potential dangers. It is little surprise that many students choose to come out of this posture earlier than required. What makes this pose so difficult for some is this vulnerability and the intense sensations that bubble up on your unprotected and open front. There are definitely specific ways to get past these sensations, to treat them equanimously and get all your benefits.

Ustrasana

CAMEL POSE

23

The technique

After your sit-up turn around on your knees and stand on them with your legs and feet parallel, hip distance apart.

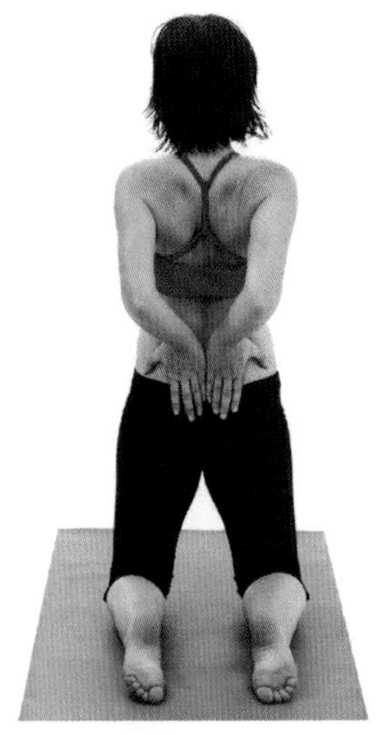

1.1 **YOUR HANDS AT THE LOWER SPINE**: Position your hands along the centerline at your lumbar spine, fingers pointing down and thumbs on the outside.

1.2 **RELAXED SHOULDERS**: Hold your shoulders away from the ears. The chin is parallel to the ground and your chest is open. Focus on yourself in the mirror.

1.3 **HIPS SQUEEZED AND FORWARD**: Now squeeze your bottom and push your hips strongly toward the mirror with the assistance of your hands. You should always aim to position your hips forward of your knees.

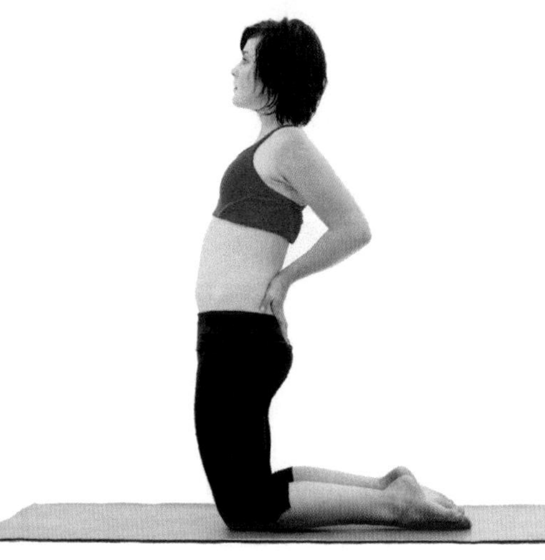

1.4 **HEAD BACK**: Take a big breath in and elongate your torso. Now drop your head back and look back towards the wall behind you. You are already in a slight backbend by virtue of your hip position and hanging head.

1.5 **NOW GO BACK**: Deepen your backbend by going back. Continue squeezing your bottom and pushing hips towards the mirror forward of your knees.

1.6 **USE YOUR EYES**: Looking back as far as you can always helps deepen your backbend. If at this point you cannot see where the floor meets the wall, then this is your pose for today and you stay here until release. Your job is to breathe, maintaining visual focus on the wall behind, or if it is all you can manage, just the ceiling, but never down your nose.

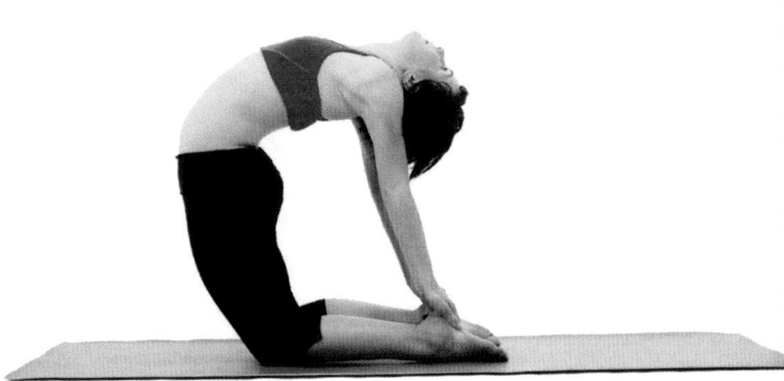

1.7 **HANDS TO ANKLES ONLY IF**: If you can see where the floor and wall meet, then in 99% of cases you are ready to proceed to the next part of Camel. Drop your right hand down to your right heel. Grab your right heel, with your thumb grasping the outside and your fingers on the inside. Now time for the left hand – thumb to the midline.

1.8 **HANG FROM YOUR ANKLES**: Now PULL on your heels as if you were hanging from them. Your arms are straight with absolutely no sensation of your hands, arms or body resting back on your feet. You are using powerful energy here to project your hips, thighs and stomach forward and very importantly, your chest up and outward.

Ustrasana

Camel Pose

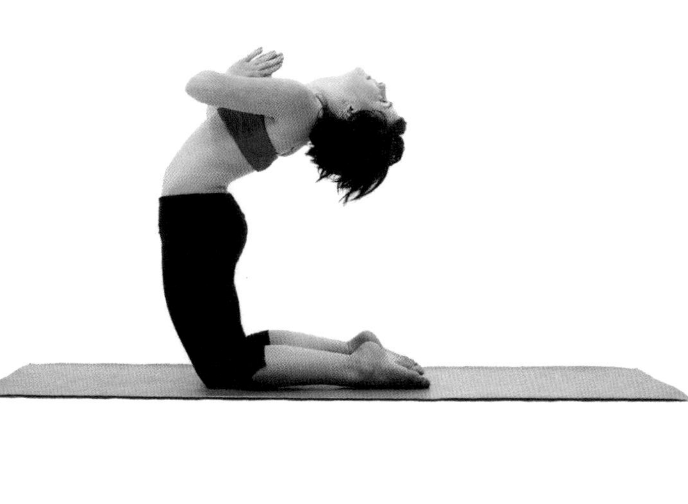

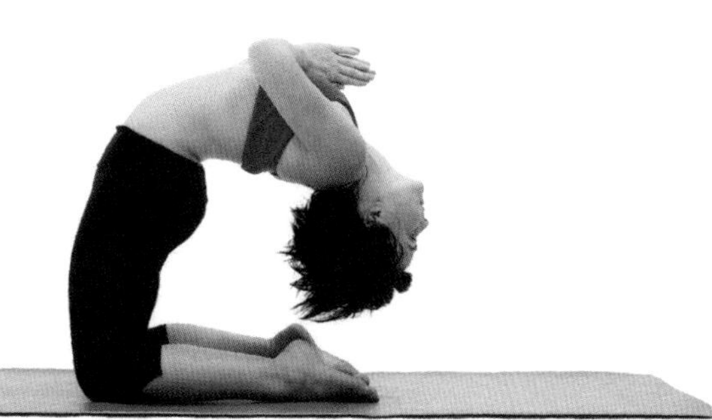

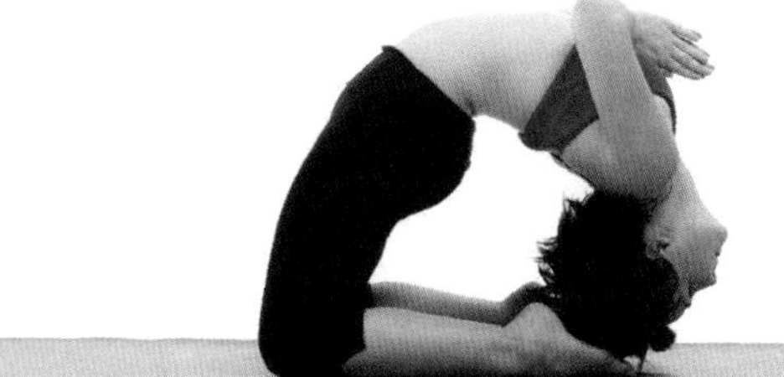

1.9 **Continue With The Basics**: Continue to squeeze your bottom; push your hips and thighs forward ensuring your thighs are forwards of your knees – no exceptions here; keep your neck soft and always keep your eyes looking back and down (imagine you can see your toes and then look for them!). Enjoy this deep arch in your spine. It provides the beautiful liberating stretch down the front side of your body, which starts at your knees, travels along your thighs, through your hips and abdomen, over your chest and gets full extension through your neck to your chin.

1.10 **A Practice Tip**: With air passages stretched and narrowed it is easy to get stuck with an anxious or panic breath at the top of your lungs. Always aim to slow and deepen the breath so you get all the oxygen you need. Draw the breath down into the belly. Keep looking back. Feel the calm.

An unusual and incredible challenge

One of the teachers I had at Bikram's Teacher Training had a feisty (and flexible) student become as calm as a sleeping cat in a matter of minutes. This student was instructed to stay in Full Camel for 10 minutes.

This inspired me to incorporate a long-hold Camel into my classes. Sometimes I offer the invitation to those game to make a personal breakthrough, to stay in one long set of their expression of Camel. The biggest barrier appears to be fear. Most have procrastinated for many classes before their first attempt. The effects are so great and instant that those same fearful students request it when I don't offer the choice.

Please only do this if invited to do so by your teacher; you need to practice THEIR class. Know however that there are no half measures. Stay in it for two sets (about 2 minutes) or not at all. No prizes for coming out early or for staying in for one set and a few seconds.

Be aware of the varied sensations. My arms tingle like crazy. Continually recommit to the basics and work on your steady breath, strength, stamina and persistence.

You really want to preserve the benefits of doing this wild backbend which can make your spine feel open and rather delicate. So be mindful and careful on exit, into Savasana and for your next sit-up. Take extra time. Consider skipping the next sit-up if you need to (I do). Avoid any kind of forward bend (Rabbit is next for that) and allow yourself to come out slowly and mindfully.

Ustrasana

Camel Pose

Second set

The second set offers you the opportunity to deepen your backbend in three ways all described below. Place your feet as before but set your knees a few inches (10 cm) further apart so your legs are positioned in a 'V' shape. With your knees further apart you will notice how your floor support is wider and you can get deeper into your hips.

2.1 **Deepen Your Backbend**: Most students follow this technique. Proceed as in set 1, with your knees further apart as described above. Your hips will open more and your backbend will be greater. Take note of how much further back on the ceiling or down the wall your eyes rest.

2.2 **The Interim Pose**: This is for those who easily grasped their feet and saw the floor behind them in the first set. Knees are set further apart. Allow your head to go back on your soft neck. Now bring your hands into prayer position at your sternum. Keep your hips strong for support and start your backbend.

Go back remembering to use your visual focus to lead you. Look for your feet. You might like to try wiggling your toes. This helps you locate them in your peripheral vision and focus your attention in the right direction.

Your hips will no longer be forward of your knees so focus on abdomen and chest lift. It may take a few classes to gain confidence in your abilities and your growing strength now that your hands are not on your feet. You must be comfortable enough to come up from this pose with the strength of your back and the push through your hips, allowing your head to come up last. This feels very rewarding.

2.3 **Progressing To Full Camel**: Being able to glimpse your toes in set 1 is a sign that you may be ready for Full Camel. Start moving backwards with your hands in prayer position. Release your hands in front of your shoulders, palms forwards. Continue to arch your spine. Reach your hands down and behind your head in an attempt to lay your hands on your feet (or firstly the floor) with your thumbs on the inside.

One day, your head will land between your feet and your chin will be on the floor! Wow. Yogis who get into Full Camel pose say that it is easy for them and they can stay there a long time. Always use the first set to practice the basic Camel position with the hands pulling on the feet for best leverage.

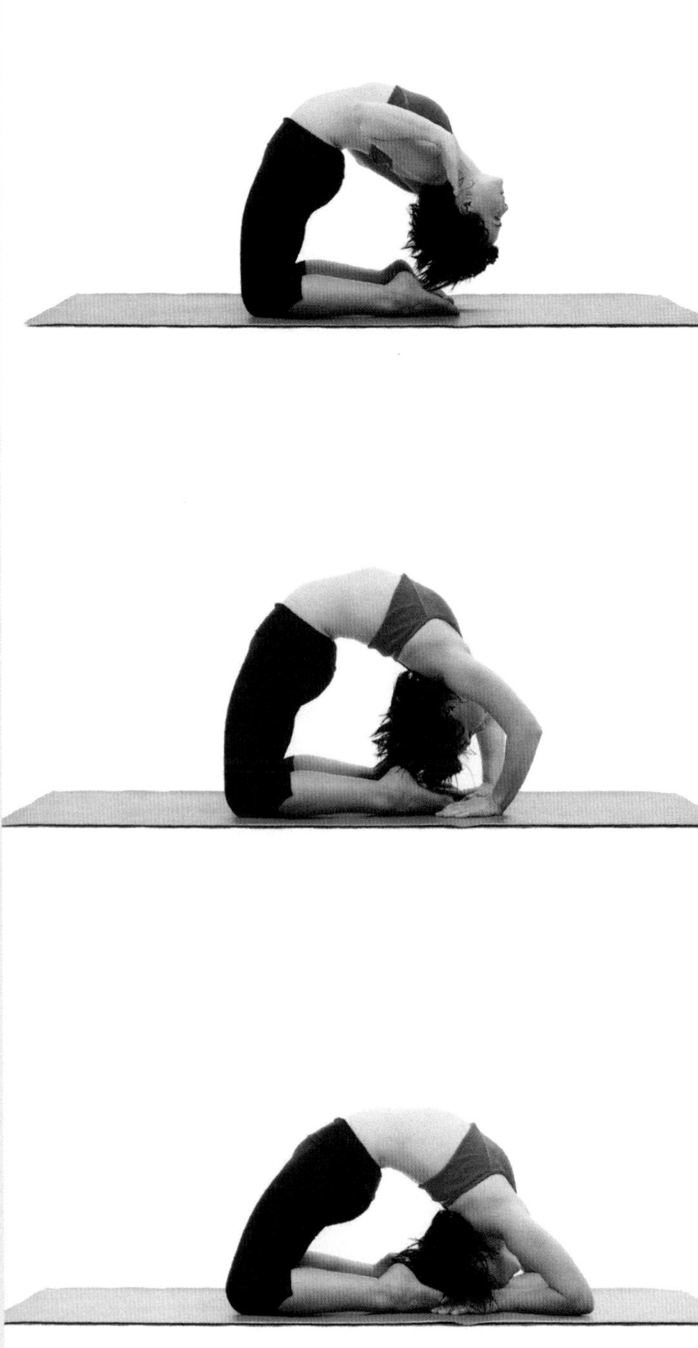

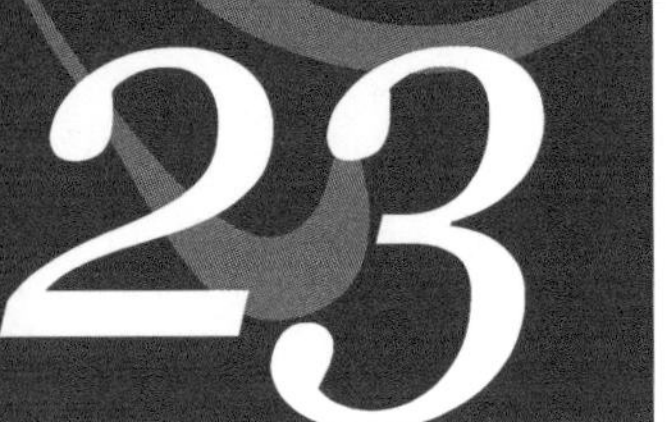

Ustrasana

Camel Pose

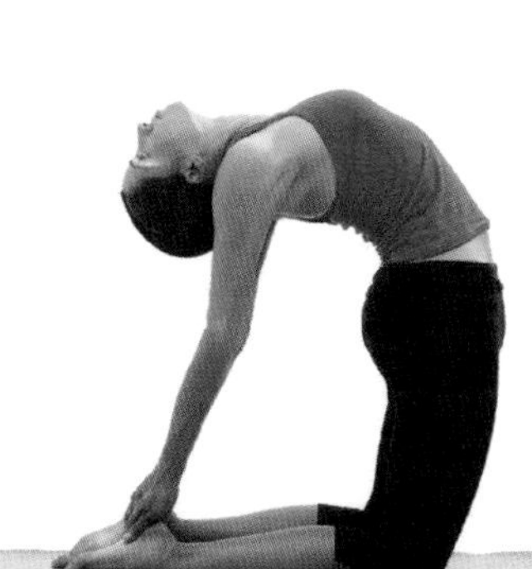

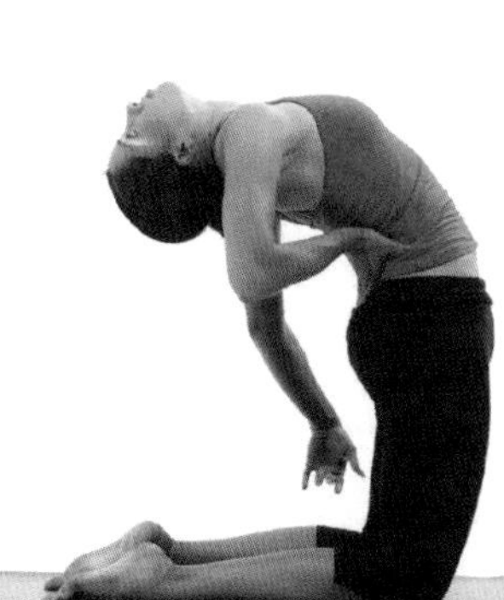

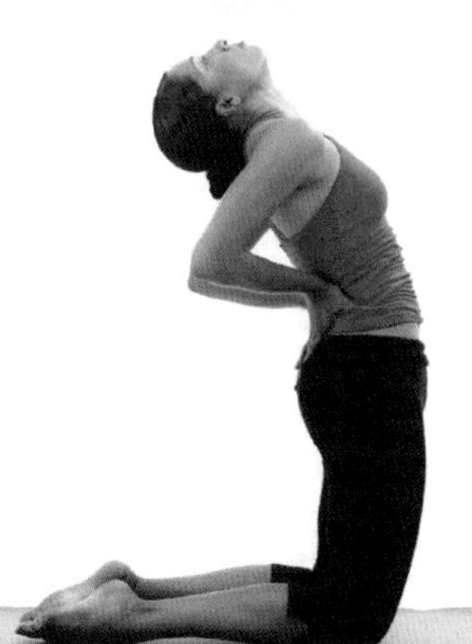

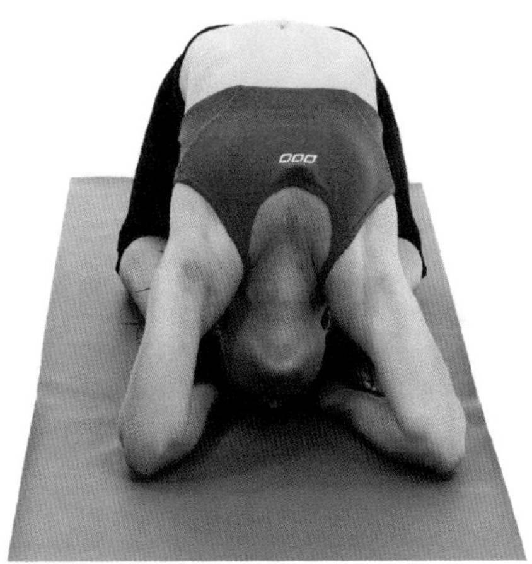

Release

a. Keep your head back, look back.
b. Bring each hand onto each hip.
c. Squeeze your bottom.
d. Project yourself forward, neck soft, head back.
e. Bring your head up last.
f. Make contact in the mirror.
g. Lower yourself down onto your heels.
h. Your back stays straight in a neutral position.
i. Never fall into a forward bend.
j. Spin onto one hip, turn around, extend legs and lie down in Savasana.

In the Interim and Advanced poses exit with your hands in prayer as you project yourself forward with the power in your hips and back. Your head comes up last.

When you exit you will be ready to counter this backbend with a mighty big forward bend, but not until after your Savasana.

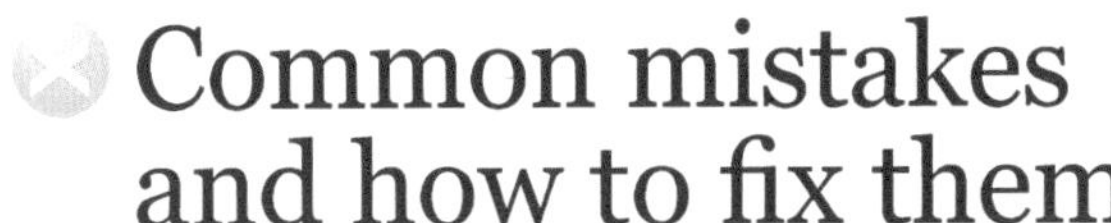

Common mistakes and how to fix them

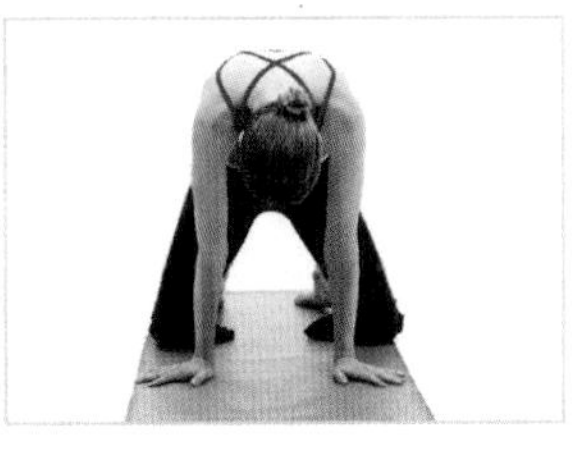

Forward bend is incorporated in the exit: UNDER NO CIRCUMSTANCES should you exit from the pose and slump forward, back rounded, with your hands on the floor. Often students slump onto their forearms and take their head to mat. Simply be mindful. You are coming out of a backbend. Countering your pose before Savasana is going to negate your hard work and rob you of benefits. Head up last. Lower your vertical body to your heels. Spin to one side without rounding forward. Extend your legs and lie down avoiding forward bending as much as possible.

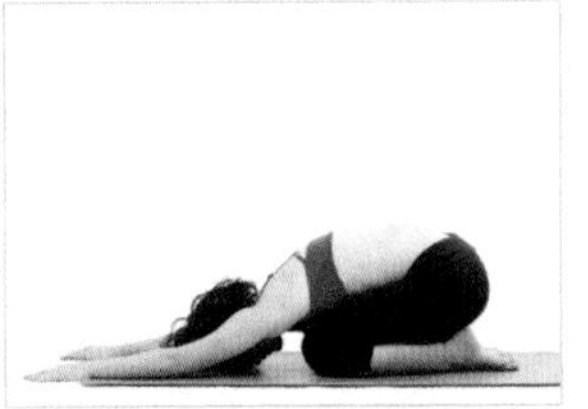

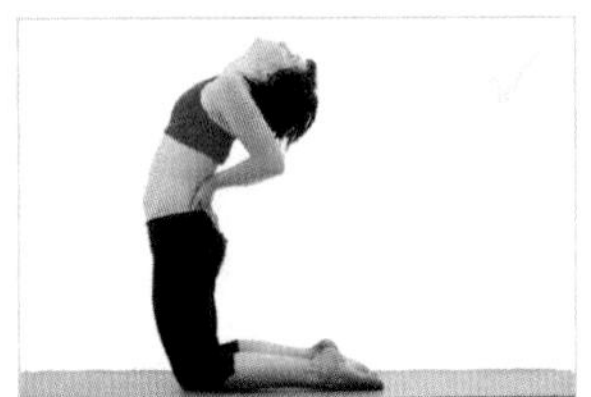

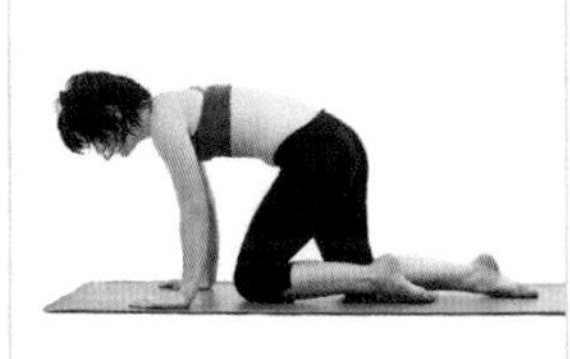

Crawling to your position on the mat: Many teachers request that students turn around and come to the top of the towel. This is not technically a mistake, but then neither does it add any value. It requires a lot of effort to turn and then crawl up to the top - not to mention having to crawl back down afterwards which often entails committing a big mistake; a forward bend before Savasana.

When you exit the sit-up, turn around and simply kneel where you find your knees, probably in the middle of your towel! Your activity and energy expenditure will be minimized and movements will be smoothly efficient. It makes absolutely no difference to the actual pose outcome, except of course you don't have to crawl back and forth to the middle of your mat. You turn, plant your bottom, extend your legs and lie down!

Unsure whether to stay with hands on hips or proceed: If unsure as to whether you should try to grip your heels, remember to look for where the wall and floor join and then proceed! Often on first attempts students are not very confident. If you are not feeling safe, then ask your teacher to support your hips so that you can go back confidently, one arm at a time. This will remove the possibility of undue or damaging twisting movements, or strain of the back or neck as you search and reach for your feet.

If you had help for the entry then make sure (for the first time) your teacher is there to pull forward on your hips for your exit. Even with exit assistance you must practice proper technique: Leave your head back, bring one hand then the other onto each hip, and project yourself up with your head coming up last.

Holding your neck up: Lifting the head tenses, rather than stretches the front side of the body. It works against your outcomes in this pose. Keep your head heavy on your relaxed neck.

Hips behind the knees: When you go into your backbend your hips should always be pushed forward of the knees (unless you are progressing beyond the hands to feet position). Your backbend is better supported and you come up with greater ease and safety.

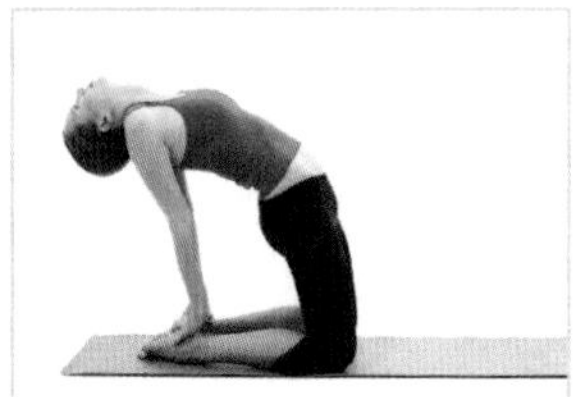

Leaning on your heels: If your knees are closer to the mirror than your hips this means you have placed your hands on your heels and are leaning weightily backwards on your heels.

You can feel quite heavy and often students introduce neck and body tension by lifting their heads. So do some more classes before trying to grab your heels again. See below for an exception.

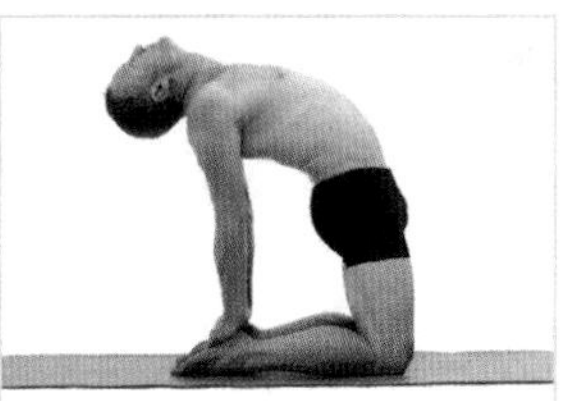

***An odd exception for students with tight lats**: Those with tight latissimus dorsi usually have to bypass correct technique to bring hands to feet. The feet take all the weight, the head doesn't fully drop back and the hips are behind the knees.

However if you can soften your neck completely then bring hands to heels on the second set. Pull on your feet to experience a chest-opening, lats-lengthening bliss in a stretch that you cannot get anywhere else. The hip position is not optimal so you will be unable to fully pull forward from your heels. However the benefits of stretching and lengthening your torso is incomparable and will go towards countering all the problems associated with tight lats and shoulders in other poses.

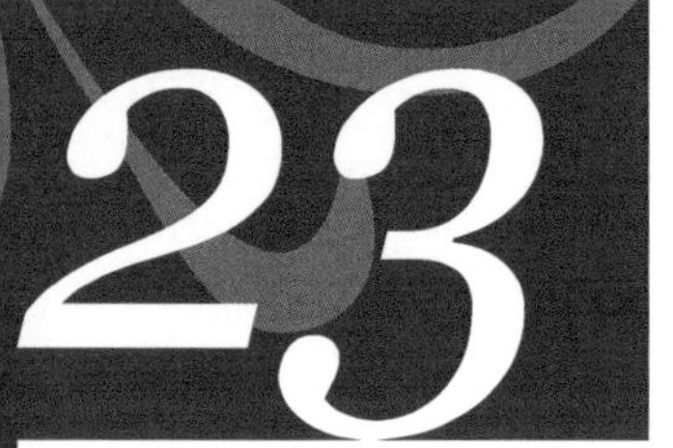

Ustrasana

Camel Pose

Resting on your heels: Even flexible students (who have correct hip position forward of their knees) will, at some point place their hands on their heels and then rest.

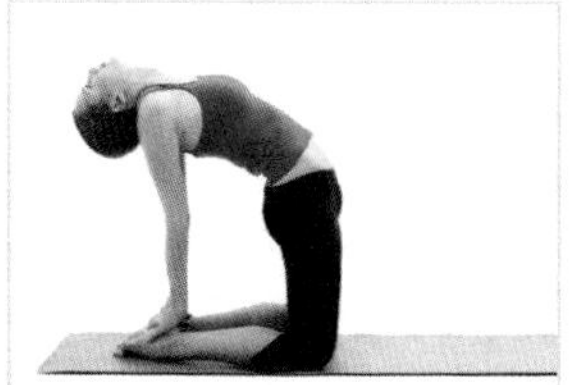

The aim is to pull hard as if you were hanging from your heels. Your feet are relaxed as you pull on your heels with straight stretched arms to create traction. Enhance your pose by pushing your chest up and squeezing your hips and thighs forward.

Allowing your eyes to change their back-of-the-room focus: Many don't realize the pivotal role the eyes play in Camel. Due to its strenuous nature it can be difficult to maintain focus on your task and in response the eyes often wander. If you look 'down your nose' then somehow you become more aware of and focus on the often intense chest or throat sensations. The breath usually quickens, strain is created in the neck, students give up, exit early, and may even fall forward.

Instead of allowing your eyes to wander – which can change depth of pose – keep them looking back and down the wall. Work your visual endpoint, remember it and try to go beyond it second set. Continue looking back and work to calm your breath.

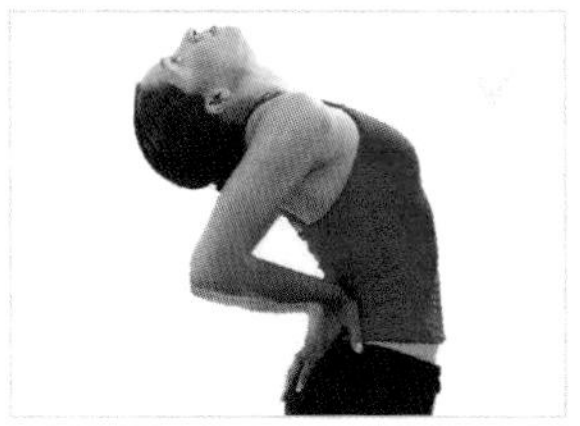

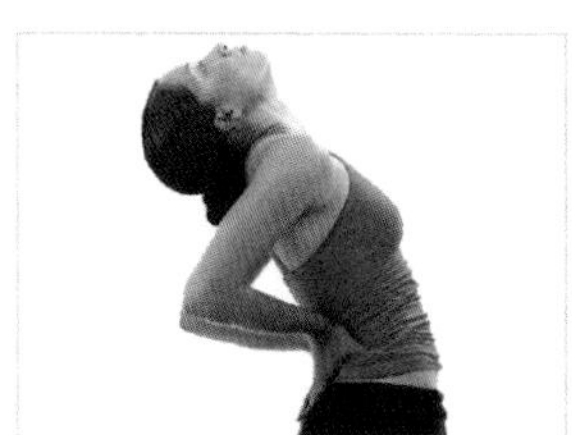

Allowing intense feelings to dominate your experience: With the strong feelings often swirling around the solar plexus, chest and throat areas, our visual focus tends to drop – down the nose towards the chest – in an attempt to connect with our emotional body. Coming out early from the pose is a result of succumbing to these intense feelings.

Newer students may only have access to a shallow breath and this can intensify the reactions. Overriding the strong compulsion to look down makes it possible to breakthrough limiting behavioral patterns and will take strength, courage and determination.

True enlightenment through meditation is brought about by awareness of and not connection with your feelings. Observe and honor your sensations, yet go beyond them. Your job is not to dwell on and react to them but simply be aware. Practice mindful control of your breath.

I often suggest to individuals who seem to be on the edge of a breakthrough that they simply see how much further down the wall they can look. A slower calmer and deeper breath will also help. If your primary aim is to stay in without coming out early then you will be well on the way to not only rid yourself of whatever block you came with, you will prove to yourself that you have stamina in spades!

Hunching shoulders: Hunching causes neck and shoulder tension and obviously cannot help you. This reaction could be due to a number of factors:

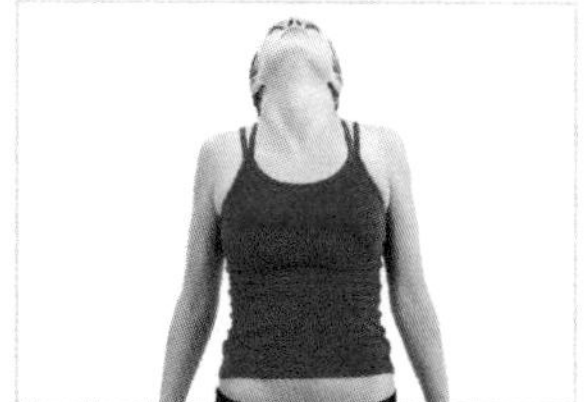

a) Unfamiliarity with the pose.
b) Fear creating an unwillingness or lack of courage to look back.
c) You may have placed your hands on your back but your shoulders are rounded forward. When you attempt to drop your head back there is neck resistance.
d) Existing injury has you trying to protect your neck from experiencing pain.

Try small shifts of your hand positions to see if this is the culprit. Allow your neck to be soft. At some point you are simply going to have to let go.

However if you do have real pain that goes beyond discomfort then you may need some help. Start with a solid set-up of your lower body. Look up and consciously go back to an appropriate point where you experience discomfort and no pain; where you can feel your shoulders can stay down and your neck long.

You can get some help from your teacher. Once or twice may be all it takes for your trust to grow and allow full neck relaxation. It may only take the edge of your teacher's hand placed at the bottom of the neck against which the head can rest. After that it will be easier and you can go it alone.

Ustrasana

Camel Pose

Hands placed wrongly: Some students place their hands on the side of their hips or even with their fingers pointing up. Fingers face down and parallel if possible. If they are lower than your hips then you won't have the support. Place them at the lumbar area.

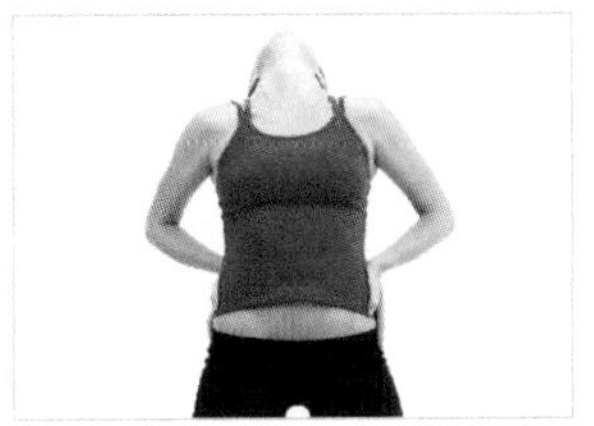

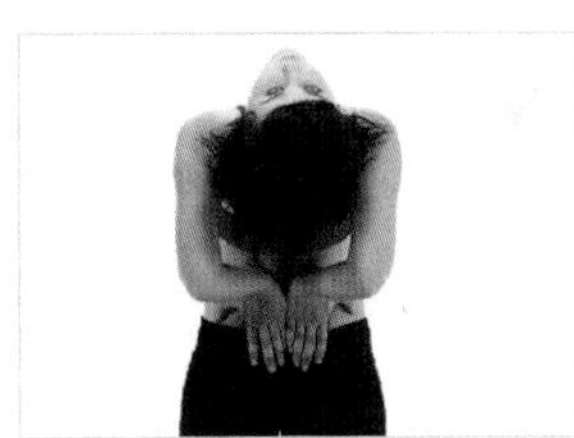

Bottom is soft: You will set up this pose by squeezing the bottom and then push the hips forward. When you inhale length into your torso you will feel the muscles at the top of the hips release a little. This will help create the right support for your back while giving you good flexibility in the lower spine. A soft bottom means you lose the support. Over-stabilized hips create less flexibility and less opening. So start with squeezed hips and remember to elongate the torso to let go of the right muscles for this backbend.

No time is more important than on release, to push your tightened hips forward and help you propel yourself safely out of each of the described varieties of this challenging pose. In this way your head can stay securely back on your relaxed neck and you avoid involving your neck and abdominal muscles to exit. It is only in the Full Camel position where your bottom may need to relax. Recommit your muscles on the way out.

Knees too close together: When your knees are close or touching then your support, balance and safety are reduced. Widen your knees to shoulder/ hip width.

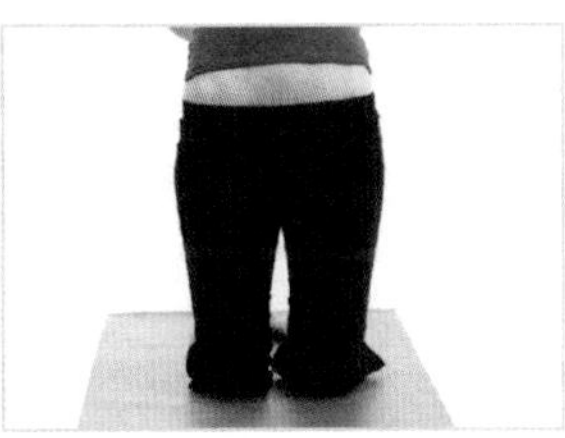

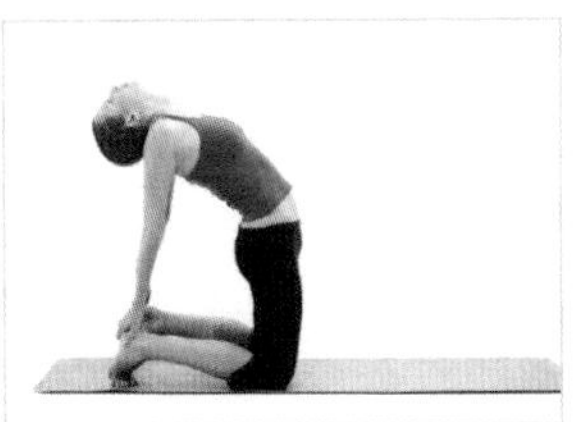

Feet are flexed: Flexing your feet, engages your calves, creates tension in the area and usually takes your focus away from the task at hand. Your feet should be on the floor extended back with the tops of your ankles stretching (if possible) and your toes relaxed.

Breath is too shallow: Breathing too fast or shallow keeps the air exchange up at the top of the lungs and oxygen delivery is greatly impaired. When the breath becomes panicked students come out early. Notwithstanding that you may find it difficult to breathe in this position, try to calm your breath, slow it down so that you can focus on it more. Take your awareness to your gaze and breathe deeply into your belly, letting it move towards the mirror on every inhale.

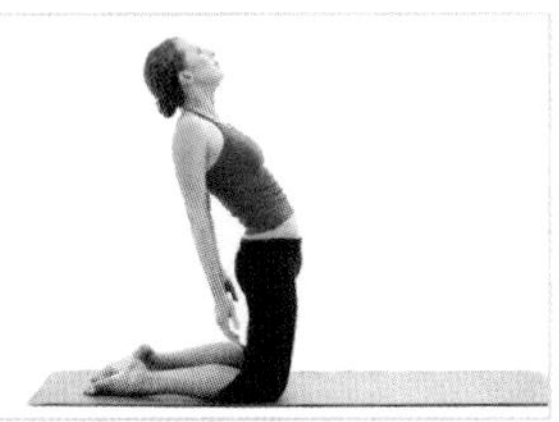

Head leads the charge on exit: If you bring your head up first then you are using the muscles in your head and neck to bring you out. Muscle strain is a likely outcome. Plus you rob the neck of softening and opening benefits. Please keep your head back, focus on supporting your body with your hands, propel yourself forward with your squeezed bottom and hips.

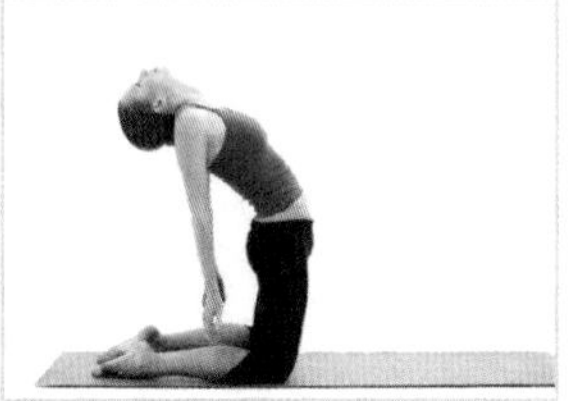

On exit, the back is unsupported: Don't release your hands from your lower back to exit. This is especially important for those whose hands either pull on the heels or remain on the hips during the pose. For those progressing toward Full Camel however, your release will generally be with hands in prayer position. Your hips play a big part in supporting you for release. Each hand comes from heel to hip in turn. When you let go of your heels you should propel forward because of the insistent forward movement of your squeezed bottom.

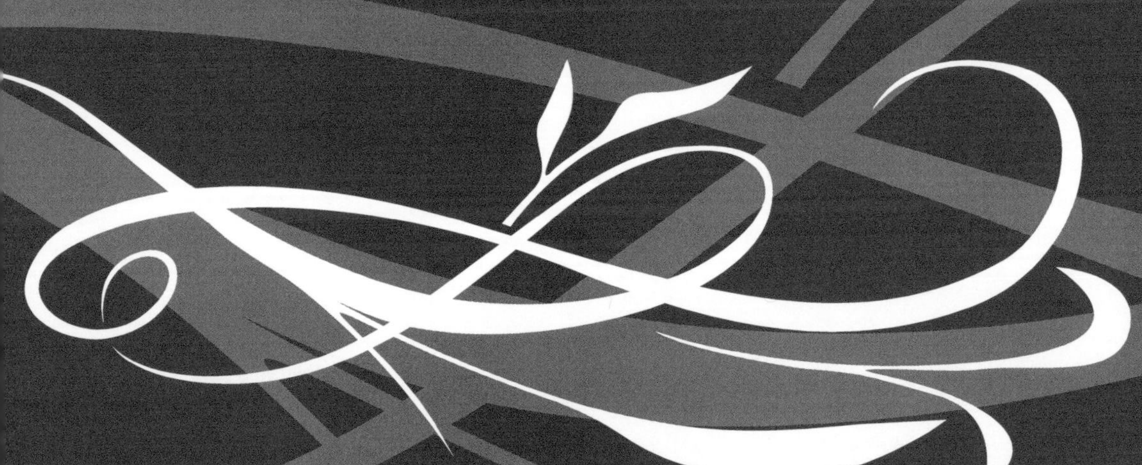

Sasangasana

More people would learn from their mistakes if they weren't so busy denying them.
—Harold J. Smith

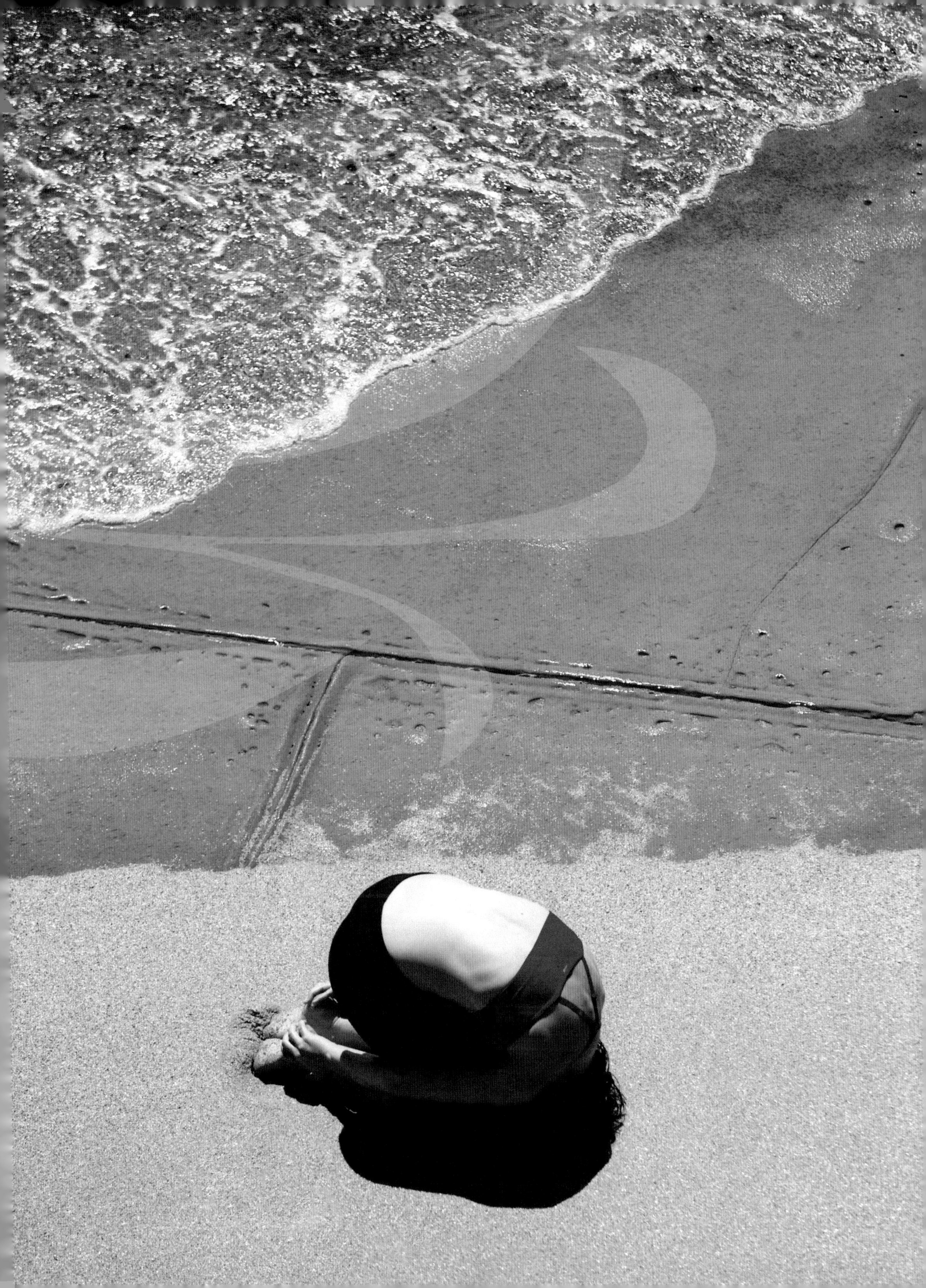

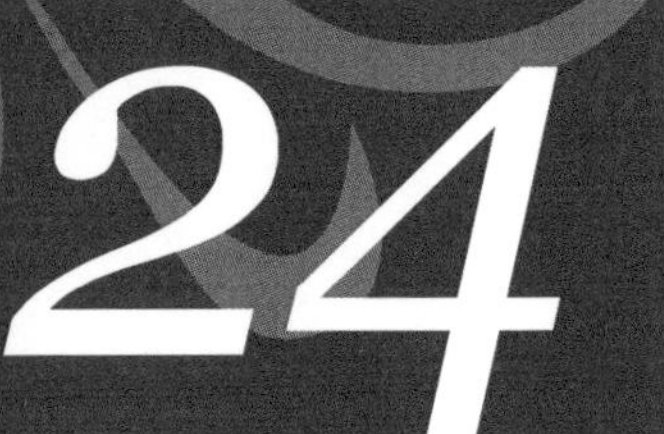

Sasangasana

Rabbit Pose

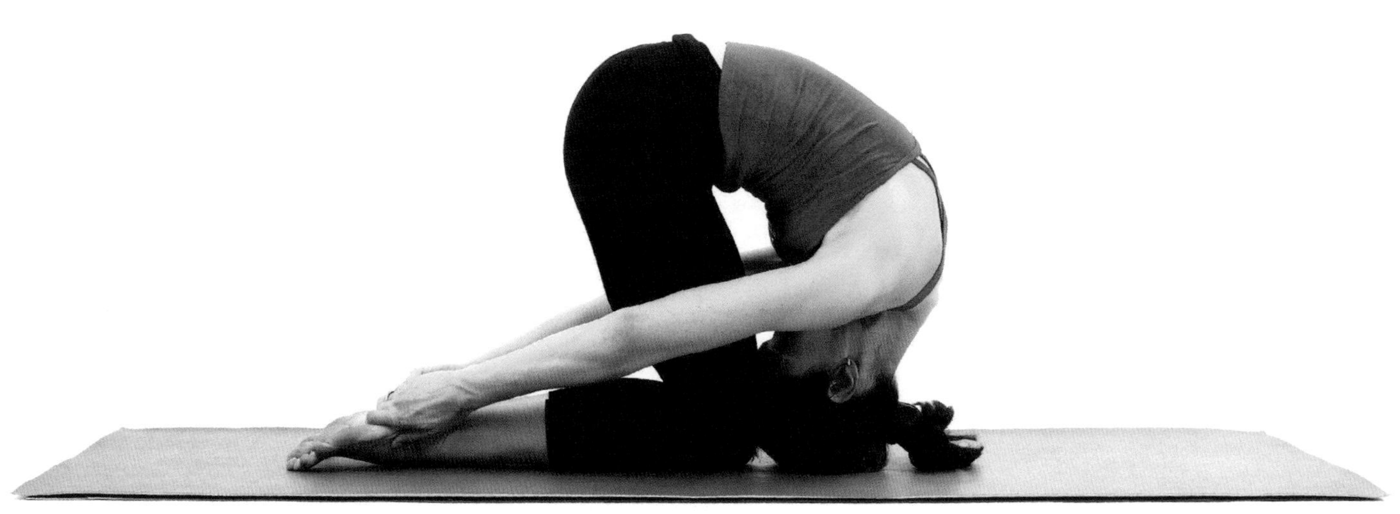

The essentials

Rabbit is perhaps the most extreme forward bend pose in hot yoga. It creates great compression of the organs in the abdomen and thyroid area, regulating metabolism, while enormously opening up the spine and neurological pathways of the central nervous system.

It is the perfect counterpart for Camel and also requires a fully warmed spine for safety. This is a complicated pose. Because of this, everyone needs close attention regardless of yoga experience. Being 'good' at Rabbit is not a function of how good you look, your flexibility or how far you can get. It is about how the right technique can give you the benefit outcomes that you seek.

What makes this pose so difficult to get right?

Spinal safety is a serious issue. Learning how to regulate the pressure on your neck is crucial. Looking around while in this pose is definitely dangerous.

In Rabbit pose it would seem that one leans on the head. This could not be further from the truth. There is contact with the head on the ground but it is more a stabilizing support to prevent imbalance and to stop rolling too far. The real pressure is from the knees down to the ankles, the pull of the hands on the feet, and the upward push of the spine towards the ceiling.

Living in a resort town I have taught thousands of students visiting from other studios. It never ceases to amaze me how many of them still do Rabbit incorrectly and dangerously, despite being longstanding regular hot yoga goers. The number is enormous. Whether they are misinterpreting the directions, or receiving poor instruction I can never be sure. Their relief is obvious when simple tweaks remove the struggle.

Sasangasana

Rabbit Pose

The technique

After your sit-up turn and sit on your knees and heels about a foot (30cm) from the back of your mat. Make contact with yourself, ready to proceed.

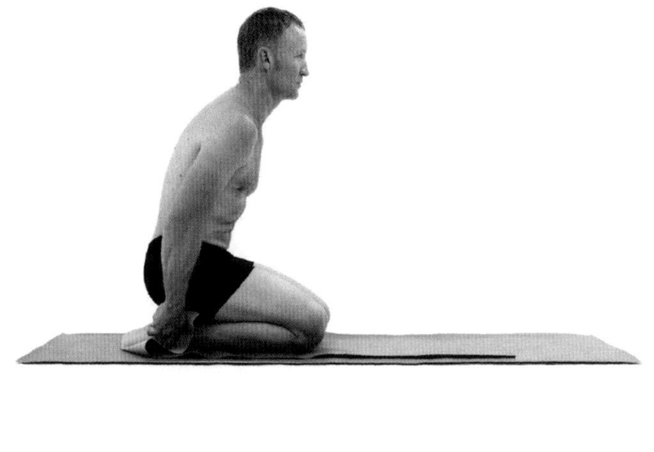

1. **Wrap And Grip Your Heels**: To start, wrap the corner of the towel over each heel and place your hands so that your i) thumbs are on the outside ii) fingers are on the inside iii) palms and insides of your elbows are oriented towards the mirror and the shoulders are down. You may choose not to wrap your heels.

2. **Chin To Chest, Eyes down, Ready To Curl**: Inhale, draw in your abdomen, glue your chin to your chest to look into your heart. You must never, ever untuck your chin from the get-go until you release. The exception worthy of mention is if you have fused cervical vertebrae (see note below).

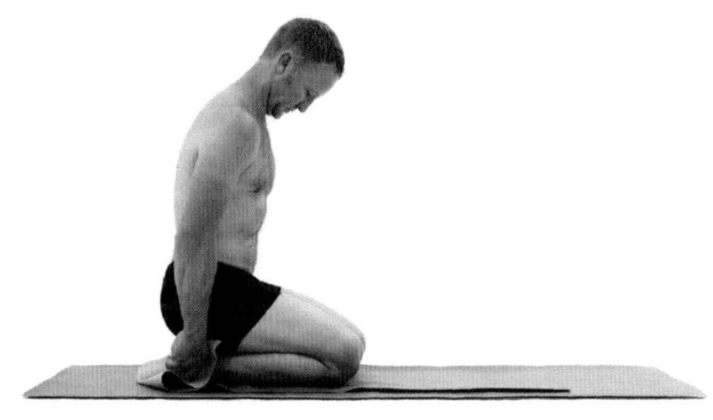

3. **Curl Down**: With your chin and abdomen in you will already start to feel your spine curve, rounding out toward the back wall as you allow your pelvis to tilt. Exhale and commence your curl down into a nice tight ball enhanced by your tight chin tuck and visual focus. Allow each vertebra to open up as you curl. Maintain a constant positive grip as you pull on the feet to slow the descent and stop you diving to the floor.

4. **Forehead To The Knees**: Your forehead lands as close to the knees as possible (except with cervical spine fusions). You will find your forehead touching somewhere at your knees or your eye sockets fitting neatly at the front of the knees. The top of your head may or may not be touching the floor depending on your individual body geometry. It is totally acceptable to have some space between your forehead and your knees as long as the chin is tightly tucked and you curl tightly.

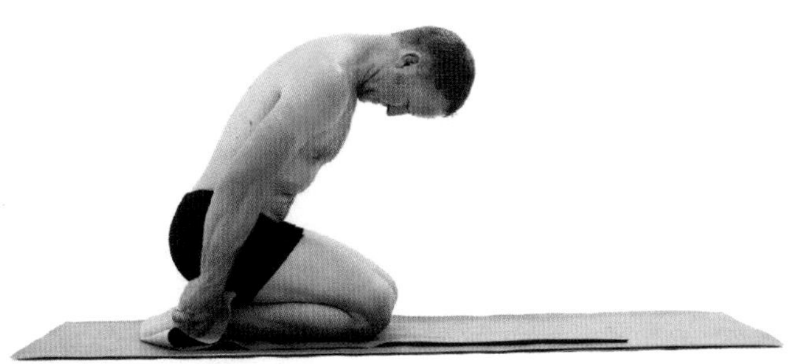

5. **Re-Grip Your Feet And Keep Them Relaxed**: With your body and legs in closer proximity you are in a better position to grip your feet correctly. Few students can maintain a good grip from set-up. Draw your fingers around the back of your heels and use your hands to grab or squeeze them firmly. Make sure that your feet are relaxed. The tops of your feet are extended on the floor. They simply stay put and are non-reactive to the pull by the hands.

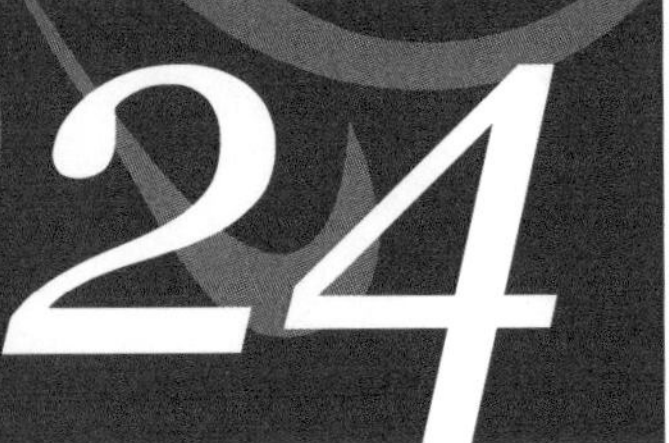

Sasangasana

Rabbit Pose

6. **Breathe, Pull, Lift And Roll**: Take a big inhale. On your exhale, pull on your heels, and roll forward. This pivoting movement around your knees will ideally lift your hips up so that your thighs are vertical and parallel to the mirror. The pull on the feet has to be constant so that the movement of the spine is upwards and opening, rather than downward and into a dangerous compression of the neck into the floor.

7. **Feel Stretch, Not Compression**: Best case scenario is the predominant feeling of the stretch across the lower thoracic and lumbar spine– indicating the upward and outward opening of your back through traction. Feeling an even stretch across the whole back is also acceptable. If you feel no stretch, or a big stretch ONLY across the shoulders then you are doing this pose wrongly. The good news is it is relatively easy to fix: See below.

8. **Knees Close To Your Forehead**: Walking the knees forward to touch the forehead is actually wrong instruction. It only works for a small proportion of people. Forehead to knee contact is not essential and can actually cause problems. More important is to approximate forehead to knee while maintaining traction in the arms and body. Never lessen the space if it bends the arms, loses the traction or tightens the body. Otherwise you must reverse the move. Work on maintaining the pull on your feet with straight arms for support and safety. Avoid pressing your head into the floor. Keep the chin tucked and rest your head on the mat.

9. **Shoulders Up Toward The Ceiling**: Relax the shoulders away from the ears and decompress the neck. There is no shrugging. The pull comes from a stretch in the arms: It emanates from the shoulders

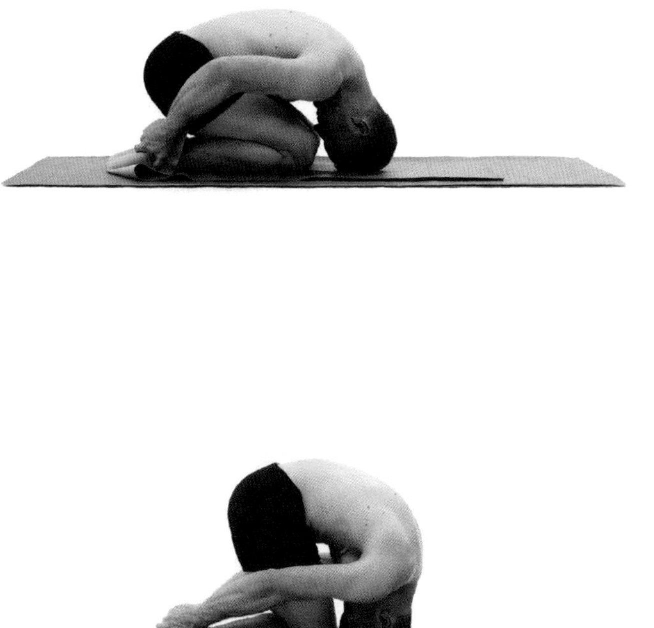

forehead lands on the knees for this more flexible student

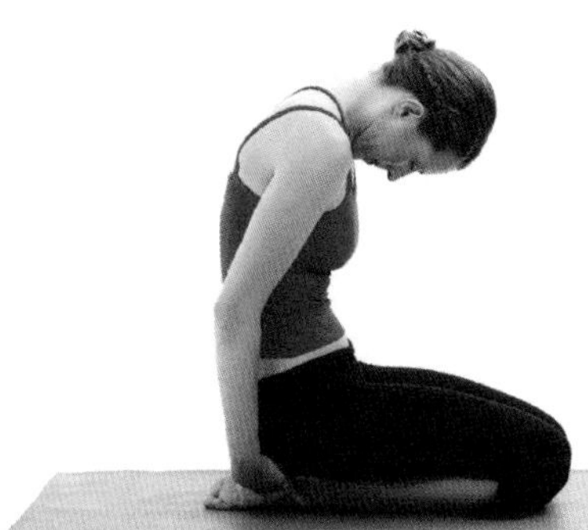

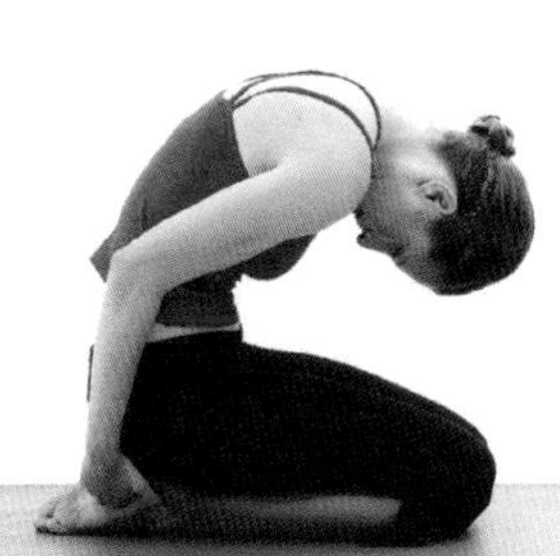

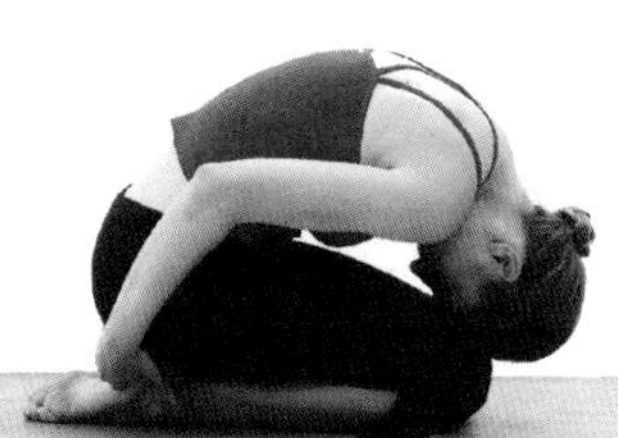

Sasangasana

Rabbit Pose

but is NOT powered by them. 'Climb' the inner part of the arms up the thighs to preserve optimum position or to fix your shoulders mid-pose.

10. **Push Down Knees And Shins**: Every force has an equal and opposite force. So when you are pulling on your feet, you are pushing the floor away from you with your knees AND YOUR SHINS. Imagine your drawn in abdomen touches your spine: This will help you round your spine more and lift your hips up further.

11. **Heels Together**: Move your heels together to improve grip, alignment, pose depth and safety. Your heels and shins will align squarely to the floor. This removes twisting elements which adversely affect traction. With correct alignment the arms' pull against the heels is easier and the push down is more effective through the shins. Your hips raise higher in response.

12. **Keep Breathing**: This is an intense position which lasts around 30 seconds. Learn to breathe calmly and deeply so you can harness the energy to work hard, create the traction and open the spine.

In summary, here are your main actions:

a) Tuck your chin firmly to your chest.
b) Relax your un-hunched shoulders and feet.
c) Pull on your heels, feet together.
d) Roll forward to lift your hips.
e) Push your knees and shins as hard as you can into the floor.

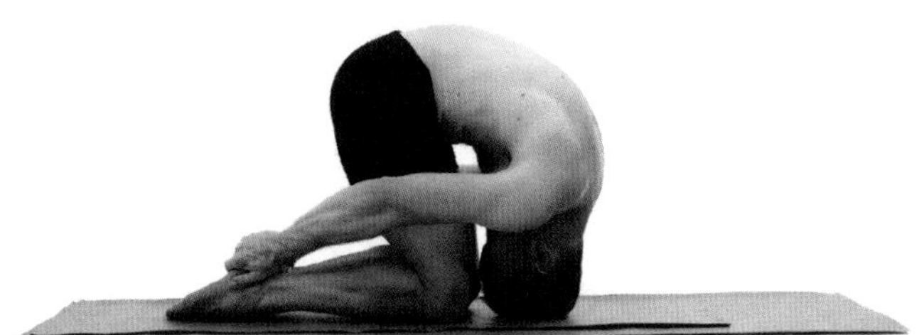

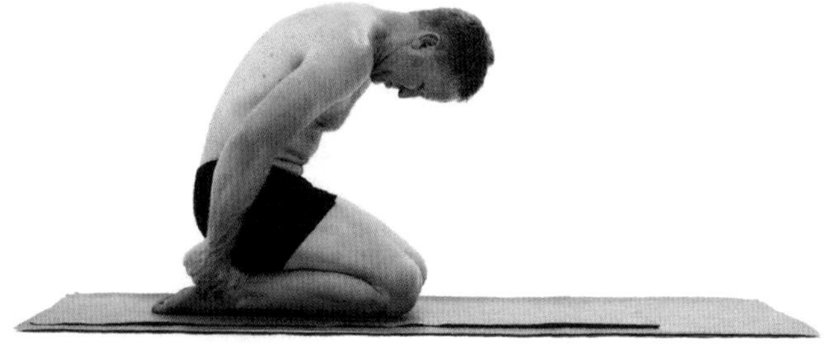

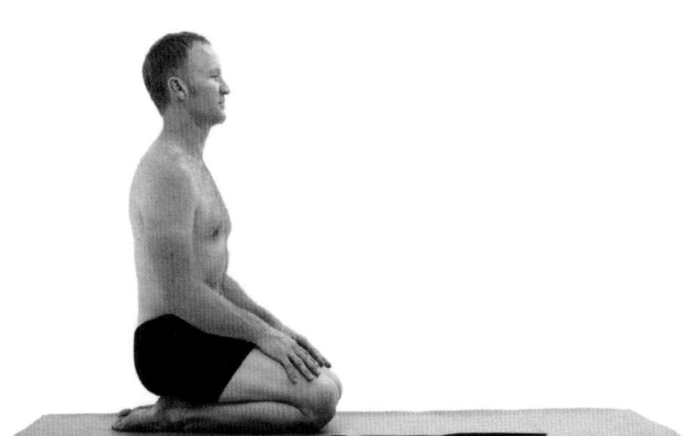

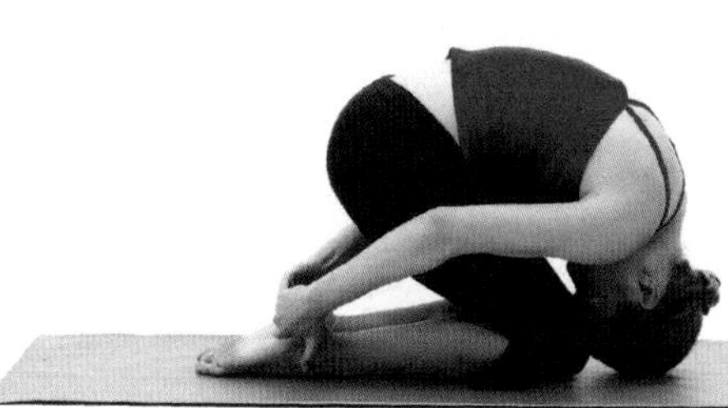

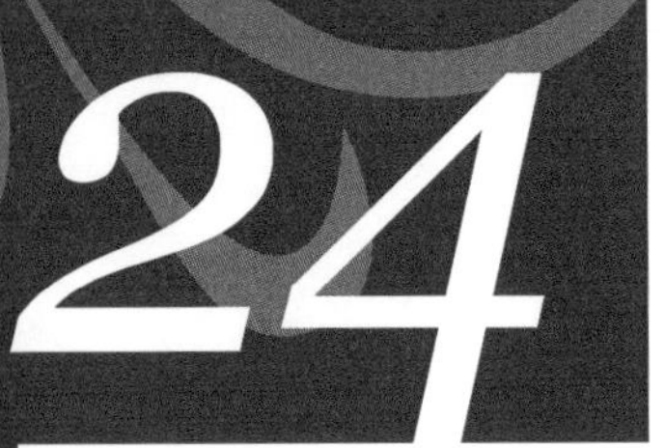

Sasangasana

RABBIT POSE

Release

Going into and out of this posture mindfully (as if mirroring the entry) is extremely important here for spinal integrity. Maintain the pull on the heels and your chin tucked. Inhale as you roll up, pivoting around your knees, to bring your hips to your heels. Your chin comes up last. Make sure you finish the pose, make contact in the mirror, then mindfully, move onto one hip, turn around and lie down in Savasana.

Common mistakes and how to fix them

Can't grab your heels: Don't fret! Most students cannot grab their heels in final grip until they have moved partway into the pose. It is very much dependent on each person's arm length, flexibility, bulk and ease of sitting in readiness for the pose.
So the initial seated grips have the following range:

- Some cannot even sit on their heels and have difficulty in reaching their feet at all through the pose.
- Some cannot even touch their feet whilst kneeling.
- Some can get their hands to the side of their feet.
- Some can get their thumbs into position.
- You are on easy street if you can get your thumbs to the outside and feel like you are sitting on your hands.

Although not ideal, gripping your heels after your head is already on the floor may simply be what you have to do. If you cannot manage any grip at all, consider rolling your towel up under your ankles. You should be able to pull on the towel from the side of the feet to create some traction in your body.

Difficult to get to the floor with grace or ease: The less flexible you are, or the less able you are to curl up, the more pressure with which your head could hit the floor. Perhaps, for example, you have a tight or straight lower back, tight hips, or a larger body shape. All is not lost here. Once your head is down, if you have the right grip, the chin tucked and the right pull and push elements, you can still achieve your outcomes in Rabbit.

Hands on feet, not gripping: Quite commonly I see students who have hips at half mast and forehead on the floor: Their hands lie on their feet in the right orientation but there is no grip at all. Grip the feet, tuck the chin, pull and lift.

Pushing the top of your head into the floor: If most of your weight is on your head then you are either pulling with bent arms or you are curled in position without a strong grip on the feet. Perhaps your hands are in position but your grip is feeble; you are not creating the correct pull and push forces to create the traction through the arms, legs and hips. With your hips up the weight compresses your cervical spine. Lower your hips a little, tuck your chin, re-grip your feet correctly and then pull on your heels with straight arms. Push down through the ankles and shins as you press the spine up.

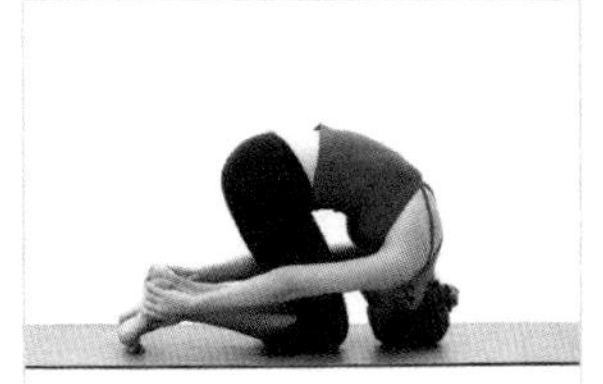

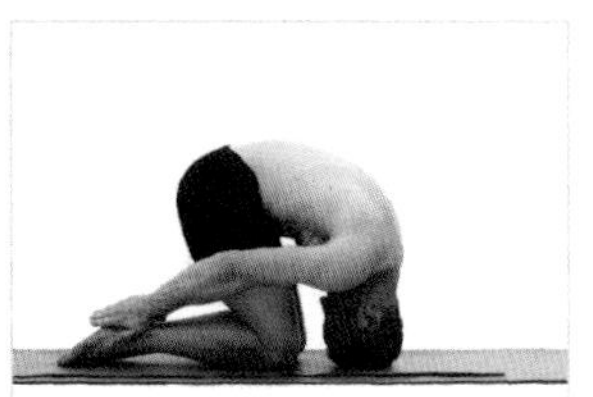

Chin away from the chest or pushing your forehead into the floor: WARNING, this is dangerous. With an exception (see below) your chin always stays in touch with your chest. Commonly students curl down and when their head encounters the floor they unlatch the chin and place the forehead squarely on the mat. They have the mistaken hope that there will be less weight on the head.

The exact opposite happens. All the weight falls forward and immense pressure is placed on the neck. The hips certainly won't lift with ease. Sometimes the feet come up off the floor! Another natural reaction to relieve this pressure is to pull with bended arms (which is the other classic Rabbit error). Tuck your chin again. Depending on your body there may or may not be a space between forehead and knees. Place your head in the position that allows straight arms to pull in traction and then pull again on your feet.

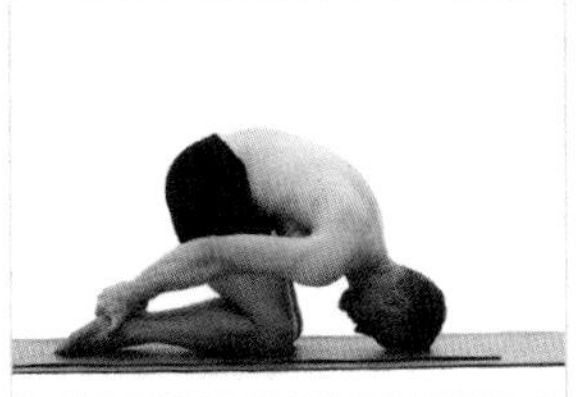

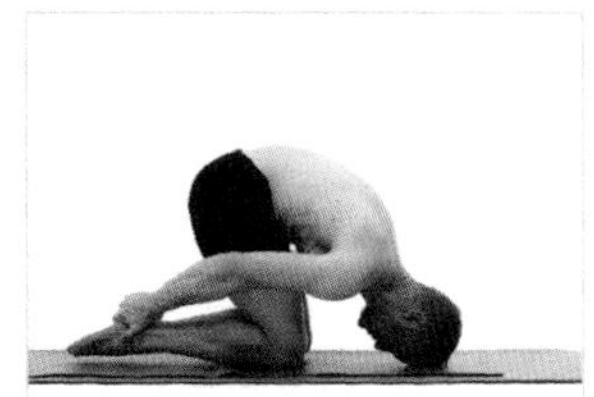

A large gap between forehead and knees: Students with very straight and inflexible lower backs (often females), or with tight hips, damaged knees or ankles tend to have a large gap between head and knees. Check that the top of the head (not the forehead) is on the floor, that you have straight arms and that traction is created with the pull. If you are feeling a stretch in the right places then all is fine. You may never get head to knee contact. Tuck the chin and pull.

Sasangasana

Rabbit Pose

Feet flexed: Never purposely flex your toes to lift your feet up off the floor. You will uncontrollably roll further forward onto your head and feel strain through your back and arms. Your feet, which have a bigger part to play than you probably realize, should always be as relaxed as possible.

Fused cervical vertebrae: Here is one proviso to the chin-tuck rule: If you have fused cervical vertebrae, then this extreme forward bending of the neck is unwarranted and could be dangerous. You will untuck your chin to an appropriate degree to lessen the leverage on your vertebrae and rely on arm strength and pushing your lower legs into the floor. I would recommend making sure you consult an authority – your specialist, your physiotherapist, someone knowledgeable you trust.

In such cases you must take a lot of personal responsibility in keeping safe. Know your condition and your limitations. I do the best I can in keeping up with all my students' conditions. However, students usually only detail their problems to the first teacher that they have. If you have an important condition, make it your business to tell each and every new teacher that you encounter. It doesn't hurt to remind them a number of times especially if they haven't taught you in a while.

Bent arms: The pull against the feet does not simply stop your body rolling forward. Together with the pushing of the lower legs into the floor and the lifting hips you create traction in the legs, hips, spine and arms. The result is an upward push of the hips and a round spine.

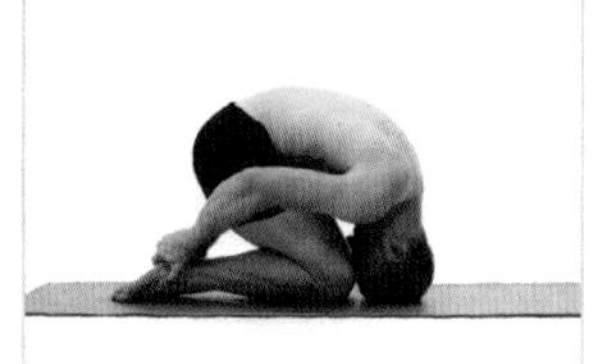

Bending the arms creates a strain and tension across the scapulae and in the shoulders. Work out whether your grip needs to be more firm around your heels. Does it work better for you with or without the towel? Check your chin tuck. In order for Rabbit to work, you must pull with your hands only, allow yourself to roll forward, and the arms must straighten.

Turning your head: If you are turning your head around, it could be that you are feeling unfamiliar or uncomfortable and are trying to observe others in the pose. You may choose to stay upright and watch others enter before entering yourself. Or ask for the teacher's guidance.

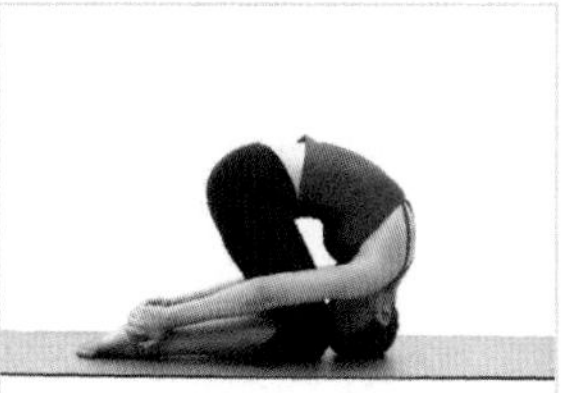

Turning your head while in this position can seriously damage the neck and put excessive pressure on the cervical vertebrae. Your vulnerable head-turning and pivoting mechanisms of the cervical spine at C1 and C2, are further put at risk. Undue compression could cause nerve or other damage. Learn the correct way and the danger signs of the incorrect approaches. Have complete attention.

Back of the head contacts the floor: If you have extremely long arms and or a very flexible neck then there is a small possibility that the back of your head makes contact with the floor. This anomaly occurs with only a very, very small number of students and causes excessive pressure on the upper spine.

The crown of the head is the furthest point to which your head should roll. Even though your forehead and knees easily contact, introduce a little distance between them to correct the contact. Or slightly move the hands to re-grip the feet less than half an inch (<1cm) further back on the heel, closer to the toes. Focus on the downward push of the knees/shins and the upward hip movement. Moving shoulders away from the ears during the pull is crucial to shifting the weight favorably away from the back of the head.

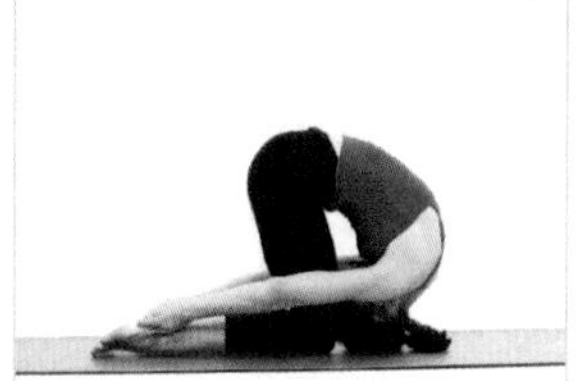

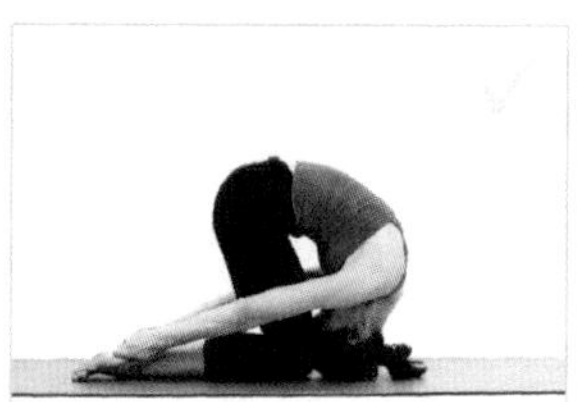

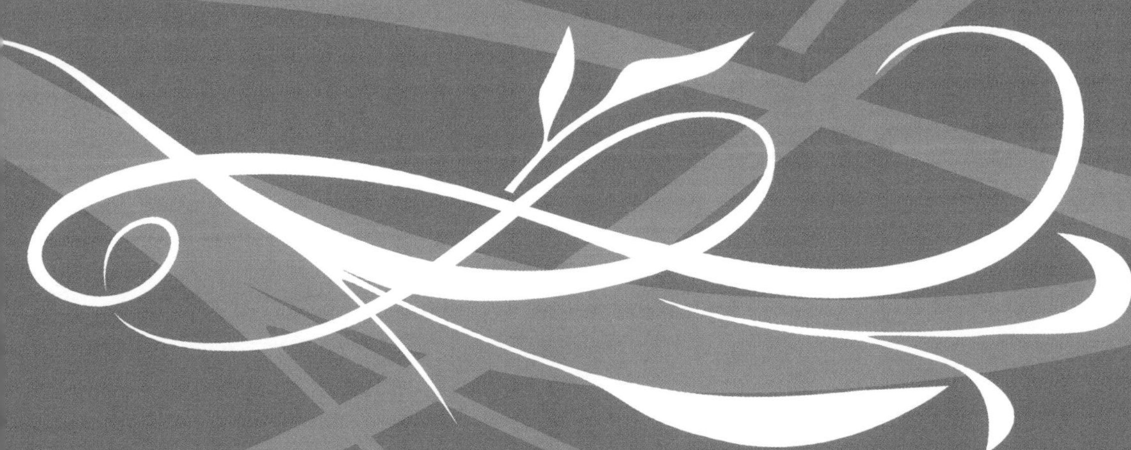

Janushirasana

If you won't be better tomorrow than you were today, then what do you need tomorrow for?
—Rebbe Nachman of Breslov

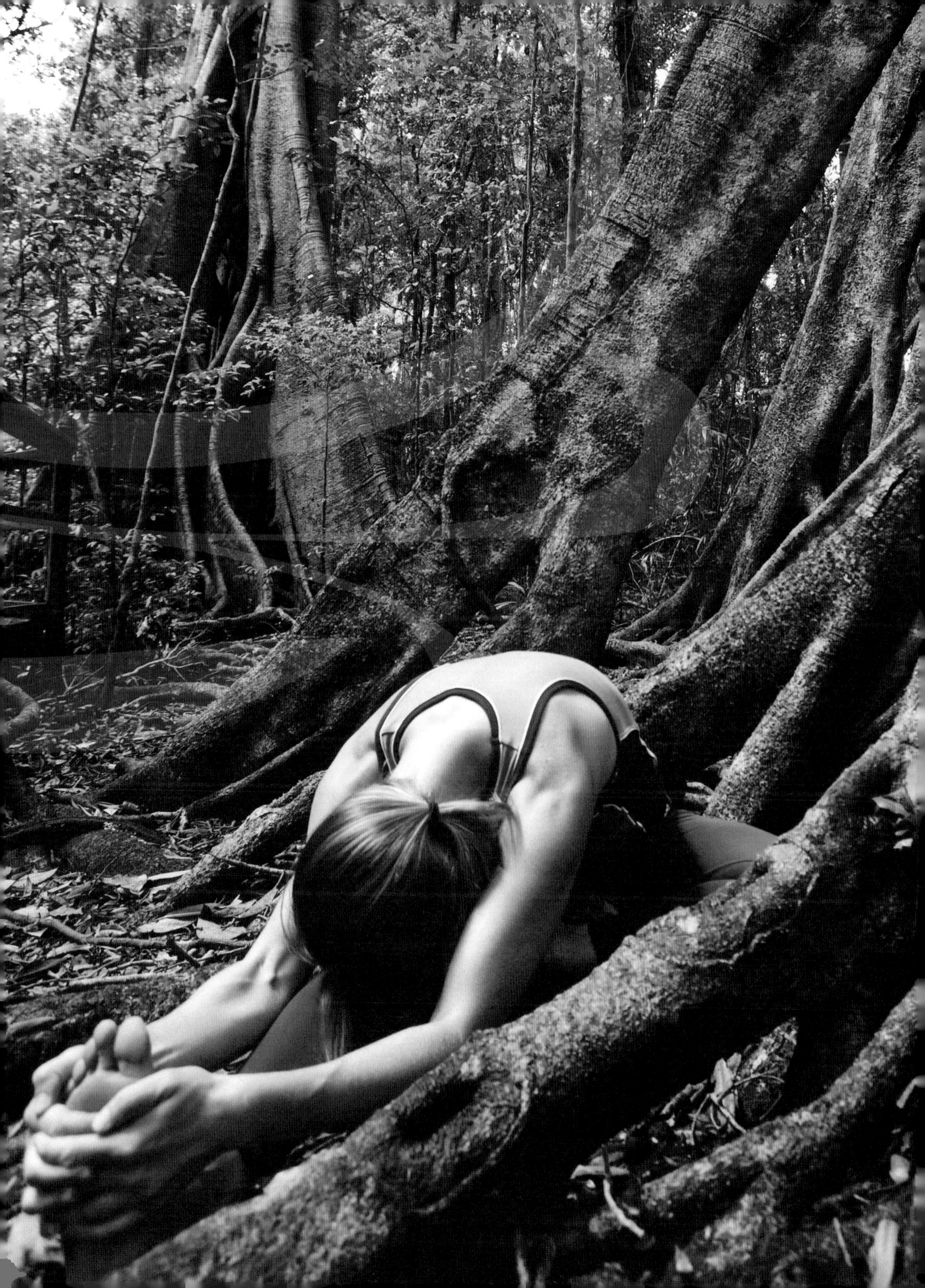

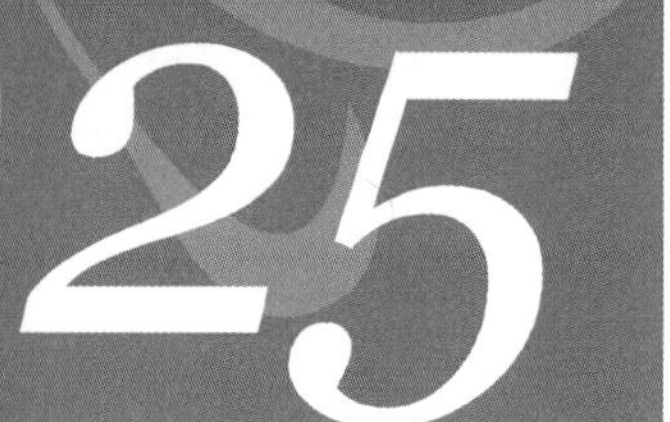

25 Janushirasana

HEAD TO KNEE POSE

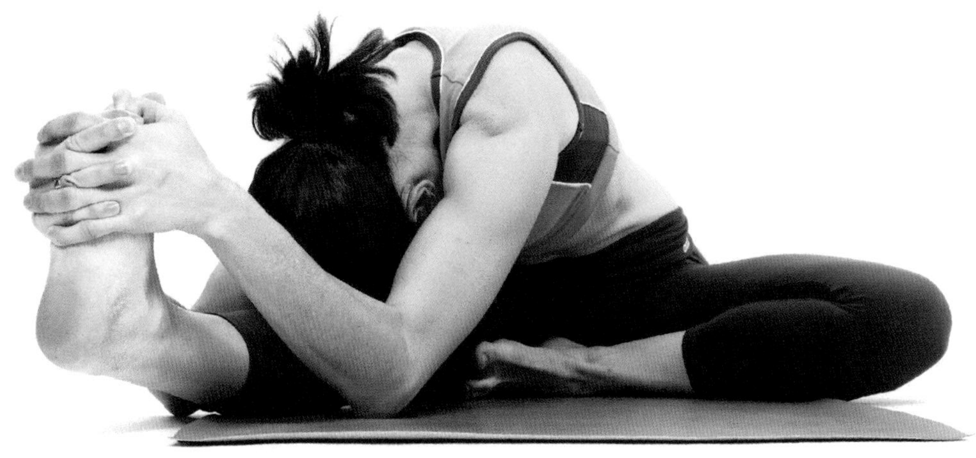

The essentials

This floor posture is the seated version of 'Standing Head to Knee' and thus requires little balance. Unlike its earlier cousin, almost everyone can get their head on their knee.

This pose is a great segue from Rabbit where you similarly continue the forward opening of your spine. You will also deeply stretch into the backs of your legs, ankles and feet, and strongly work and tone your arms into shapeliness and strength.

There are amazing forces at play to make this a very satisfying pose. Janushirasana is so much more than getting your hands on your feet or your forehead on your knee. The magic only happens once you have both working in tandem as you bring about the essential traction and stretch elements.

What makes this pose so difficult to get right?

The more inflexible, tight or injured your body, the harder this pose will be to set up. Ignoring even one of the technique elements can make it near impossible to find the tractions. Although you can fix just about anything while you are in the pose, it takes an alert and attentive student and teacher to ensure that all the boxes are checked. An error in grip, or in foot or head position, will transform this into a simple stretch without the 'sweet spot'.

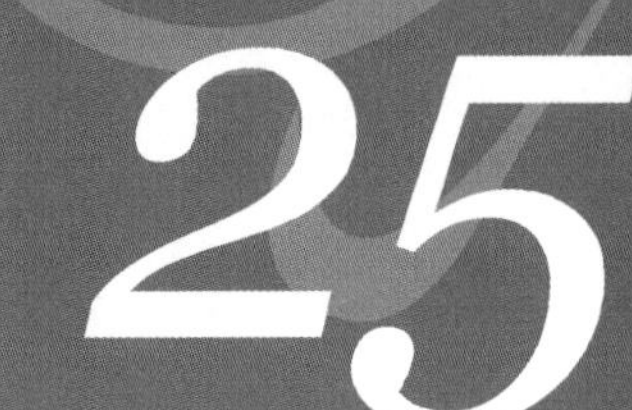

Janushirasana

Head to Knee Pose

The technique

When you come up from your sit-up please turn around and sit anywhere along your mat facing the front.

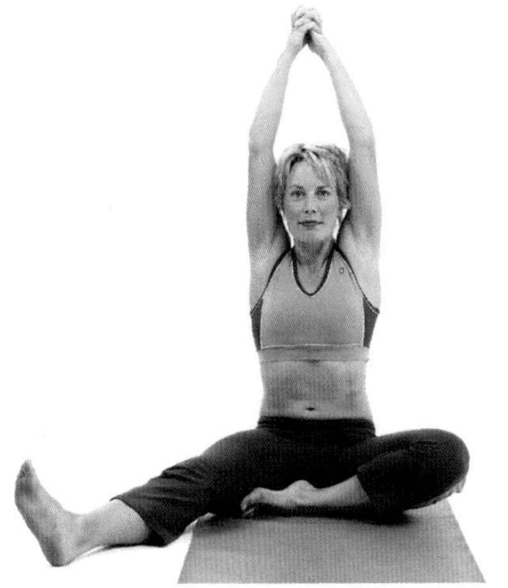

1. **Hips Square**: Sit with your hips parallel to the mirror.

2. **One Leg Bent**: Bend your left leg and draw in your foot so that your heel is at your crotch and the sole of your left foot is along your right upper thigh.

3. **One Leg Extended**: Your right leg is projecting out toward the right corner. The right foot is flexed back so that your toes are closer to the face (not pointed).

4. **Legs Have A 90° Separation**: The self-check for leg position is the hips square to the mirror and the legs at right angles to one another. Be careful not to separate the legs too much – 90° is all you need, no matter how flexible you are. You are aiming to seat your hips on the floor. Sit straight and contact yourself in the mirror and await for your instructions to proceed.

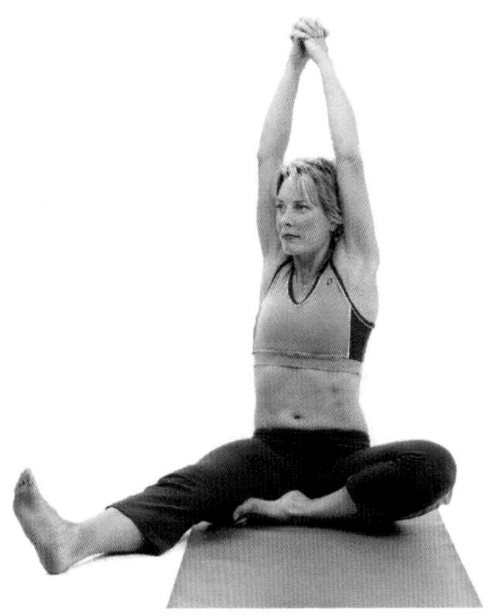

5. **Arms Up**: Inhale and bring your arms up over your head and interlock your fingers to their base. At this stage you are still sitting square to the mirror.

6. **Turn Your Body And Round Down**: Keeping your hips down, stretch some length into your torso (shoulders down and back), turn your upper body to the right. With both hips on the floor if you can, your upper body is now square to your right leg. Glue your chin permanently to your chest, draw in your abdomen and as you exhale keep your arms with your head as you round down.

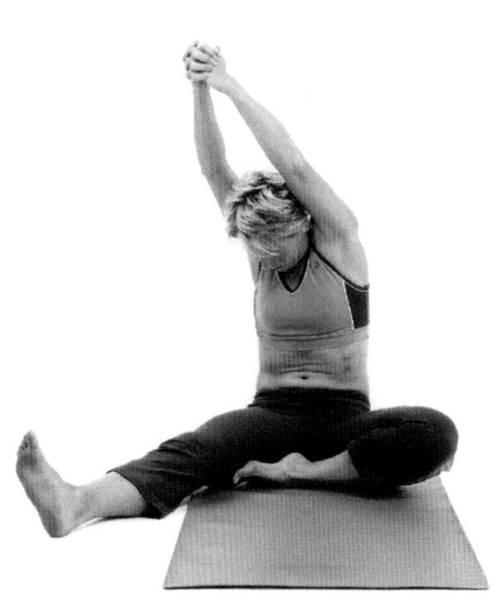

7. **Bend Up Your Knee**: Janushirasana means 'head to knee' and it is essential for contact. If it doesn't happen with a straight leg then you must bend up your leg to make it happen. Your pose depends on it. As you bend the leg, ensure that your toes stay flexed back - this will help with the hand grip (see next point). If, after your first attempt at this pose, you discover you need a bent leg to grasp your foot, then prepare for it ahead of time in future classes. As you inhale the stretch into your body, bend up your leg. You will then be able to aim for your foot without looking for it.

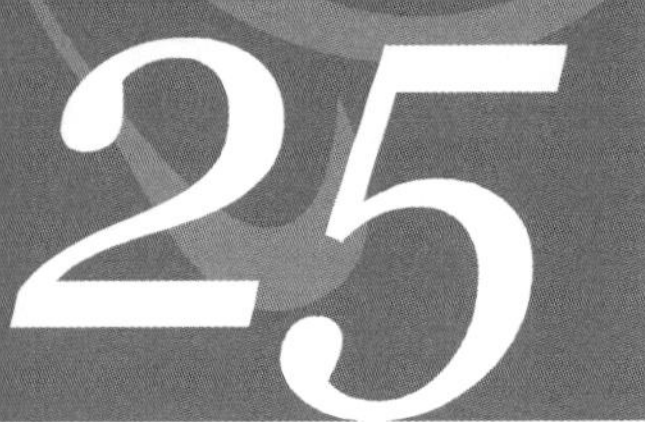

Janushirasana

Head to Knee Pose

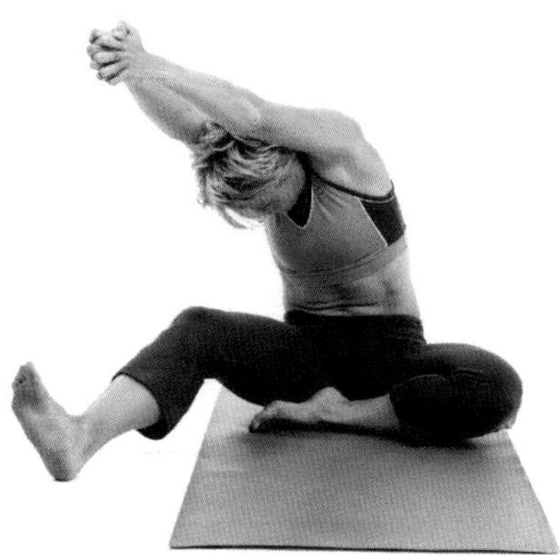

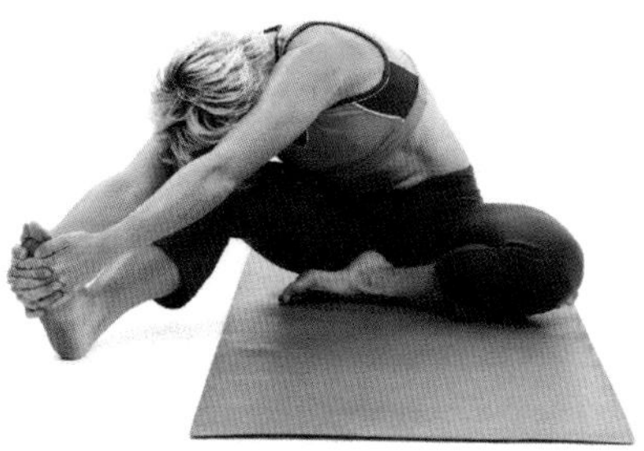

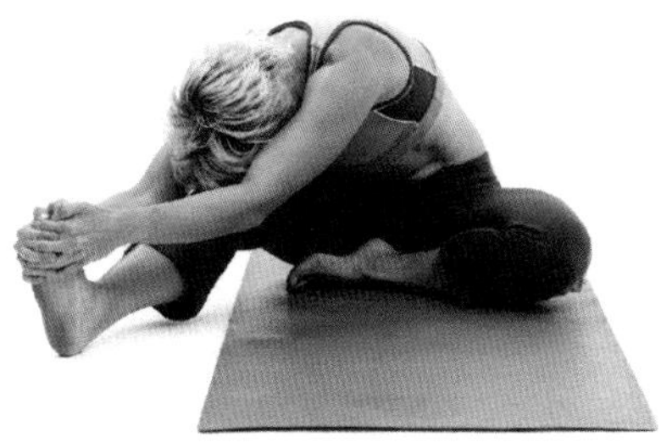

8. **Forehead To Knee, Fingers At Ball Of Foot**: On your descent with chin in, you are looking at your chest, not your toes. Bring your forehead to your knee. And, at the same time you need to bring your thumbs and still-interlocked fingers to embrace underneath and at the ball of your foot.

9. **Working In Head To Knee**: Simultaneously pull back on the toes while you push the heel away from you: Strongly work the flexion, maintain that grip and apply the pressure of the forehead on your knee. These actions lengthen the leg away from you providing stretch from flexed toes, through the heel, ankle and the back of your leg, no matter how flexible you are. Every body can get the benefits here. Remember that you must keep the following conditions in the body:

10. **Elbows Tucked In And Down**: Tuck both elbows in close to the leg. Point them below your calf muscles as if hugging them.

11. **Pull With Your Biceps**: Your arms are pulling strongly, using your biceps not your shoulders.

12. **Shoulders Down And Even**: Your shoulders are down away from the ears – in an un-hunched position. Even them out parallel to the floor.

13. **Your Bent Leg**: Have the intention of pushing your bent-in leg down to contact the floor for maximal hip opening and stability.

14. **Straighten Your Leg Eventually**: Correctly action this pose and your body will feel a very satisfying stretch: All the way from the foot through your leg and right through your spine to the neck. As the body opens, your leg will straighten; the back of your knee will eventually encounter the floor. Continue to pull on the toes, push the head on the knee and push the heel away. If your head is on the knee and leg straight, lock the knee, draw the elbows down and see if your heel can come up off the floor.

15. **Release**: Keep your fingers interlocked but release the grip and let your legs and arms relax for the exit. Then with your chin tucked, inhale as you lift out one vertebra at a time, lifting your chin up last. Reverse the entry movement so that your spine is exactly aligned along your extended leg, facing your foot. Try to keep your arms over your head and turn your body back round to the front. You are ready for the second side.

Janushirasana

HEAD TO KNEE POSE

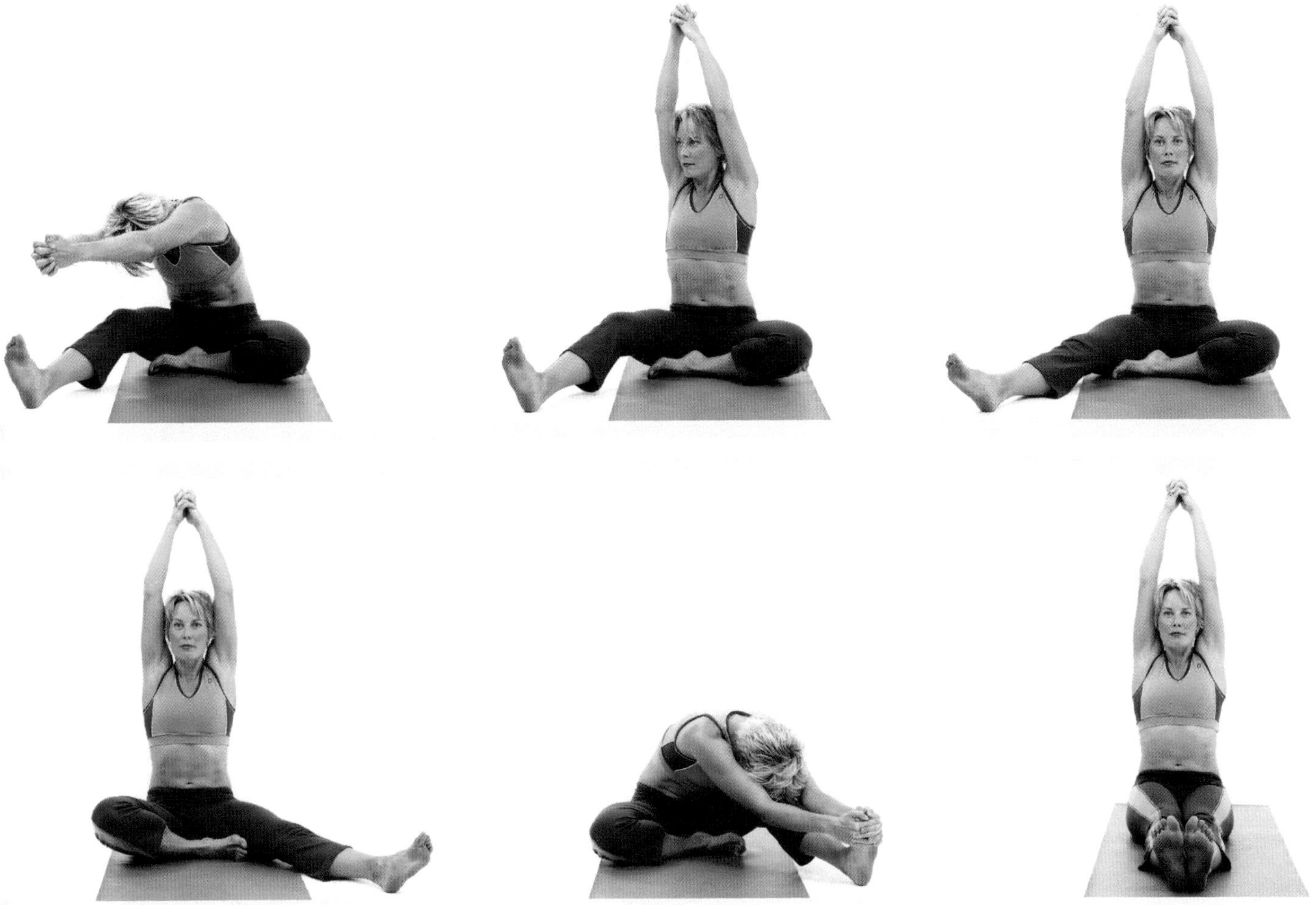

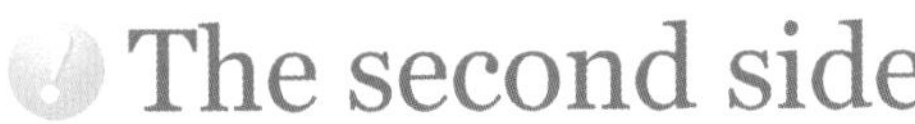

The second side

Ideally your arms are still over your head, fingers interlocked. Bring your left foot out so that it is extended out toward the left corner. Your hips stay square to the mirror. Now bring your right leg in, bent, so that the sole of your right foot contacts the inner left thigh, heel near your crotch. You may need to bring your arms to the floor to support yourself as you move your legs, especially if you have tight hips or shoulders or damaged knees. Don't launch straight down into the second side, make some contact sitting square, before twisting your torso to face your left leg.

Release

After second side of both sets you must reverse out, with your chin out last. Bring your legs out directly in front of you and face the mirror. There is no Savasana after Janushirasana. You move directly into the next pose.

Janushirasana

HEAD TO KNEE POSE

Common mistakes and how to fix them

At any stage you need to dial back to a secure position if:

- Your head pulls away from your knee.
- Your fingers are no longer interlocked fully.
- If your foot is not flexed but is pointing to the mirror.
- If your thumbs come to rest on the top of your foot instead of underneath.

Can't reach your foot: You are not alone. If after your first try you cannot reach the foot of your straight leg, then it is simply a matter of adjustment. Bend your leg up so that:

a. Your foot remains flexed, toes pointed to your nose (only the back of your heel on the ground)
b. You have your head on your knee and
c. You can get your interlocked fingers below the ball of your foot.

In order to reach the foot your leg may be bent very high with only inches between the heel and the hip. This makes descent minimal. There is nothing wrong with that. You work with your body for good alignment to get the benefits.

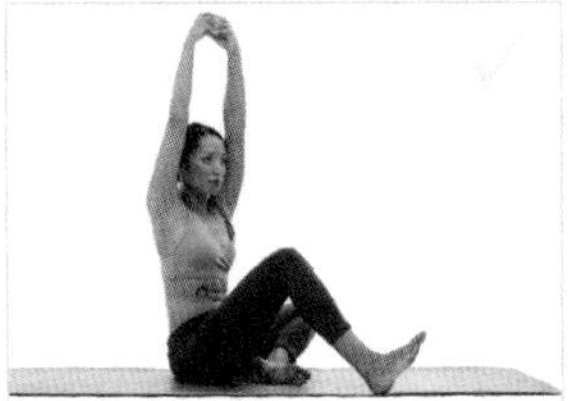

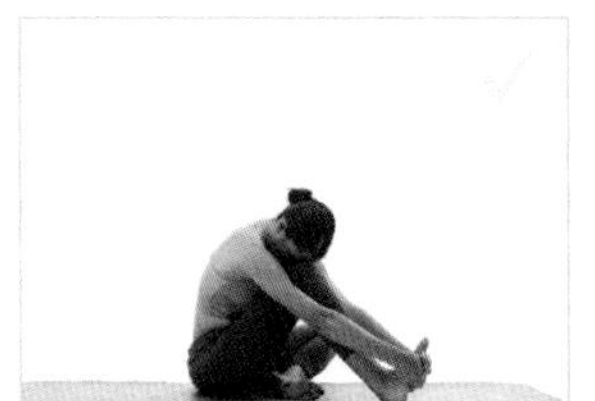

Looking for your foot: Watching one's foot while bringing the head towards the leg could be the most common error. Performing this graceful ballet-type move transforms the posture from one of rounding the spine to a spinal extension (at least at first) robbing you of the full intent of this pose. Rounding from the get-go builds on the intense forward bend and offers an intense abdominal organ compression.

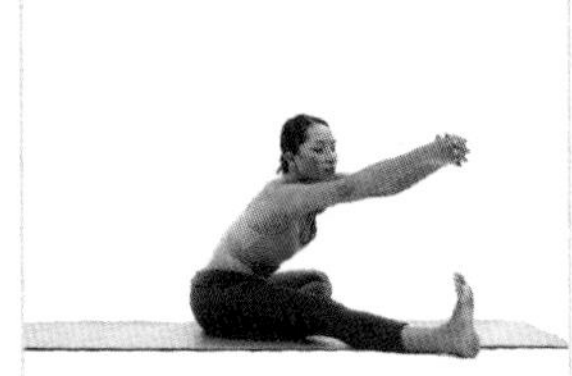

You will easily find your foot. It is right at the end of your leg, always has been. There's nothing to look for. That sounds like a joke, but so many people look for their foot as if it were a moving target. You must tuck your chin and get your forehead on your knee. You lower your hands down to below your foot for the hold.

Shoulders not square: Most often the inside shoulder is higher than the outer one. Evening out your elbows corrects the shoulders to make them parallel with the ground. You get a sense of their relative position to the floor even though you cannot see them directly. If both hips are not grounded you may find it a little more difficult to also square off your upper body.

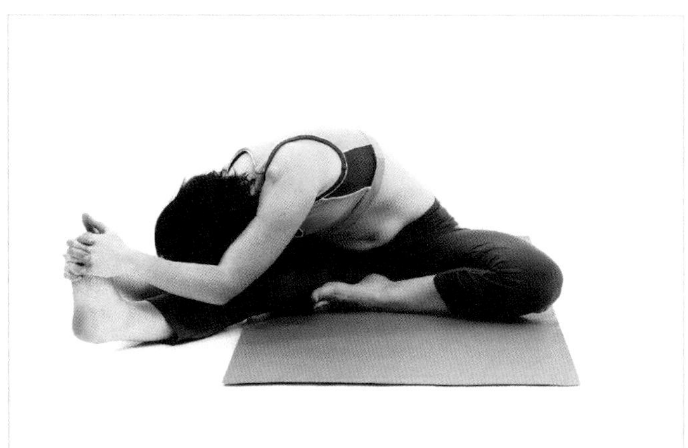

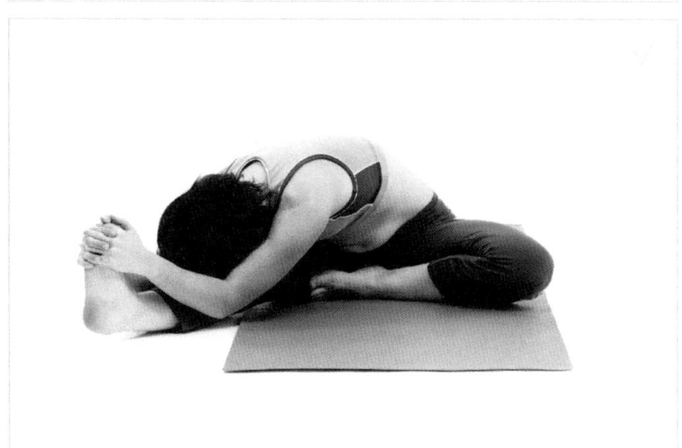

Thumbs on foot: Thumbs on top will engage the pull of the arms differently. Your shoulders will be used instead of being relaxed and your elbows will likely move out like wings instead of pointing down. Your thumbs are very strong so use them to get leverage in this pose. Pull with them placed under the foot but do not interlock them.

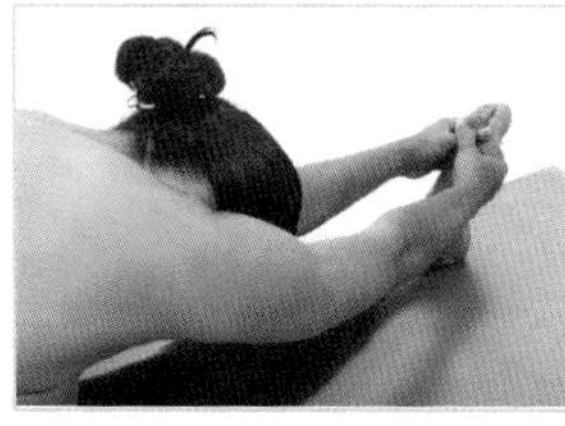

Elbows out: If your elbows are out like wings when you are pulling back on your foot then you are most likely involving at least your shoulders. Check to see if you have mistakenly placed your thumbs on top of your foot. Dropping your arms in will release your shoulders and you will be able to pull with just your biceps muscles. Tension in your upper back and neck area will resolve and you can focus on the body opening.

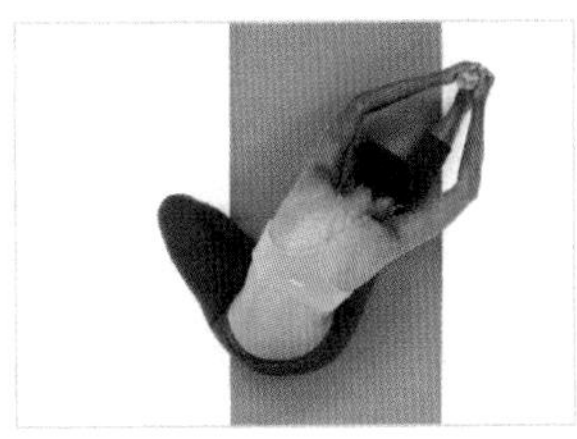

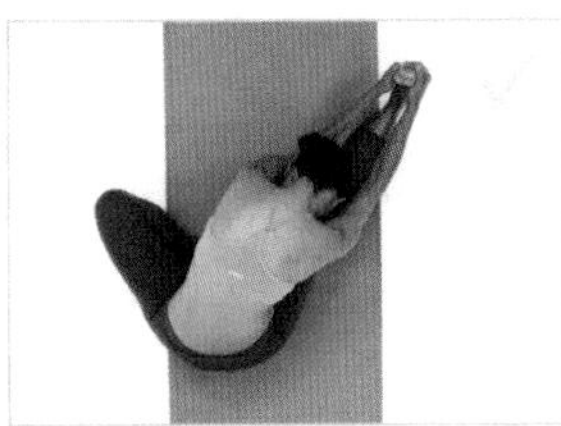

Chin on knee: As the name indicates, Janushirasana is head to knee, not head to shin, chin to shin, or chin to knee. Tuck the chin under and keep it there. Do whatever it takes including bending up the leg to gain contact. Not surprisingly, if you are very tight it can become quite difficult the higher your knee is bent, to grab the foot and get head to knee.

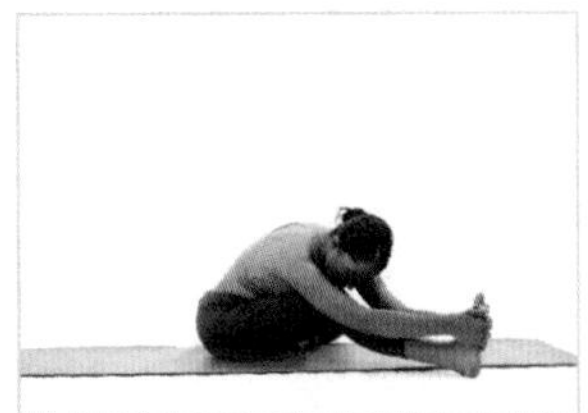

Forehead away from knee: Head to knee contact is required, not a little space between them. You need the pull against your flexed foot, opposed by an extension through the heel moving away from you. To assist this your head pushes down on your knee, together they move closer to the floor. Alter or take one of these elements away and you don't have this pose. Set up this series of active stretches well and you create the traction areas in the body. Find them and it becomes a joy, an achievement, something you can find again and again.

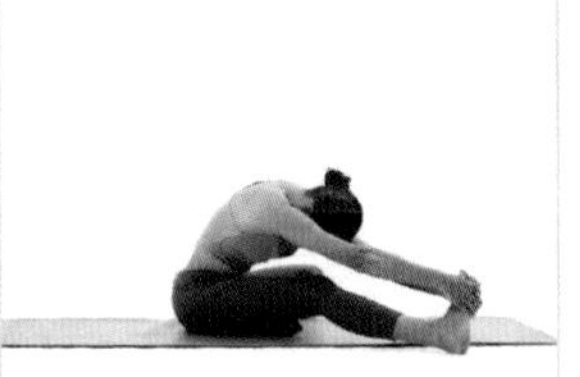

Toes pointed, heel towards hip: Quite often in an attempt to get any of the Janushirasana poses, students wrongly extend their leg by pushing the toes and ball of the foot against the hands, while drawing the heel back toward the body. The arms tend to extend and the shoulders come forward. The foot moves in a way that is opposite to that which is intended, the back of the leg contracts and there is some associated muscle strain across the mid and lower back. Somewhere along the way the student thinks they are getting the stretch.

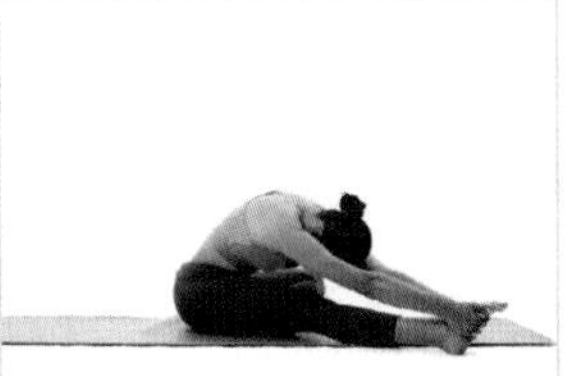

Even though it is impossible to enact, try visualizing your toes flexing back so much that they could touch your shin. Feel the extension through the back of your leg right through your forward extending heel. Regardless of how bent your knee is you will feel a deep stretch, but you need to set it up and pull.

***An adjustment for those with hip or knee problems**: Some people topple when they bend in their leg on one or both sides of Janushirasana and may even have to position a steadying hand on the floor.

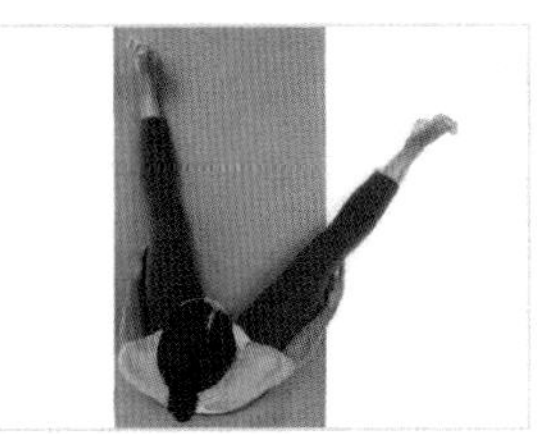

If this is you, extend your leg out as per the correct technique. Instead of bending the second leg, you may have to leave it extended directly to the mirror or bent in partway without contact of the sole to inner thigh. Be aware that if this is an asymmetrical problem you may only have to make the adjustment on one side.

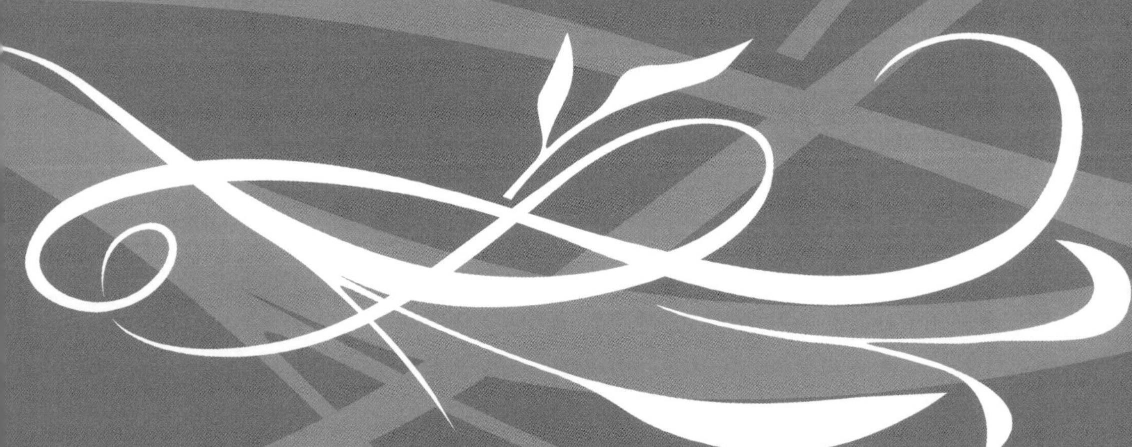

Paschimottanasana

There is only one corner of the universe you can be certain of improving, and that's your own self.
—Aldous Huxley

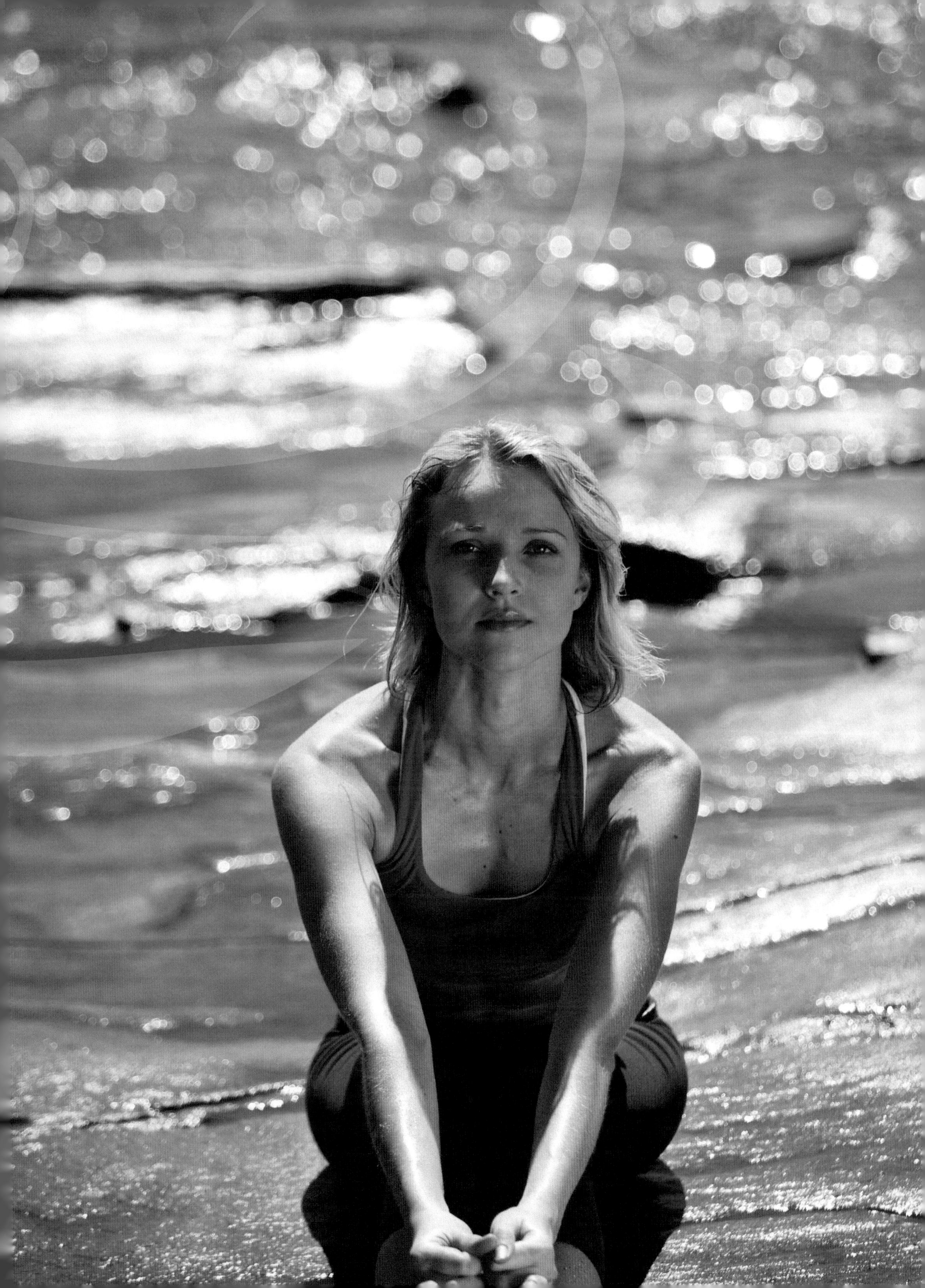

26 Paschimottanasana

Intense Stretching Pose

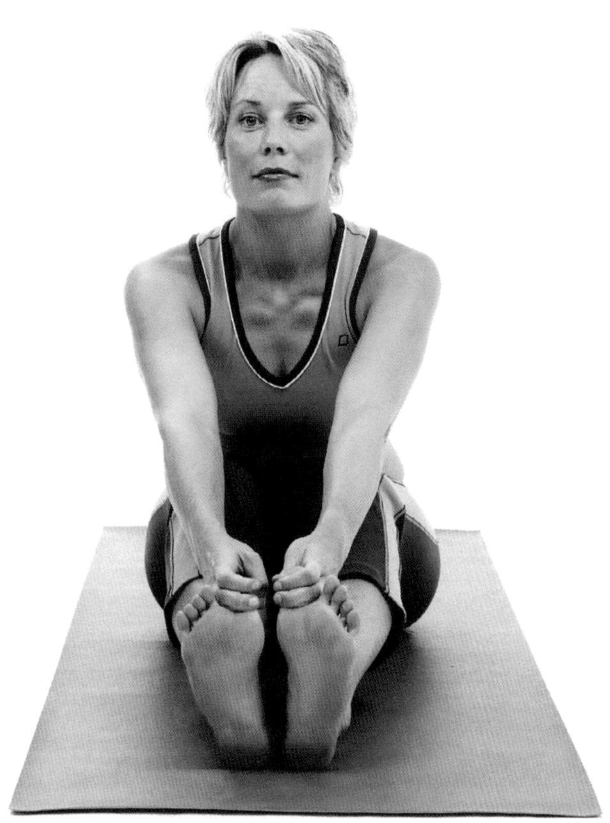

The essentials

As much as you are trying to be 'in the moment' it is hard to escape the fact that you have almost finished class at this point. Paschimottanasana is a deep long stretch for the spine, the back and the legs. Your body is warm, has little resistance to the pull and you can feel your body's tensions ironing out.

What makes this pose so difficult to get right?

Here we find ourselves heading into a pose without the contextual separation of a Savasana. As a result many students carry the same principles of the previous Janushirasana into this opposing but complementary pose. However as its Sanskrit name suggests, this is an intense straight back stretch which contributes to open the chest, lungs, and then lengthen the whole back side of the body.

It is essential to work on the premise that this intense stretch positively avoids any forward rounding component. As you will read below, I teach my students that the moment they are aware of roundness in the back they make the necessary adjustments to straighten up again.

The link between the two consecutive poses

There are definite similarities between the Janushirasana and Paschimottanasana poses making it easy to understand why there are misunderstandings. But there are definitely more differences. I have summarized all the components in the following table. The table must be used in conjunction with both pose chapters to gain full understanding of the fine details.

The feet, legs and shoulders all work in the same way for both poses. The similarity in the leg/foot/hand traction relationship is identical but the hand positions are different. Beyond that it all differs markedly.

The relationship between the two different poses

What is different?	Janushirasana	Paschimottanasana
Chin	Tucked	Extended, parallel to floor
Hands	Fingers interlocked, thumbs under foot (never on top)	'Peace fingers' grip big toes
Arms	Use biceps for strength, always keep them bent	Arms STRAIGHT if legs are bent. Arms only start to bend using biceps (not shoulders) when legs and back are both straight
Elbows	Bent	Straight. Bend them only when legs in full extension so that you can bring your STRAIGHT back to eventually lie on your straight legs
Spine	Always rounded	Always straight, extended
Gaze	Into heart or abdomen	Forward, make contact with your own eyes
Breathing	May be shorter due to compression through throat and chest.	Long, slow, deep, calming breaths. Inhale length into your body, exhale depth into your stretch

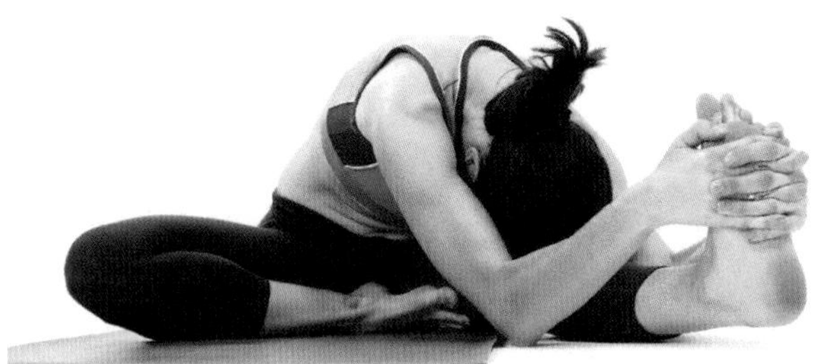

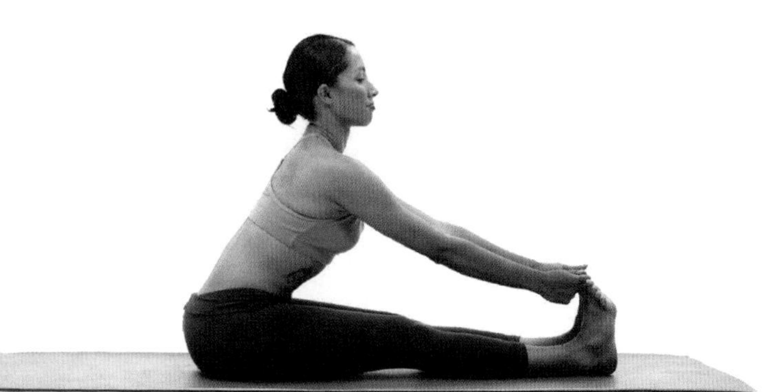

What is the same?	Janushirasana	Paschimottanasana
Shoulders	Relaxed and down	
Feet	Flexed, toes back, only back of heel contacts floor	
Legs	Most start with bent legs. Work toward having long straight, locked legs (heels may then lift up)	

26 Paschimottanasana

INTENSE STRETCHING POSE

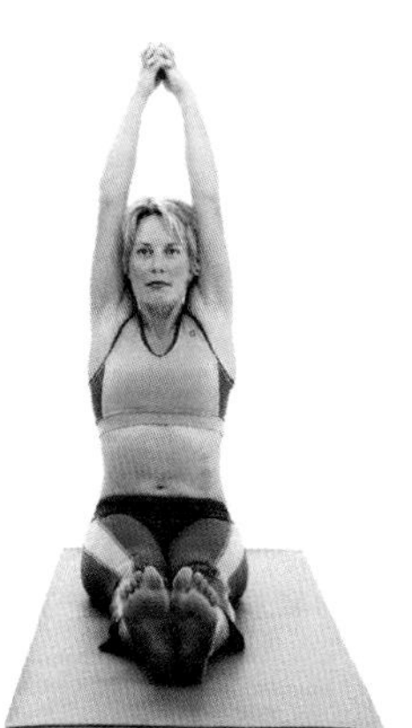
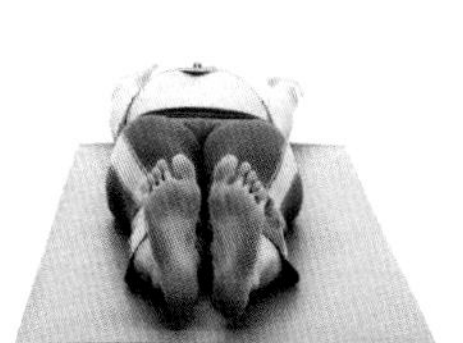
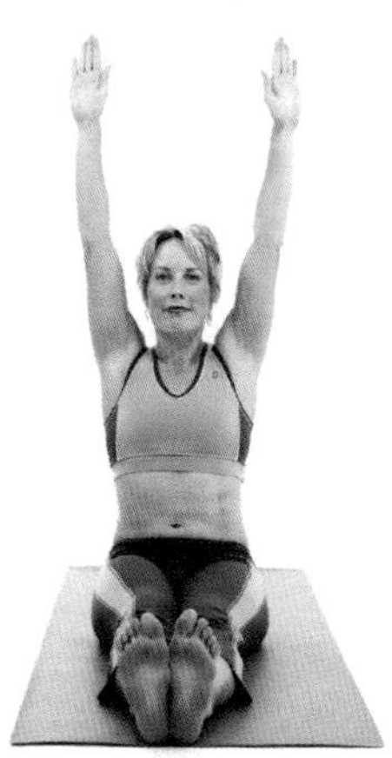
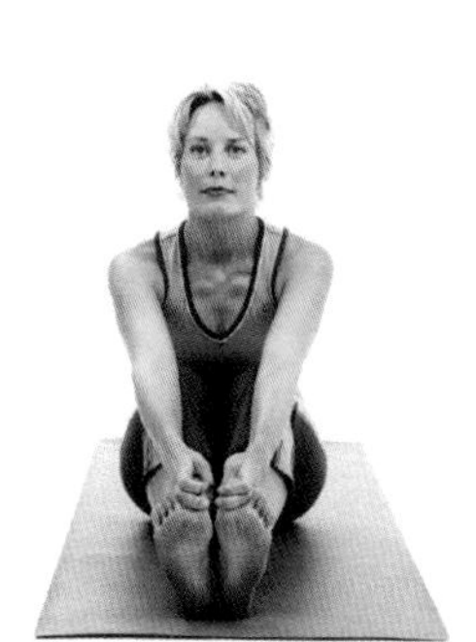

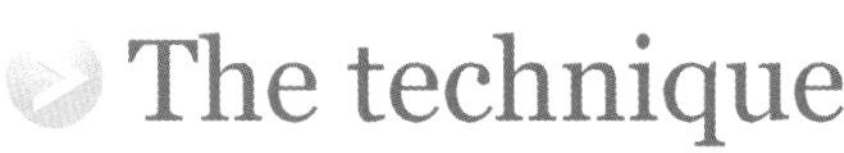

The technique

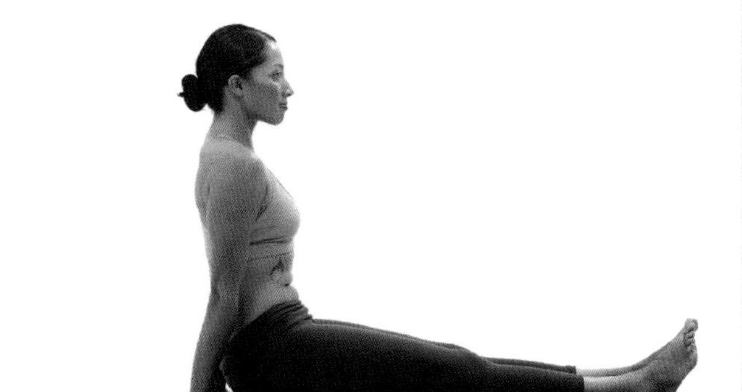

Moving from Janushirasana to Paschimottanasana

As previously indicated, there is no Savasana before this pose. After Head to Knee your legs are extended out in front. If you can, lie back bring your arms up over your head on the floor and do a sit-up. Please see the chapter on sit-ups for details.

The following is the alternative to the sit-up. Use it if you have a weak or tender lower back or have simply run out of puff!

1. Bring your legs in front of you.
2. Position your arms by your sides.
3. Place your palms on the floor adjacent to your hips with your fingers facing forward.
4. Leaving your heels on the floor, take the weight of your entire body on your hands and lift your hips up off the floor for about a half a second.

The purpose of both techniques is to squarely re-align your hips.

The set-up

1.1 YOUR LEGS OUTSTRETCHED: Your legs are together and outstretched in front of you.

1.2 BEND YOUR LEGS AND GRIP YOUR BIG TOES: Even if you can reach hands to your feet while legs are straight, bend the legs and grab your big toes. More flexible students will create a space of around 4-6 inches (10-15cm) under the knees and less flexible students about 6-12 inches (15-30cm). Grab your big toes by inserting your 'peace' fingers (index and middle) between the first and second toes.

Paschimottanasana

Intense Stretching Pose

1.3 Self-Contact And Chin Up: Make contact with yourself. Always keep your chin up parallel to the floor.

1.4 Sit Forward On Your Sit-Bones: To start the lengthening process, leave your heels where they are and 'walk' your hips back one at a time several times each side. This orients your pelvis correctly and you feel the front of your 'sit bones' contacting the floor. You should feel a small arch (a slight backbend) in your lower back due to the pelvic tilt and because you are lifting your breastbone to further pull open your chest.

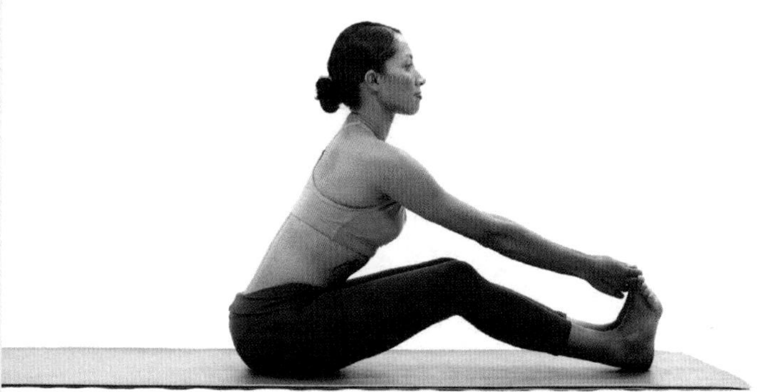

1.5 Pull Back With Straight Arms: Your feet are strongly flexed. Shoulders down and back. Create traction as you 'hang' from your toes with straight, relaxed arms, by pulling your toes back while lifting your breastbone. This will help you maintain the correct pelvic tilt and stop you rounding your spine.

1.6 The Importance Of A Straight Back: Be careful to preserve your straight back, relaxed shoulders, and forward tilted hips. It is hard to see how straight your back is by looking in the front mirror. If you do have a side mirror then take a brief look to verify. Your first priority must always be to have a straight back. So, you must bend your legs if your back is not straight. In this way you can correct discrepancies, rework the length in your back and the orientation of your pelvis.

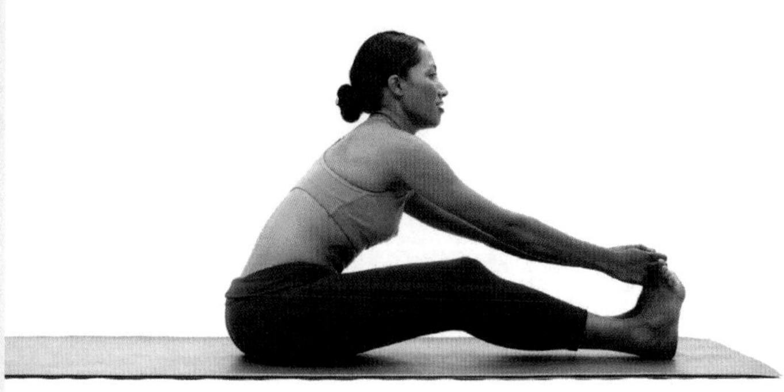

The pose

2.1 Inhale And Lengthen: Your back and arms are straight; your legs have a slight to large bend in them; your feet are strongly flexed and you have a grip on your big toes. Take a big inhale and find a lengthening stretch in your torso.

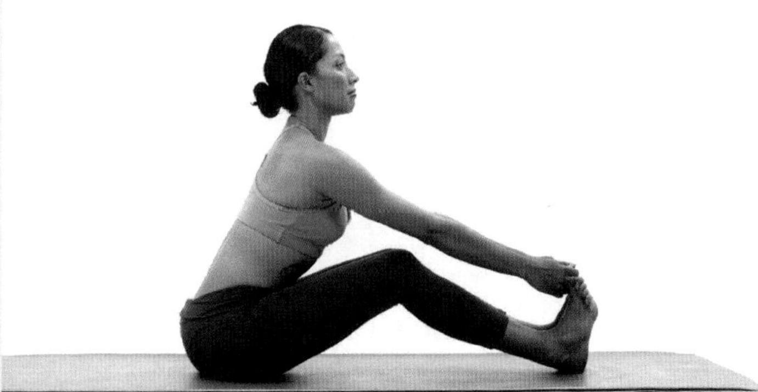

2.2 Exhale And Pull, Always Keep A Straight Back: On your exhale pull on your toes with straight arms and push your heels away from you to create immense traction. It should feel as if you have a 'hook' under your breastbone pulling your chest up: The more you pull on your toes, the more your arms stretch straight and the taller you grow. Keep your chin parallel to the floor. As you pull, simply try to straighten your legs. When you follow these directions, then no matter how bent or straight your legs, your back will always be straight and you will always get a full body stretch.

26 Paschimottanasana

Intense Stretching Pose

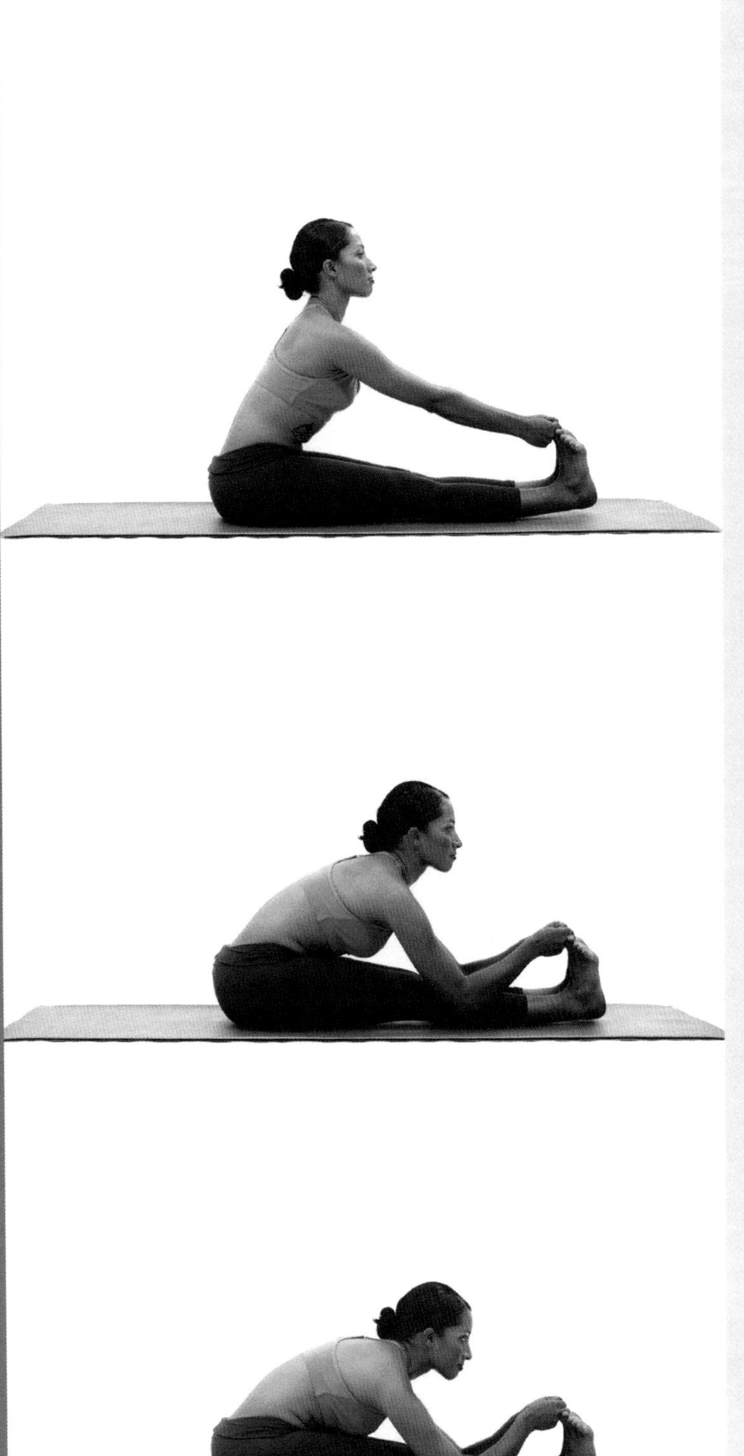

2.3 **Form A Triangle, Constantly Correct**: You have to be able to form a triangle with 3 straight sides; back, arms and legs. Anyone can sit with legs and arms straight with a rounded back. But then we wouldn't be calling this pose Paschimottanasana. If your back is rounded, back off, firstly by bending up your legs and sitting forward on your sit-bones again. Then, lift your chest, straighten your back, pull back on your toes to straighten out your arms again. If your legs are not straight then make it your intention to iron out your bent legs to form 3 perfectly straight sides of a triangle. Pull, extend, stretch, and open to create your 3 sides.

2.4 **Most Students Have Bent Legs**: The majority of any class will see more students with bent legs than straight. Have the humility to bend them up and work your straight spine into that gratifying deep stretch.

2.5 **Straight Legs? Then Lift Heels And Bend Your Arms**: With your body, straight arms and legs in a triangle formation, lock out your legs and continue to pull your toes back and get your heels up off the floor. You can now start to pull with your biceps muscles, bending your arms and pointing your elbows down. Continue to pull against your feet; heels forward, toes back. Keep the lift in your chest as you try to place one vertebra at a time along your thighs. Eventually as you lay forward on your legs your elbows will contact the floor. Naturally you will then move them out to the sides to continue the stretch.

2.6 **Forehead On Toes**: For a very small majority of students and maybe then for a small percentage of classes, the forehead (and not the top of the head) will touch the toes. Your straight body and legs are folded against each other. Your heels pull off the floor. Your elbows bend out, arms pulling strongly from relaxed shoulders. Your thumbs will move out of the way to allow contact of forehead to toes.

2.7 **Work The Breath**: Wherever you are, keep on pulling and focus on a straight back. Every inhale work the length into your torso, every exhale work the depth into the stretch, and surrender.

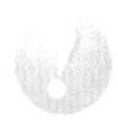

Release

On release, let go of your feet. Inhale as you bring your body back up to a central neutral position while you maintain mirror contact. Spin around and lie down on the floor for your Savasana.

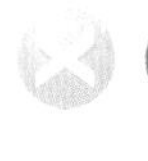

Common mistakes and how to fix them

An error in the grip: Although it doesn't actually change the outcome markedly you should not pull back on the feet with your whole hand. Over time your fingers will be strong enough to do the work and not slip. Just pull on your big toes with those two fingers. Your thumbs may or may not actually be involved in the grip.

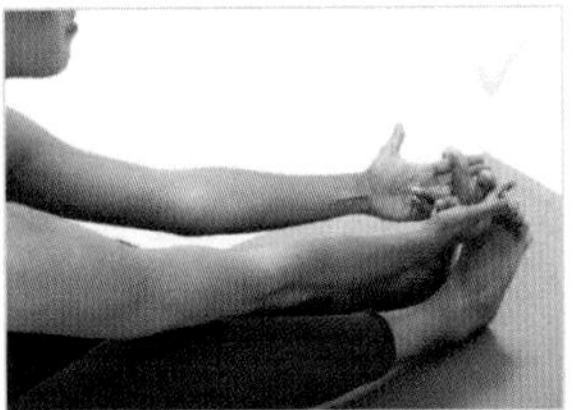

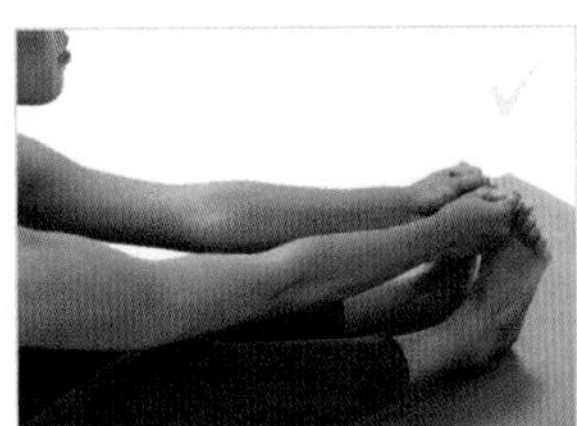

No triangle: The most common mistake is to keep the legs bent and hinge at the hips, bringing the body close to the thighs. Sometimes your back may even be straight (over bent legs) but pulled forward by bent arms, bypassing the triangle stage and creating no traction. Often students pull against pointed toes (see below).

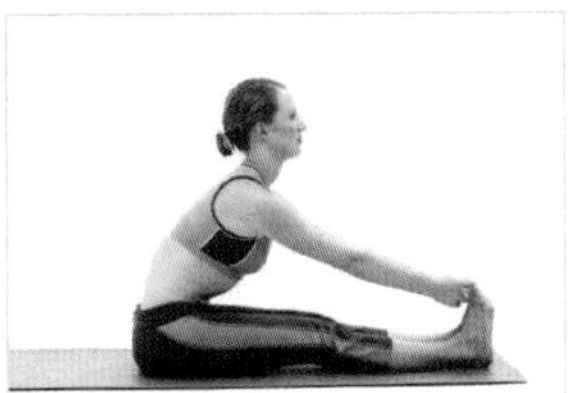

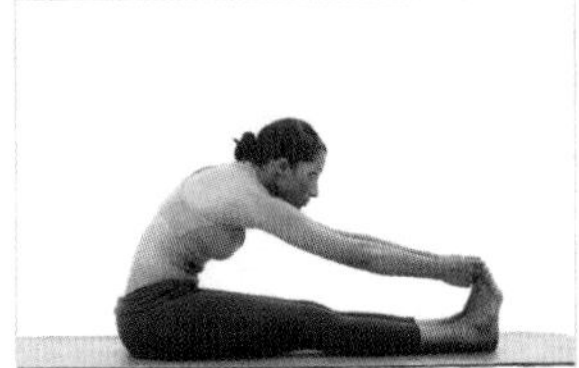

Pulling against pointed toes: In an (unconscious) effort to get the body closer to the mirror many students point their toes. Yes it provides a stretch but also risks damage to the back. The back of the leg shortens as the heels move closer to the hips. You need to fix this by simultaneously pulling your arms straight and lifting the chest. Roll forward again onto your sit-bones.

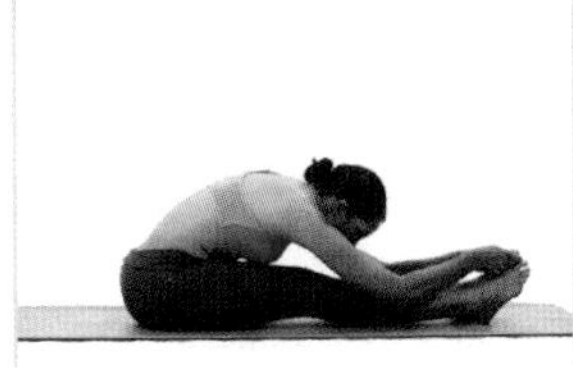

A cocktail of errors: There are no prizes for sitting there with your chin towards your toes if:

- Your back is rounded like a ball,
- Your toes are pointing towards the mirror,
- Your legs are straight,
- Your arms are bent out to the side.

There is little to no benefit if you put these above four conditions together. Students mistakenly believe that since their rounded bodies are folded in half with their chest on their knees that they are getting something right! Re-establish the basics. Straighten your arms and bend your legs, roll your hips down to sit forward on your sit-bones.

Chin drops toward the chest to some degree: Your nose should NOT at any time be on your legs. Project your chin forward. You are working through a spinal extension. The closer your chest is to your straight legs, the more of a challenge it is to keep your chin parallel to the floor. Your chin will naturally (and not at all consciously) drop in relation to the floor only when your head is very close to your toes. Therefore always try to keep your chin parallel to the floor.

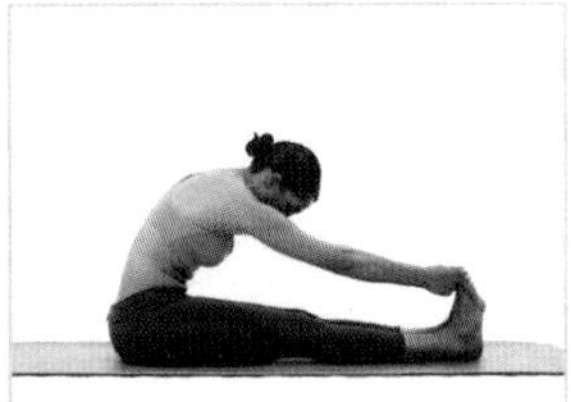

Can't straighten your legs: So what? It doesn't matter. This is yoga. You just do the best you can. Follow the guidelines. If you can't straighten your legs then you will have:

- A beautifully straight yet slightly arched back, tilted pelvis creating the stretch through both sides of the body,
- Long strong arms,
- Some measure of bend in your legs,
- And a delicious stretch through your body.

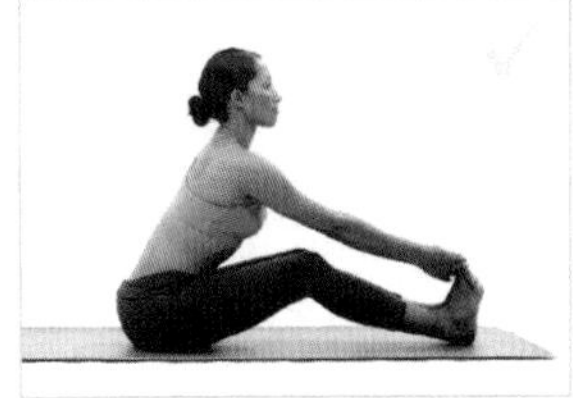

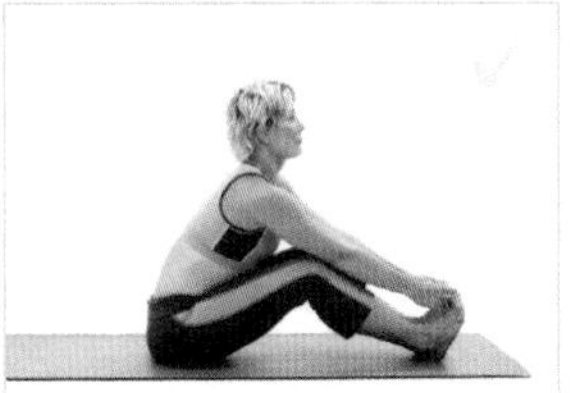

There is no rest: At no stage in this pose do you hang out.

- This is an active traction pose and not at all passive. You are working here every moment.
- So **if your legs are bent** you are accentuating the hip tilt accompanied by the up and outward movement of the chest, the push through the heels and the long straight arms.
- **If your legs and back are straight** then you keep pulling your feet back, push through the heels, and start to pull your body over your locked legs to bring your chin over your toes. It is only at this point when you are permitted to bend your arms.

Ardha Matsyendrasana

Whatever you can do or dream you can, begin it. Boldness has genius, power, and magic in it.
—Goethe

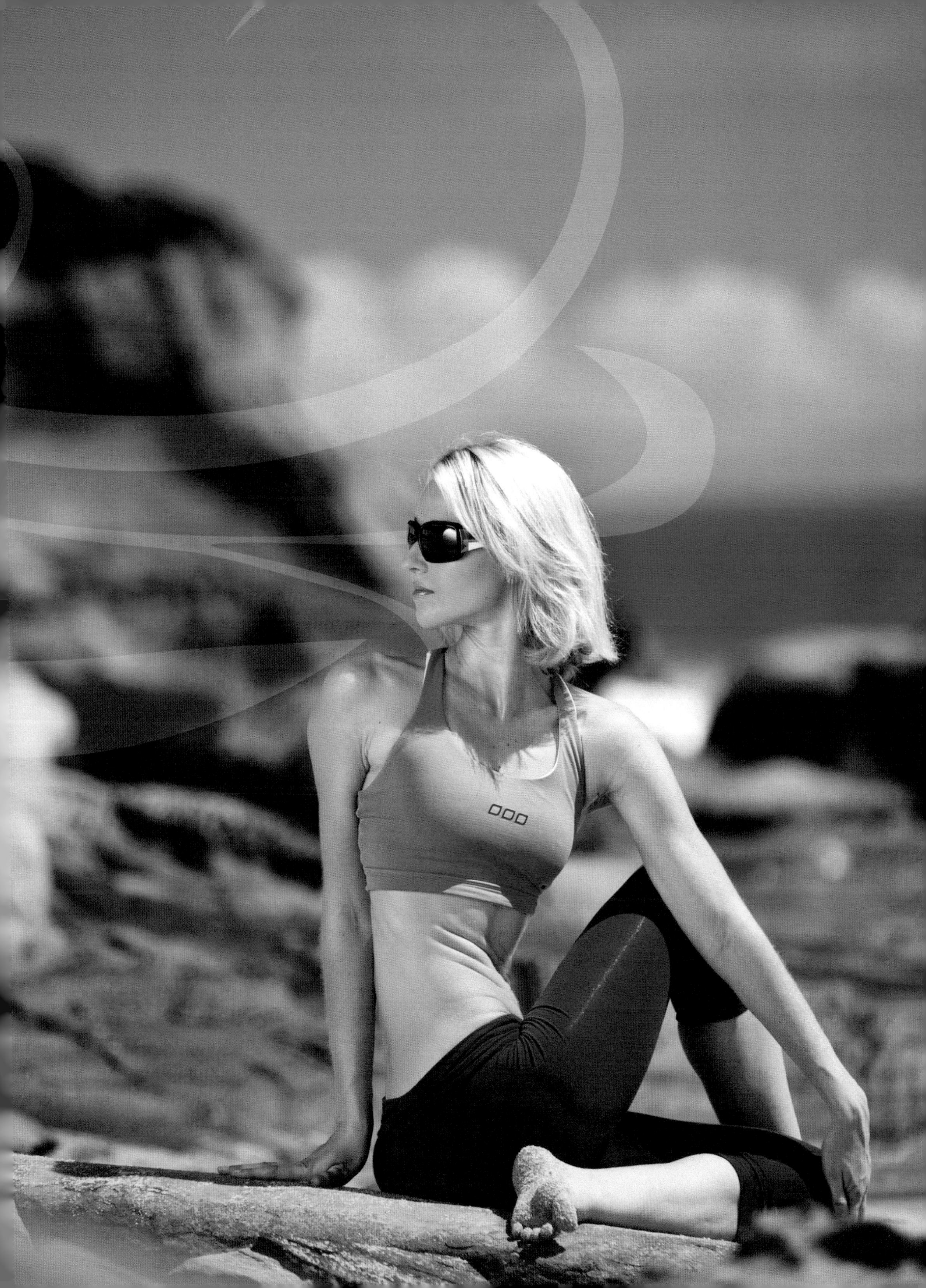

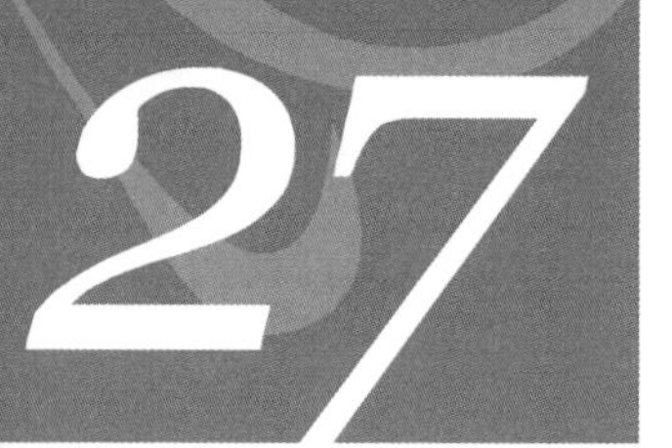

Ardha Matsyendrasana

Final Twisting Pose

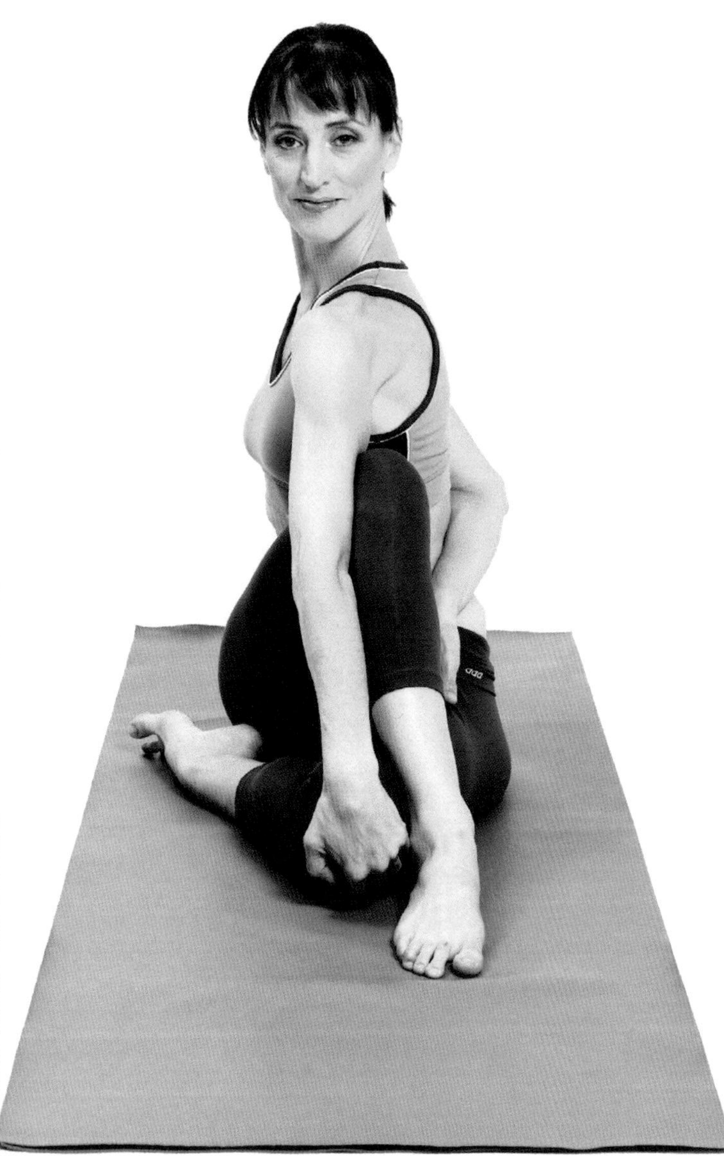

The essentials

We are almost at the end of the class. This is an intense spinal twisting pose working deep into the hips and abdominal organs, creating lateral spinal freedom, and a phenomenal stretch. It helps restore a healthy operational spine and central nervous system. This pose is so intense that we only do it once each side; there is no second set.

Although seen as a spine opener through twisting, this pose has a great deal to do with hip opening. It is through traction of the hips and upper body that this beautiful stretch is created. Seat your hips firmly and work the twist all the way up from the floor to the crown of the head. Feel the way you can effectively and literally squeeze the air out of your lungs to cleanse them.

What makes this pose so difficult to get right?

Final Twist is the second 'pretzel' position; Eagle is the other. This pose is really quite active with a number of elements to pay attention to. It all comes down to getting the right geometry and mechanics. Once we nut out your hip, leg and foot positions plus a couple of checkpoints you will find this pose simple to understand.

Ardha Matsyendrasana

27

Final Twisting Pose

The technique

After your sit-up swing around to a sitting position. In studios you commonly turn to the right to face the left wall but it is not a steadfast rule. In order to track your movements let's arbitrarily label the wall to which you face to begin, 12 o'clock.

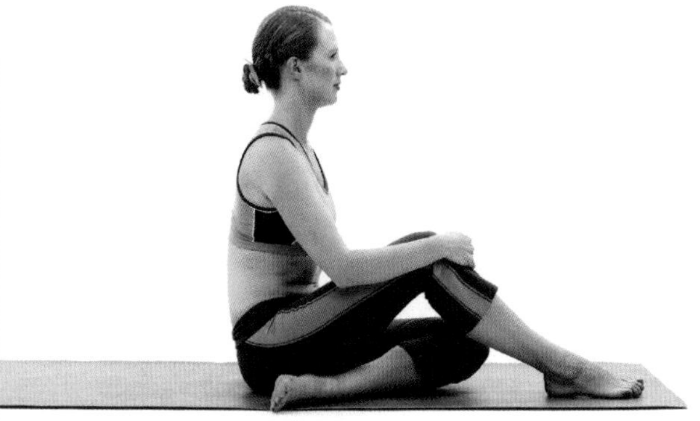

1.1 **Sit Square With Legs At 12 O'clock:** Have both legs facing 12 o'clock and your hips exactly square to the wall.

1.2 **Your Left Leg Bends In:** Draw your left leg in toward you, placing your left heel close to your right hip. Point your toes to the back wall for ankle extension. The outside of your leg lies flat on the floor with your knee at 12 o'clock (between both hips).

1.3 **Your Right Leg Bends Up And Over:** Bend up your right leg and bring your foot across the body to land to the left of your lower leg knee. Your foot is flat on the floor, toes at 12 and heel at 6 o'clock. Initially place your heel into position level with your left knee.

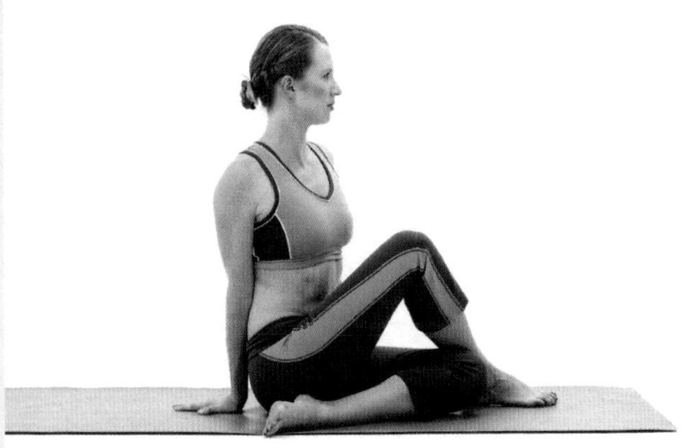

1.4 **Your Right Hand Behind:** Place the heel of your right palm on the floor centrally behind you as close as you can to your spine at the sacrum. For maximum leverage to push against the floor (see later) and to relax your shoulder, your hand is flat and your fingers are pointing toward 6 o'clock, square to your hips.

1.5 **Inhale Left Arm Up:** As you inhale bring your left arm up by your ear and on the exhale bring your arm down across your body and leg to land with the back of your elbow against your bent up (right) knee and the crease of your elbow facing your right at 3 o'clock.

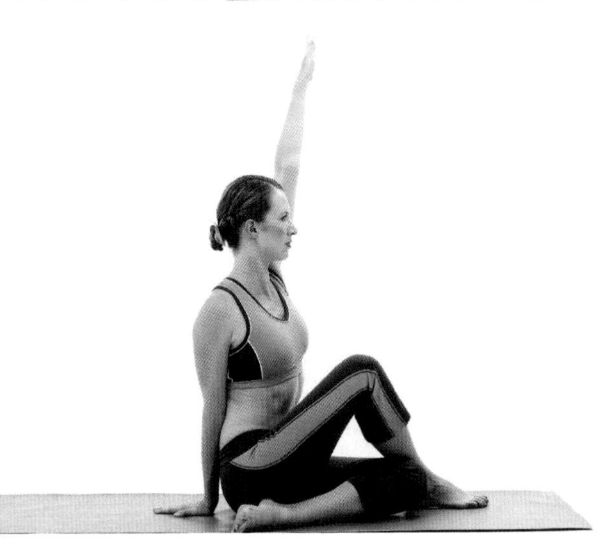

1.6 **Open Your Left Arm:** Hinge your left arm open to full extension. Your palm is also facing 3 o'clock (or to the right). Whilst maintaining some pressure of your elbow against your knee turn or hook your hand round to grab the left knee on the floor.

1.7 **You Are In Position, Facing Forwards:** Both arms are extended. One hand is now grabbing onto your knee. You are sitting squarely on your hips with one hand behind you aligned with your spine, fingers facing backwards. To start this twist pose you initially face forwards (12 o'clock).

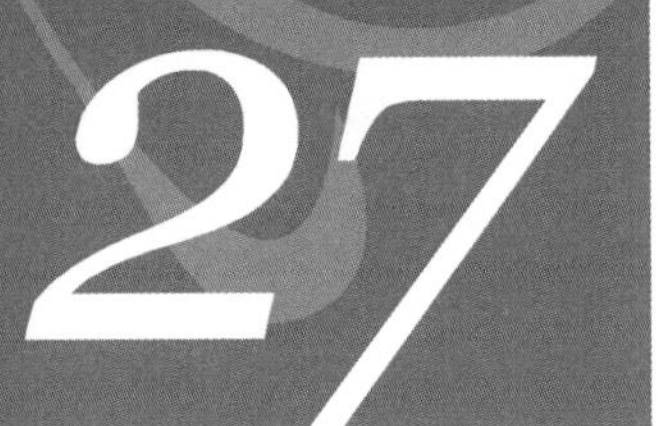

27 Ardha Matsyendrasana

Final Twisting Pose

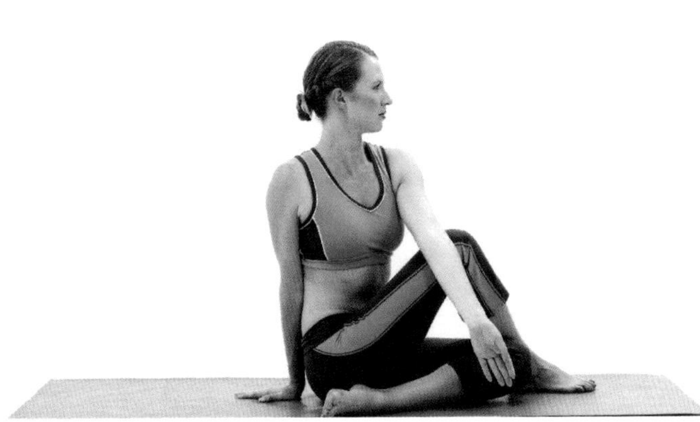

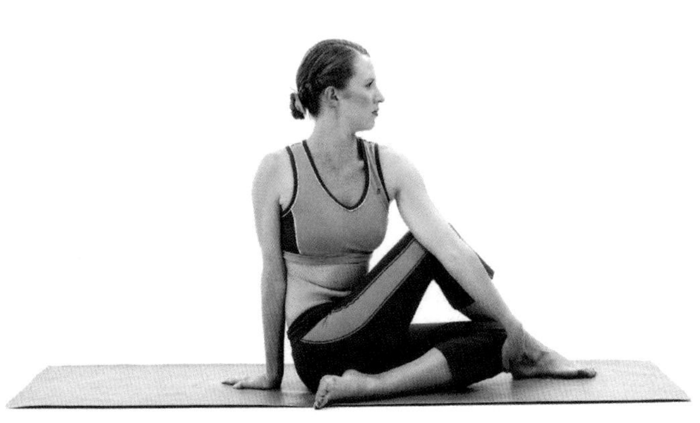

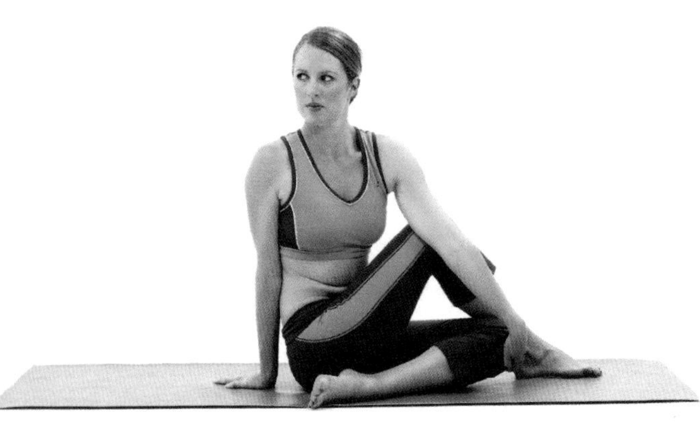

1.8 **Start The Twist, Use Your Eyes**: Look forward at a point on the wall, chin parallel to the ground. Inhale length into your torso. Then, as you exhale, push on the floor, pull on your knee and simultaneously turn your head slowly to create the twist in your lengthened spine. Where your eyes go, your body follows so use your intraocular muscles to look as far as you can over your shoulder.

1.9 **Work With Your Breath**: You have around 30 seconds of traction and breath work to facilitate deep body opening. Every inhale extend your body up creating stretch and length in the spine. Every exhale pull yourself around further with traction to twist more deeply. Each breath cycle will incrementally bring your body around further. I find that my eyes really feel the work too.

1.10 **Use Your Limbs To Create Traction**: Use your arm to pull on your front knee and, at the same time use the power in your leg to push that same knee back to the ground and feel that inner thigh stretch. That same elbow pushes your top knee back. Push the heel of the palm of the hand behind you downward into the floor.

Positioned and used correctly, the arms externally rotate. Their pull and push action against the floor and leg create the upper body traction. For optimal spinal extension and enhanced twisting, try gently stamping the front foot onto the floor and feel your breastbone lift as you turn. Your hips bed down more positively, and the spine straightens vertically allowing a more thorough lateral twist from your sacrum right through to, and including your neck.

1.11 **Ground Your Hips**: Your spine starts at the hips so always be mindful of squaring the hips. It means a greater likelihood of a straight spine, a more effective twist and greater benefit. When your right hand is behind you, your right hip has a greater tendency to rise up (the left hip rises on the second side). Push this hip down at every opportunity. Make it more effective by pressing the front foot down to also raise the chest and elongate the spine. Separately, each of these techniques works to unravel and straighten a rounded spine. Together the results are remarkable.

1.12 **Two Straight Lines**: Ideally your vertical spine deeply twists; knees and shoulders form a straight line, front to back dissecting the hips.

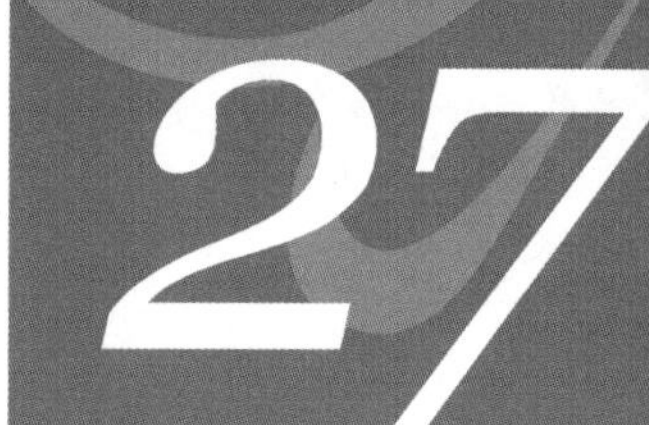

Ardha Matsyendrasana

Final Twisting Pose

Advanced pose technique

2.1 **Set Up As Normal**: Set up as normal with your hand behind you. Inhale your arm up and exhale grab your front knee. Look forward. At this point maintain your straight back with hips grounded.

2.2 **Lift Your Back Hand, Rotate Your Arm**: Lift up your back hand and bring your arm to your side. Internally rotate your arm so that your palm faces - and elbow bends - outward.

2.3 **Swing Your Arm Behind, Palm Out**: Swing your arm around behind you in an arc with your palm facing away from you. This action creates space in your shoulder. When your arm bends against your back, your hand is still facing outward.

2.4 **Grab Your Pants Or Thigh**: Reach your fingers around and grab either some material of your yoga pants or if you are very flexible or have long arms like me you can grab and pull against the tendon on the inside of your thigh.

2.5 **Look Forward, Then Twist**: Inhale some length into your spine while looking forward, then exhale as you turn and look over your shoulder. This time you are pulling against your lower knee with your outstretched forward arm, and pulling against your thigh with the arm that is behind you. Push your lower knee into the ground too.

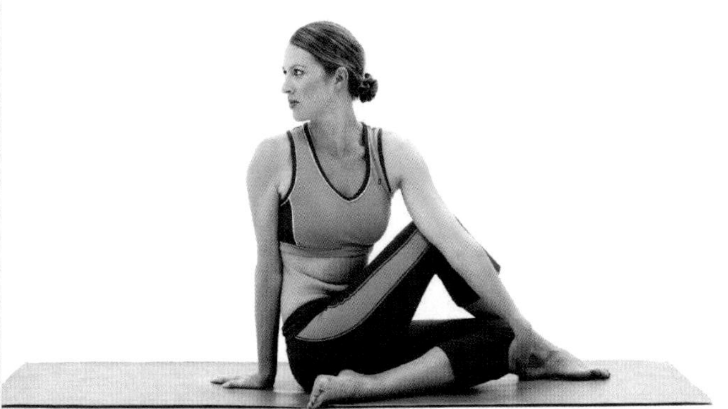

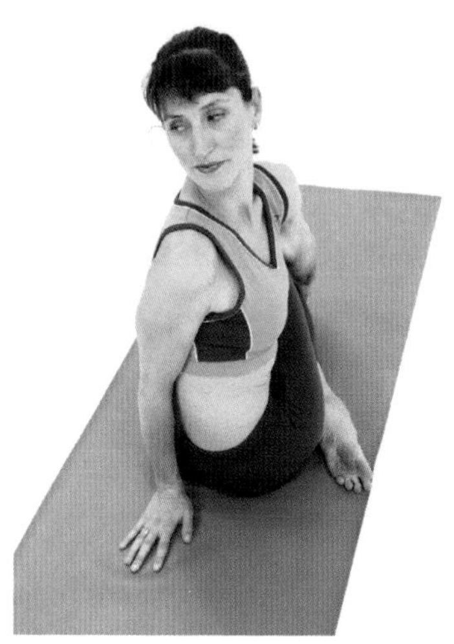

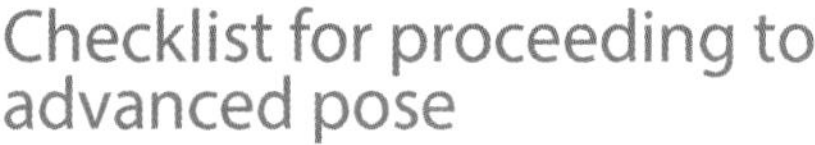

Checklist for proceeding to advanced pose

Only proceed to the advanced pose if:

1. Your twist works upwards through a vertical spine from hips which are firmly and bilaterally grounded.
2. Your front foot is securely in position somewhere between your knee and hip.
3. Your lower leg is completely in contact with and pushing into the ground all the way to the knee.
4. You are looking behind and over your shoulder. If you are practicing with a mirror in the room then on the second side you can almost look into your own eyes (I said, almost! But you can certainly see part of your own reflection). You can definitely see people in Final Twist practicing directly behind you (at 6 o'clock).

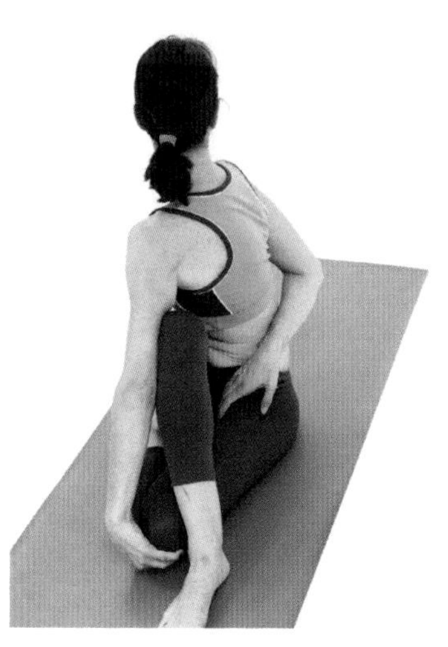

Ardha Matsyendrasana

FINAL TWISTING POSE

 Release

Before you release you take one last big inhale. Exhale fully. Try completely emptying your lungs and twist as far as you can. I often liken this pose to wringing or squeezing the water out of a wet rag. The more fully you can exhale (hint; look where you are going) the more fully you can express this cleansing twist of the spine.

Once your exhale and twist are complete:

a. Relax your eyes and start to bring your head back around to the front.
b. Release both arms; the pull on your knee and your hand off the floor.
c. Stop the push of your knee to the ground.
d. Let your lungs fill as you untwist your spine gradually and deliberately as you bring your body and head back to face the 12 o'clock position.

Don't be in a rush to turn around (or to commence the other side). Respect the integrity of your spine and come out mindfully, back upright, returning to center before commencing the left side, or getting to your Savasana. Many students let go without unwinding, in their haste to get on with the rest of the class. Protocol dictates if you are reversing what you entered into then you will end up with your head facing the 'front' again.

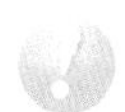 The second side

There is no Savasana between sides. So unwind your legs and lay your right leg down, hips square, knee in front. Bend the left leg up and over and place your foot down adjacent to your other knee. Continue in mirror image to the first side.

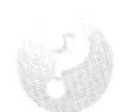 Must I face the left wall?

No! Where you face is dependent on personal choice, convenience, the space, floor coverings and mirror positions.

Facing the front mirror: There are no practical reasons to face the front mirror.

Facing the left wall: Facing left is most common and has merit. For the first side, as you twist, you will see the reflection of your entire right side, the level of your shoulders, the relationship of your chin and throat, and gain valuable proprioceptive information. You can observe whether you are leaning backwards or correctly propping yourself up using your back hand.

Facing the back wall: Facing the back wall is useful too. Sit up, then simply fold your legs into position, left under right for the first side. When you see your reflection in the mirror, you may be able to ascertain lean, get a real sense of your hips relative to the floor and what happens when you even the hips out. Watch your rounded spine straighten when you press that front foot into the floor and you push that raised hip back down!

The one disadvantage is that many get distracted by their own reflection and stop twisting. Sounds silly, but it takes some coaching to use the mirror as a corrective tool and then simply move on. Always look beyond to improve your twist. All in all, facing the left wall is the best option, with the occasional body alignment check that comes with facing the back.

 Common mistakes and how to fix them

Leaning back: If your back hand is positioned away from your body then you are probably leaning back on it rather than propping yourself up with its assistance. The traction and the twist elements will almost disappear. The problem is worse if your arm is bent. Inch your hand in as closely to your spine as possible and sit up vertically.

Front foot in wrong position: A common misconception is that the foot of the upper leg is flat on the floor close to the hip. Always start with the heel of your flat foot next to the knee. If a hip is lifted, slide the foot away from you until hip contact is maximized.

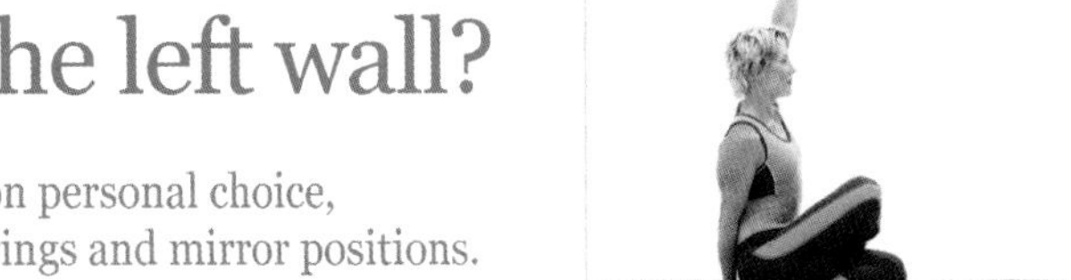

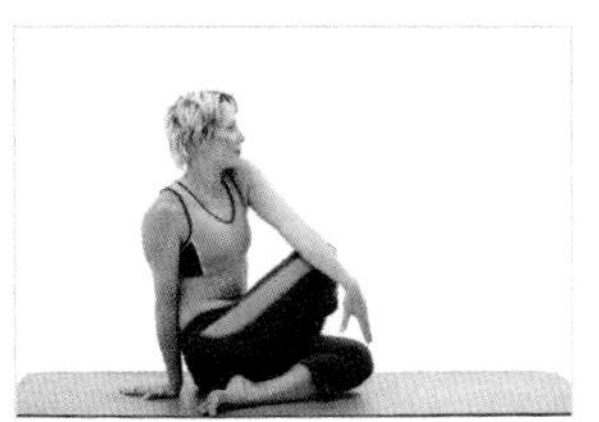

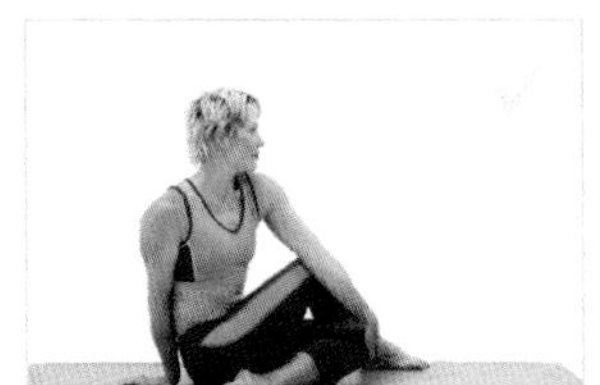

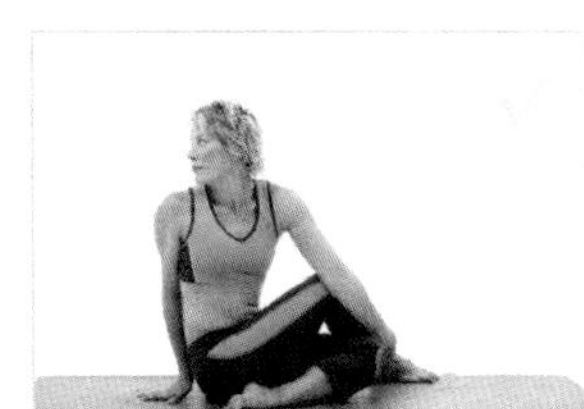

Ardha Matsyendrasana

Final Twisting Pose

***Your hand doesn't grip your knee**: See point above. You may need to slide the heel away from you. If you still can't reach the knee then reach for and pull on your towel to aid in creating the traction.

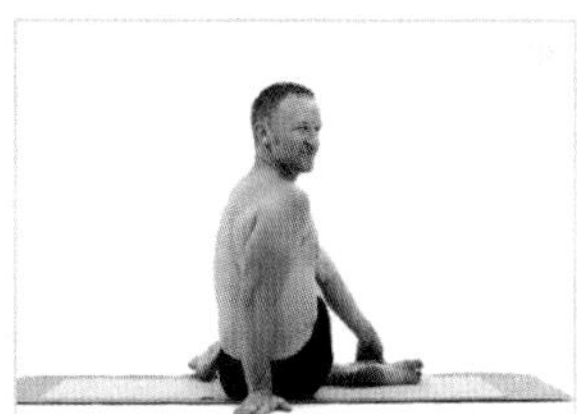

Your hand grips the knee at the shin: If your hand can only grip below the knee then the arm cannot externally rotate and create the optimum stretch. Best position for the front hand is with fingers approaching directly from 12 o'clock. Aim for this and settle for coming from between the shin and knee if that is all you can manage. A small tweak of the front heel position may be all it takes to optimize your grip.

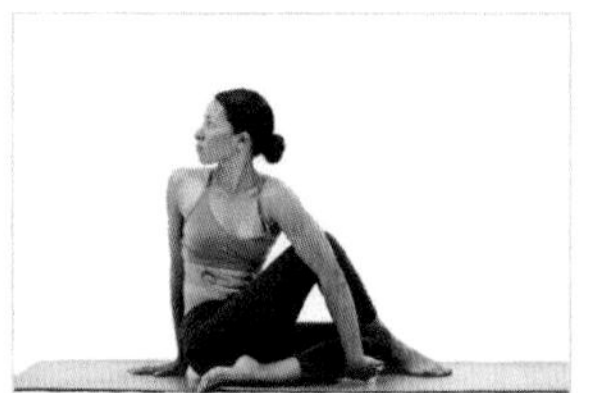

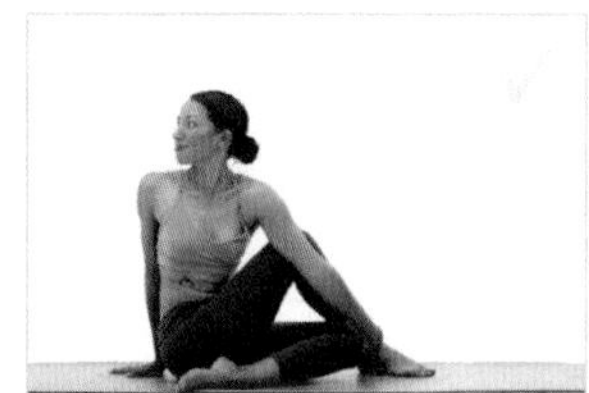

Hip misaligned and lifting: The further complication to wrong foot position is the difficulty in keeping the hips down. Adjust your lower knee to be at 12 o'clock (forward of your hips which are square to the wall). If the hip of your upper leg is already lifting markedly during set-up try gingerly advancing your heel to, or even a little forward of, your knee. Not too far or you lose the ability to create traction. Anchor your hip as best you can.

Fixing your hips can happen mid-pose: If the hip of the bent up leg rises up off the floor you are going to lose leverage on creating twist and traction. When making adjustments mid-pose be attentive to your hips' position on the floor. Pull back or advance your foot until your hips sit squarely. Use the balance of struggle versus ease to determine the position of your foot. A raised hip means advancing your heel forward. Ease in the pose with solidly grounded square hips means you should try pulling your foot incrementally towards your hip to find more stretch through your body. This can either happen during set-up or once the work has begun.

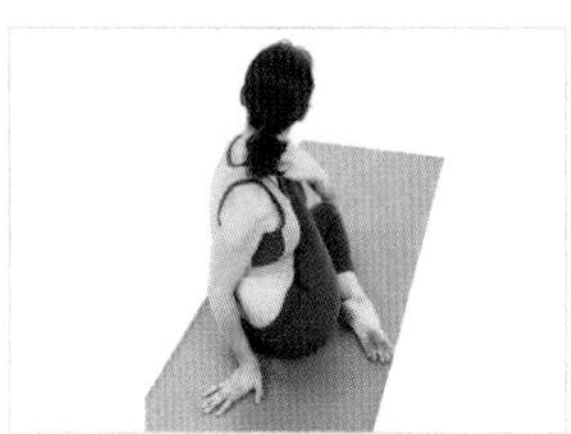

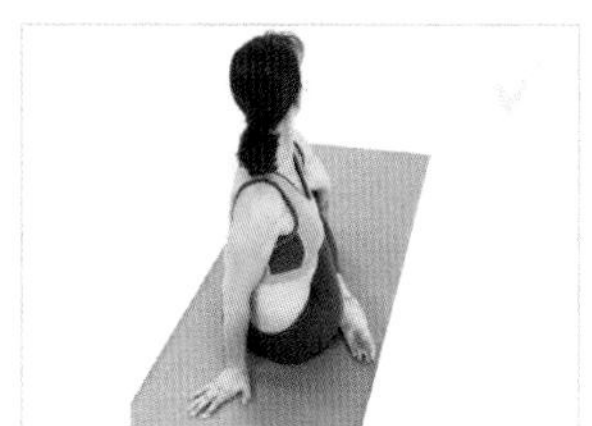

Leg positions too difficult: You may need to extend your lower leg straight if:

a. Your lower leg is in position bent and flat on the floor, but you can't get the other leg over the top.
b. You can just get your legs there but you are so tightly bound and off balance that you have no hope of placing your arms.
c. You have knee damage, or tight hips or knees restricting your movement.

Remember you should never feel excruciating pain in yoga. In these cases, extend the lower leg directly out in front of you, with your heel positioned at 12 o'clock between your squared hips. Then proceed as normal. Bring your other leg up and over and land your heel near the outside of your knee (the foot parallel with your outstretched leg). You will now be able to grab your knee and in a small percentage of cases, grabbing the towel may also be required.

Rushing in: Most students turn their heads in order to place their hands in position and then twist from there, losing valuable leverage. Get the most out of the twist by firstly setting up your limbs and then returning to face 12 o'clock. Inhale length in your torso and then turn your head as you keep the height in the spine (by pushing down with your back hand and front foot).

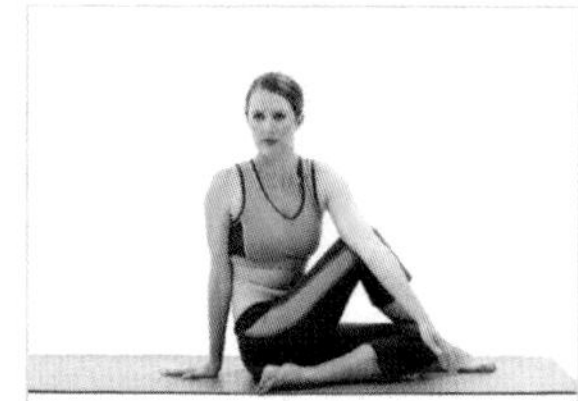

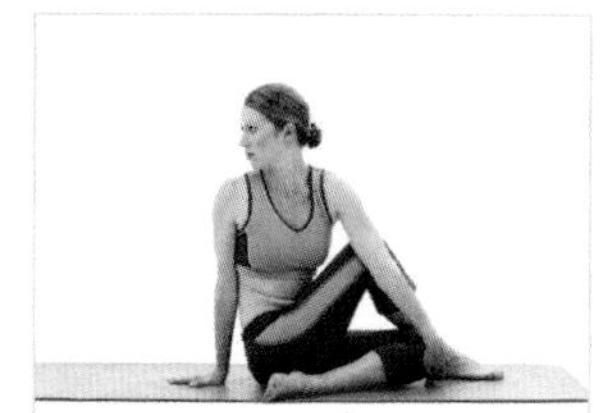

'Shaking hands' in advanced pose: If you can bring your arm behind you to grab your yoga pants then chances are you can 'shake your hands' in a grip. Even though it looks impressive it is NOT giving you what this pose is intending. Firstly the position of the forward arm is changed from a strong, open and stretching external rotation to an internal rotation. This causes the front shoulder to collapse and roll forward and down. Secondly and more importantly you lose the traction of your body against the legs. This erroneous position creates more of a forward bending twist rather than keeping your spine upright. In fact your lower leg ceases to have the impact on this pose at all as you can move it off the ground independently without affect.

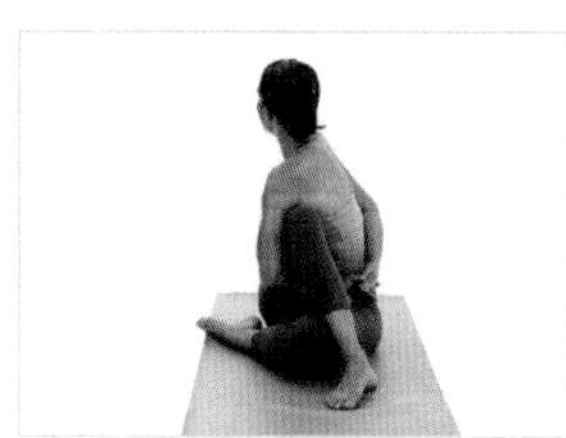

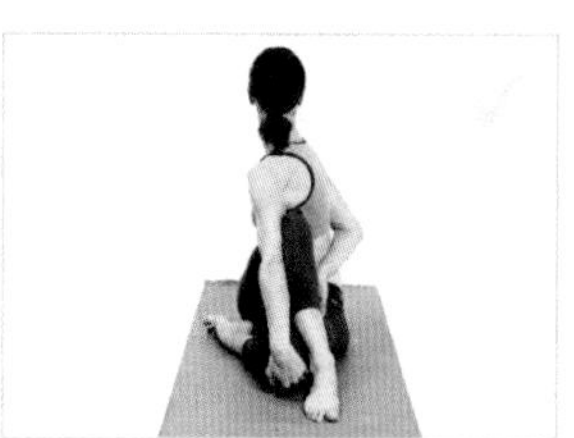

Kapalbhati Breathing

Half an hour's meditation each day is essential, except when you are busy. Then a full hour is needed.
—St. Francis de Sales

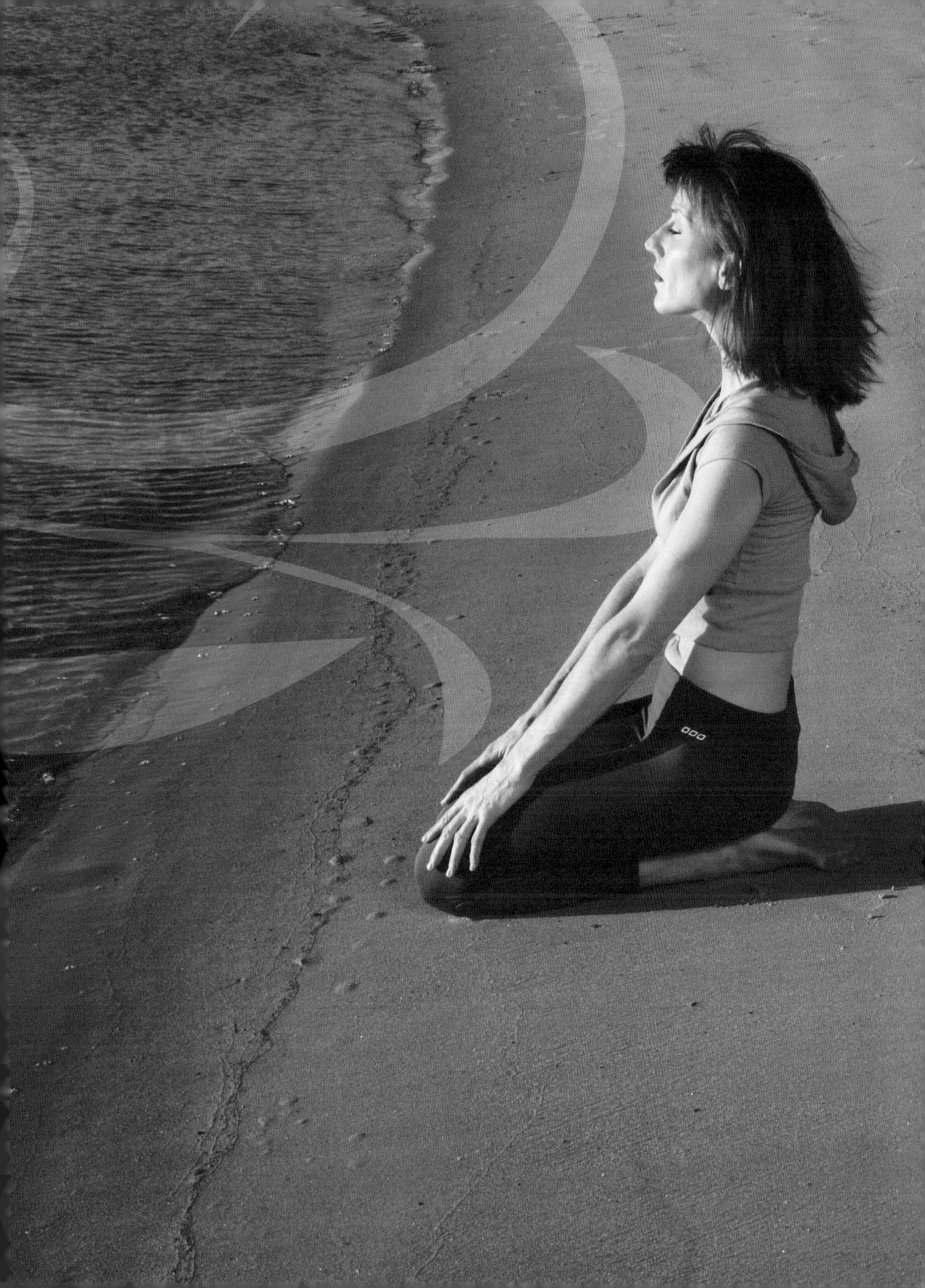

28 Kapalbhati Breathing

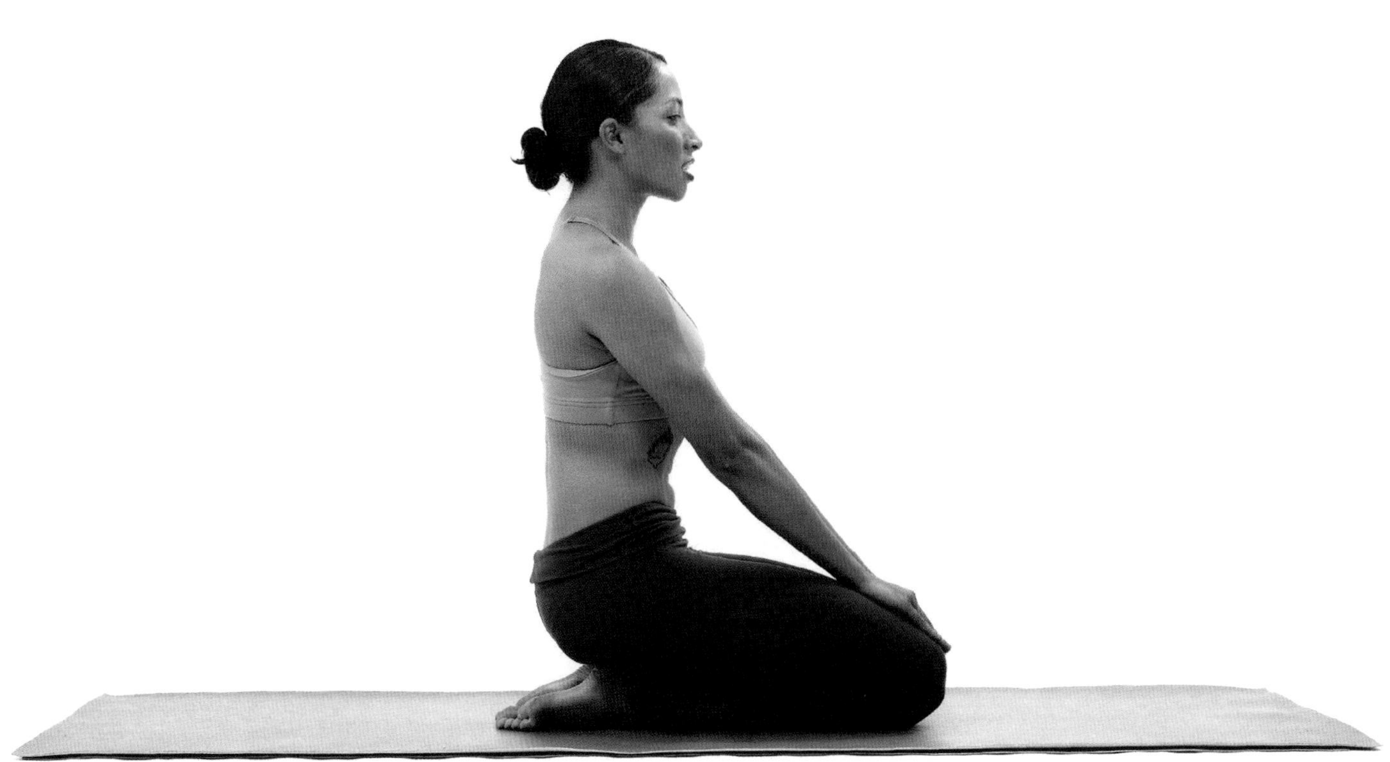

The essentials

Kapalbhati breathing is about releasing impurities, and reinvigorating the body through the breath. It precedes the very last pose of the class – your Final Savasana.

Did you know that physiotherapists encourage post-operative healing in patients, with a similar breathing exercise? It is designed to activate the lymphatic system and with the physical movement of the diaphragm, chest and lungs purges the lungs of mucus deposits that sit in the thorax.

Reassuring stuff really. The wisdom of ancient yogis adopted by the modern healing sciences.

What makes this pose so difficult to get right?

Once again this sounds like a simple posture. You take a big breath in and then breathe out 60 times in quick succession. But like everything there is a right and a wrong way.

Kapalbhati Breathing

The technique

We started with a Pranayama exercise (warming up with conscious deep breathing) and we finish with one too.

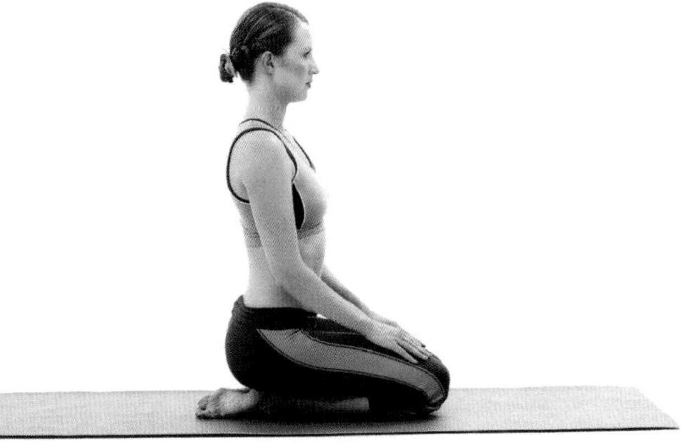

1. **Sit On Your Heels**: Come up from your Savasana and sit with hips, knees and feet together facing the front. Some will find sitting on the ankles challenging.

2. **Palms On Knees, Shoulders Relaxed**: Your arms are relaxed and may even have a slight bend. Allow your palms to rest somewhere between your thighs and knees. This lets the shoulders rest and have a neutral effect on the breathing exercise. Having locked arms with palms on knees has a negative effect. See notes below.

3. **Tuck The Tailbone Under**: A slight tuck will tilt the pelvis and create more space with which to perform the energetic exhale. The belly is not stretched but relaxed and the space 'fills' with air easily.

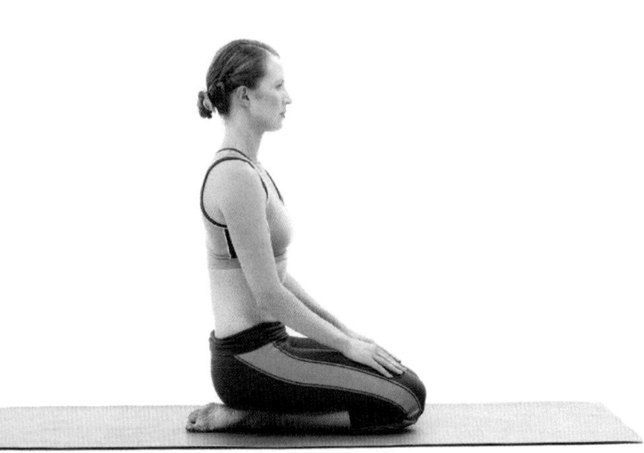

4. **Take A Big Inhale**: Close your mouth and fill your lungs.

5. **Open Your Mouth**: With your lungs full let your lips separate a little.

6. **Exhale Repeatedly**: The only conscious breathing effort required in this exercise is on every exhale. Your empty lungs, devoid of air, create negative pressure in your chest which stimulates the refilling of the lungs by drawing air in. The inhales actually happen for themselves, naturally and without thought.

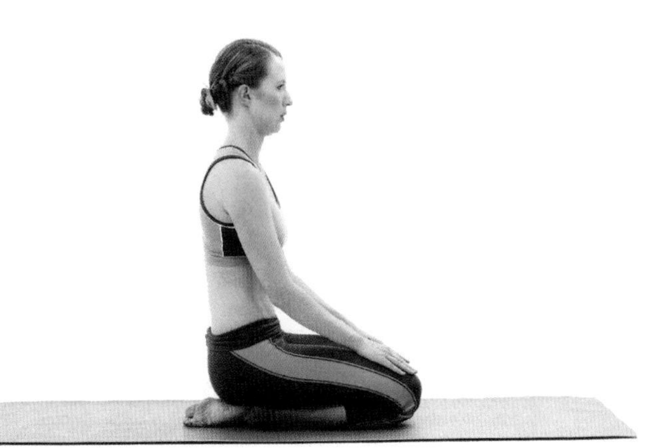

7. **Snap The Belly In Repeatedly**: Every exhale that you issue is accompanied and powered by a snapping in of the belly. This forces the diaphragm up, lungs to compress and the air to be expelled.

8. **60 Times Or So Then Rest**: On your last exhale you will naturally close and moisten your mouth and breathe as you need to during the short Savasana. The second set follows after several seconds.

28 Kapalbhati Breathing

Release

Finish your second set. It may be the end of the active poses but it is not the end of class. There is no rushing here. You may like to ritualize this time with some self-gratitude. Whatever you do is fine, just don't skip over some self-contact. Meet your own eyes and perhaps rest for a few moments in meditation before you spin around to lie down for your final and long Savasana.

Common mistakes and how to fix them

Making a 'shoosh' noise: This exercise is not about a particular noise that you can make. Many are cajoled into believing that if they make a 'ssssh, ssssh, ssssh' sound on the exhale then their exhale will be more powerful and effective. You can actually make a very loud shooshing sound with very little exhale effort.

What works far more effectively is simply opening the mouth, with the lips simply apart but not pursed there. Let your belly relax completely. Take a big inhale. Let your lips and jaws fall open relaxedly. And then repeatedly exhale:

- Using the muscles in your sucked in stomach and
- With a slight constriction in your throat to more forcibly direct the air out.
- The sound is more of a huhhh, huhhh, huhhh.

Try this following exercise for yourself:

1. Stick out your stomach, go on, push it out. Now make a 'ssssh, ssssh, ssssh' sound. You will feel your distended and tightened belly contract. These are your superficial abdominal muscles.
2. Now try to suck in your stomach strongly. Repeat the pattern of exhales and try to make the 'ssssh ssssh ssssh'. Either way, the shooshing is easy and works with or without major use of your abdominal muscles. Most of the effort is initiated in your mouth and not from where it is intended. The lungs don't fully empty right to their base.
3. Now repeat steps 1 and 2 using the huhhh, huhhh sound. Not only is it impossible with tummy out, you can feel positive that with stomach in you are using the deeper muscles to create the more forceful outward breath with the throat by slight constriction.

Shoulders jiggle: Most new students let the shoulders move up and down on the exhale making it difficult to draw the energy from the abdomen. Jiggling is usually a result of locking the arms. Relax and draw the shoulders down and back.

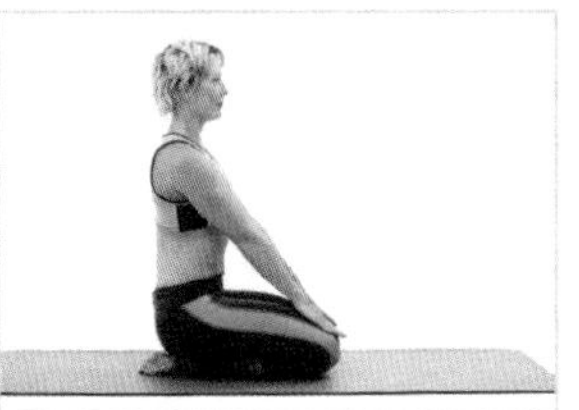

Arms are locked: Many teachers say the arms should be locked out with palms placed on knees. If you have long arms like me then you are likely to create too much stress hunching up your shoulders in an effort to have straight arms with hands precisely on the knees. I felt tension in my head and neck, and my shoulders were not in that neutral down and back position. If you have shorter than average arms then reaching your knees will also cause tension.

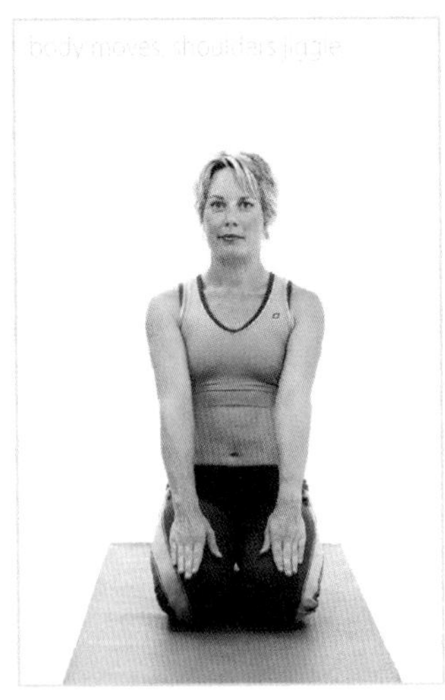

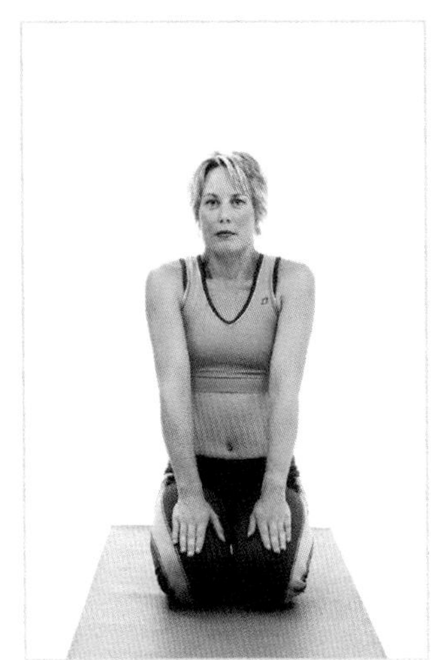

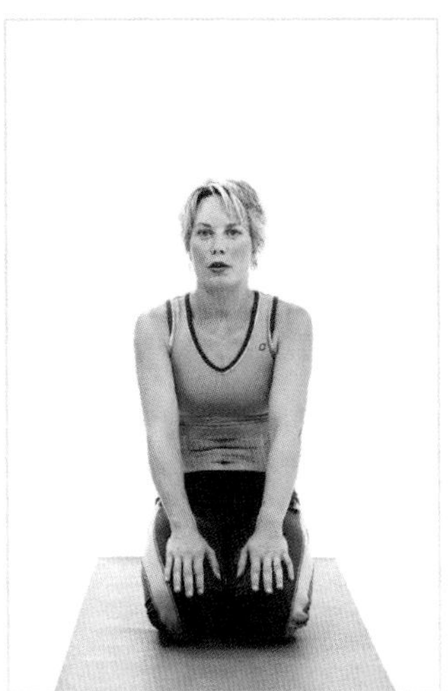

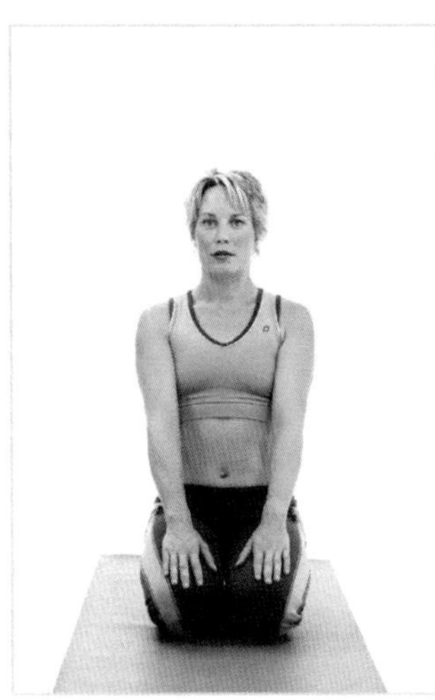

Relax your shoulders back and down. Take the tension out of your arms. You may have to introduce a slight bend at the elbows.

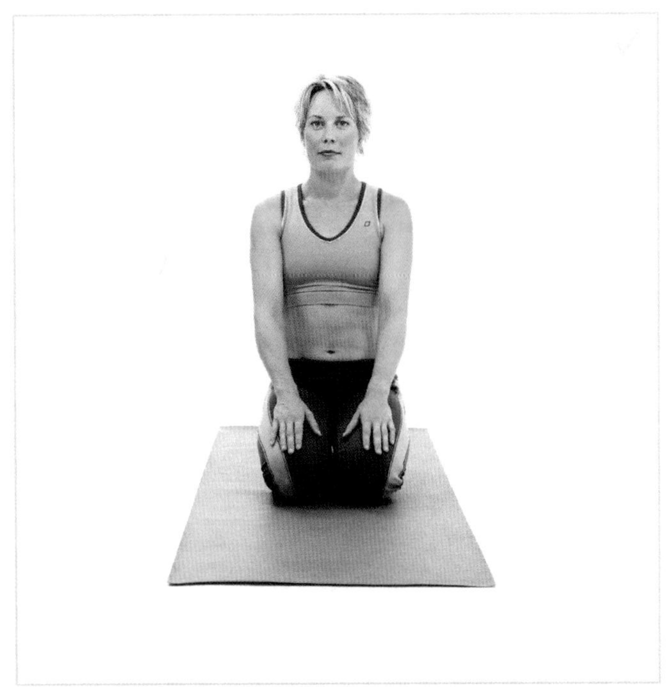

Spine rounds: When your spine is not straight the body tends to bounce with every exhalation. You simply have to sit up straight. Tuck your tailbone under.

Just not getting the abdominal movement: This is very common. Because of the unusual technique many just don't 'get' it straight away. Try diverting your attention from your eyes and instead look at your abdomen. You may even have to lift your top to see it properly. You can also place on hand on your belly. Simple and effective.

Can't sit on your feet: Try kneeling instead to get some of that ankle opening without the weight of your hips seated on top. If you can't do that then sit on your bottom, cross-legged. Be mindful however of avoiding slumping into a rounded back. Lean back a touch as you slightly pull on your knees to straighten your arms and back through traction.

Not inhaling between exhales: Occasionally a student will misinterpret the instructions and end up thinking too much. They focus on the emptying of the lungs but also stop the lungs from filling between exhales. They wonder how everyone else has such a large lung capacity! Surrender control, work on the exhales, and the inhales will happen all by themselves. The negative pressure in the lungs will allow for this to happen every time.

Slumping between sets: Keep your focus. Don't slump at the end of the first set. Just close your mouth and take a breath in readiness for the second set. Some teachers will tell you to swallow and maybe even lick your lips. All I can say to you is you need to take care of yourself. You have been breathing for as long as you have been alive! There is no special formula for the moments in between sets. Just finish. Close your mouth. Take a deep inhale and then do it again.

Final Savasana

Courage doesn't always roar.
Sometimes courage is the quiet
voice at the end of the day saying,
"I will try again tomorrow."
—Mary Anne Radmacher

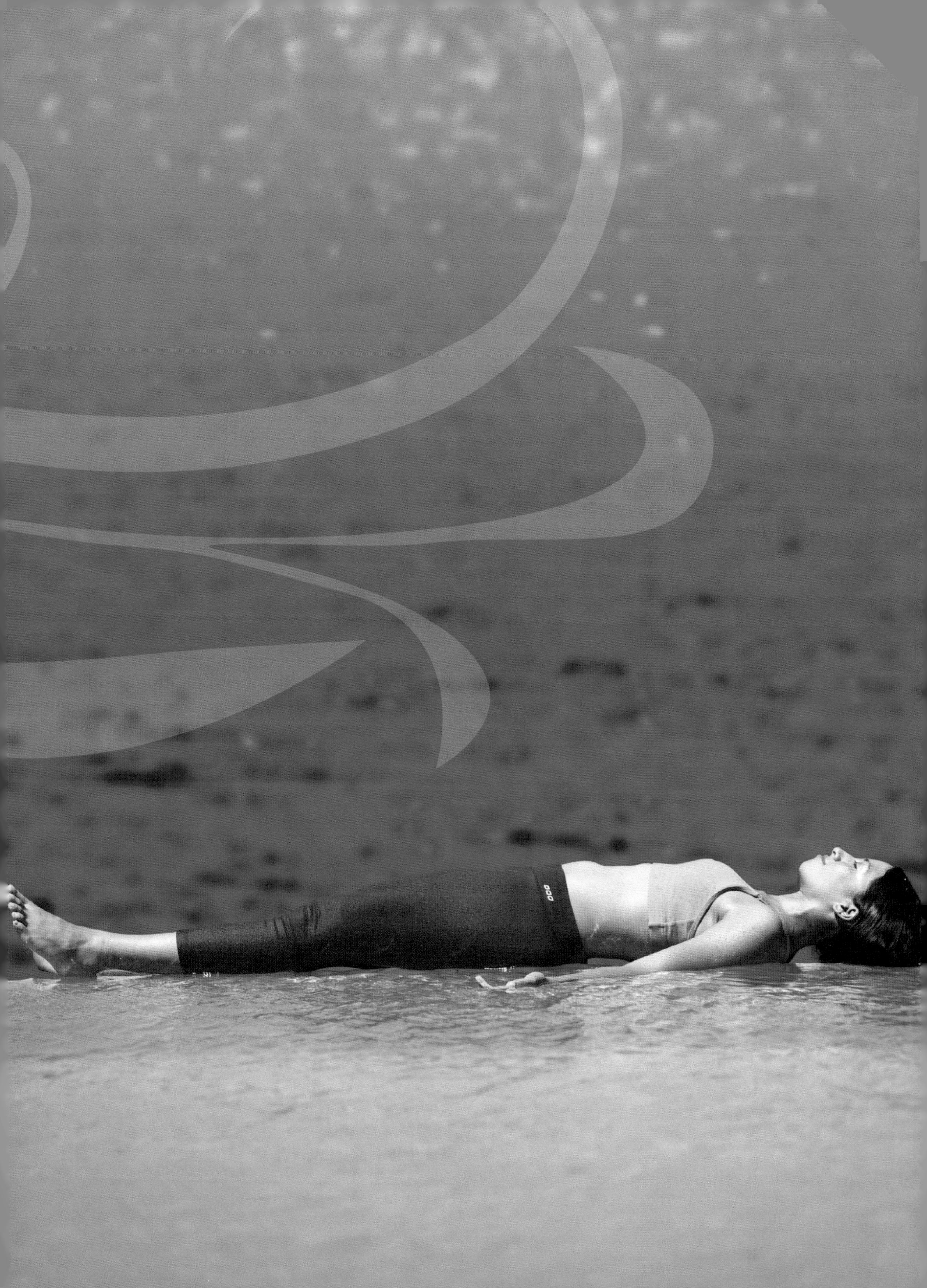

29 Final Savasana

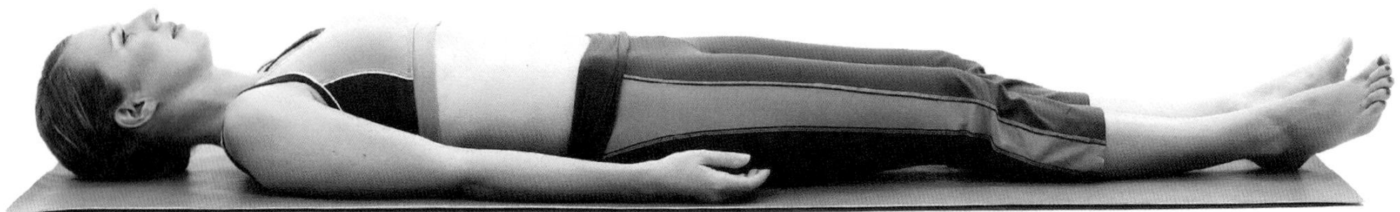

The essentials

Congratulations! You have made it to the end of class. In 90 minutes you have stretched, twisted, compressed or massaged, accessing most every cell in every system. You can now take advantage of the longest Savasana where you can release your body and mind and just be there on the floor to soak up the benefits.

Getting to this point has been no mean feat. Yet at the same time, this is just yoga. The journey is far more important than completing the class itself. What you discover on the way and how you adapt to the stresses in and out of the yoga studio is far more valuable.

The results you get are really going to be related to your intention. If you have too much ego involved then gone will be the great meditative and stress-relieving benefits. Learning focus and concentration, stamina and perseverance while letting go of your ego attachment will transform you and give you much more than just a gym-style class.

For the first few classes most people will have to be 'in their heads' to get the poses into their psyche and the thinking out of the way. After that - and because of that - it becomes the most amazing 90 minute moving meditation. There is nothing else like it. I believe that this is the most satisfying yoga workout ever.

What makes this pose so difficult to get right?

Seemingly simple, you only have to lie there. Taking time to lie completely still and to simply be will be your biggest challenge. Your time here is open ended. No pressures to continue with poses and find energy to get up off the floor. At the same time however, just lying there some feel the pressure of their everyday life lurking right outside the door.

Your biggest mistake will be getting up too early. If you are not careful you can let the frenetic nature of the world invade your thoughts and take you away from the 'now'. Or you can take advantage of giving back to yourself in a meaningful way and do absolutely nothing but breathe.

Love or hate the actual poses themselves there is nothing like the evident intense satisfaction on the faces, and in the hearts and minds of all who emerge.

Final Savasana

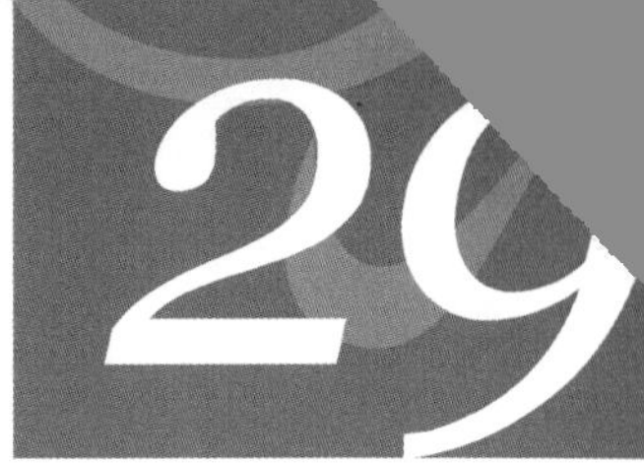

The technique

Completely Surrender

Lie on the floor in whatever way you find most comfortable. Eyes open or closed, on your back or on your stomach. Legs apart or together, arms down by your side or up by your head. Your spine has moved in all directions, your muscles are more pliable and less resistant and you may feel your body fits more snugly against the floor as you completely surrender to the pull of gravity. Let the floor hold you up. Relax the muscles in your face, around your eyes, your lips and keep your teeth apart.

Breathe Calmly

Feel your breath calm as your heart beat starts to slow down. Breathe in and out through your nose, letting your belly rise and fall, and allow fresh oxygenated blood to course through your entire body. The precise techniques of the asana themselves have allowed you to flush impurities and provide renewed nutrition to stagnant areas of your body including vessels, joints and organs. You have also sweated many impurities and improved your circulation and lymphatic systems.

You emerge refreshed, re-energized and reinvigorated – a healthier and more content you! It is as if you have pressed a reset button as your body willingly begins a process to re-regulate itself toward a state of optimal functioning.

Maybe Visualize

Many use visualizations as a handy tool to help them relax and stay still. Perhaps imagine yourself floating on water, lying in soft grass, or in sand. Maybe follow your breath with your mind's eye to relax each part in turn. Maybe feel a rising tide of relaxation lapping at your feet and moving up through your body, reaching further with each new breath. Once again, your choice.

Only thinking about your breath and cycling through and being aware of sensations in your body (no matter how subtle) is actually a more pure form of meditation and most find this more difficult than creating their own imagined journeys. It doesn't matter what you do, just stay still and enjoy your 'I' time. Your body will thank you and your mind will be quieter. Incorporate as much Final Savasana time as you can and count it as part of your whole yoga asana experience. Honor yourself and treat yourself with respect by giving yourself time to rest, breathe and just be.

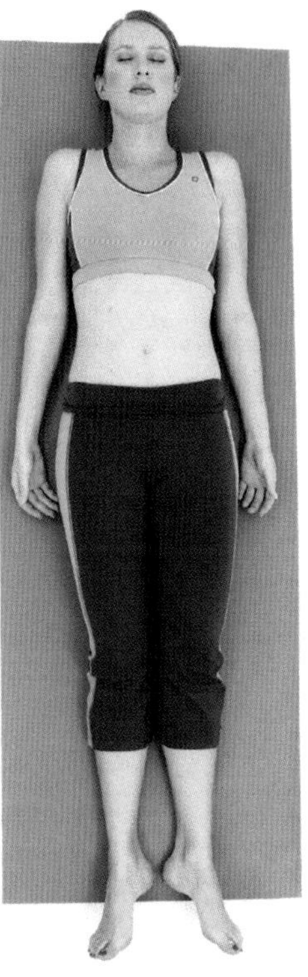

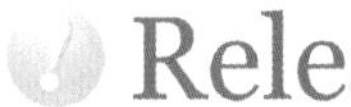

Stay as long as you can

Five minutes is minimum, ten minutes is better. If you have the luxury of time, then stay longer. Use this time to help you integrate your conscious and unconscious lessons, on physical and metaphysical levels because what you take away may not be consciously or immediately apparent.

Release

Stay on the floor until your heartbeat and breathing is back to normal. Carefully and mindfully get up off the floor. If your breathing is labored or you are still sweating profusely then you have not stayed long enough. Lie back down, or stay longer the next time.

You have now finished your hot yoga class. Stay quiet and look after yourself. Shower, change, have a cup of herbal tea, or some more water to keep your hydration up. Enjoy the rest of your day.

Embracing yoga as your journey...

There is no doubt about it. This is a challenging class. Sure, you can find harder classes, more difficult asana. After all, this is a series designed to suit all grades of yoga student from the novice to the advanced. But no matter how many times you have done this series, it is seldom 'easy'.

You will discover that, for the most part the physical poses are incidental on your journey, and it is the mental challenge that takes on the biggest significance. Ultimately it is the mind that will try to sabotage you, to stop you from going, to tell you that it is too hard. The body just wants to turn up and exercise, open up, cleanse and heal.

And yes, it can be painful, physically and emotionally. You may sometimes even ask yourself: 'Why am I doing this? Why do I put myself through the pain or the effort?' You do it because it opens up your understanding and creates awareness. You may initially just notice the obvious; the physical stuff; where you are tight or flexible; your balance; or your stamina.

However trivial those things may seem, that body awareness begins a process of self-awareness that transcends the physical to help you peel away the layers to reveal more of your true essence, dissolving mental and emotional barriers.

When you go to class you purposely place yourself under stress for 90 minutes. It is a miracle of existence that your body deals with stress in the same way and has the same reactions, whether it is physical, emotional or mental stress. Going to class teaches you how to deal with any stressful situation. Funny thing though, many students have told me that they don't care for the meditation, they just want a physical practice. This is what I love about this yoga. Everyday people learn how to meditate without intending to or even trying – their mental acuity and focus improves, the mind chatter slows down and life just gets better. These are some of the great benefits of meditation and it is all achieved by what appears to many to be a physical practice.

Some days time will seem to just fly by and you feel invincible. Other days it is a different story. Your stress training means that now it doesn't matter what surprises life offers you because you are equipped to deal with it. You understand yourself a little better and you are a little more at peace with the world.

Practicing hot yoga is a beautiful gift that you give to yourself. Be full of appreciation. Above all, thank yourself for cultivating that mental edge, for turning up at all, and then for working hard. When you finish your poses lie there, relax and get all the benefits of your class. Take as long as you need to. Your body will tell you when it is time to go. Rejoin the world out there with perhaps a different focus, an ease, a smile, a healthier, happier body, heart and soul.

Right at the beginning of this book, I spoke about the many, many students who have told me that because of hot yoga they feel happy for no good reason at all. They walk with their shoulders back and chin up, taking the world on with their smiles. They say how others notice their obvious wellbeing and want to know their secret. This is my hope for you too.

It is always my honor and my pleasure to teach and be taught by my students. Thank you for allowing me to share my knowledge and passion with you.

Namaste
Gabrielle